Author's Personal Communications with Giants of Medicine

Regarding errors in renal clearance test

Dr. John Macleod

13 Merchiston Avenue
Edinburgh, Scotland, EH10 4PJ
13/7/83

It was good of you to take the trouble to write to me about the 13th edition of Davidson.
Thank you for your kind comments.
You are, of course, correct about the typographical error on page 428. It should have been C = U × V/P; the printer omitted the division sign. This is now being adjusted.
Again many thanks for writing. With best wishes.

Regarding some clinical methods & apex beat localisation

Dr. J G Douglas

Chest Clinic, Clinic C
Aberdeen AB25 2ZN 02/11/2005
Ref: MacLeod's Clinical Examination, 11th edn

Thank you very much for your recent e-mail .... I am an editor of this edition..... I am responsible for writing much of the Respiratory Chapter and was most interested in your comments. In response:

Examining for Tracheal Shift................. Clearly this technique could also be performed with the patient standing or sitting.

Technique of Percussion – I entirely agree with your comment that to obtain the loudest percussion note ideally the other fingers, apart from the middle finger, should not touch the skin surface. Figure 4.19 is ambiguous and I will make a note of this for the next (12th) edition.

... Vocal Resonance........... However I agree that as written in the first paragraph of page 143 there is some confusion ....Again I will make a note to clarify this for the next (12th) edition.

Aegophony (page 144) .... However I agree that it's position is a little confusing and again I will make a note of this when redrafting the next (12th) edition.

Examination Sequence (page 97 .... palpation of apex beat) – I entirely agree with you that the second half of the statement under the 3rd arrow: "If you cannot feel it, ask the patient to roll on to their left side" is incorrect and references the wrong figure! I will make sure this is removed at the next reprint.

We are enormously grateful to you for your attention to detail in pointing out these points.
With best wishes. Yours sincerely.

Regarding errors in serum-ascites albumin gradient

Kurt J. Isselbacher, MD

Director, Massachusets General Hospital Cancer Center, Boston, Mallinckrodt Professor of Medicine, Harvard Medical School
Editor: Harrison's Principles of Internal Medicine, 13th edn 23/2/98

I must commend you for your astute and thorough reading of the Harrison's textbook and in addition, thank you for pointing out two obvious typographical errors. In fact, this was already done in the second printing of the 14th edition............................ *Again, many thanks for your thoughtfulness in bringing these two typographical errors to our attention.*

A compliment from Chief Editor of Harrison's book

Dennis L Kasper, MD

William Ellery Channing Professor of Medicine and Professor of microbiology and Molecular genetics, Harvard Medical School. Director, Channing Laboratory, Brigham and Women's Hospital, Boston, MA 02115
Editor: Harrison's Principles of Internal Medicine, 16th edition 7/10/2006

................I very much appreciate your interest in contributing to Harrison's. I have looked up your publications on PubMed, and I can see that you are active and productive in your field.........................., and I wish you all the best in your ongoing studies and clinical practice.
Best regards.

Regarding some queries on clinical medicine

Laurence Hunter

Senior Commissioning Editor, Elsevier
Ref: Hutchison's Clinical Methods, 22 edn
11/9/2008

Once again I am most grateful to you for taking the trouble to contact us with queries about the content of this textbook. I shall pass on to the Editors the comments and ask them to take full account of these in the revision of the book.
Thank you once again for your interest in our publishing programme.
With all good wishes.

Regarding erythema nodosum, & pulmonary stenosis

Keith A A Fox

Duke of Edinburgh, Professor of Cardiology and Head of Department, Cardiovascular Research Unit, The University of Edinburgh, Hugh Robson Building, George Square, Edinburgh EH8 9XF, 5/12/1995

Re: Davidson's Principle and Practice of Medicine: 17th Ed. 1995

On behalf of Editors of this textbook I have been asked to respond to you in view of the fact that this chapter was written by Dr. Boon and myself.

In response to your first question we have obtained source material which indicates erythema nodosum is a manifestation of acute rheumatic fever.

In conjunction with pulmonary stenosis, the only reason why the thrill may be best palpated in expiration is because of the fact that the heart moves closer to the anterior chest wall. We entirely agree that the velocity of blood flow across the pulmonary valve is increased in inspiration and this is demonstrated using echo Doppler techniques. However, for the reasons mentioned above palpation of thrill may be more obvious in held expiration when the heart and vessels are closer to the chest wall. I hope that these comments help to clarify the situation.
Yours sincerely.

Regarding contribution in "Kumar & Clark's" Textbook on Medicine

Ellen Green

Senior Commissioning Editor Elsevier, 1-3 Baxter's Place, Leith Walk, Edinburgh EH1 3AF
23/6/2005

Firstly, on behalf of Kumar & Clark, I would like to thank you for your contributions to the Online Appendix for Clinical Medicine 6e .... I hope you are pleased with the book ....
Kind regards.

In their Esteemed Opinion About the Book

Prof BM Hegde
Ex-Professor & Dean of Medicine,
Kasturba Medical College, Mangaluru (Ex-Vice-Chancellor, MAHE University, Manipal)

"Your book is an excellent replicative educational medium for exam-going students. Congratulations ....". ".......I am proud of you as you are a THINKER. May your tribe increase. Many students make you their role model. God will bless you always.........".

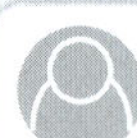

Dr AP Jain
Professor & Head, Department of Medicine,
MG Institute of Medical Sciences, Sevagram, Maharashtra

"The monograph on *Bedside Clinics in Medicine* is very well written, studded with your long experience as clinical teacher. Such monograph was a long felt need. You have really done an excellent job. The monograph will be very well received not only by undergraduate and postgraduate students but by clinical teachers as well."

Dr SB Agarwal
Professor & Head, Department of Medicine, BJ Medical College and Civil Hospital, Ahmedabad, Gujarat

"I highly appreciate the efforts, hard work and sincerity in bringing up this publication in a beautifully designed manner with rich clinical material inside".

Book review (Part I) in Journal of the Indian Medical Association (JIMA)

"........ Examinees who wish to anticipate routine questions and to avoid long embarrassing silences would do well to read these pages. .... important points have received appropriate emphasis. .... The text is closely written and the amount of information provided is truely gross. Every line and word has to be remembered. ....".

Prof (Dr) DK Hazra
Director, Professor & Head, Department of Medicine, SN Medical College, Agra, Uttar Pradesh.

"...... I have gone through this book and found it most suitable for the students. I will definitely recommend this book to the students........"

Dr PC Bhattacharyya
Ex-Professor of Medicine, Gauhati Medical College, Assam.

" .... is an excellent book for junior students in Medicine. This book, very simply written in a concised and rational manner will greatly help the undergraduate students to establish the foundation of Clinical Medicine with ease and confidence."

Dr PS Shankar
Dean, KJ Somiya Medical College, Mumbai
Book review in Journal of the Association of Physicians of India (JAPI)

Dr. Kundu has brought out a book based on bedside clinics on 26 model long cases and 74 short and spot cases oriented to clinical and oral examinations with special stress on clinical methods. .... He discusses the history, diagnosis, signs, differential diagnosis and management in the form of questions and answers. The answers are given in detail. .... There is an exhaustive coverage of the subject and Dr. Kundu has to be congratulated for bringing out such a wealth of knowledge. ......The book is very helpful to the students of clinical medicine while revising the subject before examination. Dr. Kundu has discussed the various questions which student may encounter during the examination and he has done it admirably".

Final year MBBS student, NRS Medical College, Kolkata.

"......It is a poetry on Clinical Medicine."

Dr PK Rathor
PG trainee, MKCG Medical College, Berhampur, Odisha.

".........I congratulate you for bringing out this book. ...."

Prof (Capt.) G Nagaiah
Professor & Head, Department of Medicine, Thanjavur Medical College & Hospitals, Tamil Nadu.

".....The book is good and very useful to undergraduates & postgraduates in Medicine .... I shall continue to recommend your book.............congratulation to the author for his concentrated effort."

Dr BT Tukol
Professor of Medicine, KMC, Hubli, Karnataka

".......*Bedside Clinics in Medicine* by Dr. Arup Kumar Kundu is a good book for undergraduate medical students. It is helpful for preparing for final MBBS Examination. Students can guess as what type of questions may be asked in the practicals. ...."

in http://stupidsid.com

"Kundu's *Bedside Clinics in Medicine*, Part I & II are mesmerising books for Medical students. Every student should possess these books to have knowledge in Basic Clinical Medicine"

Dr AP Jain
Professor & Head, Department of Medicine, MG Institute of Medical Sciences, Sevagram, Maharashtra.

"The second revised edition of *'Bedside Clinics in Medicine'* contains information at one place which postgraduates in Medicine aspire to assimilate in order to learn art and science of Medicine. Really an excellent job by Dr Arup Kundu".

Dr K Gandhi
Assistant Professor of Medicine, Thanjavur Medical College, Tamil Nadu.

".......It is so nice that all clinical problems are completed in so small a volume. ......".

Dr Kiranmoy Mitra
Ex-Assoc. Professor & Head, Department of Medicine, Burdwan Medical College and Hospital, West Bengal.

"........This is not a book but something more than that. This is self-explanative and could be one of the best books in the field of Clinical Medicine required for our students. The book is indispensable for not only undergraduates and postgraduate students but also for teachers and practitioners in Medicine as well. This book is a living Clinical Tutor".

Prof (Dr) CR Maity
Ex-Dean, Faculty of Medicine, Burdwan University, Principal, Burdwan Medical College, Burdwan, West Bengal (Ex-DME, WBMES, Government of West Bengal).

"In keeping with the expanding horizon of medical sciences and the gallant gallops of a plethora of newly emerging methodologies, Dr Arup K Kundu has very meticulously and ingenuously architectured his master creation *Bedside Clinics in Medicine*, Parts I and II. A purist pedagogue, a massive mentor, and an exemplary exponent engrossed with an expansive professional expertise and competency, he has probed deeply into several cases along with history, diagnosis and management invariably in an easy-to-understand question-answer form......... The diagnostic procedures and methodologies are nicely delineated. This book will be a constant concise companion for all, students and teachers alike, in different Indian Universities and Medical Colleges as this treasure will elicit the clinical spirit of approach from a modest conventional way to highly sophisticated method."

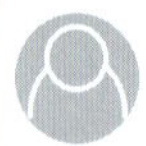

Dr V Venugopal
Professor of Medicine, Perundurai Medical College, Tamil Nadu.

I can recommend the book to my students as a ready reckoner........."

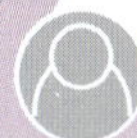

Col AS Kasthuri
Professor and Head, Department of Medicine, AFMC, Pune, Maharashtra.

"The book *Bedside Clinics in Medicine*, Part I and II is comprehensive with wide coverage of all systems and attractively produced. .... it is informative and beneficial not only to the UGs/PGs, but also to the physicians."

Dr K Ramachandran
Visiting Professor of Radiology, MG University School of Medicine, Gandhi Nagar, Kottayam, Kerala.

"....... I found that there is a wealth of information in the book which is difficult to get from other books. ....you must have gone through several journals and the whole of encyclopedia of medicine .... Congratulations."

Dr Saif Omar
Internee, Katihar Medical College, Katihar, Bihar

"....... I have been an ardent reader of both of your textbooks on clinical medicine, since the first day of my ward duty. To be very honest I have learnt more from your books than from........"

Dr Kamaalchand M
PG trainee in Pediatrics, JNMC, Aligarh Muslim University, Aligarh, Uttar Pradesh.

"....... many congratulations for writing an ultimate manuscript in medicine. ...."

Prof (Dr) PR Nath Barbhuiya (Retd.)
Professor & Head, Department of Medicine, Silchar Medical College & Hospital, Assam.

"....... *Bedside Clinics in Medicine*, Part I & Part II is a 'Treasure Island" for students of Medicine both undergraduates & postgraduates. .... The book has in fact satisfied the need of a long awaited reference book for examinee being complete by itself in all respects. ....recommend this book strongly for students of medicine........"

Dr NS Neki
Associate Professor of Medicine, Government Medical College, Amritsar, Punjab.

"....... *Bedside Clinics in Medicine*, Part I, which is highly informative, well-written with latest additions ...."

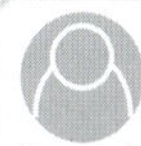

Dr Keerthana Karumbaiah K
Internee, Bangalore Medical College, Bengaluru, Karnataka.

"....... the joy of reading the book is so overwhelming that, by far, medicine has never seemed so pleasurable........ . It is unequivocal opinion that the book is outstanding and entirely removes the need to study multiple books in clinical medicine. .... For my final year exams .... the questions that were asked during discussion were entirely based upon the facts given in your book. I just had to quote them to be appreciated by the examiners........"

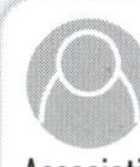

Book review (Part II) in Journal of the Indian Medical Association (JIMA)

"....... this 'made easy', if assimilated properly by the students, will help to learn many aspects of medicine. ..... The chapters on radiological diagnosis and ECG interpretations will certainly help all concerned. Emergency tackling of different cases also, will help the young professionals. ...... The book is likely to be well accepted and the second edition of the book supports that expectation."

Dr Pradeep Kumar Shenoy C
Ex-clinical fellow and registrar, Department of Rheumatology, Manipal Hospital, Bengaluru, Karnataka.

"....... its really the eighth wonder in the world. Looking back, recollecting my MD days, I repeat my words ....I owe you my MD."

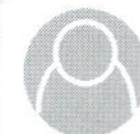

Dr Bhushan Madke
student of Indira Gandhi Govt. Medical College, Nagpur, Maharashtra.

"......I am very happy to inform you that I have got selected for MD........... I owe my success to your book, and your in time valuable suggestion and advice. You have been my behind the scene teacher and educator and inspiration.........."

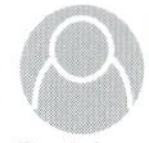

Jagroop Singh
Student of Guru Gobind Singh Medical College, Faridkot, Punjab.

".....You have donated breath to me.........."

J Mahammad Sadiq
Government Medical College, Salem, Tamil Nadu.

"I am a final year medical student. I read your book on bedside clinical examination........ The book is really wonderful. Hats of sir......"

Ramchandra Chaudhary
Student of SRTR Medical College, Ambajogai, Maharashtra.

".....I am highly impressed with clarity and concept of your book. The book is not only helpful for clinical exams but also for theory. The book is really a wonderful book....."

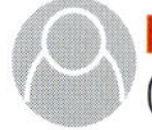

Dr Amit Sharma,
(DM cardiology student), and passed MD (medicine) from KGMC, Lucknow, Uttar Pradesh.

"Sir, its really great whatever you write, I have read your book in final year to clear exam, that helped very much to pass final prof......"

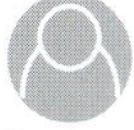

Parvathy Rajmohan
Sree Gokulam Medical College, Thiruvananthapuram, Kerala.

"First of all, thank you for writing this book. It is truly a lifesaver......"

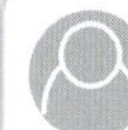

C. Manpa Phom
Intern, Agartala Govt. Medical College, Tripura.

"Sir, thanks for the wonderful book of yours of *Bedside clinics in Medicine* part I & II............ have passed my final mbbs finally and sir your book was the only book I read for my practical examination......."

Ashwin Joshi
Intern, Agartala Govt. Medical College, Tripura.

"..............I must say that the book '*Bedside Clinics in Medicine*' which you have authored is extremely useful, exam oriented and very relevant. I can vouch and say that all 180 students from final year in our college will be preparing from it, especially for the practical exam ....Highest regards and respect."

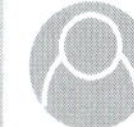

Dr. Rakesh Das
1st year PGT, Agartala Govt. Medical College, Tripura.

"....Thanks a lot to you for gifting such a nice book "*Bedside Clinics in Medicine*". Its a must read book for both UG & PGT Medicine...."

Dr Abhishek Sachdeva
DNB student, Videocon Group of Hospitals, Maharashtra.

"...........Sir your books are a great help for students learning medicine. Sir,..... I would like to tell you that its my dream to have a teacher like you some day. I also feel proud that such an amazing piece of work is done by an Indian Author."

Om Prakash Mishra
Final year MBBS student, Institute of medicine, Kathmandu, Nepal.

"First of all I would like to thank you for producing such a marvellous book, the only one of its kind, for Clinical Medicine. This book is beyond comparison. It is helping to raise the standard of clinical examinations in students' as well as doctors worldwide."

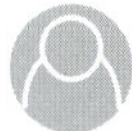

Dr Jalal Ahmed
Kasturba Medical College, Manipal, Karnataka

"Thanks for writing a great book for postgraduates ......"

Final year MBBS student, GMERS Medical College, Gotri, Vadodara, Gujarat.

"I thank you a lot for bringing out this book. I never felt medicine too interesting although I'm in final year..... credit goes to you..... Thanks sir"

Mina Aziz
Ain Shams University, Cairo, Egypt.

"Thank you for your great book. It really helped us a lot......".

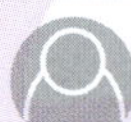

Pawon Goel
Final year MBBS student, Maulana Azad Medical College, New Delhi.

".....Here in our college your book is recommended by everyone, even the senior residents. I enjoyed your book very much....."

Gopal Yadav
MBBS 3rd year student, BP Koirala Institute of Health Sciences, Dharan, Nepal.

"Sir Namaste! Your book on bedside medicine has become a part and parcel of medical students......."

Dr Sagar Tandel
MD student, Shri MP Shah Medical College, Jamnagar, Gujarat.

"First of all I would like to congratulate you on immensely informative '*Bedside Clinics in Medicine* - Edition 7th'. You would be happy to know that we, residents, are considering it as a principle book for preparation of case presentations in our MD Medicine curriculum....."

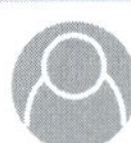

Dr Vivek Agarwala
Dept. of Medicine, GSVM Medical College, Kanpur, Uttar Pradesh.

".........I would like to congratulate you and thank you for your wonderful book and your efforts towards making the subject of medicine easier to learn for us."

Soumya Roy
Student of Calcutta Medical College, West Bengal.

"......I had been a die-hard fan of your book. Lots of respect...."

Dr Milind Patil
BJ Medical College, Pune, Maharashtra.

"I have used your book ..... during my undergraduate (MBBS) and postgraduate exam (MD) in internal medicine. Its a very good book for both exams. It saves a lot of time of students in preparing for exams. Thanks for spending your valuable time in writing such excellent book"

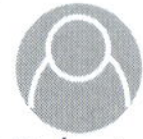

http://medchrome.com/medicalcolleges/student-life/perfecting-yourselfclinical-examination/

"Kundu's *Bedside Clinics in Medicine* — another wonder book for medicine. It has almost everything and even things found no where else. Will help students a lot. ...."

www.quora.com

"......Casewise the best in Kundu"

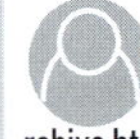

http://medcosmosbaroda.blogspot.com/2008–09–01–archive.html

"*Bedside Clinics in Medicine* by Dr Arup Kundu is really nice to crash all the viva Q-A in your clinical viva......... also it helps to clear basics.......It teaches you how to think medicine"

in www.doctorshangout.com/profile/peuishsugathan

"....Favorite medical books: Harrison's principle's of internal medicine, Kundu, de Gruchy, John Patten...."

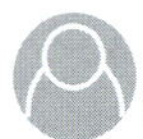

www.xmail.net/wfmustudents/medicalbooks.htm

Website in China (Weifang Medical University, Shandong, China) recommends this book for their students

mciforchina.blogspot.com/2008/08/m-c-i-screening-test-books-syllabus.html-85k

....recommended Bedside Clinics in Medicine, Part I & II for MCI screening test books for students passed MBBS from aborad.

www.quora.com

"....Kundu: the book is in question answer format. Any and all question that will ask in viva by externals in the exam comes from this book. It has part B which gives the necessary details for charts, tables, ECG, etc......"

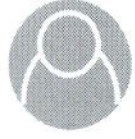

www.quora.com

"We read Arup Kumar Kundu's *Bedside Clinics in Medicine* for Medicine practicals. It has all Long, Short cases and Instruments, ECGs, X-rays, etc...."

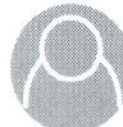

www.quora.com

".......Kundu helps you to understand the cases better and helps you to stand in good position to answer the questions"

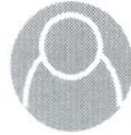

www.quora.com

".....For practical, "*Bedside Clinics in Medicine*—Kundu" (it's an unparallel clinical medicine book worth to read)......"

in www.cafemedico.com

".......I m using Kundu.........all casewise clinical study is very fine.......I really like it...."

www.quora.com

"..........Most answers in the book were based on sound concept rather than mere dumping of facts....... Level of recommendation: VERY VERY HIGH..."

in https://desimedicos.com

"........Many seniors recommend it for differential diagnosis (D/D). The book is excellently detailed. Students should go through this book .... call it best book for clinical medicine and practicals"

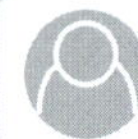

www.aippg.net

"......also Arup Kundu if you want to dash answers in ward round cases. I would recommend Kundu as a must buy over and above one basic book like Hunter....."

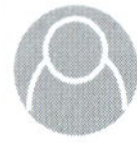

in www.doctorshangout.ning.com/ profile/DrMansi

".....Favorite Medical Books: Guyton's Physiology & Kundu's Medicine...."

Rajkishor Singh
Nalanda Medical College & Hospital, Patna, Bihar.

"I am very grateful to you that you bestow such a nice material for understanding a huge subject of medicine which made very easy for both clinical examination as well as theory exam, and best supplement for PG entrance exam. Thanks a lot"

Apildev Neupane
Final year medical student at Institute of Medicine, Kathmandu, Nepal.

".....It is a well known fact among medical professionals, that your book on bedside medicine has proved to be a holy gift to the generations of medical students in this part of the world...."

Dr Nidhish Chandra M
(DM) Rhumatology Sr. Resident, King Georage MU, Lucknow, Uttar Pradesh.

"I read your book during my MD times and was very useful as a bedside tool.......I always felt that you are teaching us from the patient's bedside. Thanks a lot for providing us with such a powerful tool...."

Abhishek Raj A
Student of Chettinad Medical College, Tamil Nadu

"..... Your book '*Bedside Clinics in Medicine* Part I' has offered the eager n thirty medical student child with in me! Kudos n power to u Sir! N may your tribe increase!...."

Part II

Ninth Edition

Bedside Clinics in Medicine

with COLOUR Photos and Clinical Integration

• X-rays • ECGs • Charts • Drugs • Specimens
• Instruments • Emergency Medicine

As per the latest NMC Guidelines | Competency Based Medical Education (CBME) Curriculum under Graduate Medical Education Regulation

- Diagnostic Aids and Analysis
- Treatment Know-how and Skill
- Extra Edge in Viva Voce

The Best Text for NExT Examinations— Thoroughly Revised and Updated

"Do not waste the hours of daylight in listening to that which you may read by night. But when you have seen, read. And when you can, read the original descriptions of the masters who, with crude methods of study, saw so clearly. To study medicine without books is to sail an uncharted sea, while to study medicine only from books is not to go to sea at all."

—Sir William Osler (1849–1919)
Professor of Medicine, Oxford, UK

Other Books/Chapters by the Same Author

- *Bedside Clinics in Medicine*, Part I (9th Ed), 2024
- *Kundu's Practical Medicine* (2nd Ed), 2024
- *MCQs in Internal Medicine* (6th Ed), 2022
- *Pearls in Medicine for Students* (3rd Ed), 2024
- *Memorable Memoirs of a Medico* (on Amazon portal), 2023

Chapters in:

- *API Textbook in Medicine*, 8th Ed, 2008
- *Postgraduate Medicine*, 2009
- *Rheumatology: Principles and Practice*, 2010
- *Medicine Update*: 2010–15, 2017, 2018, 2021–24
- *Progress in Medicine*: 2016, 2019, 2020, 2023, 2024
- *Manual of Rheumatology*: 5th Ed, 2018; 6th Ed, 2024
- *Rheumatology Clinics: Clinical Scenarios*, 2024
- Online appendix of "Kumar & Clark's", *Clinical Medicine:* 6–10th Ed

Biography (Author)

Included in Marquis Who's Who in the World 2014, 2015 and 2016
Who's Who in Science and Engineering 2016–17, and in
Wikipedia & WikiVisually

'Gifted Teacher' Awardee in 2022 (by Association of Physicians of India)

Fellow/Member of

- Fellow, Indian College of Physicians (India)
- Fellow, Royal College of Physicians (Edinburgh)
- Member, New York Academy of Sciences (USA)
- Member, International Advisory Panel of "Kumar & Clark's" textbook, *Clinical Medicine*, 7–10th Ed (Edinburgh)
- Life-member, Association of Physicians of India (API)
- Life-member, Indian Rheumatology Association (IRA)
- Life-member, Indian Medical Association (IMA)

Part II

Ninth Edition

Bedside Clinics in Medicine

with COLOUR Photos and Clinical Integration

• X-rays • ECGs • Charts • Drugs • Specimens
• Instruments • Emergency Medicine

As per the latest NMC Guidelines | Competency Based Medical Education (CBME) Curriculum under Graduate Medical Education Regulation

Arup Kumar Kundu MD FRCP FICP MNAS
Ex-Visiting Faculty and Consultant Rheumatologist
IQ City Medical College
West Bengal, India

Formerly
Professor, Department of Medicine and
In-charge, Division of Rheumatology
NRS MC, KPC MC, IQ City MC, and
RG Kar Medical College, West Bengal, India
and
Author of five other books with chapters in different books on medical sciences
Thirty years of teaching experience in Govt and private medical colleges
UG and PG examiner in different Indian Universities
Prestigious 'Gifted Teacher' Awardee in 2022 by API
Mentor and Instructional Coach, pan-India for teaching in MBBS, MD, DNB

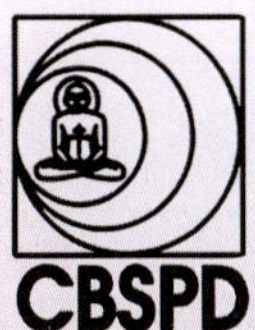

CBS Publishers & Distributors Pvt Ltd

New Delhi • Bengaluru • Chennai • Kochi • Kolkata • Lucknow • Mumbai
Gujarat • Hyderabad • Jharkhand • Nagpur • Patna • Pune • Uttarakhand

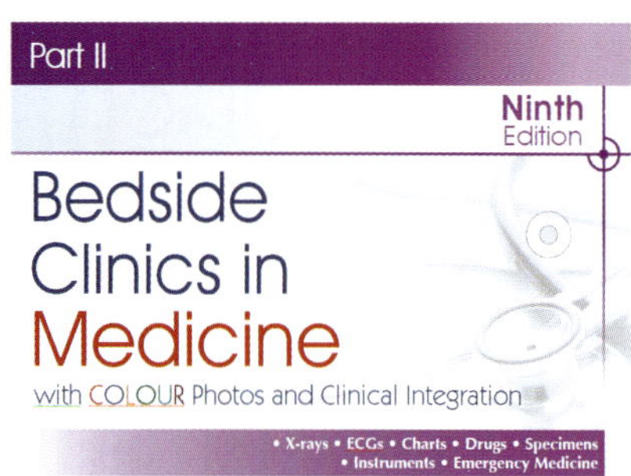

ISBN: 978-93-5466-859-3

Ninth Edition 2024
Reprint 2025
First Edition 1999
Second Edition 2000
Third Edition 2003
Fourth Edition 2006
Fifth Edition 2010
Sixth Edition 2015
Seventh Edition 2020
Eighth Edition 2022

Published by Satish Kumar Jain and produced by Varun Jain for

CBS Publishers & Distributors Pvt Ltd

4819/XI Prahlad Street, 24 Ansari Road, Daryaganj, New Delhi 110 002, India

Ph: 011-23266838, 23289259 Website: www.cbspd.com
e-mail: delhi@cbspd.com

Corporate Office: 204 FIE, Industrial Area, Patparganj, Delhi 110 092, India

Ph: 011-49344934 Fax: 011-49344935
e-mail: publishing@cbspd.com; publicity@cbspd.com

Branches

- **Bengaluru:** Seema House 2975, 17th Cross, K.R. Road, Banasankari 2nd Stage, Bengaluru 560 070, Karnataka, India
  Ph: +91-80-26771678/79 Fax: +91-80-26771680 e-mail: bangalore@cbspd.com
- **Chennai:** 7, Subbaraya Street, Shenoy Nagar, Chennai 600 030, Tamil Nadu, India
  Ph: +91-44-26680620, 26681266 Fax: +91-44-42032115 e-mail: chennai@cbspd.com
- **Kochi:** 42/1325, 1326, Power House Road, Opposite KSEB, Power House, Ernakulum 682018, Kochi, Kerala, India
  Ph: +91-484-4059061–67 Fax: +91-484-4059065 e-mail: kochi@cbspd.com
- **Kolkata:** 147, Hind Ceramics Compound, 1st Floor, Nilgunj Road, Belghoria, Kolkata 700056, West Bengal, India
  Ph: +91-33-25330055/56 e-mail: kolkata@cbspd.com
- **Lucknow:** Basement, Khushuma Complex, 7 Meerabai Marg (behind Jawahar Bhawan), Lucknow 226001, UP, India
  Ph: +91-522-4000032 e-mail: tiwari.lucknow@cbspd.com
- **Mumbai:** PWD Shed, Gala No. 25/26, Ramchandra Bhatt Marg, Next JJ Hospital Gate No. 2, Opp. Union Bank of India, Noorbaug, Mumbai 400009, Maharashtra, India
  Ph: +91-22-66661880/89 e-mail: mumbai@cbspd.com

Representatives

- **Gujarat** 0-9879558667
- **Hyderabad** 0-9885175004
- **Jharkhand** 0-9811541605
- **Nagpur** 0-8692091830
- **Patna** 0-9334159340
- **Pune** 0-9664372571
- **Uttarakhand** 0-9716462459

Printed in Goyal Offset Works Pvt. Ltd., Haryana (INDIA)

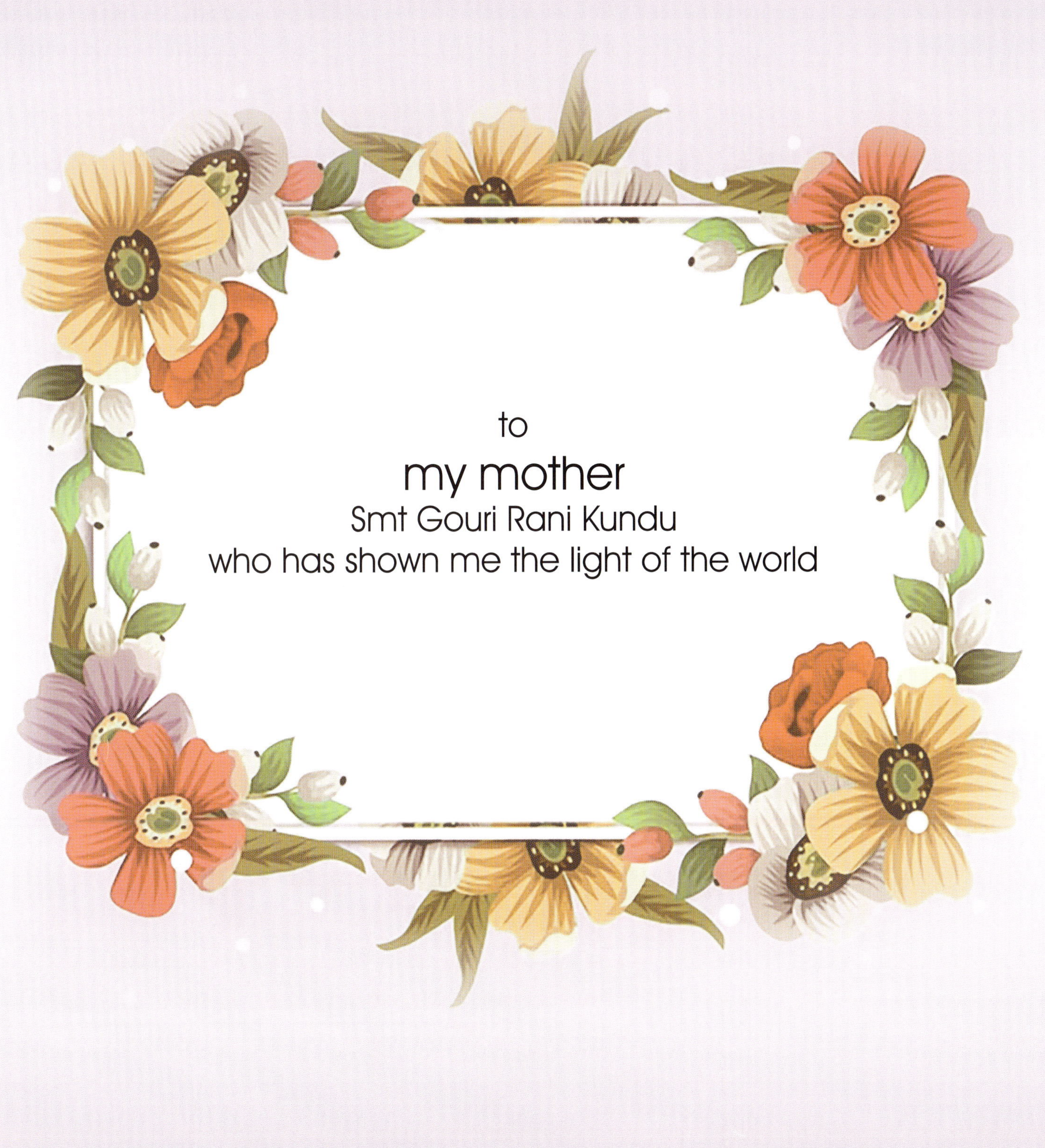

to

my mother

Smt Gouri Rani Kundu

who has shown me the light of the world

Preface to the Ninth Edition

I have great pleasure in presenting the Ninth Edition of '*Bedside Clinics in Medicine,* Part II'. The first Edition was published in the year 1999, and thereafter it was revised and edited from time to time in order to bring the same as current and up-to-date. In view of the wide acceptance of the previous editions by the medical fraternity, by the God's grace, I have ultimately succeeded to bring out the present edition of the book in a new lay-out. The overwhelming success of previous editions motivated me to bring out the new edition. Virtually all the chapters have been rewritten, appreciably revised and updated, maintaining the previous style and tradition intact. This Part II book, along with *Bedside Clinics in Medicine,* Part I, is now known by medical students all over as 'Magic Books in Clinical Medicine'.

It is a mammoth task for the students to read and remember all the current complicated medical facts and data to keep pace with the present era of information. As radiology, ECG, instrumental procedures, specimens, data analysis, different drugs and emergency medicine (i.e. **'Table-works'**) are integral parts of investigation, diagnosis and treatment, I felt committed to my students to rebuild the book with different modern clinical practices.

For more than three decades, working as a teacher and examiner in medicine, it is my belief that today's students lack clinical orientation and this is why I have attempted to write this book dealing with common clinical problems/investigations along with some fundamental information and a huge collection of invaluable facts. This new edition sketches step-by-step details of all data, approach, values, analysis, reasons behind, investigations and logical management in a question-answer format with a lucid language. The present edition deals with different must-know areas in clinical medicine which a student is expected to know at the end of his/her clinical training in medical school. I clearly emphasize that the book is a companion to the textbook and a reference manual not only to the undergraduates but postgraduates, residents, junior teachers, practicing physicians will also be highly benefitted if they read the book thoroughly. It is my strong belief that the book is a key companion to the students appearing for medicine practical examination.

This type of book with rich clinical material, which is rarely available in the market, has now become the need of the hour. All the chapters of the book are dealt with commonly encountered questions in viva-voce and practical examination in general medicine with their logical answers. The book is clear, concise and comprehensive in all respect, and contains many tables, figures, diagrams, X-rays, ECGs and charts for data analysis. The problem-solving attitude of the monograph will definitely help students in viva-voce, practical, as well as in their theoretical examination, and also in their professional life in future. This ready-reckoner handbook with a learning-revision tool is full of valuable tips from beginning to the end, and that is why students are advised to read the manual between the lines.

I feel happy and jubilant as the book is nicely accepted by academicians, students, eminent teachers and leading physicians from different corners of the country and abroad. Like the previous editions, healthy suggestions, feedbacks and constructive criticisms will always be appreciated by the author with gratitude.

I have immense pleasure in placing on record my appreciation for Mr Satish Kumar Jain (Chairman and Managing Director) and Mr Varun Jain (Director) of CBS Publishers and Distributors (CBSPD), New Delhi for publishing and distributing the book in India and abroad with great care. Mr SK Verma of CBSPD (VP, Marketing & Distributions) needs special mention who has guided me in every step of this long journey. Mr YN Arjuna (Senior Vice-President, Publishing, Editorial and Publicity) helped me by his constant input and encouragement, which have had a significant impact on the final texture of the text. I am also thankful to my wife Bijoya, son Dr Abhishek and daughter Ushasi, who have assisted me by their constant encouragement and support, and I remain indebted for their tolerance, patience and understanding during the preparation of the book.

Arup Kumar Kundu

arup2158@gmail.com

arup_kundu@hotmail.com

Preface to the First Edition

With the advancement of time, the subject of medicine is expanding astonishingly. It seems difficult for the undergraduate students to cope up with the mammoth subject. This compelled me to write a book dealing with model cases oriented to oral and practical examinations with special stress on clinical methods—the '*Bedside Clinics in Medicine*, Part I'.

As radiology, electrocardiography, urine examination, instrumental procedures, emergency medical management and drugs are integral part of diagnosis and treatment, I feel obligated to my students to write a new book which deals with those subjects. I have tried to cover the subjects thoroughly to give a vivid idea on radiology, ECG, etc. and to assist the students in economic and selective reading prior to final examination. Though basically meant for the undergraduates, the postgraduates and the practicing physicians will also be benefitted if they pry into it.

Bedside Clinics in Medicine, Part II would not have been completed had it not been for the patient understanding of our family, especially my wife Mrs. Bijoya Kundu who helped me throughout the making of this book, my parents, my daughter Ushasi and son Abhishek, who were deprived of their father's company for long long hours and days.

Finally, I am, really thankful to Mr. Kaustuv Paul of Crest Publishers for keeping me under constant pressure to write this new monograph, Mr. Kajal Saha for laying out the computerized drawings, and to the staff of Abhinaba Mudrani who have helped me in every step to complete the work. I also express my thanks to Dr. Sunetra Mukherjee, PGT in Radiodiagnosis and Dr. Sujoy Ghosh, PGT in General Medicine for providing me with X-ray plates. Healthy suggestions and constructive criticisms regarding the book will be highly appreciated and duly acknowledged.

In conclusion, I can not forget the constant encouragement given by my beloved students. I am greatly indebted to all of them.

Arup Kumar Kundu

Perspectives

In 1816, Rene-Theophile-Hyacinthe Laennec invented the stethoscope — the single instrument that came to symbolise the bedside physician and the tool used by the clinicians for almost last two centuries.

The term patient is derived from the Latin word 'patiens', or 'to suffer'. A 'patient' is one who feels sick physically or mentally, and consults doctor for relief of his ailments. In clinical medicine, patients hold the key position. Naturally, it is the task of the physician that he should do the needful for the recovery of the patient. The target of medical practice is to relieve sufferings.

To relieve the sufferings of the patients, a doctor should ascertain at first, the nature of illness from which the patient is suffering from. In other words, the doctor has to diagnose the existing disease. Physical diagnosis makes the bridge between the study of disease and the management of illness. Clinical diagnosis is an artistic science, based on three kinds of medical information:

i. Communication with the patient (i.e. the history taking),
ii. Physical examination, and
iii. Investigations.

Clinical medicine deals with the first two parts of diagnosis, i.e. 'clinical examination' of a patient consists of history taking as well as physical examination. These are the most important parts and it starts as soon as the patient comes to the doctor. At no point can **history taking** (medical events that have already taken place) be considered as 'wastage' of time; in most of the cases, the diagnosis can be made with history alone. History taking is an art, which a doctor should learn over years by repeated practice. A physician should be an attentive listener and be friendly to the patient. Regarding history taking, it is my advice to the students of clinical medicine that they should try to disprove Ben Berston's comment, who told 'A funny thing happens to medical students on their way to becoming physicians; they forget how to hold a conversation'. An appropriate history guides the patient's management in a proper direction. While examining the patient, an experienced doctor not only 'sees' but also 'uses all of his senses' and gradually develops the keen 'power of observation' which is known as 'clinical eye' or 'clinical acumen'. These insights cannot be acquired in a short-cut way and there is no rule of thumb in it. To learn this, one has to go to the bedside of the patients for years together, to make keen observations, to examine them thoroughly and sympathetically, and to try to 'associate' different observations and findings. Gradually the person develops the inherent 'knowledge of correlation' with the help of clinical eye. This is why, Hippocrates commented, 'A great part, I believe, of the art of medicine is the ability to observe. Leave nothing, combine contradictory observations and allow yourself enough time'. *An experienced clinician not only hears but listens, not only sees but observes, and not only touches but feels.* One, who has sharp clinical eye, becomes successful in life in the long run.

Traditionally, the process of **physical examination** (clinical state at that given time) is divided into four parts like looking (inspection), feeling (palpation), tapping (percussion), and listening (auscultation). From our student days we have learned to determine 'where is the lesion' as well as 'what is the lesion' derived by physical examination to arrive at a definitive diagnosis; this is also true to the students of this generation too. It should be realised that inspection/palpation/percussion/and especially auscultation are skills acquired over years of training. We know that our professional progenitors relied more on power of smelling (sweetish musty odour of hepatic coma) and tasting as well (the sweetness of urine in diabetes mellitus), but these facts have lost their importance in today's modern medicine. A sincere and meticulous physical examination combined with in-depth as well as sound knowledge of internal medicine will help the physician to determine the most probable cause/causes of the patient's present ailments. At the beginning, a student should have an open mind (observe, listen and create). It is wise to consider the patients as living pages of books, and instead of examining from 'head to feet', I should rather advise students to examine patients from 'head to toes'.

Another important part of clinical medicine is doctor-patient relationship. It has got immense value in ultimate recovery of the patient. By the way of 'conversation' and physical examination, one sympathetic doctor gains confidence and wins trust of the patient. This should never be neglected. Whenever the confidence of the patient is achieved, it becomes easier for the doctor to get his cooperation to examine the painful areas or even the diseased private parts of the body. In a non-cooperative patient, diagnosis may be much more difficult and delayed.

Investigations help the doctor confirm the diagnosis made by clinical examination. Of course, clinical diagnosis by physical examination has limitations. No doubt, in many cases one has to take the help of newer and sophisticated investigations to arrive at a definitive diagnosis. Recently, there is a boom in investigational facilities like polymerase chain reaction (PCR), ELISA (enzyme-linked immunosorbent assay) test, ultrasound, CT (computed tomography) scan, NMR (nuclear magnetic resonance) scan, PET (positron-emission tomography) scan, and SPECT (single-photon emission computed tomography) scan where the patient is being fragmented into systems, organs, tissues, cells or even the smallest DNA, and very often these facilities erode the confidence of the clinicians concerned. Nowadays, a large section of doctors feel that clinical examination is not at all essential and diagnosis can be made easily with the help of sophisticated investigations only. But this is not at all true. The laboratory should be used as an aid for confirmation of diagnosis and the final approach should be to 'treat the patient', not the laboratory reports. Try to prepare yourself with a patient-oriented mindset, rather than laboratory-oriented mindset. One confident doctor should never disregard his own clinical findings; moreover, newer investigations are often very costly and out of reach of most of the patients of a developing country like India. It seems we have reached an era of intellectual bankruptcy where the doctors ask for 'all investigations' than to ask for 'rational investigations'. A long time back, Alvan R. Feinstein remarked, 'Clinical judgement depends not on knowledge of causes, mechanisms or names of disease but on a knowledge of patients. The background of clinical judgement is clinical experience; the things that clinicians have learned at the bedside is the care of sick people'. I do think that clinical judgement and insight are inborn faculties which increase with experience.

In spite of these facts we cannot ignore the importance of 'chemical' diagnosis and contribution of physics in medicine, e.g. the discovery of X-ray by Wilhelm Roentgen or ECG (electrocardiogram) by Willem Einthoven. So question arises, will this computer and sophisticated newer technology replace the physician's task of performing physical examination? The answer is simply 'no'. The computer necessarily deals with the cold literal aspects of words, whereas the doctors are trained to search for hidden meanings. To the question, 'is your pain continuing at the present moment'? — the mechanical computer only records 'yes' even when the patient shows agony while responding. The doctor reads far more to the patient's response to 'yes'. Moreover, detailed questioning and physical examination frequently build the first emotional contact between the doctor and the patient. Can a computer be sympathetic to the patient regarding his illness? Or can a fascinating electronic gadget replace the excellence of Giant Clinicians like Battista Morgagni, Leopold Auenbrugger, Rudolf Virchow, RTH Laennec, Sir William Osler, Adolph Kussmaul and Joseph Jules Francois Felix Babinski? A human brain created the computer, and thus a slave can neither demonstrate physical signs of the disease in a patient nor can interpret the complexities encountered to have a definitive diagnosis. It has to be remembered that technology cannot be a substitute for clinical examination or the doctor-patient bond, which heals before any medicine. An internet cannot replace examination of patients at the bedside. So there is reason to believe that clinical medicine will ever persist as a basic diagnostic method and investigations will remain as 'complementary' to the clinician.

Medical knowledge is not masterable. Unlike physics or chemistry, medicine is not a pure science. Half of what is true today will be proven to be incorrect in the next five years, and unfortunately we do not know which half that is going to be. The question arises whether medicine is a science, or an art, or an art based on science? The scientists say that medicine is sometimes considered a science, and sometimes an art, and the object of medical science is to study disease. I think medicine is an art based on science; medicine is supposed to be a scientific study whether its practice is an art. However, I should say that medicine is a philosophy, the elicitation is the art and its interpretation is the science. Today, every senior doctor is shouting in every corner of this globe that the art of clinical medicine is dying in the present teaching set-up with high-tech gadgets. I also think that they are mostly true; today, doctors are more powerful but more deaf. Medical students are advised to revive the dying art of medicine and to be good artists with sufficient scientific knowledge.

It is worthwhile to mention here that lack of clinical skills may be called as 'hyposkillia'! The physicians with deficiency of clinical skills cannot take proper history, cannot perform physical examination, cannot manage the patient with proper assessment and reasoning, and posses poor communication skills. So, a proper training is essential in initial days of medical curriculum as today's medical students are the practicing physicians of future. At first, a student learns from his teacher and then 'experience' teaches him. The term 'doctor' came from the Latin word '*docere*', which means 'to teach'.

In the beginning of their clinical training, the students should also remember these golden words: '**there is no substitute for watchful eyes, alert ears, and tactful fingers in a logical mind**' as Hippocrates told 'eyes, ears, nose and palpating fingers are the gems of a physician, while intact brain is the necklace'.

Contents

Abbreviations

ABG	Arterial blood gas
AFB	Acid-fast bacillus
AGN	Acute glomerulonephritis
AIDS	Acquired immune deficiency syndrome
AI/AR	Aortic incompetence/regurgitation
AKI	Acute kidney injury
ALL	Acute lymphoblastic leukaemia
AMI	Acute myocardial infarction
AML	Acute myeloid leukaemia
ANA	Antinuclear antibody
ARDS	Acute respiratory distress syndrome
ARF	Acute renal failure
AS	Aortic stenosis
ASD	Atrial septal defect
ATD	Antituberculosis drugs
AVM	Arteriovenous malformation
BAL	Brochoalveolar lavage
BHP	Benign hypertrophy of prostate
BMI	Body mass index
BP	Blood pressure
BT	Bleeding time
°C	Degree Celsius
CAD	Coronary artery disease
CCF	Congestive cardiac failure
C/F	Clinical features
CKD	Chronic kidney disease
CLD	Chronic liver disease
CLL	Chronic lymphocytic leukaemia
CML	Chronic myeloid leukaemia
CMV	Cytomegalovirus
CNS	Central nervous system
C/o	Complains of
COPD	Chronic obstructive pulmonary disease
CP angle	Cerebello-pontine angle
CPR	Cardiopulmonary resuscitation
CRF	Chronic renal failure
CRP	C-reactive protein
CT	Clotting or coagulation time
CT scan	Computed tomography scan
CVA	Cerebrovascular accidents
CVP	Central venous pressure
CVS	Cardiovascular system
CXR	Chest X-ray
D/D	Differential diagnosis
DIC	Disseminated intravascular coagulation
DKA	Diabetic ketoacidosis
DVT	Deep vein thrombosis
ECG	Electrocardiogram
EF	Ejection fraction
EPS	Extrapyramidal system
ESR	Erythrocyte sedimentation rate
ESRD	End-stage renal disease
°F	Degree Fahrenheit
FEV1	Forced expiratory volume in one second
FNAC	Fine needle aspiration cytology
FUO	Fever of unknown origin
GBS	Guillain-Barré syndrome
GERD	Gastroesophageal reflux disease
GFR	Glomerular filtration rate
GH	Growth hormone
GTT	Glucose tolerance test
Hb	Haemoglobin
HBV	Hepatitis B virus
HCV	Hepatitis C virus
HD	Hodgkin's disease
HIV	Human immunodeficiency virus
HLA	Human leucocyte antigen
HOCM	Hypertrophic obstructive cardiomyopathy
H/o	History of
HSP	Henoch-Schönlein purpura
IBD	Inflammatory bowel disease
IBS	Irritable bowel syndrome
ICP	Intracranial pressure
ICS	Intercostal space
ICU	Intensive care unit
IE	Infective endocarditis
IHD	Ischaemic heart disease
IHSS	Idiopathic hypertrophic subaortic stenosis
IIT	Increased intracranial tension
ILD	Interstitial lung disease
IM	Intramuscular
INR	International normalised ratio
IV	Intravenous
IVC	Inferior vena cava
JIA	Juvenile idiopathic arthritis
JVP	Jugular venous pressure
LA/RA	Left atrium/right atrium
LAF	Left atrial failure
LAH	Left atrial hypertrophy
LFT	Liver function test
LMN	Lower motor neurone
LV/RV	Left ventricle/right ventricle
LVF	Left ventricular failure
LVH	Left ventricular hypertrophy
MCL	Midclavicular line
MCTD	Mixed connective tissue disease
MDR	Multi-drug resistance
MI/MR	Mitral incompetence/regurgitation
MND	Motor neurone disease
MS	Mitral stenosis
NAD	No abnormality detected
NHL	Non-Hodgkin's lymphoma
NPH	Normal pressure hydrocephalus
NSAIDs	Non-steroidal anti-inflammatory drugs
OC pills	Oral contraceptive pills
PAH	Pulmonary arterial hypertension
PA view	Postero-anterior view
PCR	Polymerase chain reaction

PDA	Patent ductus arteriosus
PFT	Pulmonary function test
PND	Paroxysmal nocturnal dyspnoea
PPI	Proton-pump inhibitor
PSS	Progressive systemic sclerosis
PUO	Pyrexia of unknown origin
RA	Rheumatoid arthritis
RAH	Right atrial hypertrophy
R/E	Routine examination
RHD	Rheumatic heart disease
RNTCP	Revised National Tuberculosis Control Programme
RTI	Respiratory tract infections
RVF	Right ventricular failure
RVH	Right ventricular hypertrophy
SBE	Subacute bacterial endocarditis
SLE	Systemic lupus erythematosus
SOL	Space-occupying lesion
SPA	Spondyloarthropathy
STD	Sexually transmitted diseases
SVC	Superior vena cava
TB	Tuberculosis
TC/DC	Total count/differential count
TI/TS	Tricuspid incompetence/stenosis
TIA	Transient ischaemic attack
UMN	Upper motor neurone
USG	Ultrasonography
UTI	Urinary tract infection
VATS	Video-assisted thoracoscopic surgery
VPB	Ventricular premature beat
VSD	Ventricular septal defect
WHO	World Health Organisation
WNL	Within normal limit

Chapter 1

Instruments and Bedside Procedures

"The greater the ignorance, the greater the dogmatism."

— **Sir William Osler** (1849-1919), Baronet, Canadian physician and professor of medicine, an author, medical philosopher, historian and teacher—could well be considered the most influential figure in the history of medicine—*'Father of modern medicine'*

RYLE'S TUBE (NASOGASTRIC TUBE)

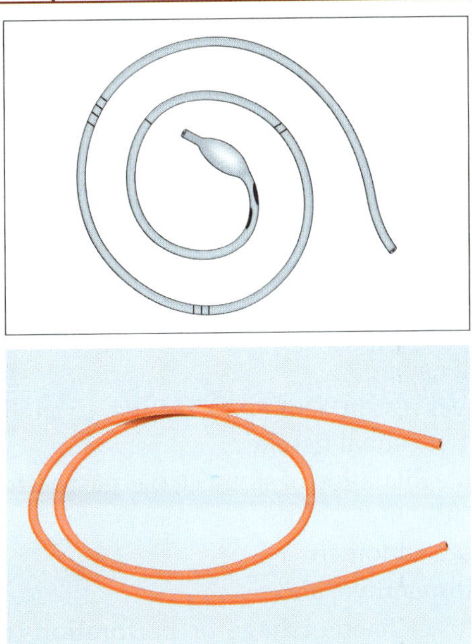

Fig. 1.1: Ryle's tube (polythene and rubber) showing markings

Q. Description (Fig. 1.1):

It is a fine bore flexible red rubber or polythene (transparent) tube with external circumference of 8 mm and length 105 cm. The blind bulbous tip contains a lead shot inside the tube to facilitate passage of the tube into the oesophagus (it is heavy and thus easier for the patient to swallow the tip). The lower end of the tube is perforated by a number of side holes at different levels to allow easy suction of gastro-duodenal contents. There are four black circular markings in the body of the tube as mentioned below:

a. *First mark (single circular mark):* Placed at a distance of 40 cm from the tip and indicates the distance from upper central incisor teeth to cardiac orifice of stomach.

b. *Second mark (two circular marks):* Indicates the distance between upper central incisor teeth and body of stomach (50 cm).

c. *Third mark (three circular marks):* Indicates the distance between upper central incisor teeth and pylorus (57 cm).

d. *Fourth mark (four circular marks):* Indicates the distance between upper central incisor teeth and first part of duodenum (65 cm). It means the tube has reached duodenum when the fourth mark is seen at the teeth.

The base (open end) is usually plugged by a conical plastic cap, and is used to fit with the nozzle of a syringe to push or to draw materials from the stomach. Ryle's tube is usually sterilised by keeping in boiling water for 30 minutes or by gamma ray irradiation.

The tip is made blunt to avoid trauma during introduction. If the perforations near the lower end are placed at same level, the tube may be easily torn during manipulation and if blocked (with openings at same level) by food debris or sticking to the mucosal surface of stomach, it would hamper suction of gastro-duodenal contents. Ryle's tube is available in different sizes like 4–18 French (tube with smaller diameter is used in children; adult size is 16–18 French). Instead of lead shot, polythene tube usually contains 3 radio-opaque metal balls.

Q. How to be sure that the tip has reached the stomach?

It is confirmed by the following methods:

1. Apply a 50 mL syringe at the open end of Ryle's tube. Inject air into the tube by pushing the piston with a single rapid thrust and simultaneously auscultate over the epigastrium. A gurgling sound confirms the position of the tube in the stomach.
2. Aspirate the gastric contents; the contents come out freely if the tube is in the stomach. Acidic nature of the

gastric contents may be confirmed by litmus paper test.

3. Fluoroscopy or straight X-ray of the abdomen shows the exact position of the tip of the tube as the tip contains lead shot or radio-opaque material.
4. Colorimetric capnography done to assure the postion in a mechanically ventilated patient.

- If the tube is passed falsely into the respiratory tract (trachea),
  a. The patient complains of a choking sensation.
  b. Violent cough appears and persists for a long time.
  c. Air comes from the open end with breathing.
  d. Yield of aspiration becomes nil.

In this situation, take out the tube immediately and try to reintroduce it cautiously.

Q. Why this nasogastric tube is named after 'Ryle'?

So far too many varieties of nasogastric tubes have been discovered but the tube designed by the physician, John Alfred Ryle (1889–1950) of Guy's Hospital Medical School is the most acceptable and commonly used type.

Another nasogastric tube: **Levine's tube** is longer, made of Portex and without the lead shot at the tip.

Q. How the Ryle's tube is introduced?

The patient is first explained about the procedure in order to obtain maximum cooperation. Ask the patient to lie flat in bed with extended neck. Remove the dentures, if present. In the nose, a more patent nostril is selected and properly cleansed, and lubricated with lignocaine jelly (2%). At first, check patency of the tube. Lubricate the tip of the sterilised tube with liquid paraffin or glycerine, and introduce the tip gently through one nostril (manually, mould the lower end of the tube a bit curved for easy passage through nasopharynx). As the tube reaches the oropharynx, the patient may start coughing once or twice and may even try to throw the tube by pulling it with his hands. Reassure the patient and ask him to swallow the tube, and to facilitate swallowing, one or two teaspoonfull of water may be poured into the mouth. With patience, the tube will gradually pass into the stomach by gentle push. Be sure that the tube is in the stomach and not within the trachea (see above). Take care in case of a comatosed patient, where the protective cough reflex is lost and the tube may be falsely introduced within the trachea without any alarming sign.

Lastly, the base (open end) of the tube is kept adhered to the forehead by a leucoplast and the open end is usually plugged (except in intestinal obstruction where the open end is kept open to allow continuous drainage). In a restless patient, hands should be tied.

Conventionally, the tube should not be kept for more than 48 hours. After 48 hours, the tube should be smeared daily with some antiseptic solution by withdrawing it only for 2 inches (the part lying within the nose), and then reintroducing it.

- Do not force the passage of Ryle's tube, if persistent resistance is felt.
- In repeated failure, try a smaller gauge tube.

Q. Different uses of Ryle's tube?

A. Diagnostic

1. To confirm and evaluate upper GI haemorrhage (i.e. in haematemesis or melaena).
2. Fractional test meal (gastric analysis)—virtually obsolete nowadays.
3. To isolate AFB from gastric juice in a child who is suffering from pulmonary tuberculosis (children usually swallow their sputum), or the patient who cannot expectorate sputum; searching for malignant cells in gastric carcinoma.
4. For forensic purpose—detection of cause of death in a suspected case of poisoning by subsequent chemical analysis of gastric aspiration (e.g. barbiturate, organophosphorus, copper sulphate, alcohol, etc.).
5. To aspirate duodenal secretions for analysis of:
   a. Pancreatic functions,
   b. Detection of typhoid carriers, and
   c. Detection of *Giardia lamblia* infestation.
6. To diagnose gastric outlet obstruction (gastic aspirate will exceed 200 mL after overnight fasting).

B. Therapeutic

1. Nasogastric feeding (*see* the next question).
2. Nasogastric suction in:
   a. Acute intestinal obstruction to relieve abdominal distension,
   b. Bowel rest in acute pancreatitis, Crohn's disease and intestinal fistula,
   c. Acute dilatation of stomach (i.e. gastric decompre-ssion),
   d. Acute abdomen,
   e. Postoperative, and
   f. GI tract haemorrhage or perforation (paralytic ileus).
3. Gastric wash or lavage done in:
   a. Pyloric stenosis,
   b. Non-corrosive poisoning, drug overdose, and
   c. Severe hiccough (i.e. bowel irrigation by ice-cold water or sodi-bicarbonate solution).
4. Medication in comatose patient or critically ill patient.
5. It can be used as a tourniquet (tourniquet is a device, made of latex tube, which is commonly used to stop the flow of blood through a vein or artery).

- **Gastric lavage is contraindicated** in a) Corrosive poisoning (Ryle's tube may perforate the oesophagus in acid or alkali poisoning), and b) Kerosine oil, paraffin or petrolium poisoning (gastric lavage increases the chance of development of lipoid pneumonia). Ryle's tube should not be used in severe fracture of base of the skull as there is a rare chance of intracranial introduction. Nasogastric feeding is unsuitable in stricture of upper GI tract and patients with high risk of aspiration (e.g. kerosine oil).

- The **two main indications for use of Ryle's tube** are: a) aspiration of gastric contents, and b) nutritional supplementation of the patient.
- Left lateral position of the patient facilitates the recovery of gastric juices through Ryle's tube.
- Insert a cuffed endotracheal tube before performing gastric lavage in unconscious patients.

Q. Indications for Ryle's tube feeding:

1. Unconscious patients (e.g. CVA, hepatic encephalopathy, diabetic ketoacidosis, cerebral malaria, encephalitis, meningitis, head injury) or critically ill patients.
2. Inability to swallow, e.g. after facio-maxillary injury or surgery, bulbar palsy.
3. Patients who are reluctant to take food orally, e.g. severe anorexia, anorexia nervosa, etc.
4. Neurogenic dysphagia, nasal regurgitation in polymyositis or dermatomyositis.
5. In patients with burns.

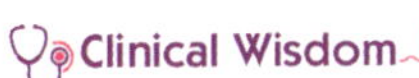

Previously used intragastric milk drip in acute exacerbation of chronic duodenal ulcer is not practised now as milk may increase gastric acid secretion and release of gastrin, stimulated by direct effect of milk protein and calcium.

Q. Complications of nasogastric intubation:

1. Rhinitis and pharyngitis; ulceration in oesophagus may develop.
2. Epistaxis (from nasal injury during introduction).
3. If the tube enters into trachea, aspiration pneumonia and even death may result.
4. Blockage of the tube.
5. If the tube is kept *in situ* for a prolonged period (e.g. in bulbar palsy), it is often difficult to take out the tube (the Ryle's tube may be coiled spontaneously inside the lumen of stomach).
6. Perforation of pharynx or oesophagus (chance increased in presence of oesophageal disease).
7. Chance of respiratory tract infections in prolonged intubation (thus, chest physiotherapy is necessary).

Q. Stomach wash (gastric lavage) tube: What is it (Fig. 1.2)?

It is a special wide-bore tube of 75 cm in length, and with an attached funnel (may have a plastic or wooden mouth gag, which prevents biting of the tube by teeth) at the proximal end to wash (gastric lavage) poison, alcohol or overdose of drug. It has a black ring at 45 cm from the tip which indicates the distance between upper central incisor teeth and cardiac end of stomach. This tube is used for stomach wash and is kept in emergency room of every hospital (adult size: 36–40 French). The complications encountered are aspiration, laryngospasm and bradycardia.

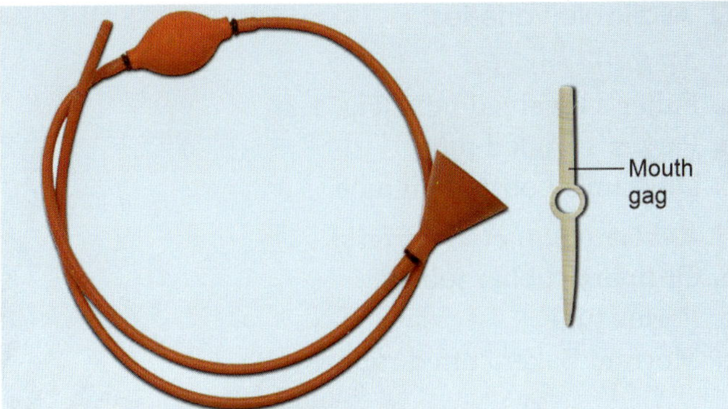

Fig. 1.2: Stomach wash tube (Ewald's)

Q. Hypochlorhydria and hyperchlorhydria:

A. Hypochlorhydria or achlorhydria:

1. Aged persons >60 years.
2. Pernicious anaemia.
3. Gastric malignancy.
4. After proton-pump inhibitor therapy.

B. Hyperchlorhydria:

1. Zollinger-Ellison syndrome.
2. Systemic mastocytosis.
3. Hyperparathyroidism.
4. G-cell hyperplasia.

Note

Read corrosive poisoning, drug overdose, haematemesis in details.

TRACHEOSTOMY TUBE (Fig. 1.3)

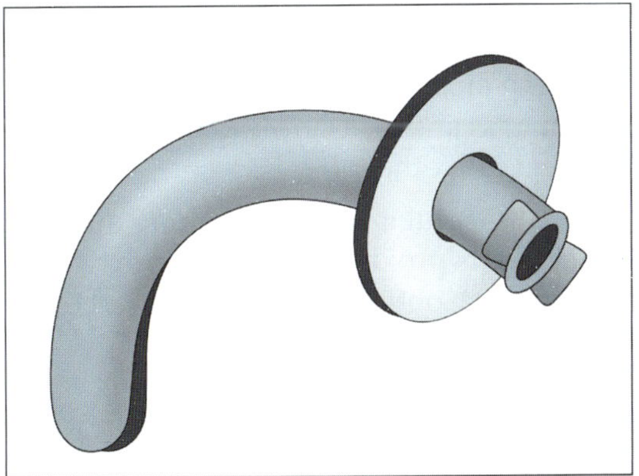

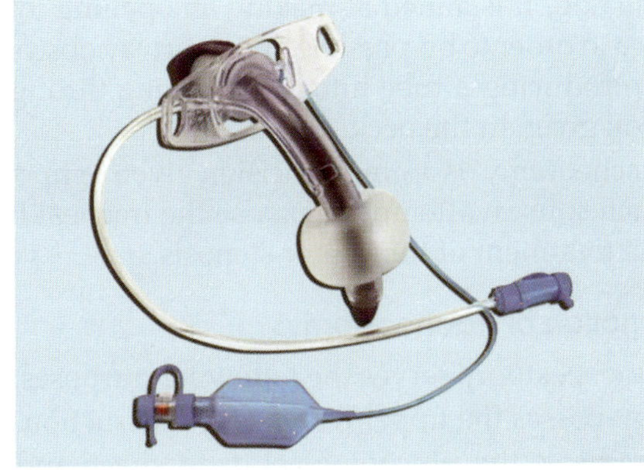

Fig. 1.3: Fuller's bivalved tracheostomy tube

Q. Available varieties:

A. Metallic variety:

a. Fuller's bivalved tube (Fig. 1.3).
b. Parker's angled tube.
c. Durham's Lobster tail tube.

B. Rubber (synthetic) variety:

a. Ordinary rubber tube.
b. Portex tube.
c. Morrant Baker cuffed rubber tube.

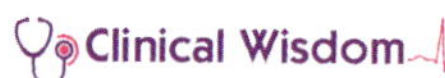

Plastic or silicone tubes are increasingly popular because they are softer, less irritant and there is less crusting of secretions.

Q. Types of tracheostomy tube:

A. Metallic, or portex or rubber.
B. Cuffed (i.e. a balloon at the distal end of the tube, which can provide a seal between the tube and tracheal wall, if inflated) or uncuffed.

- Cuffed tracheostomy tube prevents aspiration, keeps the tube in position and prevents gaseous leak while on positive-pressure ventilation.
- Metallic tube is used in permanent tracheostomy, e.g. following laryngectomy.

Q. Description of Fuller's tracheostomy tube:

It is the commonly used type. It consists of one outer and one inner tube.

Outer tube: The curved tube is split distally into two thin blades which can be easily approximated. As the blades have spring-like action, it acts as a tracheal dilator. Proximally, the outer tube contains a rounded shield bearing an opening on each side through which threads can pass and is fastened to the back of the neck of the patient to fix the tube.

Inner tube: It is a tube with an opening and made for air passage. At its proximal end, there are two rings for easy handling. An obturator is the third part of the tube.

Q. What is tracheostomy?

'Tracheostomy' is an operation for temporary relief of a patient who is suffering from acute upper airway obstruction. It is aimed at making an opening into the trachea in order to by-pass the upper airway obstruction and introducing a tube into that opening through the incision given in the neck.

'Tracheotomy' is a simple incision given temporarily on trachea in an attempt to expose the tracheal lumen for the treatment of tumour or stenosis.

Q. Function of tracheostomy:

The tracheostomy serves the following purposes:

1. It by-passes the upper respiratory obstruction.
2. It reduces the physiological dead space and thus improves efficiency of respiration.
3. It diminishes airway resistance, i.e. strain of respiration is reduced.
4. It helps in removing the excess bronchial secretions.
5. Insertion of a cuffed tracheostomy tube helps in application of positive-pressure ventilation.

Q. Common indications for 'emergency' tracheostomy:

The principal indication is upper airway obstruction like:

1. Laryngeal diphtheria (pseudomembrane obstructs the larynx).
2. Impacted foreign body in the larynx.
3. Acute laryngeal oedema (oedema glottis resulting from anaphylaxis or inhalation of irritant gases) with cyanosis.
4. Tetany (in case of laryngysmus stridulus) or tetanus (laryngeal spasm).
5. Acute bulbar palsy (e.g. poliomyelitis, GB syndrome, rabies, myasthenic crisis).
6. Ludwig's angina.
7. Spasm of vocal cord (tabetic laryngeal crisis) in tabes dorsalis (not seen nowadays).

Q. Common indications for 'planned' or 'elective' tracheostomy:

1. As a preliminary step in different operations in larynx.
2. To relieve obstruction in a case of laryngeal carcinoma.
3. In respiratory failure (paralysis of intercostal muscles), i.e. for long-term ventilation, this is aimed to reduce the dead space. Apart from this, intermittent positive-pressure ventilation may be applied through a cuffed endotracheal tube inserted via a tracheostomy, in patients suffering from respiratory paralysis with or without bulbar palsy (particularly when the respiratory paralysis is likely to last for more than 2–3 days)—facilitation of ventilation support.
4. Bronchial lavage.
5. Incompetent larynx with aspiration.

Q. Different types of tracheostomy:

It depends on the position of isthmus of the thyroid gland.

a. *High tracheostomy:* Opening done above the isthmus (it has the risk of injuring cricoid cartilage, followed by stenosis).
b. *Median tracheostomy:* Opening done at the level of the isthmus (choice in acute emergencies).
c. *Low tracheostomy:* Opening done below the isthmus (some physicians prefer this method).

Q. Common bedside features of laryngeal (or upper airway) obstruction:

The patient presents with:

1. Restlessness with hyperactive accessory muscles of respiration.
2. Dyspnoea and even orthopnoea.

3. Cough (croupy cough is seen in diphtheria).
4. Stridor.
5. Central cyanosis.
6. Intercostal suction.
7. Signs of exhaustion.

Q. How the tube is introduced?

The two tubes are separated. Press the two cusps (blades) of the outer tube and try to appose them, and now introduce it with its concavity directed downwards. The blades will open up and will act as a tracheal dilator. Tie the outer tube round the neck with a thread. Then introduce the inner tube through the outer one and place a piece of wet sterile gauze over the opening of the tube. The advantages of double tubing are:

a. When the inner tube is taken out for cleaning, the outer tube serves the purpose.
b. Bivalved outer tube helps to avoid the use of an additional tracheal dilator.

Q. Precautions taken during the period of intubation:

1. The metallic tube is kept for a short period, usually not more than 24 hours to avoid necrosis of trachea which may lately give rise to tracheal stenosis. This should be replaced by rubber tracheostomy tube.
2. The rubber tube may be kept up to a desired period.
3. Precautions are taken so that the tube remains patent. Intermittent suction may serve the purpose.
4. Strict asepsis is maintained. A sterile gauze piece soaked in 1:1000 acriflavine solution or povidone-iodine solution is commonly used over the opening of the tube.
5. Systemic broad-spectrum antibiotic is used to prevent respiratory tract infections, as and when necessary. Good nursing care with strict asepsis is maintained.

- The inner tube should be removed every four hours for cleaning purpose. The excess of secretions should be removed (by suction) with a soft rubber catheter. Mucolytic aerosols or humidifiers are often used to liquefy the viscid secretions. The rubber tracheostomy tube can be kept usually for 2–3 weeks.
- Once the patient can sleep for a night with the tube plugged, it is then possible to remove the tracheostomy tube.
- The tracheostomy tube is sterilised by immersing in concentrated lysol solution.

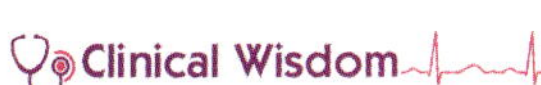

Explain the procedure (if possible) and obtain **written informed consent** from the patient or relatives in all invasive procedures like tracheostomy, lumbar puncture, bone marrow aspiration, liver biopsy, etc.

Q. Postoperative complications:

1. Bronchopneumonia.
2. Mediastinal emphysema.
3. Mediastinitis (i.e. mediastinal infection).
4. Pneumothorax.
5. Pressure necrosis of anterior tracheal wall by inflated cuff.
6. Blockage of the tracheostomy tube (in improper toileting).
7. Tracheal stenosis or collapse of the tracheal rings; collapse of the lung.
8. Tracheo-oesophageal fistula.
9. Erosion of innominate artery.
10. Difficulty in decannulation ('decannulation' is the method of removal of tracheostomy tube by which tubes of progressively smaller diameter are introduced in order to adapt the patient to breathe through the normal airway, as the patient often forgets to breathe normally when tracheostomy tube remains for a longer period).

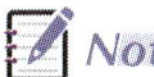
Note

Read steps of tracheostomy operation from standard ENT textbook. Read diphtheria and bulbar palsy in details.

SIMPLE RUBBER CATHETER

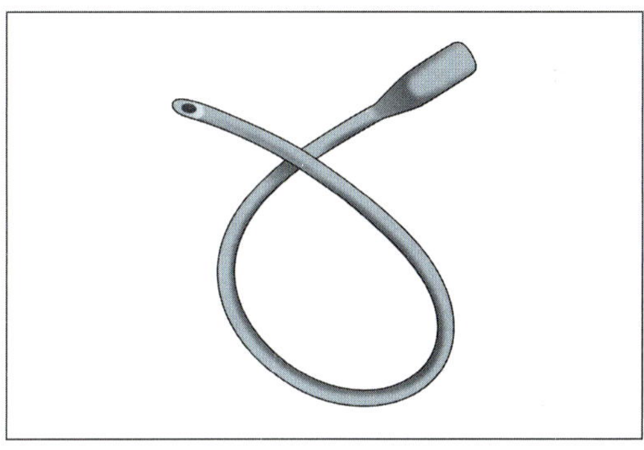

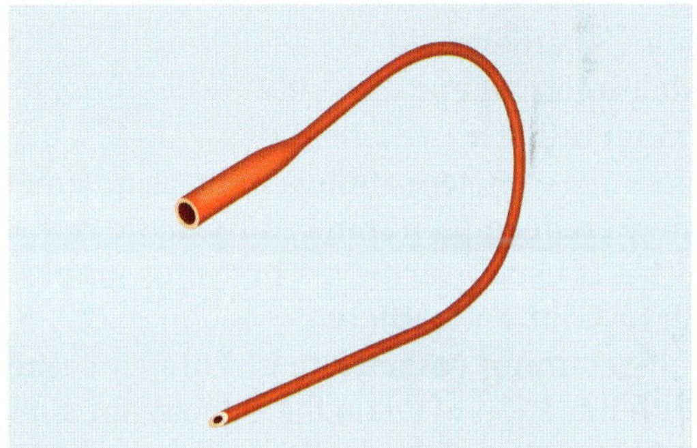

Fig. 1.4: Simple rubber catheter

Q. Description (Fig. 1.4):

1. Simple tube made of India-rubber or latex-rubber, and is also known as Robinson or Nelaton catheter.
2. There is a channel throughout the whole length of the tube.
3. Blunt and rounded tip with perforation (eye); the other end is open.
4. Number of size (available in different sizes) is printed on the catheter.

- The catheter is sterilised by keeping in boiling water for 30 minutes or by gamma ray irradiation.
- Catheters made of 'latex' make it biologically inert as far as possible. 'Silicone' catheters are preferred when required to be kept for a longer time or patient is allergic to latex.

Q. Different uses:

1. To relieve acute retention of urine.
2. To differentiate retention of urine from anuria.
3. To obtain urine specimen for examination in an unconscious or comatose patient.
4. To differentiate pelvic lump from bladder swelling.
5. Before or during delivery (child birth).
6. To monitor the urine output or to measure the residual volume of urine.
7. To prevent urinary incontinence in neurogenic bladder.
8. Used prior to cystography (to introduce dye in the urinary bladder).
9. For bladder wash or irrigation (by acriflavine or silver nitrate solution).
10. As a drainage tube.
11. As a tourniquet (to produce haemostasis or to make the veins prominent).
12. As an oxygen tube, i.e. used as a nasal catheter.
13. In infants, it may be used as a feeding tube.

- Simple rubber cathater is used for catheterisation 'just once' only.

Q. Mention common 'medical causes' of catheterisation:

Urinary catheters are of three types:
1. Simple rubber cetheter (intermittent self-catheter)
2. Self-retaining catheter (indwelling catheter):
   a. Gibbons catheter
   b. Foley's catheter
   c. Malecot's catheter
3. Condom catheter (*see* later)

Temporary catheterisation is done as an emergency measure to relieve pain induced by acute retention of urine. This is usually achieved by using simple rubber catheter or **Gibbons catheter**.

A self-retaining catheter (e.g. **Foley's catheter**) is used with intention to retain the catheter for a few days (Fig. 1.5A). They are basically used in patients with benign hypertrophy of prostate (BHP) who are unfit for prostatectomy, neurogenic bladder and in patients who are mostly bed-bound (e.g. hemiplegia or paraplegia). **Malecot's catheter** is not used as an urethral catheter; the wings of the catheter provide increased drainage and as such it is used for drainage urine after renal or bladder surgery, pus from empyema thoracis or to relieve a patient of pneumothorax (Fig. 1.5B). A 'haematuria catheter' is a three-way catheter (used in haematuria) with an extra channel for irrigation. The 'medical causes' are:

1. Coma or unconsciousness due to any cause, e.g. CVA (*hemiplegia*), diabetic ketoacidosis, encephalitis, hepatic coma, cerebral malaria.
2. Meningitis (tuberculous commonly).
3. Compressive myelopathy (caries spine), acute transverse myelitis, spinal injury, anterior spinal artery thrombosis, i.e. in *paraplegia*.

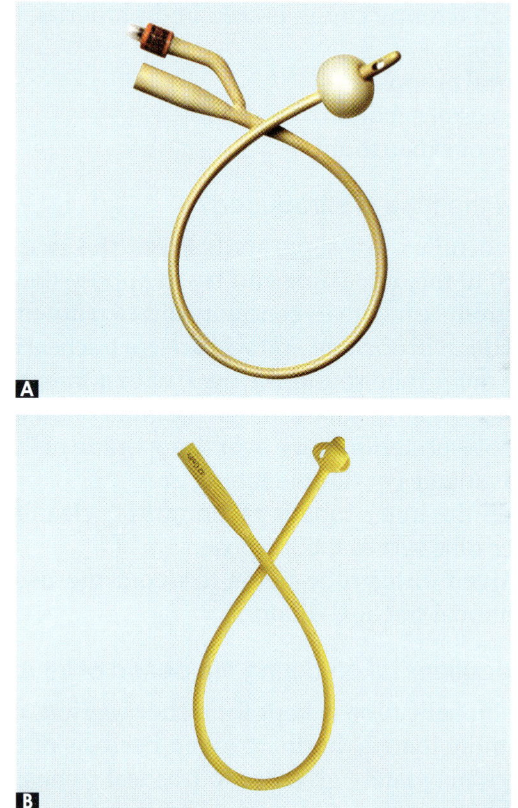

Fig. 1.5: (A) Foley's catheter; (B) Malecot's catheter

4. Poisoning: Opium, dhatura, organophosphorus or drug overdose (sedatives).
5. Snake bite (especially Viperidae group).
6. Sometimes, catheterisation is done in acute nephritis, nephrotic syndrome, renal failure and patients in intensive therapeutic unit (ITU) to measure the actual urinary output.

- Common surgical indications are BHP, vesical calculus, bladder injury and carcinoma of prostate.
- **Suprapubic cystostomy** (in hypogastrium) is done when urethral passage is narrow or blocked (e.g. severe prostatic enlargement), post-bladder and urethral surgeries, or for long term bladder drainage.
- Recurrent UTI is a relative contraindication for catheterisation.

Clinical Wisdom

Foley's catheter is named after American urologist Frederic Foley, who designed it in 1929. The balloon inside should be inflated by sterile water, and not by saline or air.

Q. Contraindications of catheterisation:

1. Recurrent urinary tract infection (UTI).
2. Meatal stenosis.
3. Rupture (suspected) of the urethra.
4. Stricture of the urethra.

Q. How to catheterise the urinary bladder?

Maintenance of strict asepsis is very important.

1. The procedure should be explained to the patient. The catheter is sterilised properly (or already done by manufacturers). The physician should follow strict

antiseptic and aseptic measures—hand washing by soap and spirit, and wearing sterile mask, gown and gloves. The local part (urethral meatus) of the patient is cleansed meticulously by any antiseptic solution.
2. The tip of the catheter is lubricated by liquid paraffin and introduced per urethra while the left hand is holding the shaft of the penis erect, in case of males; 2% lignocaine jelly may be used to reduce pain during introduction.
3. Oulflow of urine confirms proper introduction while evacuation of the bladder is done gradually.
4. The free end of the catheter should not touch the urine contained in the kidney-tray as contaminated urine from the container may be sucked into the bladder by negative intravesical pressure after evacuation.
5. The catheter is taken out after evacuation is over or may be kept for some time by proper adhesion on the thigh by leucoplast; if repeated or prolonged catheterisation is necessary, a self-retaining catheter (e.g. Foley's catheter) should replace simple rubber catheter.

- For self-retaining catheters in adults, it is better to choose the 'medium size' (neither too large nor too fine). A 14 Charriere catheter is a good first choice in an adult (catheters are sized using the system invented by Joseph FB Charriere). A Charriere's French scale was used to describe the external diameter of a catether. Adult sizes of catheter: 14–24, Children 8–12.
- *Large size catheter:* Used in postoperative bladder irrigation, haemorrhage in bladder and pyuria.
- *Small size catheter:* Used in urethral strictures and bladder neck obstruction.

Q. Risk of rapid evacuation of the bladder:

Rapid evacuation may be dangerous due to development of:

1. Reflex shock.
2. Haematuria as a result of rupture of engorged and dilated submucous veins of the bladder.
3. Reflex anuria (rare).

Q. Initial steps to relieve acute retention of urine:

1. Reassurance.
2. Alternate application of hot and cold over the hypogastrium.
3. Produce the hissing sound of a running tap (to initiate childhood reflex).
4. Apply hot hip bath.
5. Inj. carbachol—2 mL, IM may be given to initiate the reflex; parasympathetic stimulation enhances evacuation of urine.
6. Lastly, try catheterisation.

Q. Differentiation between retention of urine and anuria:

A. Clinically: On inspection, hypogastrium looks distended in retention of urine. Now percussion of the hypogastrium is done from above downwards where retention will produce a dull note and in anuria, normal tympanitic note of abdomen is elicited. Moreover, application of pressure over hypogastric swelling produces desire for micturition in retention of urine.

B. By catheterisation: In anuria, no urine comes out after introduction of a simple rubber catheter; urine comes out after catheterisation in a case of retention of urine.

Q. Complications of catheterisation:

1. Urinary tract infection or UTI—urethritis, cystitis (the most common); catheter fever.
2. Catheter trauma to urethra and bladder, and bleeding.
3. Haematuria after sudden and rapid evacuation.
4. Shock (reflex)—rare.
5. False passage (rare).
6. Blockage of the lumen of catheter leading to retention of urine.
7. Long-term catheterisation may be associated with urethral ulceration, stricture formation, formation of vesical calculus or calculus formation at tip of the catheter.
8. Perforation of urinary bladder.

- An indwelling catheter invariably leads to urinary tract infection (UTI) within days or weeks. This can be minimised by regular bladder wash done by saline or dilute chlorhexidine solution, and changing the catheter once in 2–3 weeks. The patient is strictly advised not to pull the catheter by his hands
- In urine leakage around Foley's catheter, think of smaller catheter size, smaller balloon size, spasm of urinary bladder or UTI.

Q. What is a urosac bag (Fig. 1.5C)?

This is a calibrated bag, usually of 2-litre capacity, which collects urine drained by a self-retaining catheter. The bag is disposable and sterile. It has two tubes: one is connected with the urinary catheter and the other is used to empty the urosac. The urosac is usually tied with the iron rod of the bed.

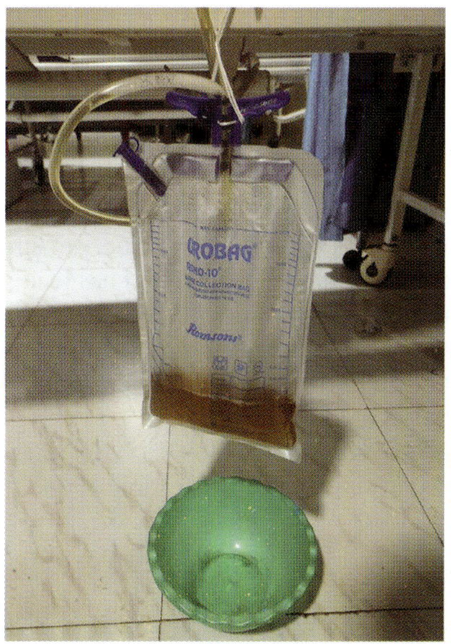

Fig. 1.5C: Urosac

Q. Common causes of anuria:

A. Pre-renal:

1. Shock, sepsis (septicaemia), haemorrhage (massive).
2. Dehydration due to any cause (e.g. acute gastroenteritis) or severe vomiting.
3. Crush syndrome.
4. Burn (extensive).
5. Intravascular haemolysis, mismatched blood transfusion.
6. Congestive cardiac failure.
7. Acute pancreatitis.

B. Renal:

1. Acute glomerulonephritis, rapidly progressive glomerulonephritis (RPGN).
2. Acute renal failure (ARF) or acute kidney injury (AKI).
3. Acute papillary necrosis (diabetes, phenacetin-induced, sickle cell disease).
4. Diffuse cortical necrosis.
5. Complete renal arterial and venous obstruction.
6. Chronic renal failure (produces anuria terminally)

C. Post-renal:

1. Reflex anuria (calculus in one ureter may produce reflex obstruction of the other ureter).
2. Ligation of the ureters (accidental) or bilateral ureteric obstruction by clots, stones or crystals.
3. Ureteric obstruction due to retroperitoneal fibrosis or malignant infiltrations around the ureters.

- Clinically distended bladder, enlarged prostate and hydronephrosis point towards post-renal cause of ARF.

Q. No urine comes out after catheterisation—reasons behind:

In this situation, one should think of:

1. False passage.
2. Eye of the catheter remaining above the urine level in the bladder—a little adjustment of the catheter brings out urine.
3. Catheter is blocked.
4. Dealing with anuria instead of retention of urine.

- An oxygen tube may be used as a rubber catheter though it is very thin. Don't confuse a simple rubber catheter with the Ryle's tube (Ryle's tube is longer, and has lead shot or metal balls at the tip).
- A **suction catheter** (extracts secretion of body like mucus and is connected with a suction machine) looks like a simple rubber catheter.
- Self-retaining catheters (Foley's, Malecot's) are usually encountered in surgery practical examination.

Clinical Wisdom

Keep the urosac bag lower than the bladder so that urine does not flow back up into the urinary bladder.

BONE MARROW ASPIRATION NEEDLE

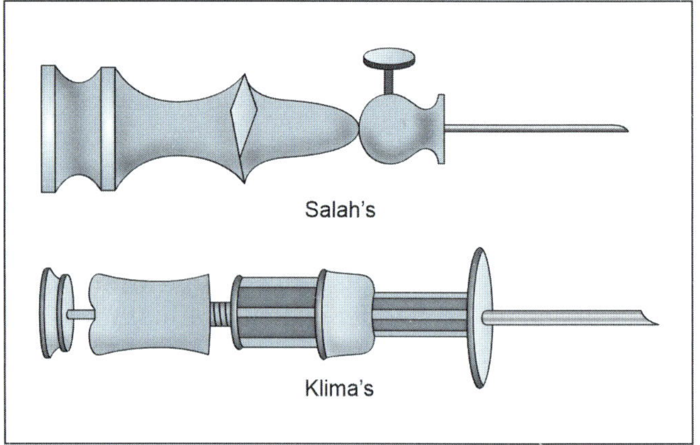

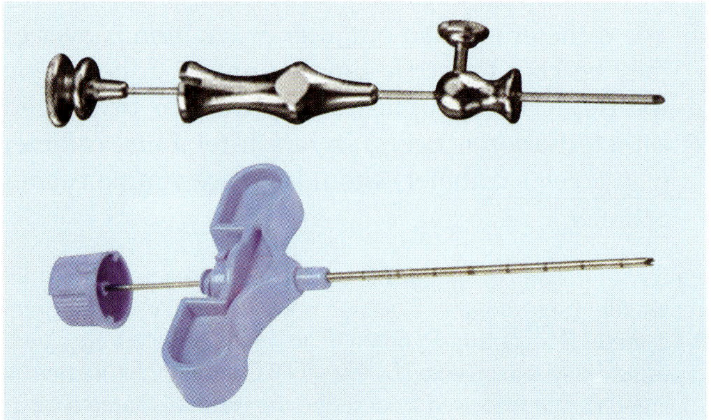

Fig. 1.6A: Sternal puncture needle (Salah's and Klima's variety)

Q. Use:

It is used for bone marrow aspiration. Often it is loosely termed as sternal puncture (SP) needle.

Q. Description:

The needle consists of three parts:

1. *The needle proper:* It is a stout wide bore needle (length is 5 cm); the needle is shortly bevelled at one end, and the base of the stylet or the nozzle of a syringe fits in the other broad end.
2. *The stylet:* It keeps the needle patent during introduction. When kept inside the needle proper, it helps to know whether the tip of the needle has entered into the marrow cavity or not. The base of the stylet contains a small projection for better fixation with the needle proper.
3. *The adjustable guard:* The adjustable screw guard prevents over-penetration of the needle. The plane or flat surface of the guard should look down to the chest wall of the patient.

   The SP needle is made of steel. There are two types: 1. Salah (commonly used) and 2. Klima.

   The two varieties differ in the design, especially in the type of the guard. Klima's variety contains an adjustable guard on the stem of the needle proper; it has a central screw (not projected from the side like Salah's variety). The neede is sterilised by immersing in concentrated lysol solution.

Clinical Wisdom

Bone marrow biopsy is of two types:

a. Aspiration biopsy (by Salah's or Klima's needle) **(Fig. 1.6A)**, and

b. Trephine biopsy (by Jamshidi's needle).

Q. Sites of puncture:

1. *Body of the sternum:* 2nd or 3rd piece of body on either side of midline (manubrium sterni is less cellular). According to haematologists, this site is not recommended at present for safety purpose.
2. Posterior iliac crest (an ideal and safe site for all) **(Fig. 1.6B)**.
3. Upper part of the medial surface of tibia, just below the tibial tuberosity.
4. Spinous process of lumbar vertebrae (rarely used).
5. Ribs (rarely used).
6. Any site of bone infiltration or tumour (in disease).

No. 2 (above two years of age) and No. 3 (below two years of age) are the ideal sites of puncture in children because these sites contain sufficient marrow material and are without any risk of injuring great vessels. In adults, all the sites may be used for puncture.

Marrow aspiration from posterior iliac crest is less painful and less hazardous. It is also preferred in elderly (especially osteoporotic individuals), patients receiving sternal irradiation (sternum may not yield marrow) and in repeated marrow aspiration. In obese persons, sternum is the preferred site.

Q. Indications of bone marrow aspiration:

1. *Anaemia:* Hypoplastic anaemia (hypocellularity of bone marrow), megaloblastic anaemia (megaloblasts), sideroblastic anaemia (ringed sideroblasts) and other unexplained anaemia.
2. *Leukaemia:* Confirmation of different leukaemias, especially subleukaemic and aleukaemic leukaemias.
3. Pancytopenia, or thrombocytopenia, or abnormal cell morphology in peripheral smear.

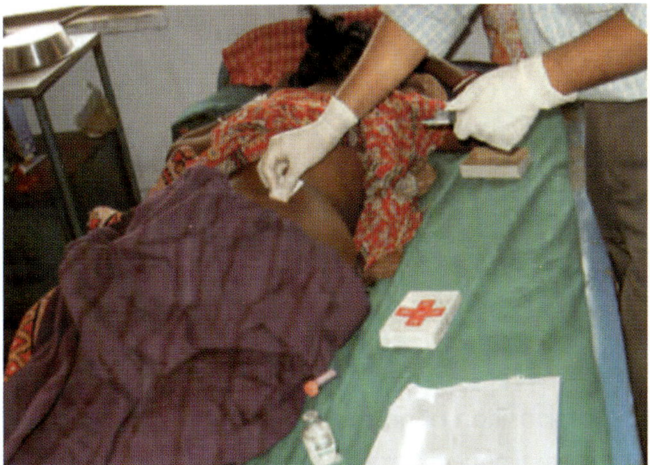

Fig. 1.6B: A patient of acute leukaemia is undergoing **bone marrow aspiration** from posterior iliac crest

4. *Kala-azar:* Demonstration of LD bodies confirms the diagnosis (chronic or acute).
5. Multiple myeloma
6. Hypersplenism.
7. Bone marrow transplant (therapeutic use)
8. Miscellaneous—secondary carcinoma of bone (bony metastasis), myelofibrosis, polycythemia, immune thrombocytopenic purpura (ITP), lymphoma (mainly for staging purpose), agranulocytosis, AIDS, lipid storage disease (Gaucher's disease), carcinomatosis and other myeloproliferative disorders.

In clinical practice, bone marrow aspiration is usually carried out in unexplained anaemia, unexplained hepatosplenomegaly, unexplained lymphadenopathy and in cases with pyrexia of unknown origin (PUO).

Q. Contraindications of bone marrow aspiration:

1. Local sepsis or infection; osteomyelitis
2. Coagulation disorders like haemophilia or severe thrombocytopenia (platelet count <20000/mm^3); or hepatic disorders (relative contraindications).
3. Very poor general condition/restless patient.

- Always measure the platelet count, BT, CT and prothrombin time before aspiration. Usually thrombocytopenia (i.e. platelet count <100000/mm^3) is not a contraindication.

Q. How the sternal puncture tray is prepared?

1. Spirit, iodine, sterile gown, mask and gloves for antiseptic purpose.
2. 2% lignocaine solution as local anaesthetic.
3. 2 mL glass syringe with needle for local anaesthesia,
4. Sterile SP needle with stylet.
5. 2 mL metal syringe or record syringe (the piston and nozzle are made of metal) for aspirating marrow material.
6. Cotton, sterile gauze, gauze-holding forcep.
7. 6 pairs of glass slides.
8. Blotting paper or pipette.
9. Benzoin solution and leucoplast.

Q. Procedure of bone marrow aspiration:

A. Sternal puncture:

1. Local antiseptic and aseptic preparations are taken (spirit-iodine-spirit). Skin is shaved over sternum in hairy chest. The physician should wash his hands, and wear sterile mask, gown and gloves, and should stand on the right side of the patient.
2. The patient is sedated by inj. diazepam 10 mg or inj. pentazocine 30 mg, IM given 30 minutes before the procedure.
3. The patient lies supine. Reassure the patient and explain him what you are going to perform. Keep the prepared SP tray by the side of the patient.
4. The skin and the subcutaneous tissue down to the periosteum (periosteum is very sensitive to pain)

are anaesthetised by 2% lignocaine injection and during the procedure, the depth from the skin to the periosteum is assessed.

5. The guard is adjusted at a distance which is equal to the depth of the skin and the subcutaneous tissue (varies with the build of the patient) plus 0.5 cm extra length (this is the thickness of cortex of the sternum). The stylet is now put within the needle, and by boring or drilling movement the needle is pushed through the skin vertically down (the needle is held at right angles to the bone) till the medulla is reached.
6. As soon as the bone marrow as reached, the stylet is removed and a metal syringe is attached to the needle. Now as the marrow is aspirated, the patient complains of excruciating suction pain; 0.2 mL of bone marrow is sucked out gently. The needle with the metal syringe is then removed as a whole. The aspirated marrow is dropped immediately over the properly cleaned slides to prepare films.
7. Sufficient pressure is given over the puncture site for 2–5 minutes to assure haemostasis. The puncture site is now sealed with tincture benzoin and the patient is advised to take rest for at least 30 minutes. Pulse and BP are monitored half hourly for 4 hours, and analgesics may be advised to relieve pain; nothing per mouth (NPM) is given for 4 hours.
8. Usually 6 pairs of glass slides are given in the tray. Remove the blood or fluid part from the slide by tilting the slide, or by means of blotting paper or pipette. Marrow films (marrow is granular) are now prepared like blood films (or two slides containing marrow material are apposed and slided over). After drying, the slides are stained (usually with Leishman's stain).

- Aspiration of more than 0.2 mL of material will unnecessarily dilute the marrow (as blood comes) and reduce the concentration of marrow cells. If no marrow is obtainable from a site, a different site may be chosen.

B. Iliac crest puncture (Fig. 1.6B)*:* Safest, the patient lies in prone position on a pillow placed beneath the pelvis.

C. Lumbar spinous process puncture: Easy procedure. Patient sits or adopts lateral decubitus position. The needle is introduced perpendicularly and a bit lateral to the midline.

Q. How to recognise that marrow material is present on the slide?

As the marrow is granular, the surface of the film will appear uneven.

Q. How to be sure that marrow cavity has reached?

This is diagnosed by:

1. Sudden loss of resistance.
2. The needle remains in vertical position without any support.
3. The tip of the stylet is smeared with red granular marrow material when removed from the needle.
4. Reintroduction of the stylet will produce pain.
5. Suction by the syringe produces severe and intense pain (most reliable proof), and is due to irritation of pain carrying nerve fibres surrounding the marrow cells.

Q. Complications of bone marrow aspiration:

1. Over-penetration (if posterior table of sternum is penetrated, aorta and its branches and other vital mediastinal structures may be damaged)—cardiac tamponade and pneumothorax may develop. It may happen with very soft bones.
2. Haemorrhage (haematoma) and bone pain.
3. Shock.
4. Infection (osteomyelitis).
5. Sudden death due to accidental injury to vital organs.

Q. Causes of dry tap:

Failure to obtain marrow may be due to:

1. Faulty technique.
2. Myelosclerosis or myelofibrosis (marrow replaced by fibrous tissue).
3. Marrow aplasia or hypoplasia (marrow replaced by fat).
4. Gross marrow hyperplasia—may be seen in leukaemia.
5. Carcinomatous infiltration of the bone marrow (tightly packed with infiltrates).
6. In marble bone disease (osteopetrosis), bone marrow may not be penetrated.

- These cases actually demand trephine biopsy.
- 'Bloody tap' is the bone marrow which is greatly diluted with blood.

Q. Examination of the bone marrow film:

Following are examined under the microscope:

a. The cellularity of the marrow.
b. Type and activity of erythropoiesis.
c. The number and type of:
    1. Developing WBC.
    2. Megakaryocytes.
    3. Plasma cell.
d. Myeloid-erythroid ratio (M:E).
e. Presence of:
    1. Parasites (LD bodies) or any organism.
    2. Foreign body; tumour cells or any abnormal cell.
    3. Fatty and fibrous tissue.
    4. Iron (content).

- Normal M:E = 3:1 or 4:1

Q. Composition of normal bone marrow:

The normal bone marrow is composed of haemopoietic cells (nucleated cells 20000–1 lac/mm^3), blood vessels, reticulum, fatty tissue and nerves.

Q. Criteria for ideal site in bone marrow puncture:

1. Superficial bone (i.e. easy accessibility).
2. Not close to any vital structure.
3. Thin cortex with more cancellous tissue.

- **Trephine biopsy** needle is used where aspiration of bone marrow is unsuccessful (myelofibrosis, myelosclerosis) or unhelpful (malignant infiltration) or in diagnosis and assessment of osteomalacia/ hyperparathyroid bone disease. Jamshidi-Swain (marrow) biopsy needle has a distal cutting edge. The posterior iliac crest is preferred for performing trephine biopsy.

LIVER BIOPSY NEEDLE

Q. Types:

There are three types of needle used for biopsy of liver:

1. Vim-Silverman's biopsy needle (commonly used; it is a cutting needle) **(Fig. 1.7A)**.
2. Menghini's aspiration biopsy needle (fragmentation of liver tissue is better, low cost, quicker).
3. Sheathed 'Trucut' needle (modified Vim-Silverman's needle).

Q. Description:

Vim-Silverman needle has three parts **(Fig. 1.7A and B)**:

1. Outer hollow needle: It guides the inner split needle.
2. Inner split needle: It brings out the liver tissue.
3. Solid stylet: It keeps the needle patent during introduction.

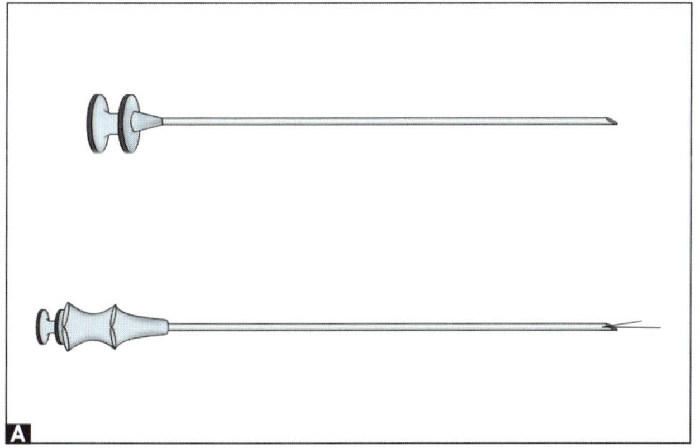

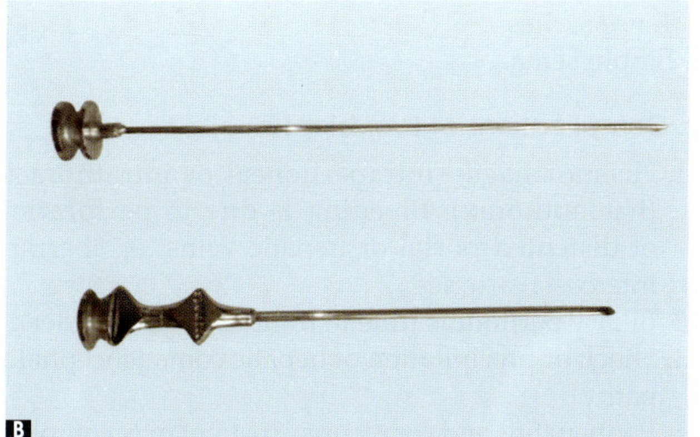

Fig. 1.7: (A) Liver biopsy needle (the solid stylet; and outer hollow needle with inner split needle within); (B) Actual photograph

Q. Indications of liver biopsy:

Liver biopsy (i.e. percutaneous removal of liver tissue for histological diagnosis) is done to diagnose the suspected cases of:

1. Cirrhosis of liver (the most common).
2. Carcinoma of liver (primary or secondary).
3. Chronic hepatitis (to diagnose, and to determine the grade and stage).
4. Portal hypertension of any aetiology.
5. Alcoholic liver disease, drug-induced hepatitis or cholestasis of uncertain origin.
6. Storage and metabolic disorders, e.g. glycogen storage disease, haemochromatosis, Wilson's disease, amyloidosis.
7. Infective or granulomatous diseases, e.g. tuberculosis, brucelosis, leptospirosis, amoebiasis, sarcoidosis.
8. Lymphoma (operative liver biopsy for staging), myeloid metaplasia.
9. Unexplained hepatomegaly or jaundice, or elevation of liver enzymes; pyrexia of unknown origin.
10. Post-hepatic transplantation (to assess for rejection and intensity of recurrence of disease).

Q. Contraindications of liver biopsy:

A. Absolute contraindications are:

1. Hepatic encephalopathy (i.e. severe hepato-cellular failure).
2. Bleeding diathesis: Abnormal blood clotting mechanism (thrombocytopenia, haemophilia).
3. Suspected hydatid cyst of liver (may precipitate anaphylactic reaction after puncture of the cyst).
4. Passive venous congestion of liver (i.e. in the presence of congestive cardiac failure).
5. Subphrenic abscess (right).
6. Right-sided empyema thoracis or pleural effusion, septic cholangitis or peritonitis.
7. Haemangioma of liver.
8. Dilated biliary channels (may lead to biliary peritonitis).

B. Relative contraindications are:

1. Massive ascites.
2. Severe and protracted jaundice.
3. Severe obstructive airway disease.
4. Non-cooperative patient (i.e. inability to hold breath).

Clinical Wisdom

Liver biopsy should not be performed if the platelet count goes below 80000/mm^3 and bilirubin above 20 mg/dL. In massive and tense ascites, specimen of liver tissue may not be obtained (as liver is displaced medially, it impedes penetration by the biopsy needle, or the biopsy material may be lost in ascitic fluid) or may lead to continuous oozing of fluid.

Q. Prerequisites for liver biopsy:

1. **Prothrombin time** should not be more than 3 seconds prolonged over control values (if control prothrombin

time is 16 seconds, then patient's value should not be >19 seconds to have a safe liver biopsy). BT (bleeding time) and CT (clotting time) should also be measured.

2. Try to rule out hydatid cyst of liver, subphrenic abscess, empyema thoracis or haemangioma of liver by prior ultrasonography. Take the H/o any bleeding tendency (e.g. from thrombocytopenia) before attempting liver biopsy.
3. Rule out protracted deep jaundice.
4. Ascites, if present, should be drained before liver biopsy is done.
5. Patient's blood group should be known; arrange for blood transfusion to combat any post-biopsy bleeding. If prothrombin time is high, try to normalise it by giving 10 mg of inj. vitamin K daily by IM route for consecutive 3 days before performing liver biopsy; correct thrombocytopenia with platelet transfusions or coagulopathy with fresh frozen plasma. Sedation before biopsy is not routinely advocated because it may interfere with patient's cooperation.

Q. How the liver biopsy tray is prepared?

1. Spirit, iodine, sterile gown, mask and gloves for antiseptic purpose.
2. 2% lignocaine solution as local anaesthetic.
3. Sterile liver biopsy needle.
4. 2 mL glass syringe with needle for local anaesthesia.
5. Sterile gauze and cotton.
6. Specimen containers (empty vials) with preservative solution (formol-saline).
7. Benzoin solution.
8. Leucoplast.

Q. Procedure of performing liver biopsy:

A. Vim-Silverman's needle:

1. Patient lies flat near the edge of the bed as far as possible. One pillow under the head and one under the patient's lower part of thorax may be placed for the purpose of expansion of thoracic cage.
2. The physician should wear the sterile gown. Standing on the right side of the patient, the physician cleans the local part by antiseptic solution.
3. Idealy, the biopsy site is 2–3 ICS below the upper border of liver dullness, which should be assessed beforehand. Local anaesthetic solution is usually infiltrated at the 8th or 9th ICS in the midaxillary line (skin, subcutaneous tissue and parietal pleura are infiltrated).
4. The outer hollow needle with the solid stylet is introduced through the 8th or 9th ICS in the midaxillary line at the end of expiration or with the patient breathing quietly (it is not always possible for the patient to hold the respiration) till is felt to enter the liver. The direction of the needle is slightly posterior and cranial to avoid the injury of gall-bladder.
5. Now ask the patient to hold breath for few seconds (ask the patient to practice holding of breath before the procedure is started). Remove the stylet quickly and introduce the inner split needle through the outer needle. The outer hollow needle is advanced completely, and the outer needle plus the inner split needle is rotated as a whole through 360° (as Vim-Silverman's needle is a cutting needle).
6. The whole needle is now withdrawn. The puncture site is sealed with tincture benzoin.
7. The biopsy tissue captured by the inner split needle is kept in the preservative solution of biopsy container for histological examination.
8. After-care—rest in bed for 24 hours is essential. Observe the pulse, BP and respiratory rate every one hour for next 24 hours. The patient is advised to lie on right lateral position for first 4 hours and no food is given per mouth for that period. Give analgesics, sedatives, antibiotics whenever indicated.

B. Menghini's needle: This needle is attached with a syringe, which is filled-up with 3 mL of sterile saline solution. Insert the needle through 8th or 9th ICS, and flush it with 2 mL of saline to clear the needle of any skin fragment. Now aspiration by the needle starts. Asking the patient to hold breath in expiration, the needle is quickly pushed to liver substance and then withdrawn quickly applying negative pressure to the syringe. Following steps are as per Vim-Silverman method.

- The hepatic biopsy tissue is usually sent for histopathology, cytology, frozen section or culture examination. In selective cases of Wilson's disease or haemochromatosis, copper and iron contents are measured, respectively.

Q. How to be sure that needle has gone within the liver?

After introduction of the outer needle with the stylet, take off your hand from the needle, and ask the patient to breathe in and out very slowly. If the needle is within the liver, it starts moving with respiration.

Q. 'Dry' (tap) liver biopsy or biopsy failure:

1. Faulty technique.
2. Very tough hepatic tissue (e.g. cirrhosis of liver).
3. Tense ascites.
4. Emphysema.

Q. Complications of liver biopsy:

1. Haemorrhage—intraperitoneal or intrathoracic (haemothorax). Bleeding is due to perforation of distented portal or hepatic veins, or aberrant intercostal arteries.
2. Biliary peritonitis (due to trauma in gallbladder).
3. Shock or precipitation of hepatic coma (encephalopathy).
4. Perihepatitis and/or pleurisy (patient may complain of severe pain in the right hypochondrium and right shoulder, and hepatic/pleural rub may appear).

5. Haemobilia—bleeding from damaged hepatic vessel into bile duct.
6. Intrahepatic arteriovenous fistula formation.
7. Intrahepatic haematoma or laceration of liver.
8. Transient bacteraemia, septicaemia.
9. Anaphylaxis (if hydatid cyst is punctured).
10. Small pneumothorax (right), puncture of intra-abdominal viscera.

- Nowadays, USG or CT-guided biopsy reduces the rate of complications. Actually, if the performer is skillful and the patient is carefully selected, the rate of complications is less.

Q. Criteria for ideal biopsy tissue:

It is surprising that a small biopsy tissue is the representative of changes in the whole liver. The biopsy tissue should be 2–4 cm long and should weigh 20–40 mg. Naked eye appearance of the biopsy tissue often gives clue to diagnosis, e.g. chocolate-coloured in Dubin-Johnson syndrome or green-coloured in biliary cirrhosis.

Q. What is trans-jugular liver biopsy?

When the patient suffers from massive ascites, coagulation disorder, small liver (from cirrhosis commonly) or is really uncooperative, a special Trucut needle is inserted to perform the biopsy through a catheter which is already placed in the hepatic vein, via the jugular vein. The extra advantage of this method is the measurement of the wedged hepatic venous pressure.

- Liver biopsy is done by 4 methods: 1. Percutaneous (by Vim-Silverman's needle), 2. Trans-jugular, 3. Laparoscopy, 4. Laparotomy (if done for some other reason).
- The modern 'biopty gun' (Biopter) is a modified Trucut needle.
- The **'Trucut' needle** is less injurious to Vim-Silverman's needle, and is disposable. The 'Trucut' needle (may be called as **tissue biopsy needle**) may be used for taking biopsy from liver, kidney, pleura. It has a trocar and canula, and the trocar is longer than the canula. It is also a cutting needle; the cutting needle comprises a 11.5 cm long pointed needle with a 2 cm notch close to the tip, enclosed by a cutting sleeve of 2 mm diameter. Trucut needle is less traumatic and yields a better specimen. Menghini's needle is less injurious than others, so far the complications are concerned; and the success rate is approximately 75%. The success rate of Vim-Silverman's needle is high (approximately 95%).
- Liver biopsy needle may be used in pleural biopsy in the absence of Abram's or Cope's pleural biopsy needle. The needle is sterilised by immersing the separated parts in concentrated lysol solution.

Clinical Wisdom

Fine needle aspiration cytology (FNAC) is less reliable than excisional biopsy of any tissue. The technique usually obtains only a suspension of cells from within a mass. Cytology from unexplained mass of lymph nodes, thyroid, breast, bone, or pleura/liver/abdomen (USG or CT-guided) is examined by a skilled histopathologist. Though not full-proof, FNAC is very often the investigation of choice in early malignancy where the primary investigations do not yield any result.

LUMBAR PUNCTURE NEEDLE

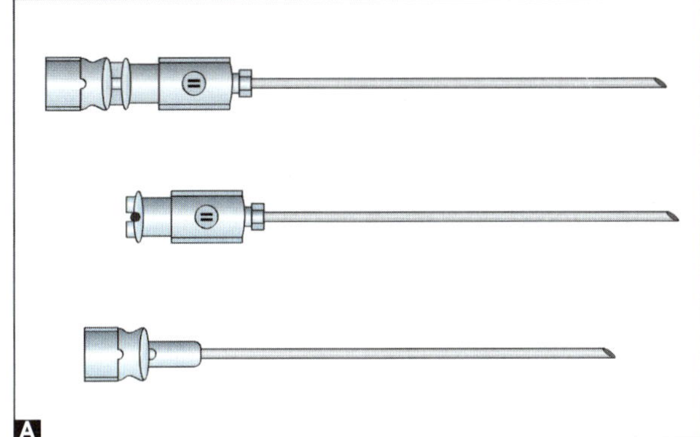

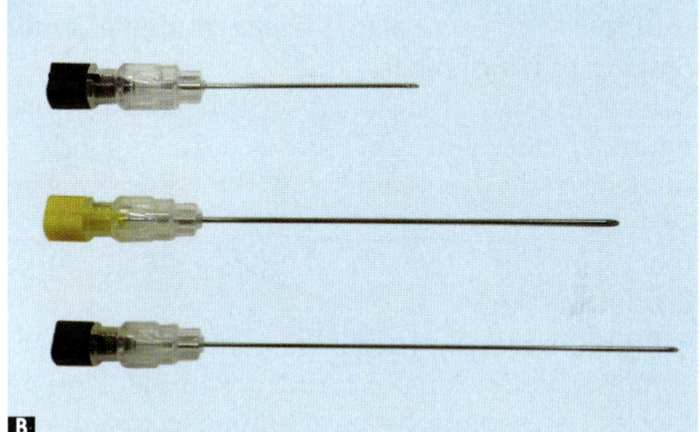

Fig. 1.8: (A) Lumbar puncture needle (the complete set, the needle proper and the stylet presented sequentially); (B) Actual photograph

Q. Description (Fig. 1.8A and B):

This is a sharp, slender, malleable narrow-bore needle and consists of two parts like:

1. *The needle proper:* It is made of platinum-irridium or German alloy, and gives the needle its malleability (nowadays, malleable steel is being used). The needle is round, slender, cannulated with a shortly bevelled tip and the usual length is 10–12 cm. The base of the needle fits with the knob (or projection) of the stylet and thus locks the stylet with the needle proper. The hole in the base allows the nozzle of a syringe for intrathecal injection.
2. *The stylet:* It maintains the patency of the needle, i.e. prevents blockage of the needle proper. The knob (or projection) present at its base fits well with the groove present at the base of the needle proper. The length of the stylet should be such that if should not protrude through the bevelled cutting edge of the needle proper.

- The needle is sterilised by immersing the separated parts in concentrated lysol solution or by gamma ray irradiation. The needle is made malleable for finer adjustment during manipulation.

Q. What is lumbar puncture (LP)?

It is a manoeuvre by which a temporary artificial communication is made with the CSF pathway and the exterior (at lumbar region). It is a simple method to collect CSF sample.

Q. Indications of lumbar puncture:

A. Diagnostic purpose:

a. Meningitis (bacterial, tuberculous, viral, fungal or carcinomatous).
b. Subarachnoid haemorrhage (SAH)—especially if CT scan of brain is normal.
c. Encephalitis or meningoencephalitis.
d. Meningism.
e. Unexplained coma—where the diagnosis cannot be reached by other investigations.
f. GB syndrome (albumino-cytological dissociation) or multiple sclerosis (isolated rise in gammaglobulin).
g. Staging of lymphomas.
h. *Miscellaneous:* PUO, unexplained dementia, neurosyphilis, neurosarcoidosis, Behcet's syndrome, or neoplastic involvement of the central nervous system.
i. Queckenstedt's test for diagnosis of spinal subarachnoid block.
j. CT myelography (done in a suspected case of compressive myelopathy to diagnose the level of spinal block), cisternography or pneumoencephalography (done to demonstrate cerebral atrophy; obsolete in the era of CT or MRI scan).

Clinical Wisdom

LP is done cautiously in a suspected case of spinal subarachnoid block (Froin's syndrome) as it may aggravate the neurodeficit.

B. Therapeutic purpose:

a. Intrathecal administration of drugs, e.g. methotrexate in acute lymphoblastic leukaemia (previously streptomycin was administered in tuberculous meningitis); in lymphoma.
b. Spinal and epidural anaesthesia, especially in operation of lower adbomen, lower limbs or in perineal surgery **(Fig. 1.8C)**.
c. To relieve intracranial tension in normal pressure hydrocephalus (risky and not used commonly) or benign intracranial hypertension.

Clinical Wisdom

While using a drug intrathecally, at first withdraw equal amount of CSF by LP needle and then push the drug slowly with strict asepsis.

- LP is not done routinely in CVA (cerebrovascular accidents) patients except in case of subarachnoid haemorrhage; LP should be avoided in infants, if possible.

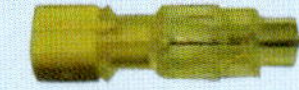

Fig. 1.8C: Spinal needle for spinal anaesthesia and spinal analgesia

Q. Contraindications of lumbar puncture:

1. **Papilloedema** or any other feature of **raised intracranial tension** (may precipitate cerebellar pressure cone syndrome—so, ophthalmoscopy is a must before performing lumbar puncture).
2. Local sepsis, skin infection or bed sore (may lead to meningitis, arachnoiditis).
3. Gross bony deformity in lumbar region or any congenital lesion like meningocele.
4. Restless patient/non-cooperative patient/very low general condition/bleeding diathesis/suspected spinal cord compression or spinal canal stenosis, or suspected posterior fossa tumour.

Q. What is 'cerebellar pressure cone syndrome' or 'cerebellar coning'?

It is the tentorial herniation or tonsillar herniation through foramen magnum leading to sudden death due to compression of medullary vital centres (i.e. as a result of descent of cerebellar tonsil). The syndrome develops if lumbar puncture is done in the presence of raised intracranial tension (e.g. brain tumour). The patient suddenly becomes drowsy, with positive neck stiffness and dilaled pupil; Cheyne-Stokes respiration/irregular slow respiration → decorticate posturing → bilateral Babinski's sign → apnoea → bradycardia → coma and death may supervene.

Q. How the lumbar puncture tray is prepared ?

1. Spirit, iodine, sterile gown, mask and gloves for antiseptic purpose.
2. 2% lignocaine solution as local anaesthetic.
3. Sterile LP needle with stylet.
4. Sterile plain glass test tubes (three).
5. 2 mL glass syringe with needle for local anaesthesia.
6. Sterile gauze and gauze-holding forcep.
7. Benzoin solution with cotton.
8. Leucoplast.

Q. How the lumbar puncture is performed ?

1. The patient is first explained the procedure to obtain full cooperation. Lumbar puncture is best done when the patient is kept in one lateral position (right or left) at the edge of the bed with the knees drawn-up against the abdomen and head flexed (actually an assistant helps in approximating the chin of the patient with his knees). The flexion posture helps in increasing the interspinous space on which the success of LP depends; LP may be done in sitting posture of the patient (e.g. in lumbar spondylosis).
2. The puncture is usually done between L_3 and L_4 interspace, 1/2″ on either side of the midline (**puncture site**—join the highest points of iliac crests by a line and it will pass through L_4 spine; puncture the space just above this line). The spinal cord ends at the lower border of L_1 vertebra and thus there is

no risk of injuring the cord. A space above or below may also be used in a desperate situation.

3. The physician washes his/her hands and wears gloves. Then the puncture site is properly cleansed with spirit-iodine-spirit from centre-outwards and above-downwards. The site is now infiltrated with 2% lignocaine solution upto ligamentum flavum.
4. Reconfirm the puncture site. Keeping the bevelled end upwards, the LP needle with the stylet in position, it is introduced a bit obliquely in upwards and forwards direction towards patients umbilicus, keeping it parallel to bed (oblique introduction will not cause any injury to the theca), by cork-screw movement. The ligamentum flavum is pierced and the destination of spinal subarachnoid space is indicated by sudden loss of resistance (penetration of the dura matter), and is actually confirmed by CSF coming out drop by drop when the stylet is withdrawn (the needle passes through the skin, interspinous ligament, ligamentum flavum, the dura and the arachnoid matter). If CSF does not come out, slightly rotate the needle or introduce it inwards slightly. If the CSF still fails to come, withdraw the needle and introduce it again.
5. The rate of flow of CSF is noted and is collected in three sterile test tubes each containing minimally 10 drops to maximally 2 mL.
6. The stylet is reinserted and the LP needle is withdrawn. The site is now sealed with tincture benzoin solution and leucoplast.

- Manometric study may be done prior to collection of CSF. The CSF pressure rises and falls with respiration and heart beat, and rises on coughing.

Q. Management of post-lumbar puncture period:

1. The patient is kept in bed for next 8–24 hours under observation.
2. Plenty of water to drink (to prevent post-lumbar puncture headache).
3. *Foot end of the bed is raised* with no pillow below the head (to prevent post-lumbar puncture headache).
4. Analgesics are given, if headache appears.

Q. Complications of lumbar puncture:

1. Traumatic puncture (trauma to vessel, nerve, intervertebral disc).
2. Post-lumbar puncture headache or low-tension headache.
3. 'Coning' or cerebellar pressure cone syndrome.
4. Breaking of the needle.
5. Introduction of infection (meningitis, arachnoiditis).
6. Bleeding (due to puncture of para-vertebral venous plexus).
7. Low backache.
8. Aggravation of root pain and signs of cord compression (in the presence of spinal cord tumour).

Q. What is post-lumbar puncture headache?

This usually occurs in patients where LP is done with normal intracranial tension. Headache (bifrontal and/ or occipital) appears within 4 hours, stays for a few hours to days, and is enhanced on assuming sitting or standing posture. It is due to low intracranial tension produced as a result of:

a. Withdrawal of CSF, and
b. Continuous leakage of CSF through the puncture site in the theca.

Low tension exerts traction on the meningeal blood vessels (pain-sensitive) and results in headache.

The headache (usually a dull ache) may be avoided by adopting these preventive measures:

1. Using a narrow-bore LP needle (i.e. guarded lumbar puncture).
2. Not withdrawing over 10 mL CSF.
3. Oblique introduction of the needle (transverse introduction 'divides' or 'tears' the fibres of dura and ligamentum flavum but oblique introduction 'separates' the fibres, and thus chance of CSF leakage is less if the needle is introduced obliquely).
4. Slow withdrawal of CSF.
5. The patient is kept lying flat in bed for 8–24 hours with foot end of the bed raised. Putting the patient in prone position may relieve headache.
6. Treatment of headache is done by drinking large amount of water, consuming caffeine and application of NSAID.

- Prolonged headache is recently being treated by 'autologous intrathecal blood patch', i.e. by injecting 20 mL of the patient's venous blood into the CSF.

Q. How much CSF should be withdrawn at a time?

1. For diagnostic purpose—usually 5–8 mL.
2. For therapeutic purpose—usually 10–20 mL (the amount of drug in volume should be measured first and then the same amount of CSF is withdrawn; now the drug is pushed into the subarachnoid space after fitting a syringe with the LP needle).

Q. Thick-bore needle—advantage and disadvantage:

a. *Advantage:* Helps in drawing thick purulent material in pyogenic meningitis.
b. *Disadvantage:* Post-LP headache and cerebellar pressure cone syndrome may develop as large amount of CSF is withdrawn in a short time.

Q. What is a dry tap?

CSF does not come out through the LP needle in:

1. It is due to faulty technique (needle not in subarachnoid space), incorrect position of the patient or needle blockage. If the needle is blocked, insert the stylet again to dislodge any dural flap, if present.
2. Spinal subarachnoid block.

3. Presence of very thick pus.
4. Lumbar subarachnoid space filled up with neoplastic tissue or obliterated by adhesive arachnoiditis.
5. Obstruction near foramen magnum as a result of basal meningitis.
6. Lipoma or dermoid (may be present in a case of spina bifida)

Q. What is bloody tap?

It is due to injury of meningeal vessels resulting in 'CSF mixed with blood', which may be easily confused with subarachnoid haemorrhage (SAH). Read **Table 1.1** for differentiation.

Q. What is Queckenstedt's test?

This test detects the patency of CSF pathway. It is done along with the lumbar puncture. Rise of CSF pressure is noted which is normally >40 mm of CSF or H_2O, after the compression of internal jugular vein (negative test). If the rate of flow of CSF is not increased after either internal jugular venous compression, the test is declared positive (CSF pressure is usually detected by a spinal manometer). A positive test is obtained after complete spinal block (partial block gives negative result). **Spinal block** may result from arachnoiditis, meningioma or neurofibroma, or vertebral disease with compression.

If CSF pressure rises after compression of one internal jugular vein but not with the other, it is known as positive Tobey-Ayer test and is found in lateral sinus thrombosis.

Compression of internal jugular vein results in congestion of cerebral veins and the rise in venous pressure leads to increased pressure in CSF.

Q. Other uses of LP needle:

1. Cisternal puncture (used during myelography to delineate the upper limit of spinal subarachnoid block)—not practised nowadays.
2. Splenoportal venography (to diagnose portal hypertension).
3. Paracentesis thoracis or paracentesis abdominis.

Q. CSF dynamics and other details:

CSF is formed by the choroid plexus of lateral (major source), 3rd and 4th ventricles. CSF circulation: Choroid plexus of lateral ventricles—Foramen of Monro—Third ventricle—Aqueduct of Sylvius—Fourth ventricle in the medulla—Foramen of Magendie and Luschka—Cisterna magna and cisterna pontis—Cerebral and spinal subarachnoid space—Circulation over brain and spinal cord. CSF is absorbed into venous sinuses by arachnoid villi.

Function of CSF

CSF acts as a buffer or cushion between CNS and bones. It also supplies nutrition to nervous tissue and removes the end-products of neuronal metabolism. CSF regulates the intracranial tension too.

Normal CSF Values

a. *Amount or volume:* 100–150 mL (approximately 130 mL in adults). Daily formation of CSF is 1500 mL
b. *Pressure:*
   i. 60–150 mm of CSF (lying position), and
   ii. 150–250 mm of CSF (sitting position)

- Roughly, the normal CSF flow (pressure) is equivalent to 1 drop per second on lumbar puncture.

c. *Colour:* Crystal clear or colourless
d. *pH and specific gravity:* 7.31–7.34 and 1007 respectively, osmolality: 292–297 mOsmol/kg of water
e. Biochemical:
   i. Protein: 20–40 mg%
   ii. Sugar: 40–80 mg% (usually 1/2 to 2/3rd of the random blood sugar concentration)
   iii. *Chloride:* 720–750 mg%
f. *Cells:* 0–5 cells/mm^3 and all are mononuclear cells (70% lymphocytes and 30% monocytes)
g. *Bacteriological:* Sterile
h. *Oligocional bands:* Negative

- The CSF IgG index (normal value is <0.65) is the ratio of IgG to albumin in the CSF divided by the same ratio in the serum; though the total CSF protein is usually normal or slightly elevated, the CSF IgG index is increased in multiple sclerosis, where the abnormal CSF IgG may be oligoclonal.
- CSF ammonia (normal: 25–80 µg/dL) may be increased in hepatic encephalopathy.

Q. How the examination of CSF is done?

a. *Physical:* Pressure, colour, fibrin clot.
b. *Biochemical:* Protein, sugar, chloride concentration.
c. *Cytological:* Number and types of cells are analysed (whether polymorphonuclear or lymphocytic pleocytosis present, or not).

Table 1.1: Differentiation between traumatic and non-traumatic haemorrhage

Tests	Traumatic (bloody tap)	Non-traumatic (SAH)
1. CSF collected serially in 3 test tubes	1. First tube is bright red and the next two tubes are faintly red	1. Uniformly red
2. Supernatent fluid after centrifugation or on prolonged standing	2. Clear	2. Yellowish or xanthochromic
3. Shape of the RBC	3. Normal	3. Crenated
4. Coagulation of blood	4. Occurs	4. Does not occur

d. Bacteriological including staining and culture.

e. *Serological:* VDRL, Kahn test, Wassermann reaction may be helpful in neurosyphilis.

f. *Special:* Lange's colloidal gold curve reaction (positive reaction indicates high globulin content of CSF) is positive in tabes dorsalis (tabetic curve), GPI (paretic curve) and meningitis (meningitic curve). Polymerase chain reaction (PCR) for detection of DNA sequence of different bacteria or *M. tuberculosis* is done. Adenosine deaminase activity (ADA) is determined to rule out tuberculous meningitis.

Q. Can an IV needle serve the purpose of lumbar puncture?

Yes (in dire emergency, in the absence of LP needle). Nowadays very slender, highly malleable disposable LP needle is available which are used by anaesthetists in spinal anaesthesia **(Fig. 1.8C)**.

Q. While performing LP, how do you identify or suspect different diseases?

1. Difficulty in flexing the neck of the patient at the beginning (i.e. presence of neck stiffness): Meningitis, meningism, subarachnoid haemorrhage, cerebral malaria or meningoencephalitis.
2. Unconscious patient: Meningoencephalitis, cerebral malaria, meningitis, meningism, subarachnoid haemorrhage.
3. CSF coming out at a flow rate of >1 drop/second (opening pressure): See the causes of increased intracranial tension in the section on 'Charts on CSF'. Low CSF pressure is found in bad needle placement, partial spinal blook, severe dehydration and after repeated lumbar puncture.
4. Appearance or colour of CSF:
   a. *Clear:* Normal, tuberculous and viral meningitis, meningism.
   b. *Turbid:* Pyogenic meningitis (due to high leucocyte count), rarely in carcinomatous meningitis and subarachnoid haemorrhage.
   c. *Straw-coloured:* Tuberculous meningitis.
   d. *Haemorrhagic (red):* Subarachnoid haemorrhage, trauma, extensive cerebral haemorrhage, haemorrhagic encephalitis (rare), bleeding diathesis.
   e. *Xanthochromia (yellow):* See the section dealing with 'charts' on 'Xanthochromia'.
5. Coagulum on standing:
   a. Cobweb coagulum (forms after few hours): Tuberculous meningitis (most important cause). acute anterior poliomyelitis and neurosyphilis.
   b. Big coagulum (forms immediately or shortly after withdrawal): Spinal subarachnoid block, GB syndrome.
6. Manometry: Queckenstedt's test is positive in complete spinal subarachnoid block.

Q. Examination of CSF in different diseases—a synopsis:

A. Pyogenic meningitis:

- Pressure—High (++)
- Colour—Turbid (indicates increased cellularity)
- Total cells—Increased +++ (200–5000/mm^3), predominantly polymorphonuclear pleocytosis
- Protein—Increased (++)
- Sugar—Low (--)
- Chloride—A bit reduced
- Gram's stain—Gram-ve diplococci, or Gram +ve cocci in pairs

B. Tuberculous meningitis:

- Pressure—High (++)
- Colour—Clear
- On standing—Formation of cobweb coagulum
- Total cells—Increased ++ (200–500/mm^3); predominantly lymphocytic pleocytosis
- Protein—Increased (++)
- Sugar—Low (–)
- Chloride—Low (–) (may be due to prolonged vomiting)
- Ordinary culture shows no growth (sterile)

❍ Cobweb coagulum indicates presence of mild to moderate rise in protein along with fibrinogen in CSF.

C. Viral meningitis:

- Pressure—High (++)
- Colour—Clear
- Total cells—Increased + (approximately 150–200/mm^3); predominantly lymphocytic pleocytosis (may be mixed pleocytosis for first 36 hours)
- Protein—Increased (+) or normal
- Sugar—Normal
- Chloride—Normal
- Ordinary culture is sterile

D. Carcinomatous meningitis:

- Pressure—High (++)
- Colour—Clear or haemorrhagic
- Total cells—Plenty (lymphocytes ↑), malignant cells +
- Protein—Increased (+)
- Sugar—Normal
- Chloride—Normal

E. Subarachnoid haemorrhage (SAH):

- Pressure—High (++)
- Colour—Blood-stained, turbid or xanthochromia
- Total cells—Plenty; RBC+++, a few are crenated
- Protein—Raised (protein from blood is added to CSF)
- Sugar—Normal
- Chloride—Normal
- On centrifugation—Supernatent fluid is yellow
- Culture—No growth (sterile)

❍ In traumatic haemorrhage, CSF pressure remains normal and CSF protein content is not too high.

F. Meningism:

- Pressure—High (++)
- Colour—Clear
- Total cells—0-5 cells/mm^3 (all mononuclear cells)
- Protein, sugar and chloride—Within normal limit
- Gram's stain—Nothing could be detected
- Culture—Sterile

G. Xanthochromia:

- Pressure—Very low or nil
- Colour—Xanthochromic (yellowish)
- On standing—Formation of big coagulum
- Total cells—0-5 cells/mm^3 (all mononuclear cells)
- Protein—Increased (++)
- Sugar—Normal
- Chloride—Normal
- Queckenstedt's test—Positive (i.e. no rise in CSF pressure on compression of internal jugular vein)
- Culture—Sterile

- This last chart is of complete spinal subarachnoid block with albumino-cytological dissociation.
- Polymerase chain reaction (PCR) is helpful in diagnosis of some cases of meningitis. Though cryptococcal antigen test is very sensitive, the 'India ink test' is still valuable in diagnosis of meningitis caused by *Cryptococcus neoformans*.

Clinical Wisdom

Lumbar puncture is a very important bedside diagnostic tool though nowadays radiodiagnosis (e.g. CT or MRI scan) has gained importance over this age-old practice.

IV FLUID BOTTLE AND INFUSION SET

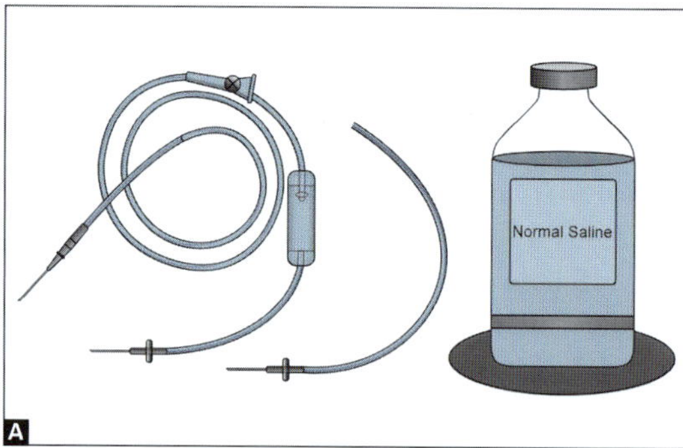

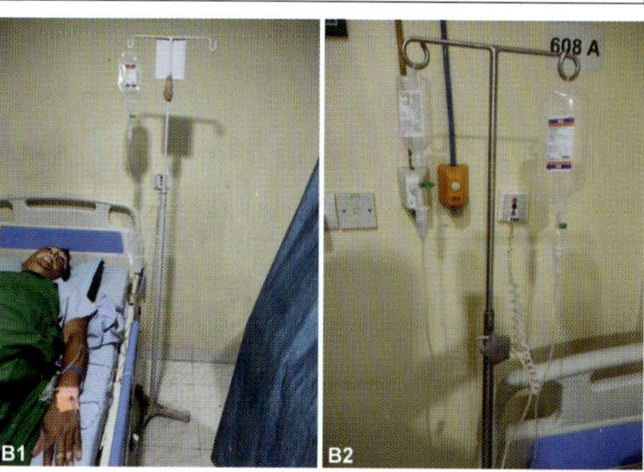

Fig. 1.9: (A) Drip tube, airway tube and the IV fluid bottle; (B_1 and B_2) Real life scenario

Q. Description (Fig. 1.9):

a. Bottle: 640 mL; made of glass or plastic. The glass bottle has a rubber stopper in the mouth with two openings (one for air entry and the other for fluid outlet). Plastic bottle has now replaced glass bottle.

B. Infusion set (i.e. IV drip set):

a. One long plastic tube (drip tube) with two needles on two sides—one enters into the bottle and the other enters into the patient's vein. A small part of the plastic tube (near the patient's vein) is replaced by a rubber tube to inject drugs by shot-push. In the middle of the tube, there is a small plastic container (Murphy's chamber) to measure the flow of the running fluid. The rate of flow of the fluid is controlled by an adjustable valve attached to the set.

b. A small plastic tube with a needle for air entry in the bottle (airway tube).

- Blood transfusion set contains a 'strainer' (to filter clots) in the Murphy's chamber. It is used for transfusion of blood and blood products (e.g. packed cells, cryoprecipitate, platelets, etc.).

Q. What is Murphy's chamber?

It is a plastic or glass chamber attached to the infusion set to regulate the flow of fluid by adjusting the number of drops coming down per minute. It has two ends: Through the inlet fluid enters into the chamber (via a glass tube), and through the outlet fluid leaves the chamber. For proper flow of fluid, a fluid level should be maintained in the chamber. If the chamber is fully occupied by fluid, it has to be reset.

Q What is a micro-drip set?

It is the same variety of IV set but contains a small calibered lumen in the Murphy's chamber. In ordinary IV set, 15 drops of fluid make 1 mL but in microdrip set 60 (micro) drops constitute 1 mL of fluid. The microdrip set is used when very small and accurate quantity (e.g. microgram dose) of a drug is delivered in IV route, e.g. dopamine, dobutamine, noradrenaline, nitroglycerine, etc.

Q. How to set-up a drip?

Indications

1. Replacement of fluids (crystalloids, blood products, different electrolyte solutions).
2. To establish an external route for administering IV medication, nutrition or blood products.

- **Crystalloids**, i.e. solutions containing solutes that can pass a semipermeable membrane → rapidly expand both intravascular and extravascular compartments; examples are dextrose, normal saline, Ringer's lactate solution, mannitol. **Colloids,** i.e. solutions containing large molecules which do not pass semipermeable membranes → expand the intravascular space more efficiently; examples are albumin, dextran, haemaccel, blood and hetastarch.

Choice of Site

Most convenient sites for peripheral cannulation are veins over the forearm, wrist or elbow. Selection of left side allows the comfortable mobility as well as different activities of right arm. If veins of the upper extremity is not available, veins of ankle or feet are used. Other sites of cannulation are subclavian or jugular vein.

Precautions

1. In patients with renal failure, there is a chance of fluid overload.
2. In patients with heart failure, problems may be alleviated by prior administration of a diuretic.
3. Proper asepsis is required to start a drip in patients who are immunocompromised or having valvular heart disease.
4. Always choose a vein with adequate calibre to maintain a smooth flow.

Procedure

1. All the clothes are removed from the site of puncture and a tourniquet is applied proximally to make the vein distended and prominent. The puncture site is cleansed with spirit properly.
2. Keeping the needle parallel to the vein chosen and with the bevelled edge facing upwards, the vein is pierced, by moving the needle, it is continued for a distance within the lumen of the vein. Now, the tourniquet is released and let the fluid from the bottle flow within the vein through the IV infusion set. The adjustable valve attached with the IV set controls the rate of flow of the fluid. The needle is fixed to the skin with adhesive tape (leucoplast) and the limb may be splinted with a wooden piece
3. Follow-up: Look for any sign of inflammation (redness, thrombophlebitis, brawny induration) at the puncture site. An IV set should not be continued for more than 2–3 days and should be replaced.

Clinical Wisdom

If no veins are visible after intensive search for intravenous infusion of fluids, a venesection or **'cut-down'** procedure may be employed in ankle, antecubital fossa or wrist in a desperate situation. Always change the puncture site (i.e. reintroduce in other site) with the appearance of first sign of inflammation (i.e. thrombophlebitis). If the drip is continued for long, pyrexia may complicate the situation. Many a time, inflammation at the venepuncture site of a drip is responsible for unexplained fever.

Q. How to change the bottle/discontinue infusion?

To change the bottle, the adjustable valve attached with the IV infusion set is locked to prevent entry of air in the tube distal do it. Now, the empty infusion bottle is replaced by a new one.

To discontinue infusion, the adjustable valve is locked; the IV needle is removed and a sterile dressing is applied over the puncture site.

Q. Different content of bottles:

1. Normal saline or isotonic saline (0.9%).
2. Glucose or dextrose solution (5%, 10%, 20%, 25%, 50%).
3. Dextrose-saline solution (DNS).
4. Sodium lactate solution.
5. Hypertonic saline (3% or 5%).
6. Ringer's lactate solution.
7. Darrow's solution.
8. Mannitol (5%, 10%, 20%).
9. Haemaccel.
10. Low molecular weight dextran (40 and 70 kDa).

- Nowadays, multiple electrolyte solutions (e.g. electrolyte R, electrolyte M, etc.) are available and contains dextrose, sodium, potassium, calcium, etc. in varying combination. Some are useful in maintaining (M) daily requirements of water and electrolytes, and others for replacement (R) of fluid loss.

Q. Use of different parenteral fluids:

I. Normal Saline

Its osmotic pressure is equal to that of plasma and this is why, it is known as isotonic saline. The fluid is also isotonic with the intracellular compartment of RBC and thus, called 'normal' saline; here 0.9 g of NaCl is dissolved in 100 mL of water (0.9%). Normal saline has the same sodium content as plasma (approximately 150 mmol/L). Nowadays, it is available in 100 mL, 250 mL, 500 mL, 1000 mL and 2000 ml plastic containers.

Uses

1. To correct salt-water depletion (e.g. diarrhoea and vomiting).
2. To correct dehydration and hypovolaemia.
3. Acts as a vehicle for IV drug administration (e.g. iron-sucrose infusion).
4. To maintain the fluid balance parenterally when oral intake is not possible.
5. In treating alkalosis.

II. Glucose or Dextrose Solution

It is available in different concentration (usually 5%, 10%, 20%, 25% and 50%).

Uses

1. Acts as a vehicle for IV drug administration.
2. To provide adequate calories to the body and to correct pure H_2O deficit.
3. Hypoglycaemic coma (high concentration, i.e. 25% or 50% dextrose solution is used).
4. As fluid and nutrient replenisher.
5. As a mild osmotic diuretic (10%).
6. A 50% solution may reduce cerebral oedema.

III. Dextrose-normal saline solution (DNS)

Usually available as 5% glucose plus 0.9% (normal) saline.

Uses

1. In patients who need additional fluid with minimal sodium intake.
2. As an initial hydrating solution to establish normal renal function.
3. In the presence of metabolic alkalosis (e.g. repeated gastric suction): Fluid loss with loss of Cl^- is compensated.

IV. Sodium lactate solution

It is available in two strengths:

a. Molar sodium lactate solution, and
b. 1/6th Molar lactate solution.

Sodium ion of sodium lactate combines with HCO_3^-, (coming from lactate) and forms $NaHCO_3$, and the blood becomes alkaline.

Uses

1. Metabolic acidosis, e.g. diabetic ketoacidosis.
2. To treat hyperkalaemia (alkalosis reduces the level of serum potassium level).

V. Hypertonic saline (3% or 5%)

Prepared by dissolving 3 g or 5 g of NaCl in 100 mL of water. The osmotic pressure of hypertonic saline is higher than that of plasma.

Uses

1. Severe hyponatraemia.
2. Syndrome of inappropriate ADH secretion (SIADH).

Hyponatraemia in CCF, cirrhosis or SIADH can be treated by a competitive vasopressin receptor antagonist entitled tolvaptan.

VI. Ringer's lactate solution (Table 1.2)

Uses

1. Fluid of choice in treating cholera.
2. Burns, severe infections, peritonitis, multiple fractures.
3. Replacing deficit of extracellular fluid (ECF) due to decreased water intake or increased excretion of water.
4. Deficiency of NaCl and K^+ with acidosis.

Electrolytes concentration in Ringer's lactate is almost the same as that of plasma.

VII. Darrow's solution (contains high potassium)

Uses

1. Treatment of hypokalaemia.
2. In the management of diabetic ketoacidosis (DKA).

VIII. Mannitol (usually 20% solution is used; available in 100, 350 and 500 mL bottle)

Uses

1. To reduce increased intracranial tension due to any cause (e.g. CVA, hepatic pre-coma).
2. To expedite the urinary excretion of toxic metabolites.
3. Treatment of acute renal failure or acute kidney injury.
4. To reduce intraocular tension (when other drugs fail).
5. Acts as a vehicle for injection potassium to treat severe hypokalaemia (e.g. hypokalaemic periodic paralysis).

IX. Haemaccel (polygeline)

Uses

1. Shock or peripheral circulatory failure.
2. To raise the BP in hypotension.
3. Priming of heart-lung machine and artificial kidney.
4. As a plasma expander while performing paracentesis abdominis in cirrhosis of liver.

X. Low molecular weight (average 40000) dextran

Uses

1. As a plasma expander. As a substitute of plasma, it can be used in burn, hypovolaemic or endotoxic shock.
2. Impending shock due to haemorrhage.
3. Prevention of peritoneal adhesions.
4. Foetal distress syndrome.

Q. Different electrolytes available for therapy:

1. Sodium bicarbonate (available as 7.5% and 8.4%; 1.5% $NaHCO_3$ is isotonic solution)
   Uses: Correction of acidosis, hyperkalaemia, as a lavage (e.g. bladder, bronchial) fluid, cardiopulmonary resuscitation.
2. Potassium (2 mEq/mL)
   Uses: In treatment of hypokalaemia (e.g. severe diarrhoea, diabetic ketoacidosis), paralytic ileus, digitalis toxicity. Glucose-insulin-potassium (GIK) regimen is useful in management of DKA and acute myocardial infarction.
3. Calcium (e.g. calcium gluconate 10%)
   Uses: Severe hypocalcaemia (e.g. tetany, hypoparathyroidism, alkalosis, hypovitaminosis D), growing children, pregnancy and lactation, patients on long-continued corticosteroids, or cardiac arrest (in diastole).

Clinical Wisdom

These electrolytes are available in ampoules and are given in a drip or shot-push (i.e. IV route).

Q. Advantages and disadvantages of parenteral (IV) fluid therapy:

Advantages

1. Rapid correction of fluid deficit.
2. All types of fluid can be given.

Disadvantages (complications)

1. Thrombophlebitis.
2. Extravasation with local cellulitis (swelling and oedema); needle blockage.
3. Haematoma formation.

4. Pyrogen reaction with fever.
5. Overloading with injudicious administration, resulting in heart failure (development of pulmonary oedema) and/or renal failure.
6. Chance of transmission of infection, if proper asepsis is not maintained.
7. Air embolism.

Table 1.2: Composition of plasma and different IV fluids (mmol/L)

Different fluids	Na	K	Cl	Lactate
Plasma	136–145	3.5–5.0	98–106	–
Isotonic saline	153	–	153	–
Ringer's lactate	130	4	110	28
1/6th Molar lactate	167	–	–	167
Darrow's solution	124	36	104	56

- Normal plasma HCO_3 level is 22–26 mEq/L.
- Normal plasma osmolality is 280–300 mOsmol/kg of water.
- Approximate **composition of plasma** (mmol/litre) Na-141, K-4, Ca-2.5, Mg-2, Cl-100, HCO_3-25, PO_4/SO_4-1, and protein/acid is 25 = 300 (approx). Na and Cl are main ions in extracellular fluid, and K and PO_4 are those of the intracellular fluid.
- Approximately 60–65% of body weight is 'total body water'. pH of blood varies between 7.38 and 7.44 (average 7.40).
- IV infusion set may also be used to remove ascitic and pleural fluid. It may be used temporarily in water-seal drainage to treat a case of spontaneous pneumothorax.
- Remember, IV fluid is 'infused' while blood is 'transfused'.

Clinical Wisdom

Calculation of rate of fluid to be infused:

1 mL of fluid = 15 drops.

Infusing 540 mL (1 bottle) in 8 hours, give fluid at the rate of 1 drop/4 sec, i.e. 15 drops/min (approx).

Infusing 540 mL (1 bottle) in 6 hours, give fluid at the rate of 1 drop/3 sec, i.e. 20 drops/min (approx).

Infusing 540 mL (1 bottle) in 4 hours, give fluid at the rate of 1 drop/2 sec, i.e. 30 drops/min (approx).

Q. Causes of metabolic acidosis (Table 1.3):

1. Diabetic ketoacidosis
2. Renal failure.
3. Severe diarrhoea.
4. Starvation.
5. Lactic acidosis.
6. Poisoning by methyl alcohol, salicylates.
7. Hypoaldosteronism.
8. Renal tubular acidosis.

Q. Causes of metabolic alkalosis:

1. Severe vomiting or vigorous gastric aspiration.
2. Cushing's syndrome.
3. Primary hyperaldosteronism.
4. Severe hypokalaemia.
5. Milk-alkali syndrome.
6. Diuretics (furosemide, thiazides).

Q. Causes of respiratory acidosis:

1. Depression of respiratory centre by disease or drugs.
2. Central sleep apnoea.
3. Sudden failure of ventilation (e.g. myasthenic crisis).
4. Chronic bronchitis, emphysema.

Table 1.3: Acid-base disorders

Disorders	pH (7.40)	Primary defect	Compensatory effect
Metabolic acidosis	Low	Low HCO_3	Low $PaCO_2$
Metabolic alkalosis	High	High HCO_3	High $PaCO_2$
Respiratory acidosis	Low	High $PaCO_2$	High HCO_3
Respiratory alkalosis	High	Low $PaCO_2$	Low HCO_3

Q. Causes of respiratory alkalosis

1. Pneumonia, bronchial asthma, acute pulmonary cedema, high altitude (due to hypoxia).
2. Exercise.
3. Anxiety, fever, salicylate overdose (due to stimulation of respiratory centre).
4. Hysterical hyperventilation.

Q. What is anion gap in 'metabolic acidosis'?

It is the 'unmeasured anions' and are calculated by subtracting the sum of plasma bicarbonate and chloride concentrations (i.e. the measured anions) from plasma concentration of sodium (i.e. the measured cations).

Anion gap = $Na^+ - (HCO_3^- + Cl^-)$

The normal anion gap is 8–10 mmol/L; most of the anion gap is due to negative charges on plasma proteins (mainly albumin), and phosphate, sulphate and organic acid anions to a lesser degree. When acid anions, e.g. acetoacetic acid or lactic acid accumulate in ECF, it results in high-anion gap acidosis.

a. *Increased anion gap:*
   1. Diabetic ketoacidosis (or ketoacidosis from alcoholism and starvation).
   2. Acute and chronic renal failure.
   3. Lactic acidosis.
   4. Ingestion of toxins or drugs (salicylate, carbenicillin, ethelene glycol, methanol).

b. *Normal anion gap (hyperchloraemic acidosis):*
   1. Diarrhoea.
   2. Intestinal fistula.
   3. Ureterosigmoidostomy.
   4. Renal tubular acidosis.
   5. Hypoaldosteronism.
   6. Ingestion of toxins or drugs (ammonium chloride, cholestyramine).

Q. How to analyze arterial blood gas (ABG) results?

A rough assessment can be done by:

pH	pH <7.35 (Acidosis)	Metabolic (↓HCO_3) (<20 mEq/L)
		Respiratory (↑$PaCO_2$) (>45 mm of Hg)
	pH >7.45 (Alkalosis)	Metabolic (↑HCO_3) (>30 mEq/L)
		Respiratory (↓$PaCO_2$) (<35 mm of Hg)

Q. Causes of hyponatraemia:

1. Severe diarrhoea, vomiting, peritonitis, burns, excess of diuretics, uncontrolled diabetes mellitus, CRF (all producing 'volume depletion', i.e. loss of both Na^+ and water).
2. Congestive cardiac failure, SIADH (syndrome of inappropriate ADH secretion), cirrhosis of liver, nephrotic syndrome, acute and chronic renal failure.
3. Adrenocortical failure, hypothyroidism, hypopituitarism, psychogenic polydipsia.

Q. Causes of hypernatraemia:

1. Diabetes insipidus, diabetes mellitus (when water loss is more).
2. Cushing's syndrome.
3. Primary hyperaldosteronism.
4. Infusion of hypertonic saline.

Q. Causes of hypokalaemia:

1. Diminished dietary intake (e.g. starvation).
2. Vomiting, diarrhoea, intestinal fistula.
3. Diuretics (e.g. loop diuretics).
4. Metabolic alkalosis.
5. Aldosteronism (primary or secondary).
6. After administration of insulin.
7. Diabetic ketoacidosis.
8. Hypokalaemic periodic paralysis.

Q. Cause of hyperkalaemia:

1. Renal failure (acute or chronic).
2. Addison's disease, hypoaldosteronism.
3. Metabolic acidosis.
4. Tissue damage, e.g. internal bleeding or muscle crush.
5. Potassium-sparing diuretic, e.g. spironolactone, triamterene, amiloride, or use of ACE-Inhibitors like enalapril or lisinopril, or angiotensin-receptor blockers like losartan or telmisartan.

- Pseudohyperkalaemia: It is the artifactual increase in serum K^+ due to release of K^+ during venipuncture (fist clenching), or marked increase in cellular elements, e.g. thrombocytosis, erythrocytosis or leucocytosis.

Q. Indications of 'blood transfusion' in medical ward:

One unit of whole blood contains approximately 450 mL of blood (in India, it is usually 350 mL).

1. *Restoration of volume of circulating blood:* Acute haemorrhage, e.g. haematemesis, melaena, haemoptysis, epistaxis, haematuria or menorrhagia of severe degree.
2. *Severe anaemia due to any cause:* Aplastic anaemia, anaemia of chronic renal failure, thalassaemia, disseminated malignancy, hookworm infestation, severe iron deficiency anaemia, AIDS.
3. *Granulocyte transfusion:* Severe neutropenia, neonatal sepsis, progressive fungal infection, chronic granulomatous disease.
4. *Platelet transfusion:* Severe thrombocytopenia or platelet dysfunction.
5. *Exchange transfusion:* Haemolytic disease of newborn, thrombotic thrombocytopenic purpura, severe falciparum malaria, poisoning (e.g. methaemoglobinaemia or arsine-induced haemolysis).
6. *Fresh blood transfusion:* In coagulation disorders, e.g. haemophilia or thrombocytopenia (e.g. idiopathic or immune thrombocytopenic purpura or ITP); Viperidae group of snake bite.

Q. What are central line and TPN?

Central line placement: A central venous catheter, known as 'central line', is often used to put medicines, blood products, fluid or nutrients right into the patient's blood through larger veins like internal jugular vein, femoral vein or subclavian vein. The central line is indicated in continuous infusion of chemotherapy, giving more than one drug at a time or hypertonic solution, nutritional support, haemodialysis, or required for long-term IV treatment (volume resuscitation). Central line is also used for taking out blood sample for testing and central venous pressure monitoring.

Total parenteral nutrition (TPN) therapy (method of feeding that by-pass GI tract) through subclavian vein is required in 'specialized nutrition support' (where oral therapy may be harmful or may not be possible) delivered in extensive small bowel disease, intestinal fistula, prolonged hyperemesis gravidarum, severe intra-abdominal sepsis, acute pancreatitis, inflammatory bowel disease, severe cachexia (e.g. cancer, AIDS), in patients on ventilation or any critical illness. This is usually done in an ITU (intensive therapeutic unit) setting. For a central venous TPN regimen, a pre-mixed (contains L-amino acids, lipids, glucose with vitamins, electrolytes and trace elements) 3-litre bag is infused over 24 hours with close monitoring.

SYRINGE (5 mL/50 mL)

Q. Description:

A syringe has two parts:

a. Air-tight piston, and
b. Cylinder with a nozzle at one end for fitting tightly with the base of a needle, scalp vein set or adaptor. The cylinder possesses markings on its outer surface indicating the volume of the drug to be delivered.

The syringe is usually made of glass. Disposable plastic syringe is for single use and is available in gamma irradiated packs. This type of syringes (5 mL) are often called 'hypodermic' syringe.

Q. Sterilisation:

1. Keeping (heating) in boiling water minimally for 30 minutes, seperating the piston and cylinder (before putting in water, loosely wrap the piston and cylinder with sterile gauze): The glass syringe.
2. Autoclaving.
3. Gamma ray irradiation.
4. Ethelene oxide.

Q. Different uses (Fig. 1.10A and B):

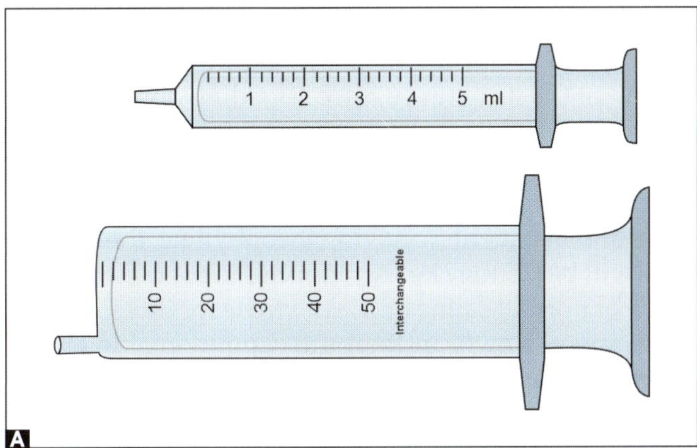

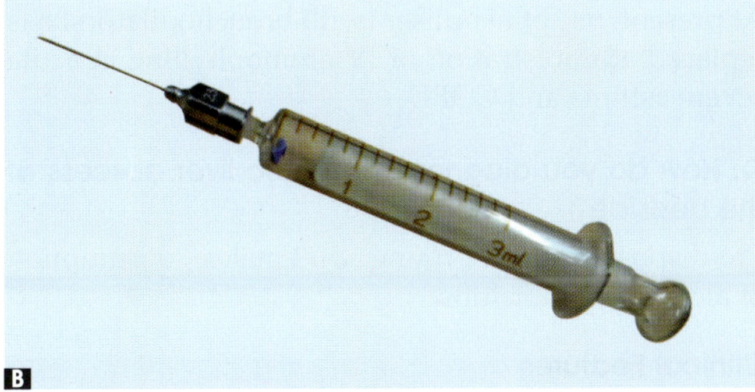

Fig. 1.10: (A) 5 and 50 mL syringes; (B) Syringe with needle

A. 5 mL Syringe

a. Collection of venous blood samples for laboratory analysis, aspiration from cyst/abscess, for myelography/IVP, etc.
b. Parenteral administration of drugs by different routes like IM (inj. tetanus toxoid), IV (antibiotics). subcutaneous (terbutaline, adrenaline, erythropoietin, adalimumab), intracutaneous (drug sensitivity, Mantoux test), intra-arterial (arteriogram), intra-articular (corticosteroid), intrathecal (methotrexate in ALL), intrapleural (for pleurodesis) and intra-peritoneal (antimetabolites).

B. 50 mL Syringe

a. Ryle's tube feeding; gastric aspiration in intestinal obstruction, pyloric stenosis, haematemesis or poisoning.
b. Aspiration of pleural and pericardial fluid, and paracentesis abdominis.
c. IV aminophylline injection.
d. Aspiration of amoebic or pyogenic liver abscess through a wide-bore needle.
e. Gastric wash by ice-cold saline in intractable hiccough.
f. Wound irrigation.

- The 'all glass' syringe is known as BD syringe (B and D stand for the manufacturer, Beckton and Dickinson). BD syringe is available as 2 mL, 5 mL, 10 mL, 20 mL, 50 mL and 100 mL syringes.
- **Venous blood collection** (Fig. 1.10C): After adopting proper aseptic and antiseptic measures, venous blood sample is usually drawn from antecubital fossa after applying a venous tourniquet proximal to the chosen site. The operator should wear double gloves as a protection against 'high risk' cases, e.g. infection with hepatitis B or C, HIV. After drawing the blood, the venepuncture site is closed by cotton soaked in antiseptic solution and leucoplast. For femoral vein puncture (lies at the mid-inguinal point medial to femoral artery), i.e. *femoral tap*, insert the needle vertically just medial to femoral artery.

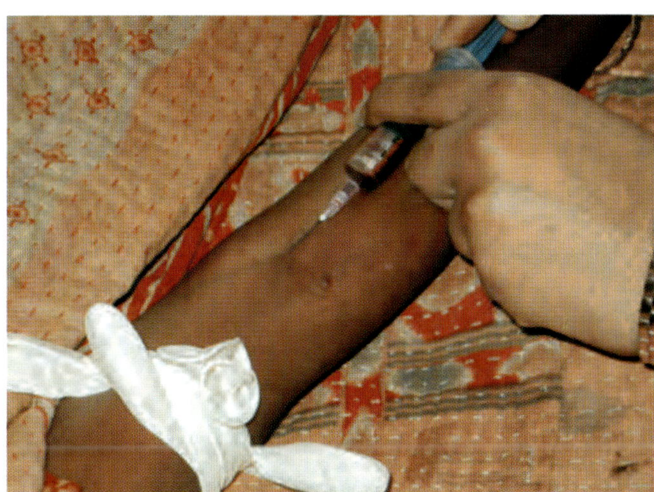

Fig. 1.10C: **Blood drawn** from right antecubital vein; a glove has been used here as a tourniquet

Q. Disadvantages of IM injection:

1. Painful.
2. There may be abscess formation.
3. Injury to the nerve may occur.
4. Muscle haematoma in coagulopathy (e.g. haemophilia) or prolonged bleeding (e.g. ITP).
5. Fibrous nodule formation at the injection site.
6. Anaphylaxis.
7. Transmission of some dreadful infection like hepatitis B rarely (in contamination).

Q. What is record syringe (Fig. 1.10D)?

Here, the cylinder (i.e. the body of the syringe) is made of glass while the piston and the long tapering nozzle of the cylinder are built of metal. Various sizes, e.g. 2 mL, 5 mL, 10 mL and 20 mL syringes are available. Autoclaving is not possible as it is partly glass and partly metallic (the syringe may be damaged by autoclaving), and thus sterilisation is done by boiling. It can be used for IM injections and bone marrow aspiration (as the piston can be locked in the body satisfactorily, the suction of the bone marrow can be well maintained).

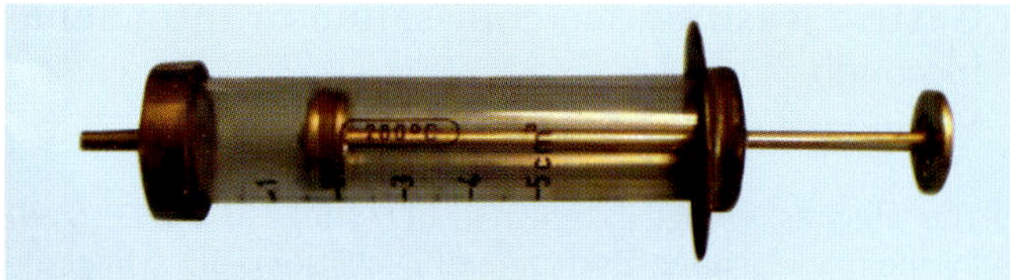

Fig. 1.10D: Record syringe

Q. What is anaphylaxis?

This is an example of immediate hypersensitivity reaction (IgE-mediated). It is a group of severe (type 1) reactions which occur in rapid succession if an antigen is injected, e.g. penicillin or sting of an insect, or rarely produced by ingested food in a highly sensitive individual. It is an acute life-threatening emergency and should be tackled immediately.

Features

Bronchospasm (wheezing), laryngeal oedema with severe dyspnoea, stridor and cyanosis, and feeling of impending doom; there is fall in BP (anaphylactic shock) and the patient may be unconscious. Swelling of the tongue, anorexia, nausea and vomiting, abdominal pain and diarrhoea may be present. Intense itching, urticaria and angioneurotic oedema (usually around the lips and eyes) may be seen. The diagnosis is purely clinical, and death may occur due to laryngeal spasm and hypotension.

Treatment

It is a potentially fatal condition and if not treated promptly, it possess a threat to life.

1. Patient lies down with head-down position. Prevent further contact with the allergen.
2. Ensure airway patency and start 100% O_2 inhalation at the rate of 4–6 litres/min. Maintain an IV line for normal saline to treat hypotension.
3. *Adrenaline:* It remains the cornerstone of therapy; 0.3–1.0 mL of 1:1000 adrenaline is injected subcutaneously (in lateral thigh) or IV; may be repeated at 10–30 minutes interval, if necessary.
4. *Corticosteroids:* Hydrocortisone 100–300 mg or dexamethasone 4–8 mg, IV, to be given immediately and every 4–6 hourly. Corticosteroids may not have any role in immediate management but may prevent delayed reaction.
5. *Antihistaminics:* Inj. diphenhydramine 25–50 mg, IV given for adult and 10–25 mg for children may shorten the duration of anaphylactic reaction. Inj. chlorpeniramine 10–20 mg IV may be given.
6. Inhaled beta agonist (slabutamol or terbutaline) may be used by nebulisation in bronchospasm; inj. aminophylline may be given as a second line drug.
7. *Treatment of shock:* Raise the foot end of the bed; start dopamine infusion. Use volume expanders (colloid solutions, e.g. dextran is preferable).
8. Assisted ventilation (IPPV) with emergency tracheostomy, or endotracheal intubation may be done, if laryngeal oedema is severe and signs of hypoxaemia are evident.
9. *Miscellaneous:* Intravenous isoprenaline, salbutamol or terbutaline may be given.

Q. How and where aminophylline injection is given?

Aminophylline is commonly given in acute exacerbation of bronchial asthma. It may be given in severe bronchospasm due to any cause (e.g. anaphylaxis, acute exacerbation of COPD).

It is also known as theophylline with ethylenediamine. Usually one ampoule of inj. aminophylline contains 250 mg of the drug (in 10 mL). A loading dose of 6 mg/kg is started, followed by an infusion of 1.0 mg/kg/hour for the next 12 hours and the reafter 0.8 mg/kg/hour is maintained. In non-smokers, maintenance dose is less and in patients receiving theophylline, the loading dose will be 0.5 mg/kg. Aminophylline is mixed in the bottle of normal saline or 5% dextrose for infusion. The drugs given slowly in IV route. Common side effects are nausea, vomiting, anorexia, seizures and cardiac arrhythmias.

Aminophyline also contracts diaphragmatic muscles. At present, use of nebuliser (with bronchodilators) has replaced administration of IV aminophylline in acute severe asthma and COPD.

Q. How do you diagnose amoebic liver abscess at the bedside?

Pre-disposing factors: Young adult males, consumption of alcohol, malnutrition.

Clinical Features

1. H/o amoebic dysentery is present in only 10% cases. Onset is usualy subacute, rarely acute.
2. The patient looks ill, mildly toxic and prostrated with a peculiar sallowness of the skin. There may be fever with chill, rigor and profuse sweating though temperature rarely exceeds 40°C; presence of emaciation. The absence of toxicity in the presence of fever is often recordable.
3. Dull and aching pain or sensation of heaviness over right hypochondrium is present. Pain increases with deep inspiration and coughing. Patient tends to turn on the left side. Pain may be referred to the right shoulder. Later on, abdominal pain becomes sharp and stabbing.
4. Intercostal tenderness (important bedside clue to diagnosis). Local oedema may be present.
5. Enlarged, soft, tender liver. A bulge may be seen in the epigastrium.
6. Jaundice is unusual.

7. Spleen is not palpable. The lower zone of right lung may show features of consolidation, pleurisy (pleural rub) or pleural effusion.

- The most common site of amoebic liver abscess is in the right lobe of liver, often postero-superiorly and is usually single. The patient may present with PUO.

Q. Indications of aspiration in amoebic liver abscess:

The needle aspirates the characteristic 'anchovy sauce' or 'chocolate' pus, which chiefly consists of liquefied nectrotic liver tissue. The pus is odourless, bacteriologically sterile, may contain few RBCs with occasional WBCs. The trophozoites of *E. histolytica* are usually absent in freshly aspirated pus but may appear in the escaping pus 4–5 days after initial aspiration. The indications for aspiration are:

1. Lack of response to 3–5 days of metronidazole treatment (i.e. failure to conservative therapy).
2. Very large abscess (>5 cm in diameter) with or without threat of imminent rupture.
3. Abscess in the left lobe likely to rupture into the pericardium.
4. To rule out pyogenic abscess, especially with multiple lesions.

- Aspiration is usually done under USG or CT guidance.
- Anchovy sauce: In real life it is a chocolate colour-like sauce made by small sea fish.

Q. Needle: Description and uses (Fig. 1.10E):

The BD needle has a bevelled end, body and shoulder. The base of a needle can be fitted directly to the nozzle of a syringe; previously available Leur Lock for fixing needle with syringe is not available nowadays. The needles are available in different sizes, e.g. No. 20, i.e. it is 1/20 inch in thickness. The higher the number, the thinner is the needle. Nowadays, disposable needles are available which are thrown away after single use.

Different uses: For IM injection (No. 22–24), for collection of blood and IV infusion (No. 18–20), for collection of blood from a donor (No. 16), and for aspiration of thick fluid from different body cavities (No. 12–14).

Sterilisation is done by boiling the needle for 30 minutes or by autoclaving.

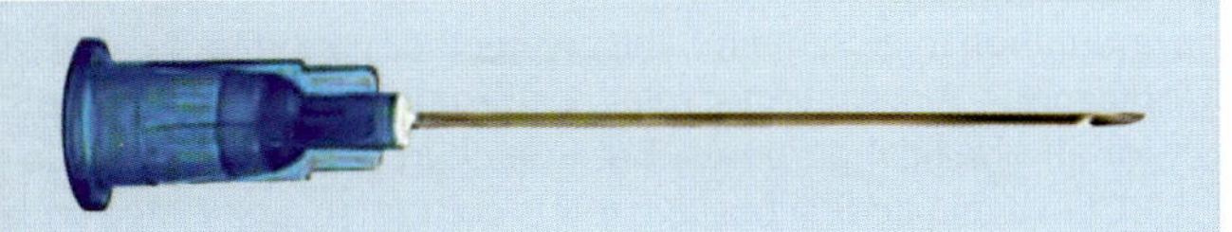

Fig. 1.10E: Hypodermic needle

Q. What is venesection?

When the veins are collapsed and venipuncture is difficult, usually the saphenous vein over the ankle is exposed to the exterior for maintenance of IV infusion by making a small incision, and is known as venesection or 'cut-down' (also *see* page 19).

Q. Arterial blood gas (ABG) sampling: How it is done?

It is done to assess the acid-base status in respiratory, renal, cardiac or hepatic failure (e.g. the blood gas analysis); also done in drug overdose/intoxication (e.g. in aspirin poisoning). Radial artery of non-dominant hand, or femoral or brachial artery is chosen for puncture. Prior to sampling, the laboratory should be informed not to delay unnecessarily. Expel the air bubbles from the 'pre-heparinised' syringe. After proper asepsis, draw the arterial blood and place the 'sample' on ice during transit to the laboratory. Haematoma formation (due to inadequate pressure haemostasis) is not uncommon.

SCALP VEIN SET

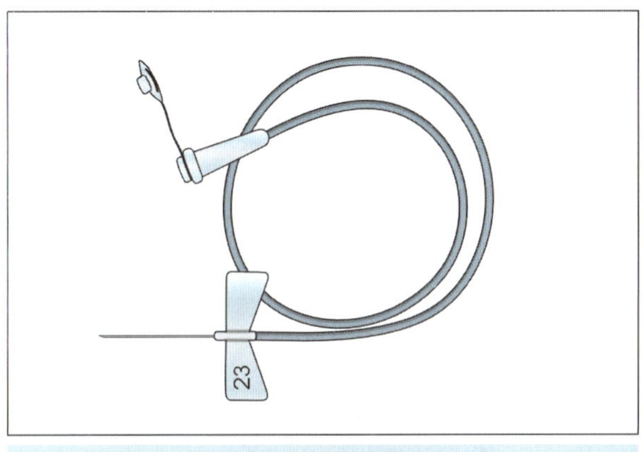

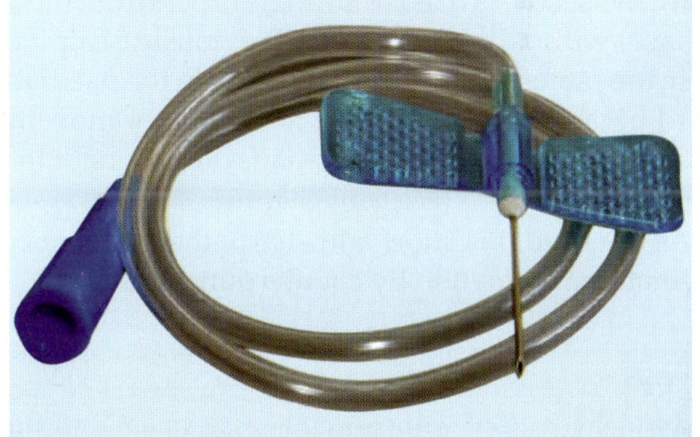

Fig. 1.11: Scalp vein set (size 23)

Description (Fig. 1.11)

1. A polythene tube: At one end, there is a fine bevelled siliconised stainless steel needle (of different size) attached and the other end is open (wider and with a cap) where the nozzle of syringe or IV set is fitted.
2. Two polythene flaps (i.e. butterfly-shaped wings) present on either side of the polythene tube near the needle: For fixation purpose by leucoplast.

The polythene tube is relatively long to be used as a heparinised channel (see below) and so much so to make the scalp vein set flexible. These are sterile and disposable needle of 18–25 G size; higher number needle possesses smaller bore.

Q. Different uses:

1. It is especially used in neonates, infants and small children where the calibre of the vein is small—can be used for parenteral fluid infusion and blood transfusion as well.
2. In adults—for the purpose of fluid infusion or blood transfusion, especially when the patient is in shock or collapsed (needle of common IV infusion set may be large in relation to a collapsed vein and thus, in that situation it may not be possible to place a big needle within the vein).
3. It may be used temporarily (making 'butterfly') for IV medication administered by shot-push (e.g. in pyogenic meningitis, SBE, septicaemia), by introducing diluted heparin (0.5 mL) within the polythene tube of the scalp vein set with the cap kept closed (i.e. acting as a 'heparinised channel'), The heparinised scalp vein set may be kept in the antecubital vein for few days for the purpose of repeated infusion. Intracath (see later) has replaced the use of heparinised scalp vein set.

Q. Why the scalp vein set is named so?

In the pediatrics ward, scalp veins may be used up to the age of 4 or 5 years for IV infusion. Usually branches of temporal vein, posterior auricular vein and veins of the forehead are commonly used as they are constant in location and large in size. The head of the child is fixed; the local skin is shaved. Putting the bevelled end upwards and maintaining the direction towards the heart, the needle is fixed at an angle of 30° (from the skin surface) with adhesive plaster. Previously, scalp veins were the preferred site for IV infusion in the paediatrics ward because it would avoid restriction of movement of limbs. Nowadays, paediatricians do not prefer to use the scalp veins as a recipient channel.

As the needle is short and sharp, there is chance of haematoma formation by counterpuncture.

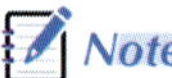

Note

Read 'dehydration' with patient's assessment and fluid replacement in details.

INSULIN SYRINGE

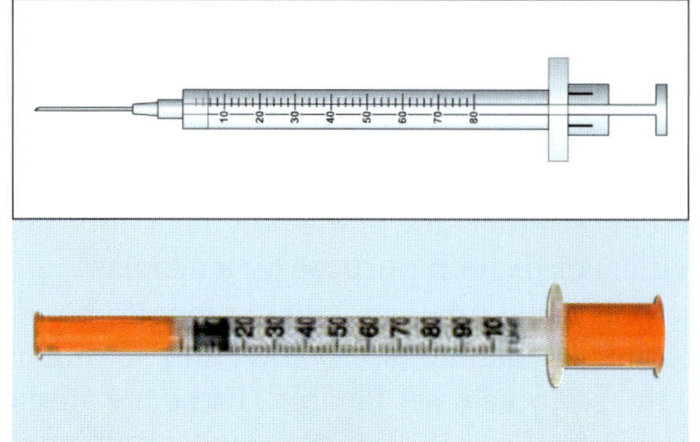

Fig. 1.12A: Insulin syringe with needle

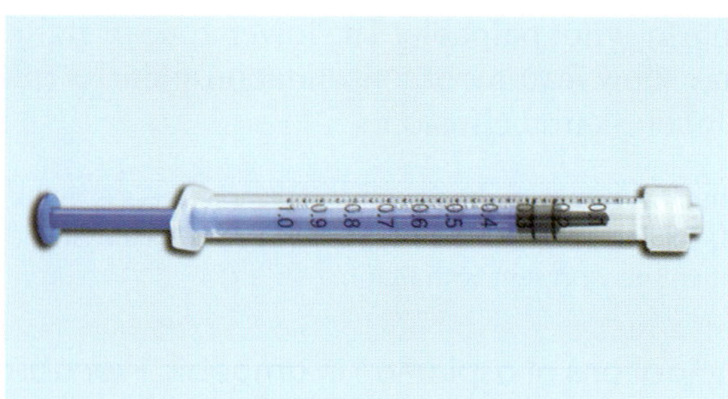

Fig. 1.12B: Tuberculin syringe

Q. Description (Fig. 1.12A):

This is a syringe with capacity of 1 mL. The cylinder has markings on its outer surface indicating the amount of insulin in units, present distal to the piston. Insulin syringe resembles tuberculin syringe though its piston is white in colour (not blue).

Insulin is available in India as 40 units/mL or 80 units/mL commonly, or 100 units/mL as available in abroad and thus, 1 mL is graduated into 40, 80 or 100 units.

Q. Different uses:

1. To inject insulin in the subcutaneous (SC) route in diabetic patients.
2. In neonates, insulin syringe may serve the purpose of a 'hypodermic syringe' for giving injections by IM or SC route. In adults, methotrexate injection in rheumatoid arthritis or inj. adrenaline in anaphylaxis may be given by using insulin syringe (by SC route).
3. Sometimes, it is used to give an intradermal test-dose on the forearm before administering a drug (e.g. test of hypersensitivity reaction before giving injection penicillin).

- A **'tuberculin syringe'** (1 mL syringe with a **blue** pistion; used for Mantoux test or tuberculin test) **(Fig. 1.12B)** may also be used in neonates for giving injection by IM or SC route. **Mantoux test** is a type IV or delayed type of hypersensitivity reaction to tuberculoprotein. One tuberculin unit (TU) is equal to 0.00002 mg International Standard PPD (purified protein derivative). Usually 5 TU is injected (0.1 mL PPD) intradermally on volar aspect of the forearm (junction of mid and upper third). The result is read after 72 hours (3rd day). If the skin 'induration' (thickening) across the transverse axis of forearm is <10 mm, the test is negative and if ≥10 mm, it is regarded as positive. The amount of erythema (redness) present is not important. A **positive test** is presumptive evidence of current (active) or prior (old) mycobacterial infection; the larger the diameter of induration (e.g. >20 mm), the greater the support for a positive diagnosis. A negative test rules out the possibility of tuberculosis for all practical purposes. But in a child below 3 years (non-BCG-vaccinated), a positive test is commonly associated with active progressive disease. It should also be remembered that the **Mantoux test may be negative** in fulminant, miliary and meningeal tuberculosis, tuberculosis with low general condition, measles, lymphoma, sarcoidosis, leukaemia and in immunosuppression (e.g. steroid therapy, AIDS, etc); technical error (e.g. SC injection instead of intradermal) may give rise to negative result.

So, Mantoux test may be positive in recent or old *M. tuberculosis* infection, non-tuberculous mycobacterial (NTM) infection or prior BCG vaccination. This test has very low specificity and sensitivity.

The WHO advocates a PPD tuberculin known as PPD-RT-23 with Tween 80. In AIDS, an induration of 5 mm or more signifies a positive Mantoux test.

- Charles Mantoux (1877–1947) was a French physician from Cannes.
- Bacillus Calmette-Guérin (BCG) vaccine, given at birth to prevent tuberculosis, was discovered in 1921.

Q. Different uses of insulin:

1. Diabetes mellitus:
   a. All type 1 DM patients.
   b. Diabetic ketoacidosis.
   c. Diabetes with pregnancy, labour and delivery
   d. In periods of stress, e.g. acute infection, major surgery, acute myocardial infarction, any acute medical illness, stroke, acute injury, or while on glucocorticoid treatment.
   e. In type 2 DM: Secondary failure of oral hypoglycaemic agents; or inadequate control with presence of complications like painful peripheral neuropathy/retinopathy; renal failure, hepatic failure or respiratory failure.
   f. Pre-renal transplantation of diabetic patients.
2. Hyperkalaemia.
3. Insulin test or Hollander's test (not used nowadays): To know the completeness of vagotomy in a duodenal ulcer patient. It is known that increase in 20 mEq/L of acidity above the basal level after injection of insulin indicates incomplete vagotomy (insulin-induced hypoglycaemia stimulates the neurogenic phase of acid secretion in stomach in the presence of intact vagus nerve).

Q. Who first used insulin?

On 23rd January 1922, Frederick G Banting (a Canadian physician) and Charles H Best (a medical student) first used pancreatic extract in Toronto General Hospital on a severely diabetic patient named Leonard Thompson. Banting received The Nobel Prize along with another physician JJR Macleod (Professor of physiology) in the year 1923 for the discovery of insulin. November 14, the birth date of Sir FG Banting, was chosen as 'World Diabetes Day'.

Table 1.4: Available insulin preparations

Preparations	Time of action		
	Onset	**Peak**	**Duration**
Short-acting			
Lispro	<15 min	0.5–1.5 h	3–4 h
Aspart	<15 min	0.5–1.5 h	3–4 h
Glulisine	<15 min	0.5–1.5 h	3–4 h
Regular	30 min	2–3 h	4–6 h
Intermediate-acting			
NPH (isophane insulin)	2–4 h	6–8 h	10–16 h
Lente	2–4 h	6–8 h	10–16 h
Long-acting			
Glargine	1–4 h	None	24 h
Ultralente	4–6 h	10–18 h	16–24 h
Detemir	1–4 h	None	12–20 h
Degludec (ultra long-acting)	30–90 min	None	>24 h
Mixtures (Premix)			
70/30, 50/50, 75/25	30 min	7–12 h	10–16 h

- Values (time of action) are highly variable among individuals. Even in an individual, values vary depending on the site and depth of injection, skin temperature and exercise.
- *Insulin combinations:* 70/30 (70% NPH, 30% regular); 50/50 (50% NPH, 50% regular), and 75/25 (75% protamine lispro, 25% lispro), 70/30 (70% protamine aspart, 30% aspart) and 50/50 (50% protamine lispro, 50% lispro) are different pre-mixed combinations used in clinical practice. NPH is Neutral Protamine Hagedorn.
- A new formulation of ultra rapid-acting inhaled insulin (Afrezza) has received FDA approval in 2014. In **diabetes with pregnancy**: drugs like metformin (in gestational diabetes with mild hyperglycaemia), glyburide (with caution) or insulin (regular, NPH, aspart, lispro) may be used.

Q. Insulin analogues (Table 1.4):

These insulin preparations are generated by modifying (i.e. changing the amino acid sequence by recombinant DNA technology) human insulin, and are useful in patients having repeated attacks of hypoglycaemia or show hyperglycaemia during some parts of the day while on regular insulin therapy. Among the six insulin analogues, three are short-acting or rapid-acting (lispro, aspart and glulisine) and three are long-acting (glargine, detemir and degludec) preparations.

Q. Insulin secretagogues and sensitisers:

Insulin secretagogues: Sulphonylureas and non-sulphonylureas (repaglinide and nateglinide). GLP-1 agonists exenatide and liraglutide (also known as 'Incretin mimetics'), and DPP-4 inhibitors sitagliptin, vildagliptin, linagliptin and saxagliptin are also insulin secretagogues.

Insulin sensitisers: Metformin and glitazones (e.g. pioglitazone).

- GLP-1 = glucagon-like peptide 1, DPP-4 = dipeptidyl peptidase-4
- Read 'oral hypoglycaemic agents' from the chapter on 'Diabetes mellitus' in 'Bedside Clinics in Medicine, Part I'.

Q. Uses of soluble or regular insulin:

1. In emergencies, it is the insulin of choice, i.e. ketoacidosis, infection, surgery, pregnancy, trauma.

2. To supplement depot insulin effects, if necessary.
3. Patients requiring >150 units of insulin/day.
4. Patients not controlled properly with depot insulins.

Q. Main types of therapeutic insulins:

1. Species	Bovine
	Porcine
	Human
2. Purity	Conventional
	Single peak
	Highly purified
3. Duration of action	Short-acting
	Intermediate-acting
	Long-acting

- Bovine insulin is more immunogenic, i.e. in relation to immunogenicity (antigenicity), Bovine >Porcine >Human insulin. Animal preparations (bovine or porcine) are no longer used.

Q. Goals of insulin therapy:

1. Alleviation of primary glycosuric symptoms.
2. Prevention of ketoacidosis and hyperosmolar coma; brings back the lost lean body mass.
3. Improvement in physical performance as well as sense of well being.
4. Diminution in foeto-maternal morbidity, foetal malformations.
5. Reduction in recurrent infections.
6. Delay, prevent or arrestation of micro- and macrovascular complications.

Q. Different insulin regimens:

1. Conventional insulin therapy (CIT).
2. Multiple subcutaneous injections (MSI).
3. Continuous subcutaneous insulin infusion (CSII).

Q. How to administer insulin?

Patient's education regarding insulin administration is important in treating diabetes mellitus.

1. Preferably, asepsis is maintained. Required dose of insulin is drawn into the syringe through a hypodermic needle.
2. A small, fine-bore hypodermic needle is now attached to the nozzle (or already attached) of the insulin syringe.
3. Preferable sites of injection are: anterior abdominal wall, upper outer arms, upper thighs or buttocks. The site is properly cleansed with spirit. Injection insulin is administered by SC route.
4. Now, a fold of skin and subcutaneous tissue is pinched-up by left thumb and index finger, and the hypodermic needle is introduced in the skinfold by right hand, from the top into the subcutaneous tissue. Insulin is injected and the needle is taken out with care (insulin leakage should be avoided).
5. Injection site is now covered and lightly pressed by a piece of cotton (rubbing should be avoided).

- The rotation of injection site should also be taught to the patient. Repeated injections in one site predispose to lipohypertrophy. Insulin injections are to be given deep subcutaneously. The sites have to be rotated so that a second injection does not fall within 1–2 cm of the previous injection site within 1 month of time. Look the injection sites for bruising, erythema or lipodystrophy.

Q. Alternative methods (i.e. other than syringe) of insulin delivery system:

i. Jet injectors.
ii. Pen devices.
iii. Insulin infusion pumps:
   a. 'Open' loop: Continuous subcutaneous insulin infusion (CSII).
   b. Closed loop (Biostator): Artificial pancreas.
iv. Nasal, oral, inhaler and rectal insulin: Not effective in practice at present.
v. Pancreas transplantation: Whole pancreas, segmental pancreas, islet transplant.

- Microprocessor based implantable pumps are now available which are more acceptable than CSII.
- 'Open' loop can be used by SC, IV or intraperitoneal route.

Q. Define brittle diabetes and insulin resistance:

a. ***Brittle diabetes:*** A small proportion of type 1 DM patients (1–2% of diabetic patients in practice) are unstable and difficult to control, and are referred to brittle diabetes. Actually, brittle diabetic is a patient whose life is constantly disrupted by episodic swings of hypoglycaemia and hyperglycaemia, whatever the cause may be and thus, it is difficult to manage. It is also known as unstable or labile diabetes.

b. ***Insulin resistance:***
   i. *Old view:* when >200 units of insulin/day are required to attain glycaemic control and to prevent ketoacidosis, it is arbitrarily said that insulin resistance exists.
   ii. *Modern view:* Daily intake of >1.5 units of insulin/kg of body weight, which is about twice the usual level necessary for full insulin replacement therapy (considering newer insulins).

- **Daily insulin production** by a normal pancreas in a healthy non-obese adult is 25–50 units.
- **Insulin resistance** is clinically diagnosed at the bedside by acanthosis nigricans, skin tags (acrochordons), central obesity, features of polycystic ovarian disease and lipodystrophy.

Q. Complications of insulin therapy:

1. Hypoglycaemia (commonest).
2. *Lipodystrophy:* Lipoatrophy (i.e. subcutaneous fat loss) and lipohypertrophy (i.e. fatty lumps).
3. Insulin resistance.
4. *Allergy:* Local, and rarely generalised.

5. Insulin oedema (rare but troublesome).
6. Weight gain, especially if the dose of insulin is increased inappropriately.
7. Sepsis.

Note

Read newer insulins from standard pharmacology or medicine textbooks.

THREE-WAY CANNULA

Q. Description (Fig. 1.13):

It is a T-shaped instrument with two inlets and one outlet. By adjustment, the outlet may be connected with either of the inlets.

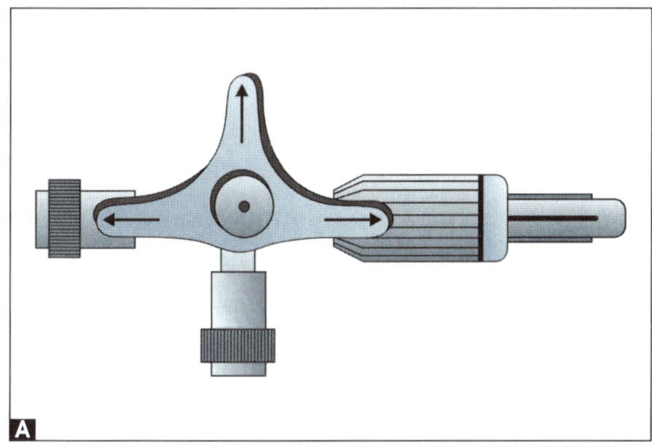

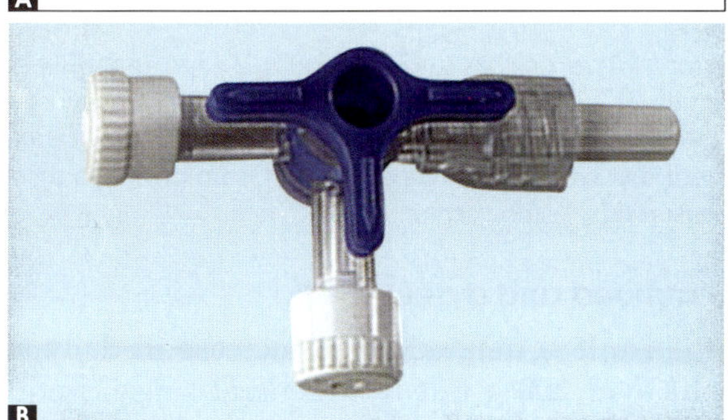

Fig. 1.13: Three-way cannula (adaptor)

Q. Different Uses:

1. To aspirate fluid from pleural, peritoneal or pericardial sac (fluid is withdrawn through one inlet by connecting a syringe with the cannula and by adjusting the screw, fluid in the syringe may be pushed into the kidney-tray via the outlet).
2. Through one inlet, IV fluid may be given (by an IV set) and the other inlet may be used for medications or monitoring central venous pressure (CVP).

ORAL REHYDRATION SALT (ORS)

Q. Presentation (Fig. 1.14):

The ORS is wrapped in an aluminium foil-packet or in a paper-packet.

Q. Indications for use:

To replace the fluid and electrolyte loss commonly as a result of vomiting and/or diarrhoea (i.e. acute gastroenteritis, cholera)—the 'oral rehydration therapy' (ORT).

Q. Composition:

As suggested by WHO (1971), the 'universal formula' is:

Ingredients	*Composition in g/litre of water*
NaCl (table salt)	3.5
$NaHCO_3$ (baking soda) or	2.5
Trisodium citrate dihydrate	2.9
KCl	1.5
Glucose (anhydrous)	20.0

Concentration in mEq/L: Na^+ 90, K^+ 20, Cl^- 80, HCO_3^- or citrate 10, glucose 111 and osmolality 311.

Clinical Wisdom

The discovery of ORS is known as 'most medical advance of the century'. In 2002, WHO and UNICEF recommended use of 'new formula ORS' or **'low osmolarity ORS'**, especially for children with acute, non-cholera diarrhoea. It prevents hypernatraemia and increased stool output, especially in infants and young children. It can also be used in adults with strict vigilance to sodium concentration in blood.

The **ingredients** (g/litre of water) are NaCl 2.6, trisodium citrate dihydrate 2.9, KCl 1.5 and glucose (anhydrous) 13.5; **concentration in mEq/L** of low osmolarity ORS are: Na^+ 75, K^+ 20, Cl^- 65, citrate 10, glucose 75 and osmolality 245.

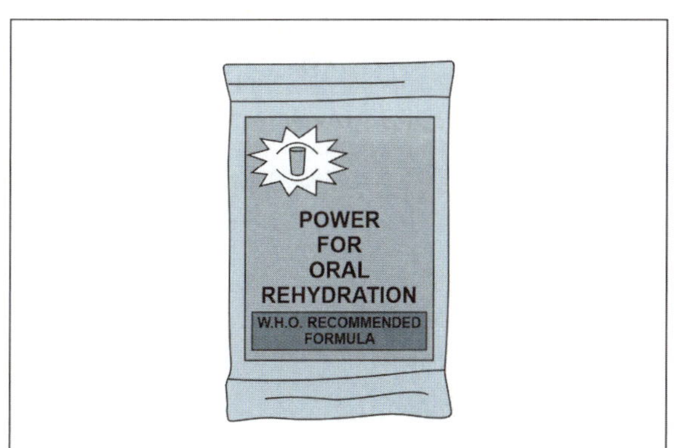

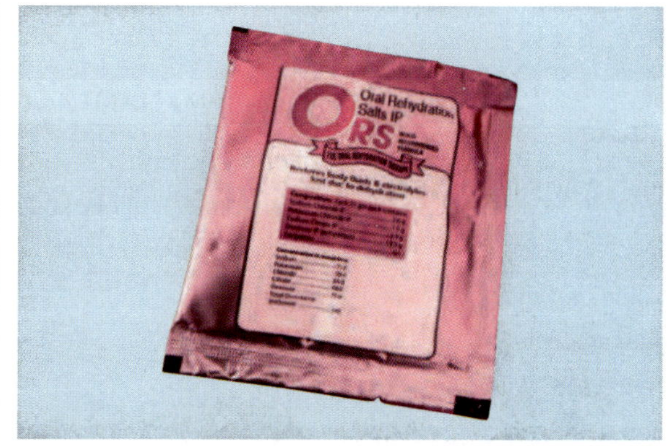

Fig. 1.14: Electrolyte sachet

Q. Method of preparation and application:

The content of the packet is dissolved in one litre of drinking water which is already boiled and then cooled, and should be used within 24 hours. It should be taken frequently as directed by the physician (depends on degree of dehydration).

Approximately, 50 mL/kg of body weight of ORS is given in first 4 hours in mild dehydration and 100 mL/kg of body weight is given similarly in moderate dehydration. Severe dehydration needs IV fluid therapy (along with ORS, 50–500 mL/kg of body weight).

Q. Advantages of use of ORS:

1. Reduces the cost of treatment (i.e. economical).
2. Easily administered at home (can be used easily by non-trained person).
3. It can be prepared easily at home by simple ingredients like sugar and common salt.
4. Practically, there is very little chance of fluid overload.
5. No pain or phlebitis (as occurs with IV fluid therapy).

Q. Disadvantages of use of ORS:

There are very few disadvantages of oral rehydration therapy like:

1. Unconscious patient (requires IV access).
2. Severe dehydration (needs IV fluid therapy).
3. Chance of fluid overload in CCF, chronic renal failure and in infants.
4. The taste may not be accepted by all (few ORS are added with rice flour and used in cholera, are really of very bad taste).
5. Patient may be reluctant to take it in the presence of incessant vomiting.

Q. Contraindications of ORS:

1. Severe hypertensive disorders.
2. Protracted vomiting.
3. Comatose patient.
4. Severe renal failure.
5. Chronic heart failure.
6. Intestinal obstruction.

Q. Principle of action of ORS:

Use of ORS is based on the observation that oral glucose (2%) enhances the intestinal absorption of salt and water (ATP-dependent pump for Na^+ absorption, i.e. glucose-facilitated Na^+ transport), even in the presence of diarrhoea.

Glucose may be replaced by sucrose (40 g of sucrose must be added as sucrose is broken down to equal amount of glucose and fructose). Cereals and other starchy foods (rice flour) may also replace glucose (starch is broken down into glucose and amino acids which facilitate Na^+ absorption)

- Fluids from cooked cereals, e.g. rice water may be used in tropics.

Q. Osmolality of blood, urine, stool and CSF:

Osmolality is the measurement of concentration of all solute particles per kilogram of solution.

Blood (plasma): 280–300 mOsmol/kg of water
Urine: 400–750 mOsmol/kg of water
Stool: 290 mOsmol/kg of water
CSF: 292–297 mOsmol/kg of water

- *Osmolality of plasma* (mOsmol/kg) = 2 [Na^+ (mmol/L) + K^+ (mmol/L)] + glucose (mmol/L) + BUN (mmol/L). Glucose and BUN are converted to mmol/L by dividing concentration in mg/dL by 18 and 2.8 respectively. Osmolality can also be measured by osmometry.

Q. Diarrhoea and dysentery:

Diarrhoea: It is defined as an increase in daily stool weight over 200 g but in a general sense, frequent passage of liquid or unformed stool is known as diarrhoea. It is divided into **acute** (lasting less than

Table 1.5: Differentiation between small bowel and large bowel diarrhoea

Features	Small bowel diarrhoea	Large bowel diarrhoea
1. Volume	Large	Small
2. Frequency	Less	More
3. Character	Soup-like, greasy	Mucinous, jelly-like
4. Colour	Light	Dark
5. Odour	Very offensive	Offensive
6. Nature	Uniformly watery	Mucoid, or watery with small pieces of fecal matter
7. Site of pain	Mid-abdomen (colicky and intermittent)	Lower abdomen (gripping and continuous)
8. Site of involvement	Small bowel or right colon	Left colon
9. Dehydration and shock	Unlikely	Common
10. Tenesmus	Absent	Present
11. Blood and WBC within stool	Rare	Common
12. Common pathogenic organisms	*Vibrio cholerae*, *E. coli*, Rota or Norwalk virus, *Campylobacter*	*E. histolytica*, *Shigella*

2 weeks—mainly the infective causes, e.g. Rota virus, *E. coli*, *Clostridium difficile*, cholera, and soon after dietary indiscretions), **persistent** (2–4 weeks) and **chronic** (lasting more than 4 weeks—chronic enteric infections, e.g. salmonellosis, giardiasis, hookworm infestation, amoebic colitis, intestinal tuberculosis, HIV infection; pancreatic insufficiency, coeliac disease, pellagra, Addison's disease, malabsorption syndrome, inflammatory bowel disease, e.g. ulcerative colitis and Crohn's disease, irritable bowel syndrome, lactose intolerance, diverticulitis, autonomic neuropathy, lactase deficiency, thyrotoxicosis or laxative abuse) types **(Table 1.5)**.

'Hyperdefecation' is characteristic of thyrotoxicosis. Frequent passage of small volume of formed stool is often associated with anorectal disorders (e.g. proctitis) or irritable bowel syndrome is known as 'pseudodiarrhoea'. Involuntary discharge of rectal contents is known as rectal incontinence, and is due to neuromuscular disorders or anorectal sphincteric disturbance (i.e. fecal incontinence).

Dysentery: Characterised by diarrhoea with blood and mucus in the stool as a result of acute inflammation of large gut, and clinically manifested by colicky abdominal pain, pyrexia and tenesmus (dysentery is basically of two types—amoebic and bacillary).

- **Tenesmus** is a feeling of incomplete evacuation with a constant desire for defecation.

Q. Mechanisms of diarrhoea in a nutshell:

a. *Secretory diarrhoea*, i.e. disruption of epithelial electrolyte transport, e.g. increased secretion of electrolytes in *V. cholerae* infection, villous adenoma of colon, etc.
b. *Osmotic diarrhoea:* Poorly absorbed solutes in lactose intolerance, maldigestion, or $MgSO_4$ or lactulose-induced.
c. *Exudative diarrhoea:* Occurs in the presence of blood and pus in the stool, e.g. IBD (ulcerative colitis and Crohn's disease) or food poisoning.
d. *Malabsorption diarrhoea:* Stool is bulky and extremely foul-smelling, e.g. in coeliac disease, etc.
e. *Motility disorder-induced diarrhoea:* Irritable bowel syndrome (IBS).

Q. What are the endocrine causes of diarrhoea?

1. Diabetes mellitus.
2. Hyperthyroidism.
3. Hypoparathyroidism.
4. Zollinger-Ellison syndrome.
5. Adrenal insufficiency.
6. Carcinoid syndrome.
7. Villous adenoma of colon.
8. Medullary carcinoma of thyroid.
9. VIPoma (pancreatic cholera).
10. Systemic mastocytosis.

Q. Common offenders in traveller's diarrhoea?

It is the passage of three or more unformed stool/ day in a resident of a developed country travelling in a developing nation. The infection is usually food- or water-borne. The common offenders are:

a. *Bacterial:* Enterotoxigenic *E. coli*, *Campylobacter jejuni*, *Salmonella*, *Shigella*, enteroaggregative *E. coli*. *Yersinia enterocolitica*, *aeromonas* spp. and *Plesiomonas shigelloides* are rare causes.
b. *Viral:* Account for minority of illness (e.g. Rota virus, Norwalk virus).
c. *Parasitic: E. hystolytica*, *Giardia lamblia* and *cryptosporidia* spp.

Q. What is food poisoning?

Any disease of an infective or toxic nature caused by consumption of food or drink is food poisoning. The most common form is gastroenteritis, following consumption of food containing preformed toxins or infective organisms that are capable to produce toxins in the intestine. The common causes are preformed toxins (e.g. *Staphylococcus aureus*), enterotoxigenic *E. coli*. *Shegella*, *Salmonella*, *Campylobacter*, viruses, *Giardia lamblia*, *Clostridium*, heavy metals (e.g. arsenic), mushrooms, certain seafoods or botulinus toxin (botulism does not produce gastroenteritis but develops into potentially fatal paralytic illness). The common symptoms are nausea, vomiting, diarrhoea (may be bloody), abdominal pain and cramping, fever and malaise. Symptoms can start as early as one hour in case of *Staphylococcus aureus*.

Q. Acute infective diarrhoea in children:

The common causes are:

1. *Virus:* Rota virus (30–40%), Norwalk virus
2. *Bacterial:*
   a. *E. coli*—Enterotoxigenic strain (30-40%)
   b. *V. cholerae* (El Tor biotype)
   c. *Salmonella*
   d. *Shigella*
   e. *Campylobacter jejuni*
   f. *Clostridium difficile*
3. *Parasites: Glardia lamblia*, *Entamoeba histolytica*, *Plasmodium falciparum* (Algid malaria)
4. *Fungi: Candida albicans*.

Clinical Wisdom

V. cholerae and *E. coli* do not invade intestinal mucosa. Diarrhoea is an important determining factor leading to malnutrition in children. Breastfeeding should continue along with oral rehydration therapy in infantile diarrhoea.

Q Chronic diarrhoea in children:

1. Cow's milk allergy.
2. Coeliac disease.
3. Chronic pancreatitis.

4. Cystic fibrosis.
5. Secondary to PEM, or viral/bacterial enteritis.
6. Worm infestations.
7. Intestinal stasis.
8. Liver diseases.

Q. How ORS can be prepared at home?

a. Two teaspoonfuls of cane sugar + a pinch of table salt + a glass of water, or
b. 6–8 level teaspoonfuls of cane sugar (i.e. 40 g of sucrose) + one level teaspoonful of common salt (i.e. 5 g of NaCl) ± few drops of lemon + 1 litre of potable water.

- 20 g of glucose is equivalent to 40 g of cane sugar (sucrose), is equivalent to 50 g of rice flour (puffed rice powder).
- Rice-based ORS gives more nutritional benefits and helps to reduce the fluid output of diarrhoeal stool.

Q. Can a green coconut (water) replace ORS?

Previously it was said by some workers in this field that oral administration of 200 mL of green coconut water (GCW) for each litre of fecal loss would serve to maintain K^+-balance in cholera patients with prolonged diarrhoea. It is known that K^+ content of GCW is high, and Na^+ and glucose contents are low in comparison to ORS. Though GCW is a readily available, cheap, sterile refreshing drink (an average size GCW contains about 300 mL of fluid), it can never replace ORS because it is not a true replica of ORS.

THE STETHOSCOPE

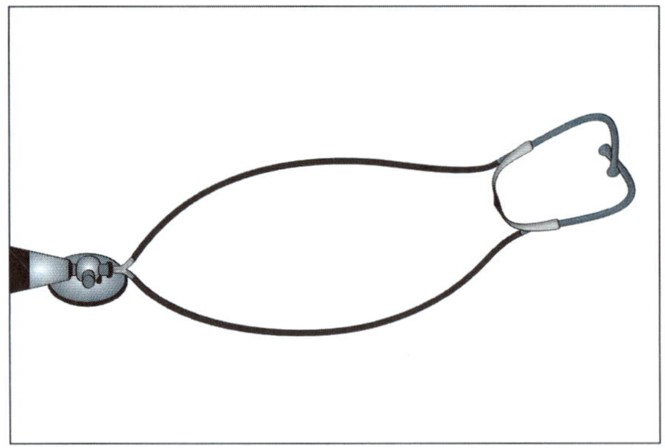

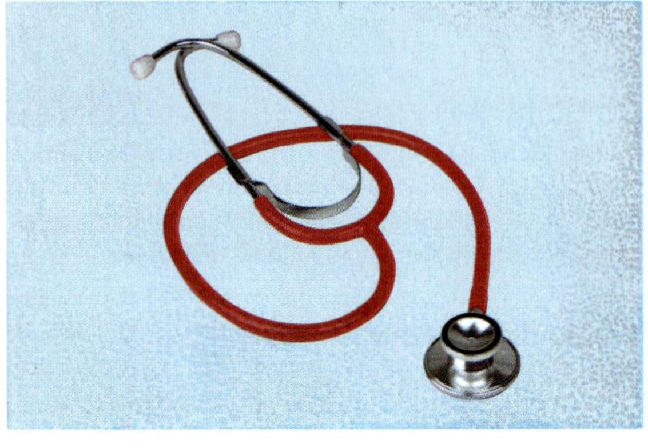

Fig. 1.15A: The stethoscope

Q. Description (Fig. 1.15A):

It has four parts such as 1. Chest piece, 2. Connecting tube, 3. Head piece, and 4. Ear piece.

1. Chest piece: Usually with a diaphragm and a bell, only one operates at a time. There is a valve that allows switching from diaphragm to bell and *vice versa*.

a. *The diaphragm:* It should be stiff and smooth to damp out low-frequency sounds, and unmask high-frequency sounds (>300 Hz). The thin plastic disc (usually having 4 cm diameter) is kept in position tightly by a metallic ring. The cardiac sounds best heard by diaphragm are, 1. All the diastolic and systolic murmurs due to different valvular lesions except mitral and tricuspid stenosis (MS/TS), 2. S_1 and S_2, and 3. Ejection click, pericardial knock, opening snap, etc.
b. *The bell:* Low-frequency sounds (80–150 Hz) are best heard by the bell. The bell (diameter of 2.5 cm) should be placed lightly on the site of auscultation (just enough to prevent room-noise leak) as firm pressure will tighten the underlying skin as a taut diaphragm (in that situation, low-frequency sounds will damp out and only high-frequency sounds are heard). The sounds best heard by the bell are, 1. Low-pitched diastolic murmur of MS and TS, 2. S_3 or S_4, 3. Foetal heart sounds, and 4. Venous hum.

2. Connecting tube: A single or double tube connects the head piece with the chest piece via a metallic connector (binaural connector) attached to the chest piece. A length of 12 inches (30 cm) is sufficient. A tall physician may add additional 3 or 4 inches. Internal lining should be smooth and is of 4-6 mm in diameter.

Long tubing attenuates high-frequency sounds. Very narrow tubes carry low-frequency sounds better, and high-frequency sounds are better carried by wider tubing.

3. Head piece: The two metal tubes of the head piece are attached together by a metallic U-connector.

4. Ear piece: The two metal tubes of the head piece end in two plastic ear pieces. Larger ear pieces are ideal as they prevent air leak. The usual stethoscope head piece is designed in such a way that the ear pieces point slightly anterioly to be in the same line with the external auditory canal.

- One should not replace the torn diaphragm with a small piece of X-ray plate because the X-ray plate is neither thin nor stiff. A beginner in medical curriculum should know every detail of a stethoscope.

Q. Criteria for a good (ideal) stethoscope:

1. *For high-frequency sounds:* Smooth, thin and stiff diaphragm.
2. *For low-frequency sounds:* Shallow bell with a large diameter.
3. Double tubing (more efficient for high-frequencies) with a metal clip which binds the tubes together.

Rene Laennec, reluctant to press his ear to chest of a young female patient, finds a solution in the wooden stethoscope

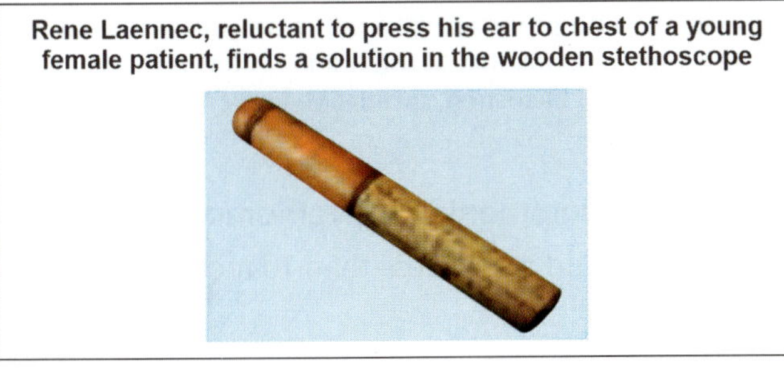

Fig. 1.15B: **Stethoscope** used by **Laennec**

4. Ear pieces should be largest possible one; soft and made of rubbery material.
5. Length and internal circumferential diameter of the connecting tubes should not cross 12 inches and 4-6 mm respectively; the inner lining of the tubes should be made smooth by 'vinyl tubing'.
6. There should be option for rotation of the metal head pieces so that ear pieces can be placed in the most comfortable position.
7. An extra pediatric-sized diaphragm and bell attached.

Q. Who invented the stethoscope?

The French physician Rene Theophile Hyacinthe (RTH) Laennec (1816) invented the stethoscope; his first instrument was a hollow wooden cylinder (Fig. 1.15B). He died at the age of 46 years (1781–1826). His idea of listening heart sounds by a roll of thick paper landed in modern stethoscope with passage of time.

Later on, his instrument was modified by Arthur Lear and George Cammann to become the binaural instrument that is used today.

Q. Different uses:

Though *stethos* means 'chest', and *skopio* means 'to examine', the modern stethoscope is used for auscultation of various parts of the body, such as:

1. *Cardiovascular system:* Heart sounds, murmur, opening snap, ejection click, pericardial knock, pericardial rub, etc.
2. *Respiratory system:* Breath sound, vocal resonance, crepitations, rhonchi, pleural rub, pneumothorax click, etc.
3. *Abdomen:* Normal peristaltic sounds, renal artery bruit, venous hum, succussion splash and ausculto-percussion in pyloric stenosis, hepatic and splenic rub, hepatic bruit, uterine souffle and foetal heart sounds.
4. *Head:* Bruit from cerebral arteriovenous malformation may be heard over cranium or closed eyes; bruit in Paget's disease.
5. *Neck:* Carotid bruit, cervical venous hum, thyroid bruit, conducted murmur of AS.
6. *Extremities:* Pistol shot sound, Duroziez's murmur, demonstration of Hill's sign.
7. Measurement of blood pressure (to listen Korotkoff sounds).
8. *Miscellaneous:* Subcutaneous emphysema, demonstration of parietal oedema.

- Worldwide, stethoscope symbolises a doctor. Stethoscope manufactured by renowned companies are Littmann, Harvey, Sprague, Leatham, etc. Besides the conventional variety, electronic, magnetic and digital stethoscopes are also available.
- Except the sounds best heard by the bell, all other sounds mentioned above are best auscultated by the diaphragm of stethoscope.

SPHYGMOMANOMETER

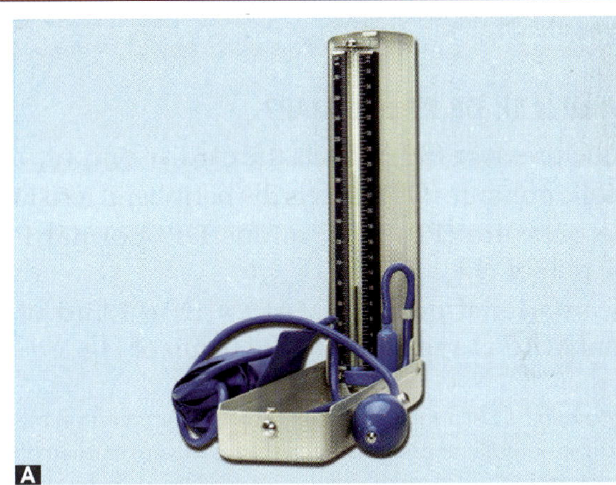

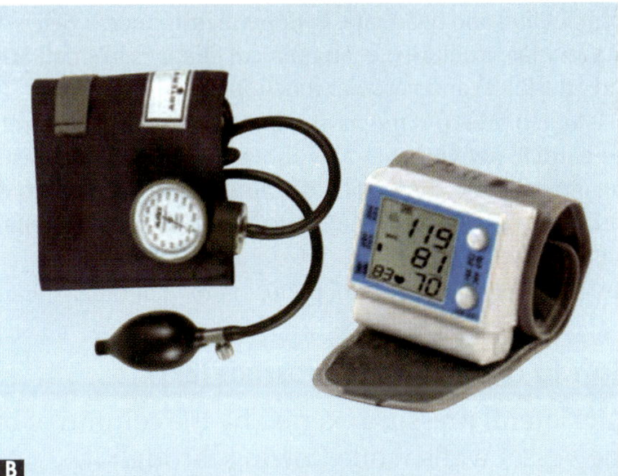

Fig. 1.16: Sphygmomanometer (A) Mercury column type; (B) Aneroid type

Q. Different uses:

They are:

1. To measure the blood pressure (BP).
2. Confirmation of,
   a. Pulsus paradoxus.
   b. Pulsus alternans.
   c. Water-hammer pulse.
3. To demonstrate postural hypotension.
4. To demonstrate Hill's sign in aortic regurgitation and low BP in lower limbs in coarctation of aorta.
5. Hess' capillary fragility test.
6. To assess the respiratory reserve (blow through the tube and observe the rise in mercury column).
7. In latent tetany (Trousseau's sign).
8. To draw venous blood.

9. As a rotating tourniquet in LVF.
10. To draw blood during blood donation.

- Sphygmomanometer was discovered by Scipione Riva-Rocci (Italy) in 1896.

Q. Types (Fig. 1.16):

There are two common types:

a. Mercury column type, and
b. Aneroid type or spring dial type (less accurate).

- Digital (electronic) BP instruments are used by lay people at home (third type).

Q. What is SP, DP, PP and MAP?

Systolic pressure (SP) reflects the cardiac output.

Diastolic pressure (DP) reflects the peripheral resistance.

Pulse pressure (PP) = SP minus DP; normal PP is 30–60 mm of Hg.

Mean arterial pressue (MAP) = DP+ 1/3rd of PP; normal MAP is approximately 100 mm of Hg.

- *Determinants of arterial pressure:* Two major determinants are cardiac output and peripheral resistance. Again, cardiac output is determined by stroke volume (it is related to myocardial contractility) and heart rate. Peripheral resistance is determined by vascular structure (i.e. anatomical changes in small arteries and arterioles) and vascular function.
- Diastolic pressure is the most important among all. SP reflects the cardiac activity over and above the peripheral resistance (i.e. indicates the constant load against which heart has to work) and thus, DP is a better guide to assess the haemodynamics in the body.
- MAP is a better indicator of perfusion to vital organs than SP.

Q. How to define blood pressure (BP)?

It is the lateral pressure exerted by the column of blood on the vessel walls while flowing through it.

Q. What is the normal BP (Table 1.6)?

It depends on age and sex of the individual, and also on many other parameters like build, exercise, posture, sleep, excitement, etc. High BP or **hypertension** is defined arbitrarily by the values which outrange the normal limits of BP as defined by British Hypertension Society or JNC-VIII. According to majority of definitions, upper limit of normal BP is 140/90 mm of Hg (<60 years). **Hypotension** is BP <90/60 mm of Hg.

Table 1.6: 2017 updated classification of blood pressure

BP category	Systolic BP (mm of Hg)	Diastolic BP (mm of Hg)
Normal	<120	<80
Elevated	120–129	<80
Stage I hypertension	130–139	80–89
Stage II hypertension	≥140	≥90

- Read JNC-VII (2003) and VIII (2014) for BP goal from any cardiology textbook. JNC stands for Joint National Committee on Prevention, Detection, Evaluation and Treatment of High Blood Pressure.

Q. Ideal measurement of sphygmomanometer cuff:

1. *Length:* Should not be less than 10 inches.
2. *Width:*
   a. Adults: 5 inches.
   b. Young children: 3 inches.
   c. Infants: 1 inch.

- Width of 8 inches cuff should be used in legs (thigh) to avoid falsely elevated BP in adults. If an adult-sized cuff is used in a child, it will falsely record low BP and if an infant-sized cuff is used in an adult, it with falsely record high BP. Obese adults require wider cuff for arms (6 inches).

Q. How do you measure the BP?

Steps

1. The patient should lie flat on his back (SP may rise after sitting or standing) and should take rest for at least 15 minutes before recording of BP (BP should be recorded with the patient taking rest in a comfortable position and thus, casual recording should always be avoided). The patient should not smoke, consume caffeine or perform exercise at least half an hour before measurement.
2. Wrap the appropriate cuff (it has an inflatable rubber bladder inside) firmly and uniformly over the arm in such a way (rubber cuff should cover 80% of arm) that the lower border of the cuff remains at least 1 inch above the elbow joint. The arm should be kept in extended position at the heart level.
3. Keep the BP instrument (or spring dial) at the level of patient's heart. The midportion of the rubber bag present within the cuff should lie over the brachial artery. Raise the pressure upto 200 mm of Hg or till the radial pulse disappears. Now start deflating, while the point of reappearance of radial pulse indicates SP by 'palpatory method'. BP is first recorded by palpation and then by auscultatory method; now place the diaphragm of sthethoscope over the brachial artery, a little below the cuff ('auscultatory method'). The cuff is inflated again and the mercury column is raised to 20 mm of Hg above the SP which was recorded by palpatory method, and then deflated slowly (2 mm of Hg/second). The BP is usually measured to the nearest 2 mm of Hg.
4. During release of pressure (deflation), following variations of sounds are heard ('Korotkoff sounds', after their discoverer Nikolai Korotkoff, a Russian surgeon, in 1905). Phase I—Sudden appearance of tapping sound (indicates SP); Phase II—Murmur-like sound replaces the tapping sound; Phase III—Gong sound replaces murmur; Phase IV—Loud sound suddenly becomes muffled: Phase V—Disappearance of all sounds (indicates DP).

Clinical Wisdom

Previouly DP was recorded by phase IV but nowadays phase V (just disappearance of sounds) is taken granted for measuring DP (interobserver variations are minimum and more closely corresponds to directly measurred DP while recording phase V). Few countries record the BP as $^{150}/_{96-90}$ mm of Hg where the SP is 150, Phase IV—DP is 96 and phase V—DP is recorded as 90 mm of Hg.

5. For recording of blood pressure in legs, wrap the larger cuff in the thigh and place the stethoscope over the popliteal artery in the popliteal fossa while the patient lies in prone position.

- Where Korotkoff sounds remain audible in spite of complete deflation of the cuff (e.g. aortic incompetence, arteriovenous fistula, pregnancy), phase IV should be used for measurement of DP. The DP may be 0 (zero) in these condition.
- In young individuals <50 years of age, DP is more important as a risk factor whereas SP is important in persons >50 years of age. SP increases continuously with ageing; in elderly persons DP may decrease.

Q. Checklists for ideal BP measurement:

1. The patient should be 'relaxed'.
2. Arm placed at heart level. Tight clothing should be removed from the arm.
3. Correct size of bladder cuff without any leak.
4. Sphygmomanometer should be placed upright; aneroid type calibrated at regular interval.
5. Confirm systolic BP by palpation of radial artery; slow deflation in auscultatory method.
6. Avoid parallax error (eye should be kept at the same level with the sphygmomanometer).
7. Record two measurements at each visit.

Q. Does any variation exist in BP of two upper extremities?

Normally, in health, there may be a difference of 10 mm of Hg observed between right and left upper limb pressure. One must think of few special situations (like thoracic inlet syndrome, aneurysm of the aorta, pre-subclavian coarctation, supravalvular AS, Takayasu's disease, atherosclerosis of aorta) in the presence of significant pressure difference between two upper limbs.

Clinical Wisdom

Normally the SP in the lower limb is up to 20 mm of Hg higher than the SP in the upper limb, but DP remains the same. Recording of lower limb BP is important in coarctation of aorta or occlusive disease of aorta (low), and aortic incompetence (high). BP should always be measured in both upper and lower limbs, and in supine and erect posture. In SI units, BP is recorded in Kilopascal (kPa) and 1 kPa = 7.5 mm of Hg (approximately).

Q. What is auscultatory gap or silent gap?

Sometimes the initial sounds (which record SP) may disappear (after initial appearance) for some period just to reappear at a lower level, and this is auscultatory gap. If a physician is not careful, he may falsely record low SP (if he misses the initial sounds and starts recording after the gap). It is why, the mercury column should be raised up to 200 mm of Hg or more at the initial part of recording to minimise errors.

Clinical importance: Observed in certain patients with systemic hypertension.

Mechanisms

1. Venous distension.
2. Diminished flow velocity in arteries.

Q. Causes of systolic and diastolic hypertension:

a. *Systolic hypertension:* Atherosclerosis, aortic incompetence, complete heart block, etc.
b. *Diastolic hypertension*: Essential hypertension, parenchymal renal disease, Cushing's syndrome, pheochromocytoma, eclampsia, etc.
c. Divergent BP (high SP and low DP), e.g. 180/30 mm of Hg is seen in atherosclerosis, aortic incompetence.

Q. Causes of secondary hypertension:

Systemic hypertension is of two types: Essential and secondary. The secondary causes are:

i. Vascular:
   a. Coarctation of aorta.
   b. Non-specific aorto-arteritis.
ii. Renal:
   a. Acute and chronic glomerulonephritis.
   b. Diabetic nephropathy.
   c. Polycystic kidney disease.
   d. Renal artery stenosis.
   e. Chronic pyelonephritis.
   f. Renal involvement from collagen vascular diseases (e.g. SLE).
   g. Chronic renal failure:
iii. Endocrine:
   a. Cushing's syndrome.
   b. Pheochromocytoma.
   c. Conn's syndrome.
   d. Acromegaly.
   e. Hyperparathyroidism.
   f. Myxoedema.
   g. Congenital adrenal hyperplasia.
iv. *Drugs:* Oral contraceptive pills, corticosteroid, carbenexolone, oestrogens, sympathomimetic amines.
v. *Miscellaneous:* Pre-eclampsia or eclampsia, obstructive sleep apnoea, alcohol, obesity, diencephalic syndrome and porphyria.

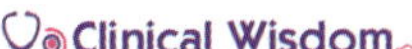

Clinical Wisdom

Essential or idiopathic hypertension comprises 80–90% cases of hypertension and rest are secondary hypertension. Secondary hypertension is a consequence of specific disease or abnormality (so, though severe diastolic hypertension may occur, they are often treatable).

Q. Symptoms of hypertension:

It is a symptomless 'silent killer' though few patients may get a signal through occipital headache or dizzy spells.

Before declaring a person hypertensive, ≥2 BP recording at each visit for 3 or more occasions are necessary.

Q. What is postural or orthostatic hypotension?

Fall of 20 mm of Hg or more in SP, or 10 mm of Hg or more in DP in upright posture than in lying down posture is postural hypotension. If the patient complains of symptoms like light-headedness, dizziness, extreme weakness, blurring of vision or syncope, even a lesser degree of fall in BP may be considered as significant. First measure the BP in lying down position and then record BP **within 3 minutes of standing.** 'Postural drop' in BP is important bedside clue in syncope, and diabetes mellitus with autonomic neuropathy.

- Postprandial hypotension, i.e. fall of systolic BP occurs within 2 hours after a meal, while the patient (old age, diabetes, parkinsonism) may feel dizzy, light-headedness or faintness.

Q. Where the BP instrument may be used as a pneumatic tourniquet?

1. Emergency control of bleeding where other methods are not available.
2. To produce a bloodless field of operation.

Q. What is 'white-coat' hypertension?

Few patients (20%, especially women) show dramatic elevation of BP when measurements are carried out by a doctor in the chamber, outdoor or indoor. Thus, often it is called as office or clinic hypertension. Contrary to previous beliefs, it may be associated with target organ damage (e.g. LVH, carotid atherosclerosis). It is an important well-known cause of refractory hypertension. It has been observed that BP recordings by a senior consultant physician is higher than recording by a junior doctor, which is again higher than the BP recorded by a nursing staff. It is believed to be due to anxiety some people experience during visit to a clinic. Accurate diagnosis requires 24 hours ambulatory monitoring of BP.

Masked hypertension—normal office or clinic BP but there is elevated home BP (opposite to white-coat hypertension).

Q. Pseudo hypertension:

In old age, there is false recording of high BP as a result of stiff and non-compliant vessels (Osler's sign). Actually, the true intra-arterial BP is lower than the BP measured by sphygmomanometer.

Q. Labile hypertension:

The patients having high BP for sometimes, but not always, are known as labile hypertensives.

Q. Paroxysmal hypertension:

This (sudden shooting of BP) is classically seen in certain patients of pheochromocytoma, and is also known as episodic hypertension. This is diagnosed by repeated recordings.

Q. Transient hypertension:

In conditions like acute glomerulonephritis, pregnancy, acute myocardial infarction or CVA, systemic hypertension may be seen for a brief period of time and may be due to stress-induced or associated with a disorder having transient phase of hypertension.

Q. Hypertensive urgency and emergency:

Hypertensive urgency: High BP without any target organ damage and thus reduction of BP can be done gradually within 24 hours.

Hypertensive emergency: Markedly high BP with impending target organ damage which needs immediate control of BP (within minutes) in order to prevent further target organ damage.

Q. Isolated systolic hypertension (ISH):

When the SP is ≥140 mm of Hg and DP remains <90 mm of Hg, it is said that ISH is present and is commonly found in old age.

Q. Accelerated and malignant hypertension:

- Accelerated hypertension: Recent and rapid increase in BP with evidence of vascular changes in optic fundi but without papilloedema.
- Malignant hypertension: Severe accelerated hypertension with DP >140 mm of Hg with papilloedema and renal dysfunction (e.g. oliguria).

Q. Refractory hypertension:

The patients whose BP, in spite of full compliance, can not be reduced to 140/90 mm of Hg, and who are on three or more drug regimen (includes a diuretic in maximal doses) are considered to be refractory or resistant. Think of:

1. Non-compliance with drug therapy (commonest).
2. Inadequate treatment.
3. Failure to recognise secondary hypertension, e.g. pheochromocytoma, renal artery stenosis, etc.

Q. Indications of ambulatory BP recording:

1. BP recording shows unusual variability.
2. To rule out white-coat hypertension.
3. Hypertension resistant to treatment with three or more drugs.
4. Syncope suggesting orthostatic hypertension.
5. Borderline hypertension.

Q. Target organ damage (complications) in systemic hypertension:

a. *Heart and vessels:* Cardiac enlargement, LVF, angina pectoris, acute myocardial infarction, arteriosclerosis, dissecting aneurysm, peripheral vascular disease.

b. *Cerebrovascular*: TIA, cerebral haemorrhage, cerebral thrombosis, hypertensive encephalopathy and subarachnoid haemorrhage.
c. *Renal:* Impaired renal function, proteinuria, CRF, ARF.
d. *Eye:* Hypertensive retinopathy, retinal haemorrhage and exudate, papilloedema (malignant hypertension), central retinal vein thrombosis, sudden blindness.
e. *Nose:* Epistaxis

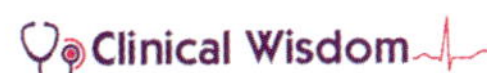

Clinical Wisdom

The purpose of treating hypertension is to reduce the risk of hypertensive complications.

Q. Classification of 'hypertensive retinopathy':

It is divided into 4 grades (Keith-Wagener-Barker classification):

- *Grade I:* Thickening of arterial wall, increased tortuosity and narrowing of arteriole though red blood column is seen; AV ratio is 1:2 (normal AV ratio is 3 : 4).
- *Grade II:* Grade I plus AV nipping and reduction of arterial calibre in comparison to vein. 'Copper wire'-like arteries seen without any visible red blood column; AV ratio is 1:3.
- *Grade III:* Grade II plus flame-shaped haemorrhages and cotton-wool exudates. 'Silver wire' arteries seen without any visible blood column; AV ratio is 1:4.
- *Grade IV:* Grade III plus papilloedema. 'Fibrous cord'-like arteries seen without any visible blood column (malignant hypertension).

- From minute to minute, BP varies with emotion, exercise, respiration, tobacco or alcohol consumption, temperature, pain, etc.
- In atrial fibrillation, multiple (at least three) BP recording with averaging is advisable.
- Blunting of the day-night BP pattern (i.e. nighttime BP is 10–20% lower than daytime BP) is seen in sleep apnoea and autonomic neuropathy. On standing, in health, SP falls but DP rises.

CLINICAL THERMOMETER

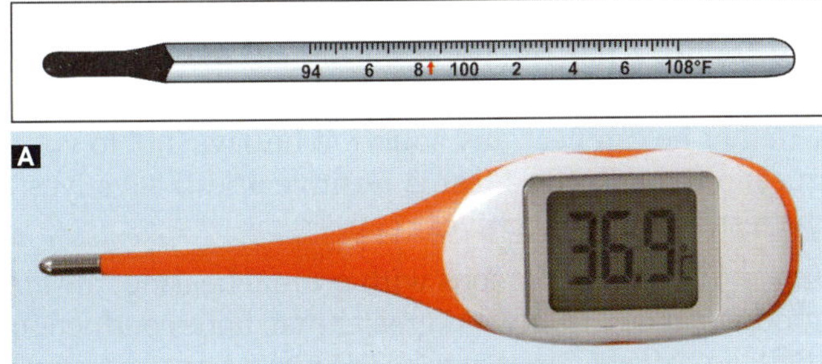

Fig. 1.17: (A) Clinical thermometer; (B) Digital thermometer

Q. Description (Fig. 1.17)

Clinical thermometer is used to record body temperature.

1. A glass tube with markings (graduations), usually 11 cm long.
2. Constricted terminal part containing mercury with the other end sealed.
3. Small lumen inside with constriction at the neck.
4. Cross-section of the body of glass tube is triangular.
5. Indication of normal temperature (98.6°F or 37°C) by an arrow-mark.

- Previously Fahrenheit scale (F) was used in the thermometer. Nowadays, temperature is recorded in Centigrade or Celsius scale (C). The formula of conversion of temperature is:

$$\frac{C}{5} = \frac{F - 32}{9}$$

- The kink inside the clinical thermometer prevents the return of mercury column when the thermometer is taken out of body. The triangular cross section (i.e. prism-like) magnifies the thin mercury line into a wider strip to help in easy reading.
- Recently, a tympanic membrane thermometer (i.e. electronic thermometer placed in the ear) is used for fast and accurate recording of core temperature. 'Digital thermometer' directly records the temperature. Lower-oesophageal temperature closely reflect the core temperature.

Clinical Wisdom

Temperature recording sites: Oral, axillary, rectal, temporal (thermometer placed on forehead) and tympanic membrane.

Q. Temperature range graduated in the thermometer:

It is 94° to 108°F in Fahrenheit scale, and 35° to 42°C in Centigrade scale.

Q. Procedure of recording temperature:

The thermometer should be washed properly with soap-water or any antiseptic solution. In hospitals, it is usually immersed in antiseptic solution. Clean with tap water before using it. Always shake the thermometer before use so that the mercury level comes below the arrow-mark. Before taking oral temperature, the patient should not consume anything hot or cold. Before keeping the thermometer inside the oral cavity, warn the patient not to bite it but to hold it by the lips while the mercury bulb is placed under the tongue.

Clean the axilla of sweat before putting the thermometer there. In infants, the temperature may be taken in groin with thigh flexed over the abdomen. The patient should not bath before recording axillary temperature.

After recording the temperature (thermometer is kept under tongue or axilla for at least two minutes), shake the thermometer again to send the mercury column beyond normal temperature. Now record the temperature in a white paper with date and time.

Q. Clinical thermometer—which type of thermometer it is?

It is a maximum thermometer. Higher temperature once attained, does not return to normal spontaneously. Clinical thermometer does not reflect the minimum temperature.

Thermometer used for weather report are made of ether or alcohol (instead of mercury), and reflects the minimum temperature. They are minimum thermometer.

Q. What is habitual hyperthermia?

In some persons, the normal temperature is above 98.6°F and is often in the range of 99°–100.5°F. Though rare, these patients run from physician to physician to allay their anxiety. The diagnosis can be made firmly after a certain period of close observation of the pateint.

Q. What is malignant hyperthermia?

In this inherited disorder, the temperature shoots from 102.2°F to 107.6°F in response to certain anaesthetics like halothane, methoxyflurane, cyclopropane or by muscle relaxants like succinylcholine. The high temperature results from muscular contraction. The situation is tackled by cooled ice, 100% O_2, fluids and diuretics (to reduce myoglobinuria and hyperkalaemia), $NaHCO_3$ (to combat metabolic acidosis), and dantrolene sodium.

Neuroleptic malignant syndrone (NMS) is probably a variant of malignant hyperthermia and is usually associated with use of neuroleptic drugs, e.g. phenothiazines, butyrophenones or haloperidol. NMS is characterised by hyperthermia, altered sensorium, muscular rigidity and autonomic dysfunction (pallor, tachycardia, sweating, labile BP). The mortality rate is high. Similar treatment as adopted in malignant hyperthermia is advocated here.

- Rectal temperature > oral > axillary or groin temperature by 0.5–1°F.
- Vide 'Charts on temperature' in the section on 'Charts' (this book) and the section on 'Abnormal temperature' in 'Bedside Clinics in Medicine, Part I' for further reading.

TUNING FORK

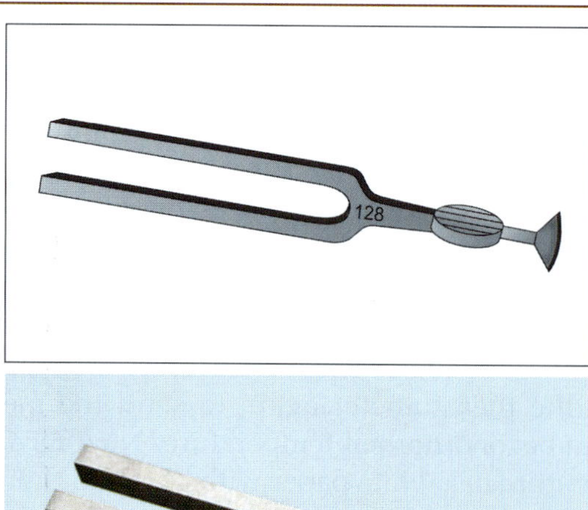

Fig. 1.18: Tuning fork (frequency 128 cycles/second)

Q. Description (Fig. 1.18):

This Y-shaped instrument has two limbs, a common stem and a disc-like base. Tuning fork produces vibration with constant frequency like 128, 256 or 512 cycles/second (Hz). The frequency is written on the instrument where the two limbs join. The tuning fork is made of steel.

Q. Different uses:

Classically the tuning fork is used for two purposes—

1. Testing of vibration sense (128 or 256 cycles/sec.).
2. Testing of hearing and quality of deafness (256 or 512 cycles/sec.).

Q. Test for vibration sense:

Vide the section on 'Charcot joint' in 'Bedside Clinics in Medicine, Part I'.

Q. Causes of loss of vibration sense:

1. Old age (physiological; even the ankle jerk may be lost in patients over 70 years).
2. Peripheral neuropathy (loss of vibration sense is an early feature in diabetes mellitus) or radiculopathy (prolapsed intervertebral disc).
3. Lesion in the posterior column (e.g. compressive or non-compressive myelopathy; classically tabes dorsalis).
4. Cortical lesion (e.g. lesion in the parietal lobe).

- Vibration sense is carried through posterior column; in diseases affecting posterior column, patient complains of ataxia (sensory ataxia). In syringomyelia and multiple sclerosis, vibration sense may be affected alone.

Q. Tests for hearing:

There are two 'tuning fork tests' which differentiate the quality of deafness.

A. Rinne's Test

A vibrating tuning fork is placed by the side of the ear to be tested. Mask hearing in the other ear by giving pressure of tragus on external acoustic meatus. Ask the patient to raise his finger when he can no longer hear any sound. After receiving the signal, the base of the fork is placed on the mastoid process and ask him again whether he can hear any sound. If he says 'no' to your question, the Rinne's test is positive and if says 'yes', the test becomes negative.

Interpretation: In persons with normal hearing, the air conduction (AC) is always greater than bone conduction (BC), i.e. AC>BC, that is to say Rinne's test is positive. If BC>AC, Rinne's test is said to be negative. So Rinne's test is positive in normal persons and in nerve type (sensorineural) deafness, and the test becomes negative in conductive deafness. It is to be remembered that in sensorineural deafness, AC>BC though both are less than normal.

B. Weber's Test

A vibrating tuning fork is placed on the centre of the vertex in the middle line. A normal individual hears the sound equally on both sides.

In sensorineural deafness, the sound is better heard in the normal or healthy ear, i.e. localisation is on the normal side. But in conductive deafness, the localisation is on the affected or abnormal side. The explanation goes like this: In sensorineural deafness, both AC and BC are reduced whereas in conductive deafness, only AC is reduced but BC is relatively increased (as ambient noise is excluded).

Interpretation: 'Lateralised' or not.

Q. Causes of deafness:

Deafness is of two types:

a. Conductive deafness—as a result of impacted wax, damage to tympanic membrane, otosclerosis, eustachian tube blockage, CSOM, etc.
b. Sensorineural deafness—due to damage of cochlear nerve and organ of Corti, presbycusis (i.e. hearing loss by natural ageing), Ménière's disease, acoustic neuroma, fracture of petrous part of temporal bone, drugs like aminoglycosides, pontine lesion, etc.

- In clinical practice, deafness is further investigated by audiometry (pure-tone) and brainstem evoked potentials in order to come to a definite aetiological diagnosis.

Q. How to differentiate between organic and hysterical loss of vibration sense?

Place the tuning fork on either side of forehead in turn. As the frontal bone is acting as a single unit, the sensation of vibration is perceived/not perceived on both sides even by the patients having organic lesion. Hysterical patients say that they can not feel the vibration on the side of 'sensory loss'.

Q. Synonyms:

Percussion hammer, patellar hammer or tendon hammer.

Q. Why the name patellar hammer?

Knee jerk was the first tendon reflex to become a regular part of the neurological examination, and this is why it is also known as patellar hammer.

Q. Parts of a hammer (Fig. 1.19):

1. Rounded (Queen square reflex hammer) or conical (triangular, i.e. Taylor hammer)—the striking end is made of rubber.
2. Shaft (plastic) with a blunt tip for elicitation of different superficial reflexes (abdominal, plantar response). The blunt tip present within the metallic shaft is seen after unscrewing two parts of the shaft.

Q. What is an ideal hammer?

A hammer with a firm and flexible shaft (made of plastic) is an ideal one.

Q. Different uses:

For elicitation of:

1. Deep reflexes or jerks (percuss the stretched tendon concerned).
2. Superficial reflexes (use the shaft with blunt tip).
3. Fasciculation (strike a big muscle).
4. Myotonia (strike the thenar eminence of palm).
5. Chvostek's sign (tap the facial nerve in front of the ear)—twitching of facial muscles are seen in tetany.
6. While percussing the chest, hammer may be used as 'percussing finger'.

 *Note*

Read all superficial (especially plantar response) and deep reflexes in details.

HAMMER

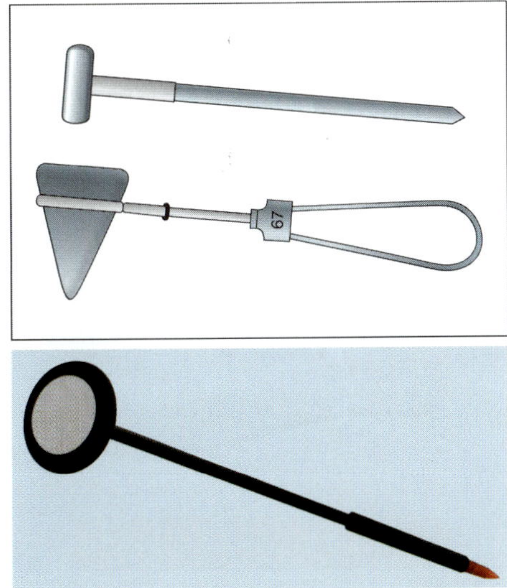

Fig. 1.19: Hammer (rounded and conical variety)

PIN

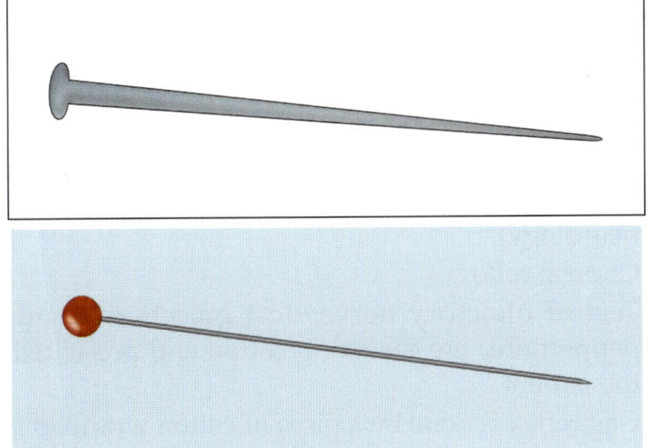

Fig. 1.20: Pin (the usual one and the red hat-pin)

Q. Different uses (Fig. 1.20):

1. Testing of pain sensation (e.g. peripheral neuropathy).

2. Testing of crude touch sensation: By the pinhead (especially in leprosy).
3. Blanching reaction in telangiectasia (with special reference to spider naevi): The pinhead is used.
4. Confrontation perimetry: With special reference to a large pin having red or white-head (hat-pin).
5. Elicitation of plantar response may be carried out by a blunt pin (in a desperate situation).

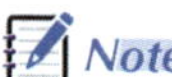
Note

Read leprosy in details.

COTTON

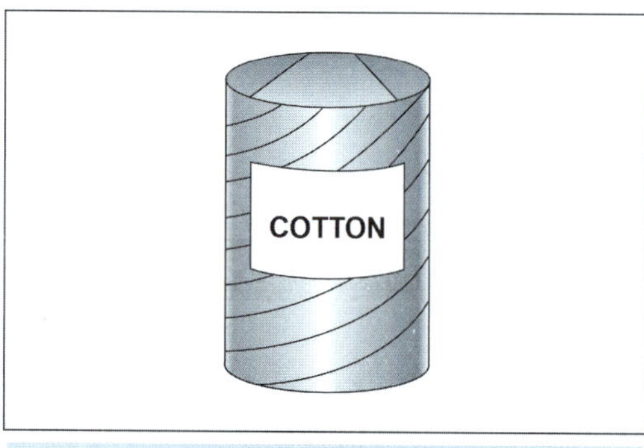

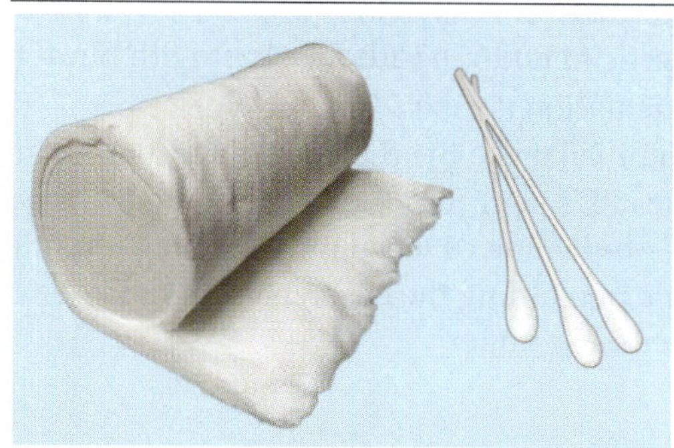

Fig. 1.21: Cotton packet and swab stick

Q Different uses (Fig. 1.21):

1. Haemostasis, wiping secretions, as a dressing material or to cleanse the local part before IV or IM injection when soaked in methylated spirit.
2. Touch sensation: When a small piece of cotton wool is twisted into a fine hair, it can be used for testing of fine touch sensation and the blunt end may be applied for crude touch sensation (with special reference to leprosy and sensory function testing in clinical neurology).
3. Corneal reflex.
4. Test of olfactory nerve: Test objects (e.g. oil of peppermint) are soaked in cotton and presented to the patient.
5. Gag reflex is done by a piece of cotton wrapped in a broom-stick.
6. For preparation of throat swab, conjunctival swab or rectal swab (see photo for 'swab stick').
7. Cortical sensation: One point localisation and sensory extinction.

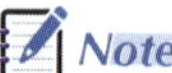
Note

Read leprosy and corneal reflex in details.

MEASURING TAPE

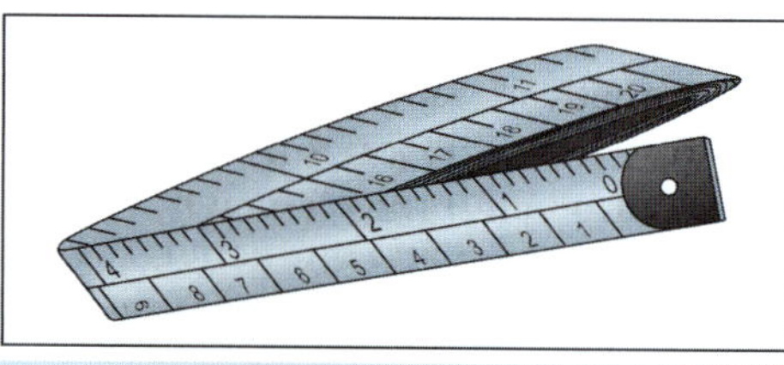

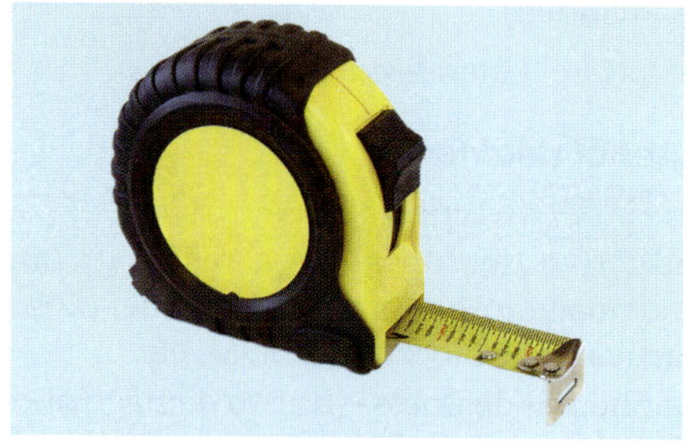

Fig. 1.22: Measuring tape

Q Different uses in clinical medicine:

It helps in the measurement of:

1. Abdominal girth in ascites (serial measurement is important).
2. Thyroid enlargement (at the most prominent part of the swelling in neck).
3. Expansion of the chest (especially in emphysema).
4. Head circumference (especially in hydrocephalus).
5. Assessment of nutrition (helpful in obesity and malnutrition).
6. To assess body mass index (BMI) and waist-hip ratio in obesity.
7. Height (e.g. cretinism, Marfan's syndrome).
8. To confirm wasting or hypertrophy of muscles.

TONGUE DEPRESSOR

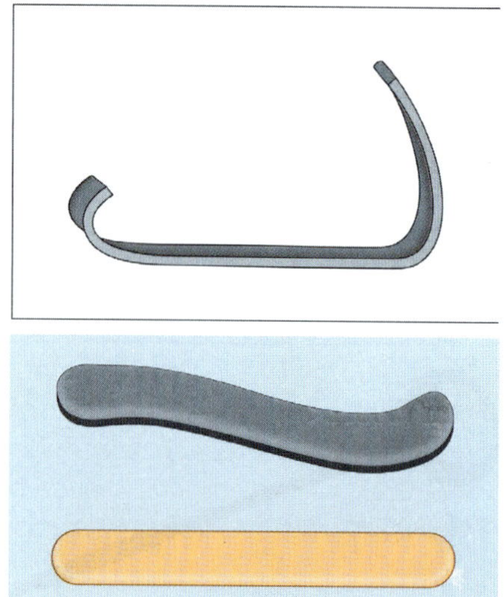

Fig. 1.23: Tongue depressor (L-shaped and straight variety)

Table 1.7: Differentiation between acute follicular tonsillitis and faucal diphtheria

Features	Tonsillitis	Diphtheria
1. Onset	Sudden	Gradual
2. Limitation of 'patch'	Only to enlarged tonsils	Tonsils and neighbouring structures like palate, pillars of the fauces may be involved
3. Toxicity	Little	More toxic than tonsillitis
4. Membrane or patch	The membrane or patch is yellowish and not adherent, and *can be easily separated* without any bleeding surface	Greyish and adherent, and *cannot be easily separated*. It leaves a bleeding surface after separation
5. Trismus	May be present	Absent
6. Cervical lymphadenopathy	+	++
7. Rise of temperature	100°–104°F	99°–100°F

Q. Synonym (Fig. 1.23)

Spatula; spatula is straight but tongue depressor is L-shaped, i.e. having an angulation with a holding part (hold by the physician) and a broader depressor part (part that depresses the tongue).

Q. Which part of the tongue is pressed?

Usually the anterior 2/3rd of the tongue is pressed. Never touch the posterior 1/3rd (gag reflex may occur) of the tongue.

Q. Different uses:

1. Examination of the throat and oral cavity (teeth, gum, cheek, tongue, fauces and tonsils, palate, oropharynx).
2. 'Spatula test' in tetanus.
3. Detection of posterior nasal bleeding.
4. Removal of foreign body (e.g. fish bone) from the tonsils, throat or posterior part of the tongue.
5. Elicitation of gag reflex.
6. Indirect laryngoscopy.
7. It helps to open the mouth for oral toilet or suction in a comatose patient; oral surgery.

Clinical Wisdom

Detection of caries teeth, gingivitis, candidial infection in buccal mucosa and tongue, patch tonsil, diphtheritic patch, aphthous ulcer, movement of palate as a part of IXth and Xth cranial nerve examination, spatula test in tetanus, Koplik's spot in measles and palatal ulcer in SLE are subjects of interest in general medicine.

Q. Causes of 'patch tonsil' (Table 1.7):

Patch or membrance seen over tonsils in situations like:
1. Acute follicular tonsillitis.
2. Faucal diphtheria.
3. Oral thrush or candidial infection.
4. Agranulocytosis.
5. Acute lymphoblastic leukaemia.
6. Vincent's angina (spirochaetes and fusiform bacilli).
7. Infectious mononucleosis.
8. Milk curd (in neonates and infants).
9. Tonsil stones (debris calcification).

- These are the causes of fever with 'membrane in the throat'.

Q. Causes of lock-jaw or trismus:

Trismus develops due to sustained involuntary spasm of masticatory muscles and is seen in: 1. Tetanus, 2. Impacted wisdom teeth, 3. Peritonsillar abscess, dental abscess, Ludwig's angina, 4. Acute follicular tonsillitis, 5. Temporo-mandibular osteoarthritis or rheumatoid arthritis, 6. Drug-induced dyskinesia (metoclopramide, phenothiazines), 7. Tetany, strychnine poisoning, 8. Parotitis, mumps, 9. Hydrophidae group of snake bite, 10. Rabies, 11. Malignant hyperthermia, 12. Hysteria.

Q. What is 'spatula test'?

In health, touching the posterior pharyngeal wall by spatula produces reflex opening of mouth. In tetanus, paradoxically mouth closes in such a way that the spatula cannot be taken out easily. Thus, spatula test is positive in tetanus.

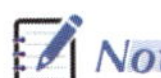 *Note*

Read tetanus, diphtheria, measles and bulbar palsy in details.

TORCH

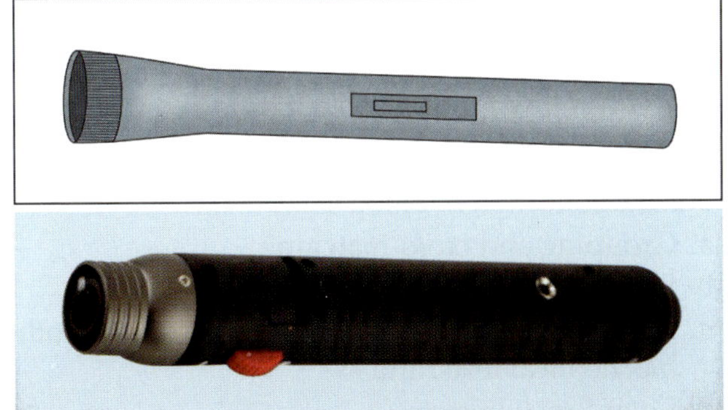

Fig. 1.24: Pencil torch

Q. Different uses (Fig. 1.24):

1. Pupillary reaction: Light reflex (bilateral fixed and dilated pupil often helps in declaring 'death').
2. Test of perception of light (PL) and projection of rays (PR) while assessing visual acuity.
3. Examination of pupil, oral cavity and throat, external ear, nose; anus, rectum and vagina.

4. Testing of photophobia (especially in meningitis).
5. Often epigastric pulsation is better seen when a torch is lighted tangentially over the epigastrium; in congenital hypertrophic pyloric stenosis, a torch is focused over the abdomen from right side of the body for better demonstration of slow peristaltic waves while the examiner looks from the baby's left side.
6. Transillumination test in hydrocele.

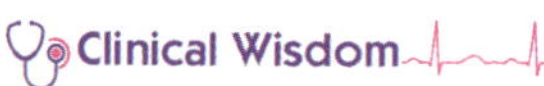

A clinician must carry a torch along with the stethoscope whether in emergency duty or in ward round. Read pupillary changes in details.

PLAIN GLASS TEST TUBE

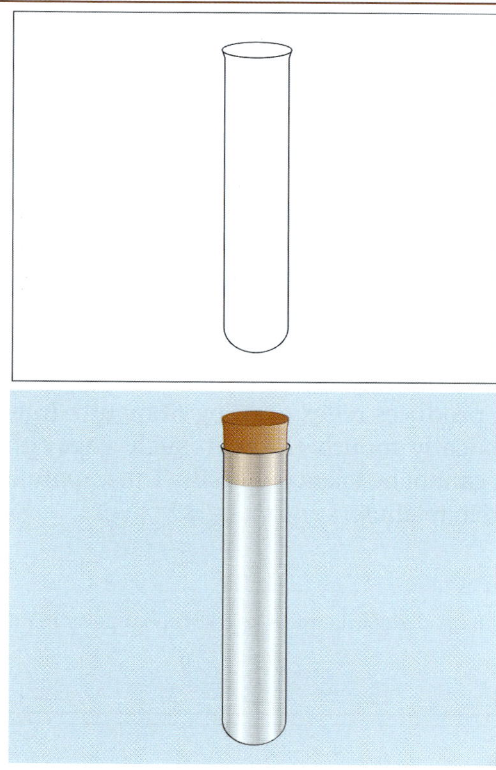

Fig. 1.25: Plain glass test tube

Q. Different uses (Fig. 1.25):

1. For the collection of blood sample for:
   a. Grouping and cross-matching.
   b. Serum electrolytes.
   c. Serum urea, creatinine, sugar, uric acid, and other biochemical tests, and
   d. Liver function tests.
2. For the collection of urine sample for routine examination (R/E) and culture-sensitivity (C/S) test.
3. For the collection of gastric juice sample for analysis/ detection of AFB in a suspected case of pulmonary tuberculosis (especially in children who cannot expectorate sputum, and often swallow it).
4. For the collection and analysis of CSF for physical, biochemical, cytological and bacteriological examination.
5. Sputum collection for Gram's staining, detection of AFB and malignant cells, RBC, etc.
6. For the collection of pleural fluid, pericardial fluid, ascitic fluid and drained pus from liver abscess for the purpose of physical, biochemical, cytological and bacteriological examination.
7. Two test tubes containing cold (5°–10°C) and hot (40°–45°C) water for assessment of temperature sensation in clinical neurology.
8. For the collection of throat swab, rectal swab, high vaginal swab, conjunctival swab or wound pus material (a sterile test tube with a cotton swab stick is used).

- The test tube should be sterilised where it is used for bacteriological examination, e.g. in 2, 3, 4, 5, 6 and 8.
- **Throat swab** examination is necessary in acute tonsillitis, diphtheria and acute rheumatic fever.

CONDOM

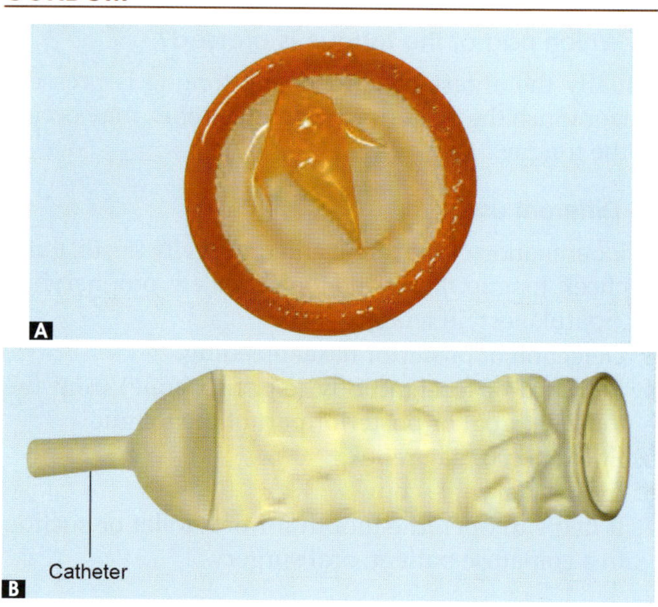

Fig. 1.26: (A) Condom; and (B) Condom catheter

Q. Description (Fig. 1.26A):

Usually it is of two kinds, i.e. latex (most widely used) and natural skin-type. Condoms may be made from other materials like polyurethane, polyisoprene, or lamb intestine. The Indian condom is usually 17.5 cm long and 4.4–5.4 cm wide. Latex condoms are preferable as HIV has been shown to leak through natural skin-type condoms.

Q. Different uses:

1. Most widely used barrier contraceptive device for males (i.e. protection for unplanned pregnancy—birth control).
2. Safe sex: Prevents sexually transmitted diseases (STD) with special reference to AIDS, hepatitis B infection, gonorrhoea, syphilis, non-gonococcal urethritis and genital herpes.

3. Often it is used for 'condom catheterisation' (prevents soiling of bed and bed-sore formation, and as the catheter is not introduced per urethra, there is less chance of development of UTI).

- Condoms are easily available, safe, cheap, durable, waterproof, disposable and having no side effects. Globally, condom is now promoted (especially in clients of commercial sex-workers) to prevent transmission of HIV infection.
- Condoms lubricated with spermicides (nonoxynol-9) are also available. A female condom is also usable, which is made of nitrile.

Q. How 'condom catheterisation' is done (Fig. 1.26B)?

Make a small nick at the tip of the condom and through it, a Malecot's or Foley's catheter is passed in such a way that the flower of Malecot's catheter rests on the nick. Now the condom is put around the penis with the help of adhesive tapes. The other end of the catheter is connected to the urosac. Condom catheterisation is valuable in (a) incontinence of urine, and (b) in comatose patients where the urinary output is to be measured.

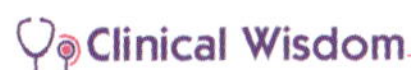

Clinical Wisdom

Charles Goodyear of America invented rubber in 1839 while first rubber condom was produced in 1855. Condoms have an expiry date. Nowadays flavoured condoms are available to make sex more enjoyable.

AIRWAY TUBE

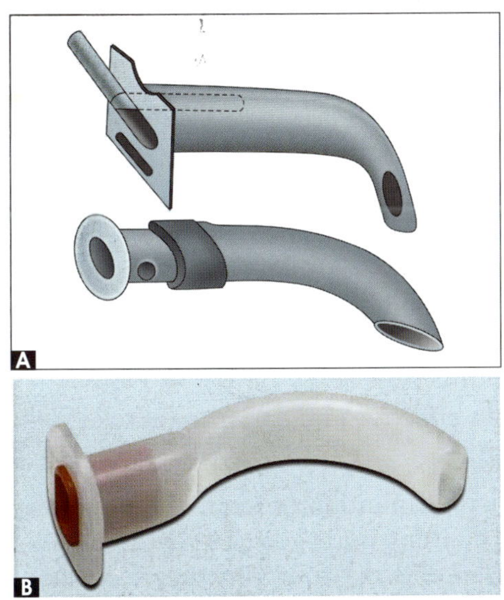

Fig. 1.27: (A) Airway tube (metal and rubber); (B) Actual photograph

Q. Available varieties (Fig. 1.27):

The slightly curved orpharyngeal airway tube is made either of:

a. Metal, or
b. Rubber.

They help entry of air into the patient's airway. This instrument is also known as 'mouth gag airway'.

Q. Different uses:

1. Unconscious patients.
2. Patients under anaesthesia.
3. During an episode of convulsions (e.g. epilepsy).

It is inserted into the mouth:

a. To prevent the tongue from falling back (the curvature of the tube is so made that it draws the tongue forwards),
b. To assist suction,
c. To prevent the endotracheal tube being bitten by the teeth during anaesthesia, and
d. To prevent the tongue bite (e.g. convulsions).

Multiple openings are present at the inner end, so that some of the openings may remain open when others are blocked by mucus plugs. Keeping the tube in boiling water for 30 minutes or autoclaving sterilises the instrument.

VENFLOW OR INTRACATH

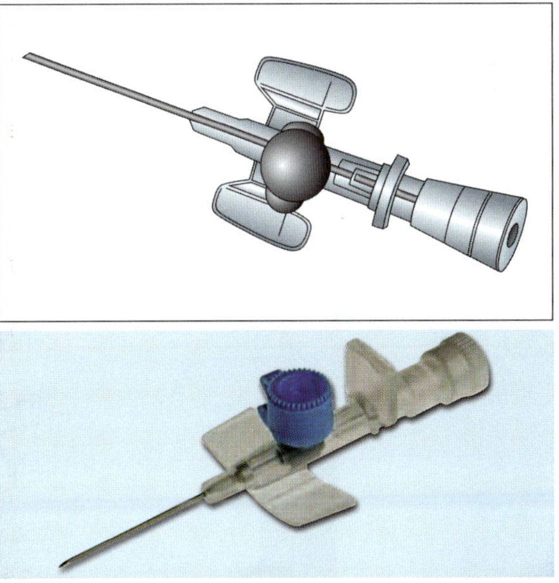

Fig. 1.28: Intracath

Q. Description (Fig. 1.28):

It has two parts:

1. *Inner:* Metallic stylet or needle (for proper guiding into the vein).
2. *Outer:* Polythene cannula or sheath.

Q. Uses:

This type of indwelling venous catheter (also known as angiocatheter) is required when the intravenous access is needed for a longer period (e.g. 24–72 hours).

Q. Procedure of introduction:

After puncturing a long vein, the whole of the intracath is gently introduced into the vein. The inner metallic needle is now withdrawn cautiously, keeping the outer polythene cannula within the vein. The polythene cannula is now ready to be connected with a venous line.

Q. Complications:

1. Counter-puncture and haematoma formation.
2. Thrombophlebitis.

Q. Advantages of 'intracath' over scalp vein set:

The intracath:

1. Can be kept within the vein for a longer time in comparison to scalp vein set.
2. Minimum chance of counter-puncture of the vein (scalp vein set often faces this hazard).
3. It produces less thrombophlebitis, and
4. There is no question of heparinisation of the channel.

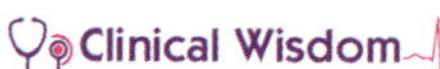

Intravenous line access is preliminary step in the management of dehydration, peripheral circulatory failure, cardiac arrest, shock and unconscious patient. The IV access in day-to-day practice is done by (i) simple IV needle, or (ii) intracath, or (iii) scalp vein set.

METERED DOSE INHALER (MDI)

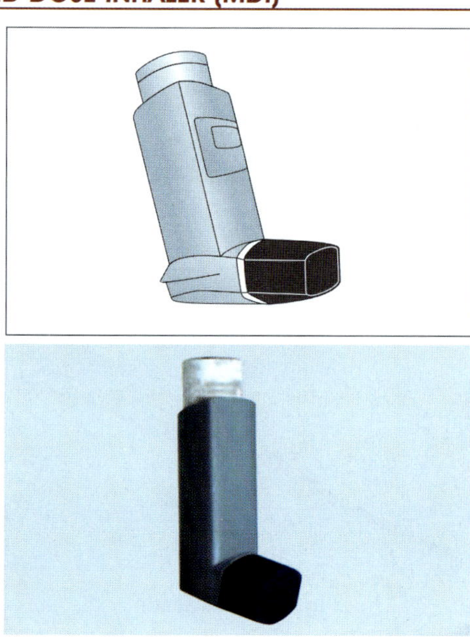

Fig. 1.29: Metered dose inhaler

Q. What is MDI?

For the past two to three decades, inhaled medicines are commonly used for bronchial asthma or chronic obstructive pulmonary disease (COPD) patients. These medicines are breathed directly into the lungs, where they are really needed. The devices used to deliver the medicine to the lung are known as '**inhalers**'. Inhalers can be of many types, e.g.

a. Spray inhaler (also called metered dose inhaler).
b. Powder inhaler (also called rotahaler).
c. Nebulisers (for giving higher doses).

The inhalers deliver drugs like β_2-agonist (salbutamol, terbutaline, salmeterol, formoterol), corticosteroids (beclomethasone, budesonide, fluticasone), anticholinergics (ipratropium bromide) or mast cell stabiliser (sodium chromoglycate) in **aerosol form** which is the preferred mode of treatment for obstructive airway disease.

Q. Description (Fig. 1.29):

This is an L-shaped tube made of plastic and consists of mouthpiece, and a tube which holds the canister (contains drug in a pressurised aerosol form) of medicines to be inhaled. The mouthpiece has a cover (cap).

Q. Method of use:

1. Take off the cap of the mouthpiece. Shake the canister 5–6 times.
2. Breathe out through the mouth, till the end of normal respiration.
3. Place the aerosol nozzle (mouthpiece) between the lips. Start to breathe in, press the canister and keep breathing in steadily, rapidly and deeply till full inspiration.
4. Remove the inhaler from the mouth. Hold the breathe for 10 seconds or as long as one find it comfortable. Now breathe out
5. After 1–2 minutes, get ready to breathe in for the second puff, if necessary.
6. Lastly, rinse the mouth with plain water (to prevent oral infections).

- As the device delivers a measured (fixed) dose of medicine, the instrument is called metered dose inhaler. In spite of good technique, only 15% of the contents are inhaled and rest 85% are deposited on the walls of the pharynx, and ultimately swallowed by the patient.

Q. Advantages and disadvantages of MDI:

Advantages:

1. Rapid onset of action.
2. Very small dose of the drug is necessary to have desired effect.
3 Very little medicine is allowed to reach other parts of the body, i.e. chances of side effects tend to be minimum.
4. It is cost-effective and easier to carry.

Disadvantages:

1. The major limitation of the mode of administration is that training and skills are required to coordinate actuation of drug from MDI (i.e. needs hand-breath coordination).
2. Pharyngeal infection (e.g. candidosis with inhaled corticosteroios) if the device is not properly cleaned at a regular interval.

Q. What is a rotahaler (Fig. 1.30A)?

Powder inhalers are devices that deliver a measured dose of medicine in a **powdered form** (i.e. a breath-activated dry powder inhaler). The transparent rotahaler breaks a capsule (rotacap) in the powdered form and the patient inhales the powder in the aerosol form through the mouthpiece of rotahaler. It is easier to use than MDI, and thus suitable for children and aged patients but needs to reload capsule each time.

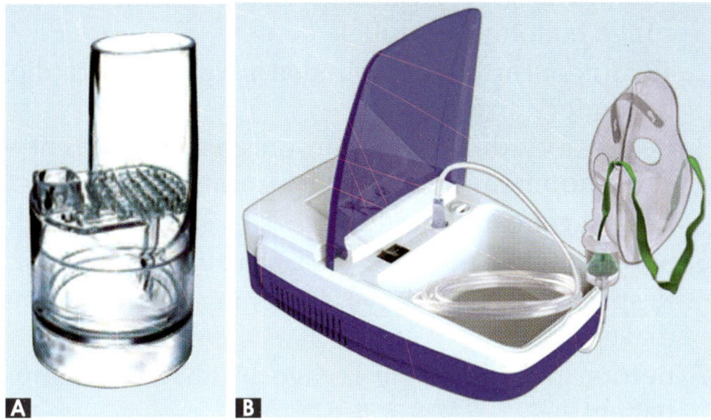

Fig. 1.30: (A) Rotahaler; and (B) Nebuliser

Q. What is a nebuliser (Fig. 1.30B)?

Nebulisers are used for giving higher doses of medication at times when breathing becomes very difficult. This is a machine that transforms the medicine (salbutamol, beclomethasone, ipratropium bromide) into a **fine mist**, which can be breathed in by normal breathing, via a facemask or a mouthpiece. The nebuliser chamber is connected to the nebuliser and oxygen mask on either side, so that nebulised drug would be inhaled along with oxygen. Its cost is more and an electrical power source is required though patient's coordination is not required and modification of doses is not difficult. Nebulisers are used in hospitals or nursing homes, for the management of acute severe asthma or acute exacerbation of COPD patients.

SPACEHALER

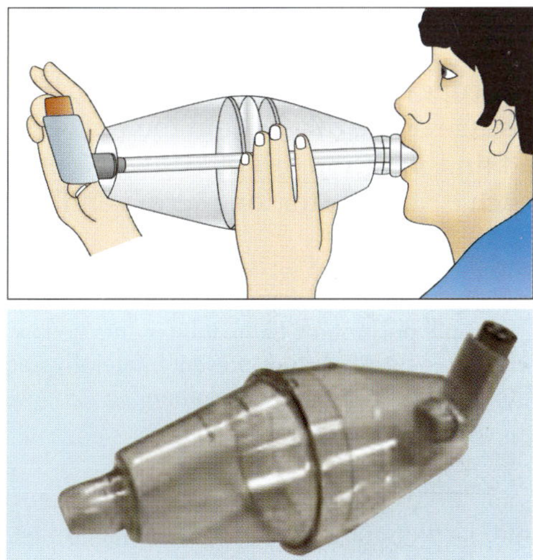

Fig. 1.31: Spacehaler

Q. Description (Fig. 1.31):

This device consists of two smooth conical plastic cylinders (one fits into the other producing a 'space'). At one end there is a mouthpiece through which the patient inhales the medicine and at the opposite end the metured dose inhaler (MDI) is placed through an inlet. It is also known as 'volumatic' or 'spacer'.

Q. Method of use:

Assemble the spacehaler by pushing the notch of one half into the slot of the other half of cylinder. After shaking the MDI well, fit it into the spacehaler. Rest of the steps are similar to the use of MDI.

Spacehalers are designed to reduce velocity of the particles so that less drug is deposited in the mouth.

Q. Advantages and disadvantages:

Advantages:

1. It makes the spray inhaler (MDI) easier to use and added to its effectiveness. The drug delivered from the MDI is not misused or lost because it is kept within a 'space'.
2. Strict coordination of the patient (i.e. aerosol activation and inhalation) is not required as the patient breathes in the cylinder.
3. Chances of development of oral candidosis with inhaled corticosteroid is reduced.
4. Low cost, portable, no electricity required (in comparison to nebuliser).
5. Useful in children and in the elderly.
6. Less drug is deposited in the mouth in comparison to MDI.

Disadvantages:

The device is big to carry in person.

- **"Nelson's inhaler"** is an earthenware steam vocal inhaler for a patient of sinusitis, cough, coryza or sore throat; singers and orators are also benefitted. The pot is filled with hot water and mixed with menthol, tincture benzoin or eucalyptus oil, when the patients inhales its vapour.

AMBU BAG

Q. Description (Fig. 1.32A):

The mnemonic AMBU stands for ambulatory manual breathing unit. It is a manual resuscitation kit for temporary CPR. A shutter valve intervenes between the bag and the face mask. Ambu bag is a hand-held device which is used to provide intermittent positive-pressure ventilation (IPPV) to patients with inadequate breathing.

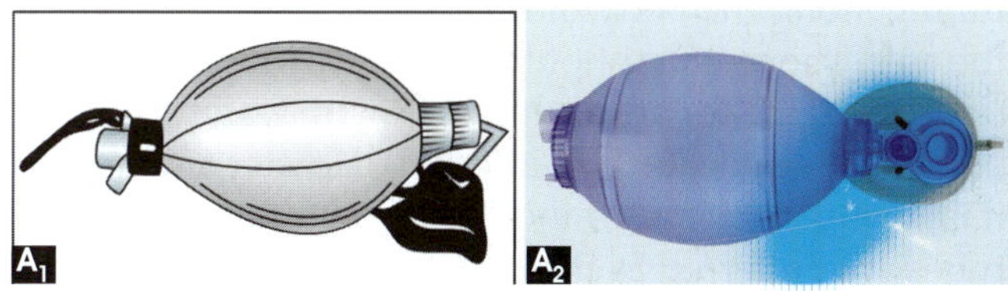

Fig. 1.32A: Ambu bag

Air (enriched with oxygen) enters into the patient's lungs through a tracheostomy or endotracheal tube after squeezing the bag. When the pressure is released, the bag inflates 'automatically' (the elastic recoil of the chest results air to leave the lungs). There is a risk of developing injury to lungs due to overstretching. This apparatus serves the purpose of mouth-to-mouth respiration.

Oxygen (face) mask (Fig. 1.32B) is a oxygen therapy device which covers the patient's nose and mouth, and attaches to an oxygen tank to deliver oxygen to the lungs. Nasal cannulas (have two prongs and sit below the nose) and face masks are commonly used to deliver oxygen to patients when needed.

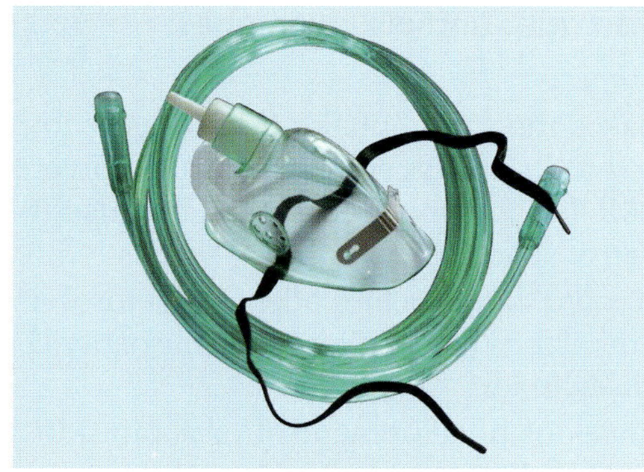

Fig. 1.32B: Oxygen mask

ENDOTRACHEAL TUBE

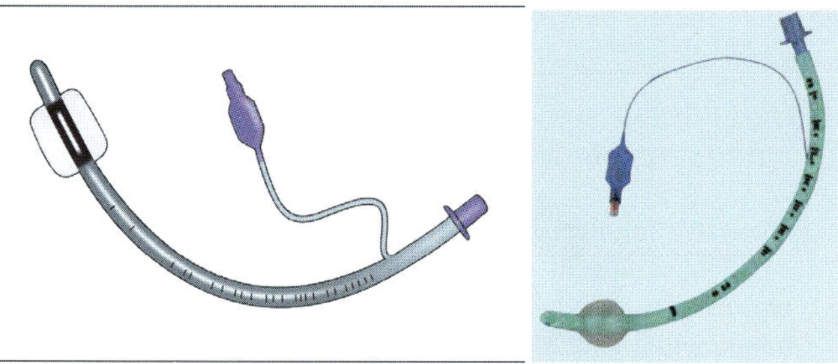

Fig. 1.33: Endotracheal tube with cuff

Q. Description (Fig. 1.33):

As the name implies, the tube is introduced within the trachea through laryngeal opening via mouth. The tube may be of polyvinyl chloride (PVC) or rubber-made. PVC variety is less irritant and can be kept for a longer period.

The endotracheal tube may be cuffed or uncuffed. The 'cuffed endotracheal tube' has a small balloon at the upper end and indicates tension in the cuff. A small tubing along the body of the tube helps in inflation of the cuff. The balloon should always be inflated with air upto 10–20 mL for an adult (never with water). The size of the tubes indicate their internal diameter and usually it is 7.5 mm for females and 7.5–8 mm for males. Cuffed tubes are preferred as they keep the tube in position.

Q. Procedure of endotracheal intubation:

It is an emergency procedure when an endotracheal tube passes from oral cavity into the trachea for providing adequate ventilation in patients with respiratory failure.

Indications

1. Acute respiratory failure as a result of COPD, massive pneumonia or respiratory muscle paralysis, in an attempt to give positive-pressure ventilation (by cuffed endotracheal tube).
2. To carry out artificial respiration in a patient of cardio-respiratory arrest.
3. Respiratory difficulty in an unconscious patient—clear the airway and prevent aspiration.
4. During general anaesthesia.
5. Severe angio-oedema of the larynx in anaphylaxis.
6. Respiratory depression in poisoning like morphine, diazepam.
7. Before giving gastric lavage in an unconscious patient.

Procedure

Pre-anaesthetic medication and anaesthesia are not required. The patient is positioned supine with neck hyperextended and chin in the midline:

a. *Oral intubation:* First, the oral cavity is cleared of secretions. The oropharynx, nasopharynx and vocal cords are visualised with the help of a laryngoscope; the lubricated endotracheal tube of appropriate size is then passed through the vocal cords and positioned in the trachea. Now the chest is auscultated for breath sounds (to confirm the air entry on both sides). If breath sounds are equal on both the sides, the cuffed endotracheal tube is then inflated with an aim to keep the tube in position, and to prevent aspiration.
b. *Transnasal intubation:* Nose as an entry point may be used in a more conscious patient. Presence of nasal polyp and deviated nasal septum make the passage of the tube difficult. Instillation of 1% ephedrine drops in the nostrils helps in easy passage of the tube through the nasal cavity. After entering the oropharynx, the procedure is the same as 'oral intubation' (i.e. a laryngoscope helps in visualisation of vocal cords and the passage of the tube within the trachea). Though it is a blind insertion, oral feeding is possible. This approach is suitable for long-term ventilation.

- After introduction, Ambu bag is connected to it and ventilation is started. Lignocaine spray, muscle relaxants and sedation can be used. Proper positioning of the tube is checked by presence of good audible breath sounds present bilaterally and absence of gurgling sounds over upper abdomen.

Clinical Wisdom

Before introduction, the cuff should be deflated first. Rubber tube is kept for 24 hours whereas the PVC tube may be kept up to 7 days.

Q. Contraindications of endotracheal intubation:

1. Trauma/injury/carcinoma or obstruction present in the upper respiratory tract.
2. Laryngospasm.

Q. Complications:

1. *Obstruction:* As a result of blockage by secretions, kinking or compression.
2. Intubation of either bronchus may lead to collapse of the lung (corrected by withdrawing the tube above the carina).
3. Tracheal dilatation as a result of overdistension by the cuff—infection—stenosis (tracheal or sub-glottic).
4. Trauma to the lips, teeth, tongue, upper respiratory tract (commonest) and vocal cords.
5. Mucosal oedema and ulceration of trachea (pressure necrosis of trachea may lead to fistula formation).
6. Aspiration during attempted intubation.
7. Dislodgement of teeth.
8. Increased intracranial tension.
9. Hoarseness of voice after extubation.
10. Long term: Vocal cord oedema, lacerations or paralysis.

- A **laryngoscope** (an endoscope for larynx) is used to pass an endotracheal tube properly as well as to visualise the upper respiratory tract upto the vocal cords.

PULSE OXIMETER

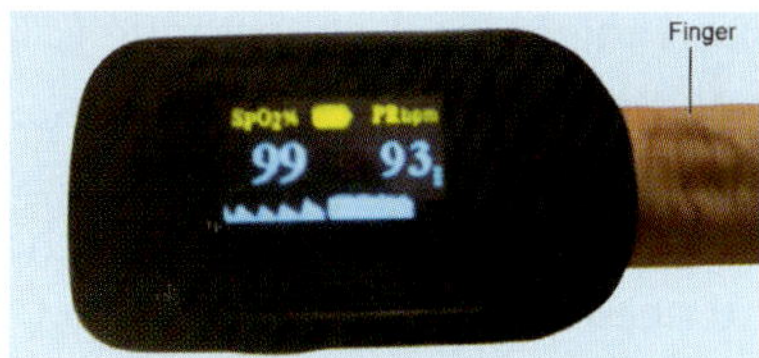

Fig. 1.34: Pulse oximeter

Q. Description (Fig. 1.34):

Pulse oximetry is a mode of non-invasive (i.e. painless) and continuous measurement of blood oxygen saturation (SpO_2). It is a small clip-like device that is attached to a body part like fingertip, toe or an earlobe. Most of the monitors also display the pulse rate. It is commonly used in emergency room and critical care setting (e.g. ICU); however, the diseases where it is commonly used are heart failure, COPD, bronchial asthma, anaemia, pneumonia or sleep disorders. Acceptable normal range of SpO_2, without lung pathology is 95–99%. It works with an electronic processor and a pair of light emitting diodes facing a photodiode through fingertip of the patient.

PROCTOSCOPE (ANAL SPECULUM)

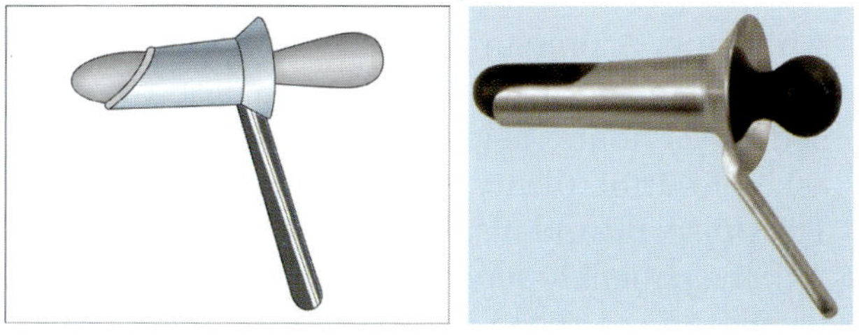

Fig. 1.35: Proctoscope

Q. Description (Fig. 1.35):

This is a 3-inch long instrument, and has two parts:

a. *A cannula (the body or flange):* One end is sharp and the other end is wide.
b. *Obturator:* The blunt end of the obturator (trocar) fits well into the sharp end of the cannula.

+

It needs a source of light (i.e. torch).

Q Different uses:

1. To visualise the anal canal for examination of fissure, internal haemorrhoids (piles), ulcer, growth, polyp, anorectal strictures, etc.
2. For injecting sclerosing agents (5% phenol in almond oil or 3% sodium morrhuate) in the submucous coat of the rectum and the anal canal through the mass of piles.
3. As a primary investigation of ano-rectal discomfort or pain.

Q. Procedure of introduction:

1. The patient is usually placed in the left lateral position (preferred with right leg flexed and left leg extended, or in the 'knee-elbow' position. Inspection outside the anus and digital rectal examination are performed to exclude any painful condition.
2. The lubricated assembled proctoscope is now pushed upwards and forwards towards the umbilicus until the anal canal in passed, while asking the patient to take deep inspirations; the instrument is then directed posteriorly (towards the sacral hollow) to enter into the rectum proper.
3. The obturator is withdrawn and the lower rectum is visulazied with the help of a torch when the light is thrown through the cannula. Now the cannula is gradually withdrawn, and the rectum and the anal canal are visualized for any pathology.

Q. Exciting factors to have internal piles:

1. Straining at defecation (e.g. chronic constipation).
2. Pregnancy, uterine tumours.
3. Portal hypertension, e.g. cirrhosis of liver.
4. Persistent straining at urination (e.g. BHP).
5. Carcinoma of the rectum.
6. Regular lifting of heavy weight.
7. Obesity.
8. Anal intercourse.

Q. Indications of rectal biopsy in clinical practice:

Rectal biopsy is done through sigmoidoscope or anoscope in:

1. Carcinoma of the rectum.
2. Hirschsprung's disease.
3. Amyloidosis.
4. Any tumour, polyp or mass in rectum.
5. Ulcerative colitis or Crohn's disease.

6. Intestinal amoebiasis, schistosomiasis (rare).
7. To determine causes of stool mixed with blood, mucus and pus

❍ **'Flatus tube'** is a stout rubber tube, which is open at both ends, and is used for removal of flatus when the tube is introduced through anus for 10–20 cm. The other end of the tube is placed in a bowl of water. It is commonly used in sigmoid volvulus, intussusception and for barium enema.

RENAL BIOPSY

Q. Indications:

1. Nephrotic syndrome (especially in adults).
2. Persistent asymptomatic proteinuria (more than 1 g/day).
3. Persistent haematuria (after extensive evaluation).
4. Acute and chronic renal failure (especially if unexplained).
5. Systemic diseases with renal involvement, e.g. diabetes mellitus, SLE, amyloidosis, Henoch-Schonlein purpura.
6. Transplanted kidney for acute allograft rejection.
7. Thin glomerular basement membrane (GBM) disease.
8. Sometimes, in rapidy progressive glomerulonephritis (RPGN).
9. To follow-up cases of glomerulonephritis (for prognosis).

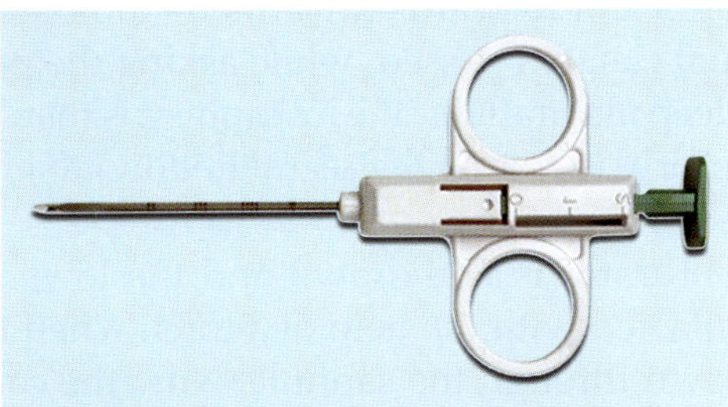

Fig. 1.36: Trucut renal biopsy needle

❍ As renal involvement may be patchy, a single biopsy specimen may not reflect the whole pathology.

Q. Contraindications:

1. Non-cooperative patient.
2. Severe bleeding diathesis.
3. End-stage renal disease (ESRD).
4. Severe uncontrolled disease.
5. Patients having solitary functioning kidney.
6. Perinephric abscess, hydronephrosis, hypernephroma or polycystic kidney disease.
7. Severe uncontrolled hypertension during the procedure.
8. Pre- and post-haemodialysis (as heparin is used during dialysis).

Q. A must before biopsy (prerequisites):

1. Renal function tests, i.e. urinalysis, serum urea and creatinine.
2. A full explanation of events is given to the patient.
3. Written informed consent of the patient or relatives.
4. A specialised centre with arrangement for ultrasonic control.
5. Normal platelet count with normal coagulation profile (BT, CT, PT, aPTT).
6. Normal or near-normal blood pressure.
7. An IVP or renogram is performed to confirm that both kidneys are functioning.
8. One unit of grouped and cross-matched blood should be in hand.

Q. Procedure of performing renal biopsy (transcutaneous):

1. Position of the patient: prone with arms abducted, with a hard pillow placed under the abdomen so that the loins are slightly raised.
2. Pre-medication (30 minutes before the procedure): By oral or slow IV injection of 10 mg diazepam.
3. The kidney is localized by USG and the biopsy site is marked with a pen. Ideally, biopsy should be done under USG or fluoroscopic guidance.
4. Strict asepsis (by sterile mask, gloves, gown and drapes) is maintained; clean the area with antiseptic solution and inject local anaesthetic (2% lignocaine solution) along the biopsy track.
5. A small nick is made over the selected site of puncture. Instruct the patient to hold the breath and the 'Trucut needle' (may refer to the section on 'Liver biopsy needle' in page 13) is introduced through the small nick (Fig. 1.36). When the needle is within the muscles, its movements are limited but as soon as it enters the kidney, its outer end sways in a wide arc with respiratory movements. Confirm this repeatedly and satisfy that the needle has reached kidney tissue.
6. The stylet is now removed and the prong is introduced through the outer coat into the renal parenchyma. A resistance to further movement is felt at this moment. The needle is advanced further over prongs so that it traps the kidney tissue incised by the prongs (the patient holds his breath during biopsy). The whole assembly is now rotated through 360° and the needle is taken out with prongs very rapidly with the trapped biopsy specimen. The biopsy tissue is sent to experienced pathologist to be examined by conventional staining (light microscopy), electron microscopy, and by immunoperoxidase or immunofluorescence.
7. After-care: A pressure dressing is applied over the biopsy site and the patient is placed on his back in bed for 24 hours (helps haemostasis). The patient is asked to drink plenty of fluids to prevent clot colic. The pulse, BP and respiration are checked regularly. Ask the patient to report any untoward symptom or haematuria (a common and natural complication). The patient is discharged on the next day with an

advice to avoid heavy lifting or gardening for next 2 weeks.

- To avoid injury to renal vessels, ideal biopsy site is usually the lower pole of kidney. Vim-Silverman's needle may be used instead of Trucut needle.
- In a bilateral lesion of kidney, preferably the left side is chosen for biopsy.

Q. Complications:

1. Microscopic haematuria (20%).
2. Profuse haematuria and clot formation leading to urinary obstruction.
3. Pain in loins, sometimes referred to shoulder.
4. Perirenal haematoma, retroperitoneal haemorrhage.
5. Bowel perforation.
6. Acute pancreatitis.
7. Arteriovenous aneurysm formation.
8. Infections causing renal abscess.
9. Shock.
10. Death (rare).

PARACENTESIS ABDOMINIS (Ascitic Tapping)

Indications:

It is a procedure to aspirate ascitic fluid by puncturing the abdominal wall. Actually they are divided into diagnostic and therapeutic indications. As a whole, they are:

1. Diagnostic paracentesis (e.g. cirrhosis, tuberculous or malignant ascites): Physical, biochemical, cytological and bacteriological study.
2. Severe abdominal discomfort or cardio-respiratory embarrassment.
3. Refractory to medical therapy.
4. Danger of strangulation of umbilical hernia, if present.
5. Paracentesis may allow better abdominal examination, needle biopsy of liver, scanning or USG.

- 2, 3, 4 and 5 are therapeutic indications.

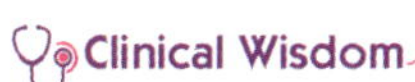

Explain the procedure to the patient and obtain written informed consent.

Q. Contraindications:

1. Cirrhosis of liver with impending hepatic coma.
2. Bleeding diathesis.
3. Severe jaundice.
4. Acute abdomen.
5. Pregnancy.
6. Very restless, non-cooperative patient (relative contraindications).

Q. Procedure of ascitic tapping:

1. At first, urinary bladder should be emptied. The patient lies supine or semi-reclined with a back-rest. He/she is reassured and explained the procedure.
2. Under strict aseptic precautions, an IV needle (large bore) is introduced (in a zig-zag track to prevent constant oozing of fluid after paracentesis) at any one of the sites mentioned below:
   a. Midway between symphysis pubis and umbilicus (bladder must be evacuated), or
   b. Junction of lateral 1/3rd and medial 2/3rd of the right or left spino-umbilical line.
3. The needle is connected with a rubber tubing which drains the ascitic fluid slowly into a collecting bag or bottle (an IV infusion set may serve the purpose). In one sitting, usually 1–2 litres of fluid may be drained over 4–6 hours. In case of cirrhosis of liver, 'large volume paracentesis' may be done by 3–5 litres of fluid aspirated in single sitting with 6–8 g/litre of salt-free albumin infusion. Diagnostic aspiration requires 20–50 mL ascitic fluid approximately.
4. After the paracentesis, the puncture site is sealed with tincture benzoin. Now the ascitic fluid is sent for physical, biochemical, cytological and bacteriological study; culture of the fluid may be done.

- Usually pre-anaesthetic medication and local anaesthesia are not required. In a restless patient, the skin and the subcutaneous tissue may be infiltrated with 2% lignocaine solution.
- In a small collection of peritoneal fluid, paracentesis may be tried in sitting posture of the patient.
- An abdominal binder may be placed, and fastened slowly and steadily as fluid starts coming out.

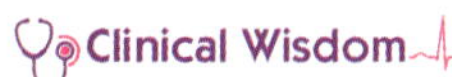

Protein loss is replaced by salt-free albumin to avoid hazardous reduction in plasma volume. To maintain the homeostasis, especially in cirrhosis of liver, it is better to run albumin (best substitute), blood, normal saline, 5% dextrose, dextran or haemaccel during paracentesis abdominis.

Q. Causes of dry tap:

Failure to obtain ascitic fluid on attempted aspiration may be due to:

1. Needle blockade by omental patch.
2. Perforation of a viscus.
3. Presence of very little fluid which could not be targeted blindly.

Q. After-care:

The patient is monitored for next 24–48 hours for development of any complication.

Q. Complications:

1. Sudden cardio-respiratory distress or shock (if appears during the paracentesis, immediately stop tapping the fluid)—i.e. haemodynamic instability due to rapid removal of fluid.

2. Vasovagal attack.
3. Introduction of infection (peritonitis).
4. Precipitation of hepatic coma (the compressed porto-caval shunts open up and nitrogenous materials reach the brain by-passing the liver may precipitate hepatic encephalopathy).
5. Perforation of hollow viscus (bladder or bowel).
6. Protein depletion (5 litres of ascitic fluid may contain 50–100 g of protein).
7. Constant oozing of fluid (especially in tense ascites or malignant ascites).
8. Haemorrhage.

Clinical Wisdom

Peritoneal biopsy is done with Cope's needle in a suspected case of tuberculous or malignant ascites, or ascites of uncertain origin.

- Previously, **trocar and cannula** were used to tap ascitic fluid, aspirate pus from amoebic liver abscess or for suprapubic aspiration of urine from urinary bladder **(Fig. 1.37)**. As this is a crude method, trocar and canula are not used now.

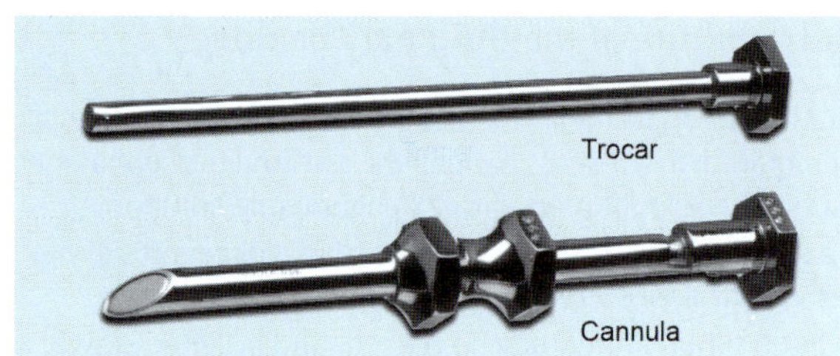

Fig. 1.37: Trocar and cannula

PARACENTESIS THORACIS (Pleural Fluid Tapping/Thoracentesis)

Q. Indications:

It is a procedure by which the chest wall is punctured to aspirate pleural fluid. The indications are:

1. *Diagnostic:* For physical, biochemical, cytological and bacteriological study of pleural fluid to come to a definitive diagnosis. Approximately, 20–50 mL of fluid should be aspirated.
2. *Therapeutic:* If there is,
   i. Respiratory distress,
   ii. Massive collection,
   iii. Bilateral pleural effusion,
   iv. Rapid collection, and
   v. Suspected secondary infection of effusion.

- Instillation of drugs (cytotoxics, tetracycline) are done in malignant pleural effusion.
- Most clinicians opine that aspiration of 1 litre of fluid in one sitting is sufficient to relieve cardio-respiratory embarrassment. Pleural aspiration needle can be used for both thoracentesis and pericardiocentesis.

Q. Contraindications:

There is no absolute contraindication. The relative contraindications are:

1. Coagulation disorders or platelet abnormality.
2. Patient with severe cough or hiccough.

Q. Procedure of thoracentesis:

1. The total procedure is explained to the patient to make him/her comfortable and relaxed. Obtain the written informed consent.
2. The patient remains semi-reclined with a back-rest, or preferably sitting and leaning forward position with arms folded before him/her and kept over a cardiac table (folded arms are placed over a pillow).
3. The site of aspiration may be:
   a. 6th intercostal space (ICS) in the midaxillary line, or
   b. 7th ICS in the posterior axillary line, or
   c. 8th ICS in the scapular line.
   d. Loculated or encysted effusion: Area of maximum dullness is the site of puncture (may require USG-guidance for actual localisation).
4. The local part is prepared under strict aseptic condition by spirit, iodine or ether. The site of aspiration is infiltrated from the skin up to parietal pleura through subcutaneous tissue with 2% lignocaine solution. The pleural aspiration needle (16–19 gauge, may be an IV needle) is inserted right angle to the skin, just above the upper border of the lower rib (nerves and intercostal vessels traverse along the lower border of the rib) to avoid injury to intercostal vessels and nerves, till the parietal pleura is punctured with a 'give away' sensation (pleural puncture may be associated with bouts of cough). The needle is then attached to a three-way cannula (adaptor), and the cannula is in turn connected with a 50 mL syringe. Application of suction in the syringe draws pleural fluid into the syringe which is pushed into a kidney-tray via the outlet of three-way cannula by adjusting its screw.
5. Fluid should be aspirated slowly and as much as possible until it is harmful for the patient (therapeutic aspiration). Few clinicians advocate not to aspirate more than 1 litre of pleural fluid on the first occasion because of the risk of development of acute pulmonary oedema.
   Repeat aspiration may be done after 3–4 days, after a check X-ray chest to note the amount of fluid remained/collected or amount of expansion of the passively collapsed lung.
6. If the patient complains of cough, respiratory distress, tightness in the chest or becomes severely restless, the aspiration must be abandoned immediately.
7. The puncture site is sealed with tincture benzoin when the paracentesis is over. The patient should be monitored for next 24–28 hours for development of

any complication. Analgesics may be prescribed to relieve pain.

8. A post-thoracentesis routine chest X-ray may be taken (to rule out hydropneumothorax, for assessment of residual fluid and for a better view of lung fields). The fluid is sent for biochemistry, microscopy, cytology and culture.

Clinical Wisdom

Appropriate site of puncture should be the area of maximum dullness on percussion or through the 'triangle of safety'. Nowadays, USG-guided aspiration is preferred.

Q. Clue to aetiological diagnosis at the time of thoracentesis:

Look for the colour of the fluid. If it is:

1. Clear—Hydrothorax.
2. Straw-coloured—Tuberculous (Fig. 1.38).
3. Haemorrhagic—Malignancy (Fig. 1.39).

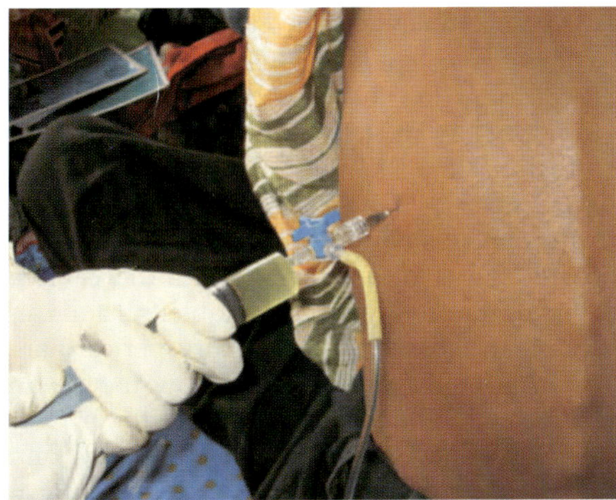

Fig. 1.38: **Paracentesis thoracis** performed with the help of a three-way cannula in tuberculous pleural effusion (aspirating straw-coloured or amber-coloured fluid)

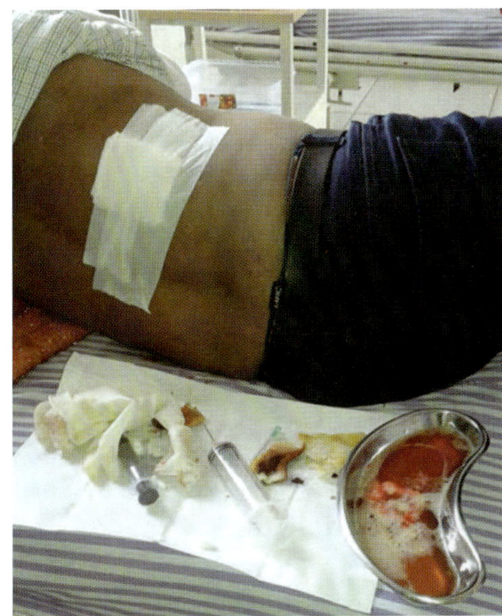

Fig. 1.39: After drainage of **haemorrhagic pleural effusion** in a patient of bronchogenic carcinoma

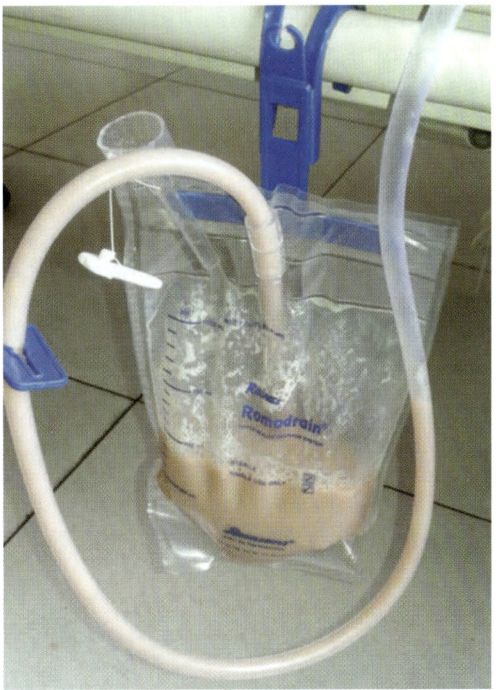

Fig. 1.40: Draining of **empyema thoracis**

4. Milky white—Chylous.
5. Thick pus—Empyema thoracis (Fig. 1.40).
6. Rapid reaccumulation after aspiration—very much suggestive of malignancy.

Q. Complications:

1. Pleural shock (as a result of vagal stimulation—Vasomotor collapse).
2. Empyema thoroacis (i.e. introduction of infection).
3. Hydropneumothorax (Iatrogenic).
4. Acute pulmonary oedema or re-expansion pulmonary oedema (non-cardiogenic)—if large volume of fluid is aspirated or the fluid is aspirated very rapidly, unilateral.
5. Air embolism.
6. Injury to intercostal vessels and nerves; injury to liver or spleen.
7. Haemothorax.
8. Cardio-respiratory embarrassment with circulatory collapse.
9. Subcutaneous emphysema.
10. Post-thoracentesis pleural pain (may develop pleural rub).
11. Late complication (rare)—intercostal artery aneurysm.

Q. Causes of dry tap:

Failure to obtain pleural fluid on attempted aspiration may be due to:

1. Empyema thoracis having very thick pus.
2. Encysted pleural effusion (needs USG- or CT-guided aspiration).
3. Interlobar or subpulmonic effusion (needs CT-guided aspiration).

4. A case of thickened pleura, tumour of pleura or massive consolidation of lung rather than pleural effusion (X-ray picture and clinical features may be misleading/simulating).

Clinical Wisdom

Pleural biopsy is done by Abram's or Cope's needle. If planned, it should be done at the first chance of pleural aspiration. Common **indications** are pleural malignancy, lymphoma, tuberculosis, and pleural effusion of unknown aetiology. Abram's needle is a punch biopsy needle which is introduced through the skin after making a small incision by a scalpel, while position of the patient remaining the same as thoracentesis. After removing the stylet, let the pleural fluid come out; the parietal pleura is punched and the needle is lastly withdrawn with a slight rotational movement. The small piece of parietal pleura (the biopsy specimen) is collected from the notch of the needle. Complications are similar to thoracentesis.

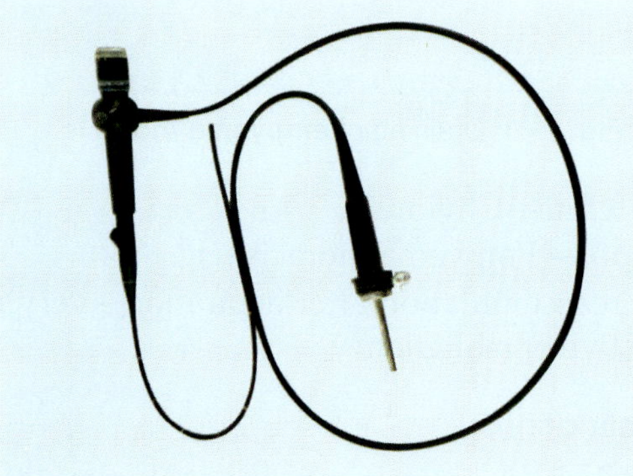

Fig. 1.41: Bronchoscope (an endoscope) for visualising the inside of lungs and airways

- A **bronchoscope** may be flexible **(Fig. 1.41)** or rigid. It is commonly used for diagnosis of bronchogenic carcinoma.

PERICARDIOCENTESIS (Pericardial Aspiration)

Q. Indications:

Removal of fluid from pericardial sac is indicated in:

1. Diagnostic aspiration (physical, biochemical, cytological and bacteriological study, culture of the fluid) of unexplained pericardial effusion: About 20–50 mL fluid is removed.
2. Therapeutic aspiration (as much as possible): If there is:
   i. Cardio-respiratory embarrassment (i.e. in cardiac tamponade),
   ii. Rapid accumulation of fluid,
   iii. Massive collection of fluid, and
   iv. Persistent collection of fluid.

Q. Procedure of pericardiocentesis:

1. The patient reclines comfortably at 45° with a back-rest. The total procedure is explained to the patient to get his/her full cooperation, and to make him/her comfortable and relaxed. Obtain the written informed consent.
2. The site of aspiration may be any one of the four:
   a. Epigastric or xiphisternal,
   b. Apical,
   c. Parasternal, or
   d. Posterior route.

   Prerequisites:
   i. At present, blind pericardiocentesis is avoided (ultrasound-guided preferred). It is recommended to be performed under ECG and echocardiographic monitoring.
   ii. Strict asepsis (sterile mask, gloves, gown and drapes) is maintained.
   iii. In an anxious and restless patient, pre-anaesthetic medication is done by slow IV injection of 10 mg diazepam. Midazolam may be given.
   iv. The skin and subcutaneous tissue of the site of aspiration are infiltrated by 2% lignocaine solution.
3. Any of the above mentioned sites may be selected but usually epigastric or xiphisternal route is preferred (usually recommended and safest route).
   a. *Epigastric or xiphisternal:* The needle (a pleural aspiration needle or an IV needle) is inserted 0.5 cm below and to the left of the xiphoid process and directed posteriorly towards the left shoulder at an angle of 45° to the skin. After piercing the skin, subcutaneous tissue and diaphragm (a resistance is felt), the needle enters the pericardial cavity. It is the safest route since it is extrapleural and carries less chance of injury to coronary, pericardial and internal mammary arteries. Now the needle is connected with a 50 mL syringe with or without placing a short rubber tube or three-way cannula in between the needle and the syringe. Application of suction in the syringe draws pericardial fluid into the syringe. The needle is further advanced slowly by about 5 cm and the aspiration continued cautiously. If the needle hurts the myocardium (if advanced too far), a crunching sensation is felt; immediately draw back the needle for 2–3 cm to place the tip of the needle again in the pericardial cavity.

      In few centres, an ECG electrode is attached with the needle by a crocodile clip. As soon as the needle touches the heart, the ECG shows a negative deflection while on slight withdrawal of the needle (i.e. needle in the pericardial cavity), ECG reflects a normal tracing. Requisite amount of pericardial fluid is aspirated in this way.
   b. *Apical:* It carries the risk of injuring the coronary arteries. In the 5th Intercostal space, the needle is inserted outside the apex beat but inside the outer edge of cardiac dullness.
   c. *Parasternal:* This route carries the risk of injuing the internal mammary artery. The needle is inserted in the left 4th or 5th intercostal space just to the left of the sternum. In a massive pericardial effusion,

the aspiration may be done in the similar way from the right side of the sternum.

d. *Posterior route:* Pericardial fluid is aspirated from below the inferior angle of the left scapula posteriorly.

4. After aspiration, the needle is removed and the punctured site is sealed with tincture benzoin.
5. After-care: Rest in bed for 24 hours is essential with nothing per mouth for first 4 hours. Hourly monitoring of pulse, respiration, BP and temperature are done for next 24 hours (clinical and ECG). Analgesics, sedatives or antibiotics are given whenever indicated. In suspected complications (pneumo-/haemothorax or pneumo-/haemopericardium), a chest X-ray may be taken.
6. Send the pericardial fluid for necessary examination in the laboratory.

Clinical Wisdom

Prior to aspiration, confirm the presence of pericardial effusion by chest X-ray or echocardiography. Before doing aspiration, facilities of cardio-respiratory resuscitation including arrangement for defibrillation should be available. Repeated and rapid collection of fluid in uraemia, neoplasia and trauma may require window pericardiectomy.

Q. How to treat cardiac tamponade?

1. It is a life-threatening condition and immediate pericardiocentesis is to be done to prevent shock and acute heart failure. Even removal of a small amount of fluid relieves the patient. It is preferably done in an ICU (Fig. 1.42).
2. In the absence of pericardiocentesis, treat with parenteral inotropic support along with IV normal saline. Diuretics and nitrates are contraindicated.

- Cardiac tamponade is a condition where there is collection of fluid in the pericardial sac, in an amount sufficient to produce serious obstruction to inflow of blood to the ventricles and thus, results in acute heart failure.

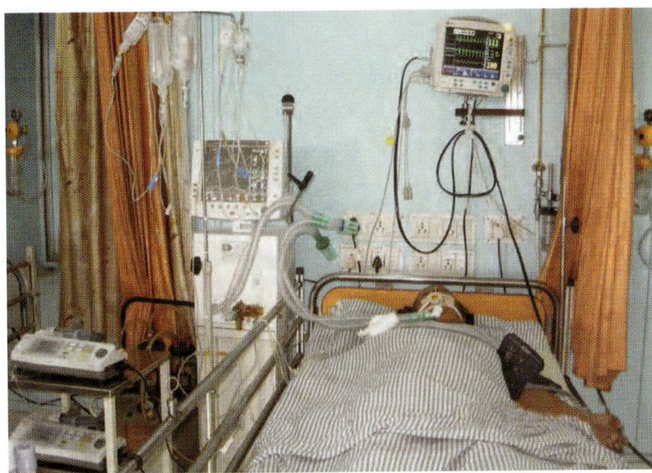

Fig. 1.42: An **ICU (intensive care unit)**, also known as ITU (intensive therapy unit/intensive treatment unit) or CCU (critical care unit) for treatment of severe and life-threatening illness by highly-trained staff

Q. Complications:

1. Vasovagal attack or shock.
2. Arrhythmias (e.g. ventricular tachycardia) and sudden death.
3. Injury to the myocardium or lung.
4. Trauma to coronary/internal mammary arteries.
5. Puncture of right atrium or pulmonary conus is rare but may be life-threatening.
6. Pneumopericardium, haemopericardium or pyopericardium.
7. Contamination of left pleural space (especially when a pyopericardium is drained in the apical route).
8. Pain in the left shoulder.
9. Injury to liver or diaphragm in subcostal (i.e. epigastric) approach.

Chapter

2

Pathology Specimens

"Declare the past, diagnose the present, foretell the future."
—**Hippocrates** (460 BC–370 BC), ancient Greek physician who lived during Greece's classical period and is considered as one of the most outstanding figures in the history of medicine—*'Father of medicine'*

Tissues are collected from different systems for diagnostic and therapeutic reasons, and these tissues are sent to a pathological laboratory for examination. The specimens are observed for the following:

Size (normal/small/enlarged), shape (normal/distorted), surface (smooth/rough/shiny), position (relations of adjacent tissues to each other), capsule (present or not; normal or thickened, opaque or adherent), colour (normal colour of the parenchyma/haemorrhagic/brown/greenish) and cut section (longitudinal, transverse or oblique cut; the normal as well as the abnormal areas). Contents: normally found or not, e.g. an abscess cavity with pus.

I. LUNG

The specimen is identified as lung by the presence of pleura, hilum and bronchovascular structures; blackish pigmentation may be distributed throughout the surface.

1. Lobar Pneumonia

There is progressive outpouring of inflammatory exudate into the alveoli in response to the irritation produced by *Pneumococcus*, *Staphylococcus*, *Klebsiella*, etc. Air in the alveoli is replaced by the exudate and the lung or part of it is converted into a solid and airless organ (just like liver). This is known as consolidation or 'hepatisation'. The lesion is divided into four stages, and one or more stages may be seen at a time. This is a progressive process starting from hilum and sweeping out to the periphery involving one or more lobes, and sometimes both the lungs.

Macroscopic (i.e. gross) (**Fig. 2.1**)

a. *Stage I or stage of hyperaemia/congestion (1–2 days):* The lung is voluminous and greyish red in colour; pits on pressure (oedema). Frothy fluid comes out from the cut surface on application of pressure.

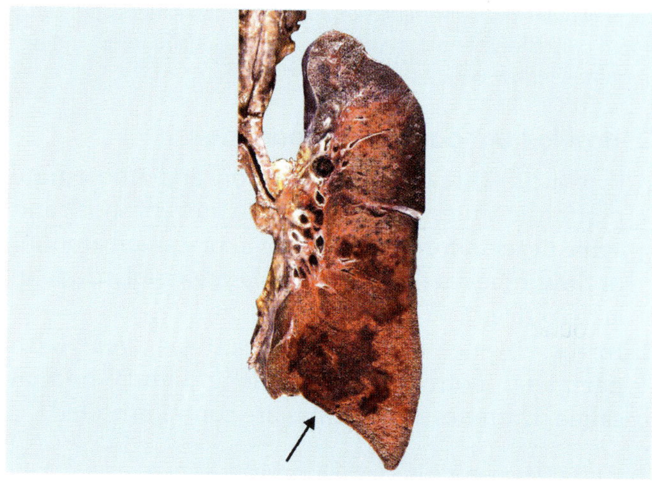

Fig. 2.1: Lobar pneumonia

b. *Stage II or stage of red hepatisation (2–4 days):* The cut surface looks red, dry, granular, friable, solid-like liver with sharp margins. The outer surface is covered with a fibrinous exudate and the cut pieces of lung sinks in water.
c. *State III or stage of grey hepatisation (4-8 days):* The cut surface looks greyish, moist, granular, more friable, airless or solid-like liver with sharp margins. The pleural exudate is thicker and the cut pieces of lung sinks in water. Bronchial lymph nodes are congested.
d. *Stage IV or stage of resolution (>8 days):* Lung is soft and translucent (like jelly). Large amount of creamy fluid may come out on squeezing.

Microscopic

a. *Stage I:* Capillaries are congested, and the alveoli contains eosinophilic fluid with few neutrophils and large number of *pneumococci*, etc. (by Gram's stain); still contains air.

b. *Stage II:* The alveolar wall is greatly oedematous and thickened. The alveolar fluid contains fibrin, RBC, and large number of neutrophils and organisms. The air is totally replaced by exudate and this is known as 'mosaic appearance'.
c. *Stage III:* The alveolar wall becomes thin; the red cells are mere ghosts, the threads of fibrin become clumped and the organisms disappear. The exudate is collected at the centre (a space left between exudate and wall). In the late stages, polymorphs are replaced by macrophages.
d. *Stage IV:* The alveoli become free from exudate. The debris and neutrophils are engulfed by macrophages; the fibrin masses shrunken.

Answer type (model): The specimen of lung is showing solidification and homogeneous grey appearance. It is the grey hepatisation of lobar preumonia.

2. Bronchopneumonia

Macroscopic (i.e. morbid anatomy)

Both the lungs show reddish brown patchy areas of consolidation with intervening normal, spongy lung parenchyma. Peural surfaces may show thin, fibrinous exudate. Bronchial lymph nodes are enlarged.

Microscopic

1. The bronchiolar wall is inflammed with congested blood vessels. The lumen of the bronchiole is filled with exudate containing pus cells, desquamated epithelium, few RBC, WBC, little fibrin and organism.
2. Peribronchiolar inflammation: Bronchiole is surrounded by a ring of alveoli filled with inflammatory exudate consisting mainly of neutrophis and fibrin.
3. Consolidated areas may alternate with area of congestion, collapse and emphysema.

Answer type (model): This is a specimen of lung from a child (as the specimen seems small) which shows several greyish patches and few bulbous patches over the lung. Both the lungs are involved; it is the specimen of bronchopneumonia.

3. Lung Abscess (Table 2.1)

Macroscopic (Fig. 2.2)

The site, size and number of lung abscess vary according to the aetiology.

1. *Site, size and number:* Not constant in aspiration or inhalation type; the abscess is usually found in posterior segment of right upper lobe or the apical region of right lower lobe (gravity dependent areas in recumbent position) as a result of vertical disposition of right main bronchus; in upright position, the common site is basal segment. It is of moderate or big in size.

   Abscess following septicaemia are usually small and present anywhere in both lungs. Post-pneumonic abscess is also found anywhere in the lungs.
2. *Gross appearance:* Usually the abscess contains yellow, foetid pus. In early stages, the abscess looks yellow with a thin red rim and feels firm. In aspiration or inhalation type, the cavity communicates with bronchus. The wall of the cavity is usually ragged and necrotic but in chronic abscess, it may be smooth due to fibrosis. Multiple small abscesses surrounding the main abscess, bronchiectatic changes, pleural inflammation (pleurisy) may be seen.

Microscopic

Acute variety shows destruction of lung parenchyma with dense polymorphonuclear and varying number of macrophagic infiltration. The blood vessels are dilated. Alveolar walls are destroyed. The chronic abscess shows a surrounding rim of fibrous tissue. Embolic abscess shows from inside outwards:

1. Zone of necrosis.
2. Zone of consolidation.
3. Zone of congestion.
4. Zone of fibrosis.

Answer type (model): It is a specimen of lung showing a big cavity in the middle part—it is lung abscess.

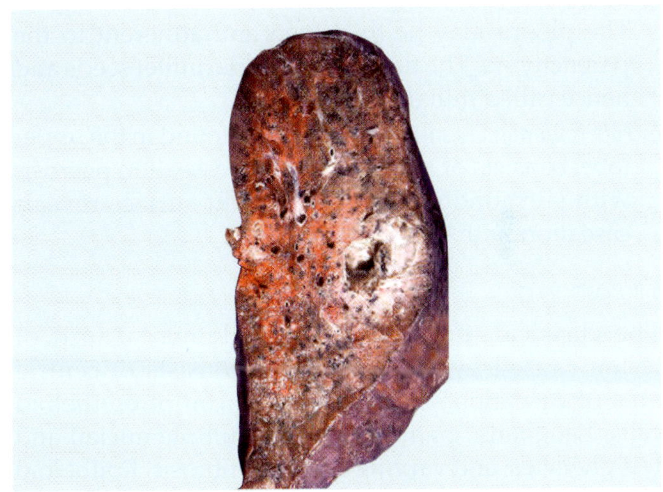

Fig. 2.2: Lung abscess

4. Pulmonary Tuberculosis (Table 2.1)

Different forms of morbid anatomy are seen in pulmonary tuberculosis which is commonly associated with overlying pleural involvement.

Macroscopic

a. *Fibroid type:* Affected areas of lungs show small, depressed, pigmented and firm (to touch) areas due to extensive fibrosis. Adjacent lung tissue may reveal emphysematous (compensatory) or bronchiectatic changes. The overlying pleura is involved with dense adhesions to the surrounding structures.

   On microscopical examination (M/E), extensive proliferation of fibrous tissue infiltrated with giant cells, epitheloid cells and lymphocytes are seen with scanty necrotic areas.

b. *Chronic fibrocaseous type:* This is the characteristic lesion of reinfection type. At the apex of the lung, the 'cavity is formed'; the walls of the cavity is smooth due to fibrosis, and is traversed by bronchioles and blood vessels. There are features of consolidation, central cavitation and caseation of cheesy material. Surrounding lung tissue may show emphysematous and bronchiectatic changes. The pleura is thickened with adhesion to parietis.

c. *Acute caseous pneumonic type:* This type of infection is seen where the virulence of the organism is maximum with least immunity present in the victim. The entire lung is converted into a solid, airless organ (like grey hepatisation of lobar pneumonia). Widespread caseous areas coalesce to form larger areas and the whole lung may appear pneumonic. 'Acute cavities' may be formed which are small, multiple with irregular lining in the walls.

d. *Miliary tuberculosis* (Fig. 2.3): The lungs are studded with multiple tubercles which are greyish translucent in appearance and usually of 1 mm in diameter; when caseation starts, they become opaque and yellowish. The tubercles are not surrounded by zone of congestion (in multiple lung abscesses, the small abscesses are surrounded by a congested zone). The pleura may be thickened and adherent to the parenchyma. The tubercles look like millet seeds and hence called miliary tubercle.

e. *Tuberculoma:* Usually solitary and is found in the upper lobe; consists of a nodular area of caseation necrosis with surrounding fibrosis. The cut surface reveals caseation with foci of calcification.

Microscopic

The classical **'tubercle'** (the fundamental unit of lesion caused by *M. tuberculosis*) consists of central area of caseation surrounded by a rim of epitheloid cells, Langhans' giant cells (with multiple nuclei) and lymphocytes, and varying degree of fibrosis. Epitheloid cells are the most characteristic cells of a tuberculous lesion.

Answer type (model): The specimen shows multiple 'sago' grain appearance in the lung—a specimen of miliary tuberculosis.

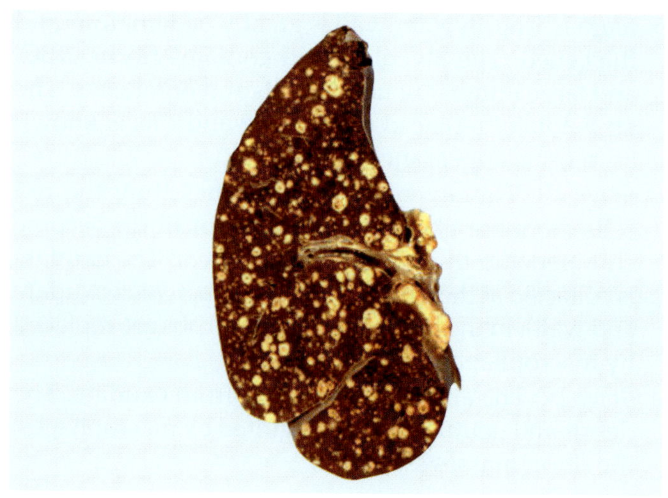

Fig. 2.3: Miliary tuberculosis

5. Bronchiectasis

It is the permanent dilatation of the bronchioles, which may be either localised or generalised.

Macroscopic (Fig. 2.4)

The affection may is unilateral or bilateral with involvement of the lower lobes mostly. The dilatation may be cylindrical, saccular, fusiform or beaded. The mucous membrane of the bronchus is hypertrophied and congested with dilated blood vessels. The lumen of the bronchus (known as bronchiectatic cavity) may contain pus. The bronchiectatic cavity may be small or big like an orange. Pneumonitis may be revealed in the surrounding lung tissue.

Microscopic

The mucosa may be hypertrophied or atrophied (lately). There is destruction of the musculo-elastic tissue of the bronchial wall (most significant) resulting in dilatation, and replacement by fibrous tissue in advanced stages. The cavity may contain pus, pus cells and RBC. Adjacent lung alveoli may reveal pneumonitis, collapse or emphysema.

Answer type (model): A cut section of specimen of lung showing multiple cylindrical or fusiform cavities, present in the lower lobe and few of them showing pus within—a specimen of bronchiectasis.

Table 2.1: Differentiation between tuberculous and lung abscess cavity

Tuberculous cavity	Lung abscess cavity
1. Usually apical or sub-apical	1. No constant site. Usualy present in the posterior segment of right upper lobe or apical region of right lower lobe
2. Wall—Usually smooth	2. Wall—Ragged
3. Contains caseous material	3. Contains pus
4. Adjacent lung tissue shows acinar lesion	4. Usually normal but may show secondary abscess
5. Hilar nodes are caseated	5. Hilar nodes are enlarged and congested
6. Caused by *M. tuberculosis*	6. Caused usually by pyogenic organisms
7. Microscopy—Structure of tubercle	7. Microscopy—Structure of an abscess

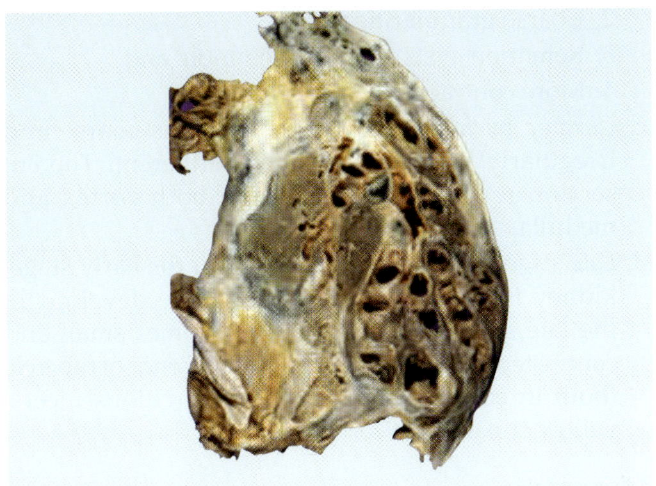

Fig. 2.4: Bronchiectasis

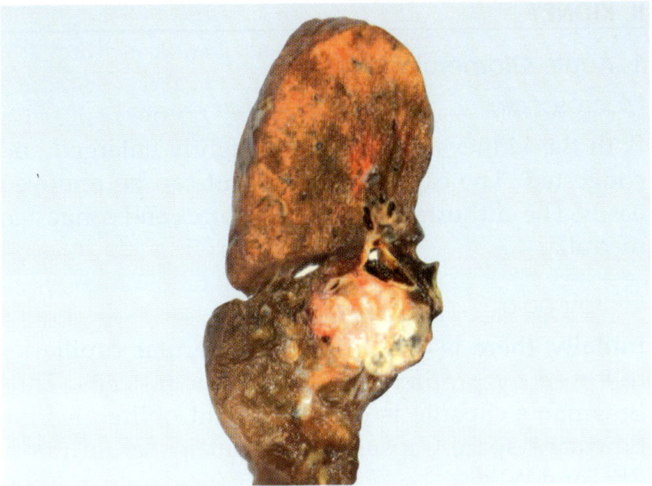

Fig. 2.6: Bronchogenic carcinoma

6. Emphysema

Macroscopic (Fig. 2.5)

The lung looks voluminous and more airy, pale and dry. Large bullae (thin-walled air spaces more than one centemeter in diameter, and are produced by rupture of alveolar walls) may develop, which are usually subpleural in location and remain along the sharp margins of the lung.

Microscopic

Large, distended, airy (clean) alveoli are seen with broken alveolar septae.

Answer type (model): A voluminous, airy, pale, dry specimen of lung with multiple sub-pleural bullae—a specimen of emphysema.

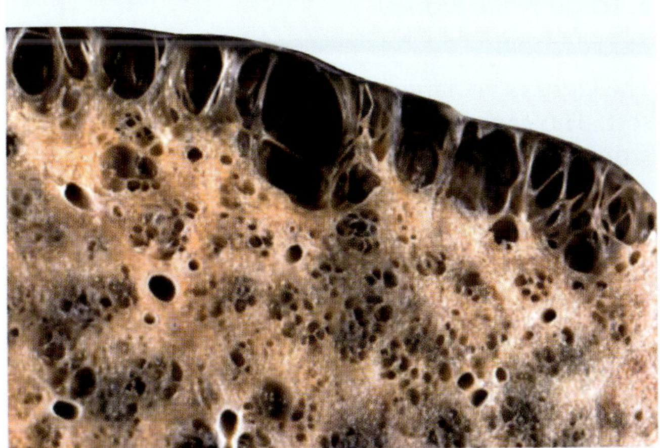

Fig. 2.5: Emphysema

7. Bronchogenic Carcinoma

Macroscopic (Fig. 2.6)

Hilar type is the commonest. Squamous cell carcinoma usually arise centrally, whereas adenocarcinoma arise from peripheral part of the lung. Commonly a 'firm, greyish-white mass' comes out of a bronchus which may produce obstruction of the bronchus by extending within the lumen or giving pressure from outside. Sometimes no growth is seen, instead a white fibrous thickening, roughening and narrowing of the bronchial wall are found. In diffuse variety, the whole of the lung may be filled with malignant deposit. The bronchial lymph nodes may be enlarged. Secondary changes in other parts of the lung result in collapse, bronchiectasis and abscess formation. The overlying pleura may be thickened and adherent to the parietis.

Microscopic

a. *Squamous cell carcinoma:* Bronchial epithelium changes into squamous type due to metaplasia and the tumour originates from this squamous cell is also known as epidermoid carcinoma. From the basement membrane, solid columns of malignant cells go downwards—the distal part of which expands and the whole appearance seems to be 'flask-like'. Large eosinophilic (irregular) cells with intracellular bridges, mitosis, and cell nests (epithelial pearl) are seen.
b. *Adenocarcinoma:* Single layered tall columner cells are seen lining the alveolar septa along with small hyperchromatic nuclei. A glandular pattern is formed by the cells which are rich in 'mucin' but sometimes the glandular structure may be distorted. The stroma varies greatly in density and amount.
c. *Anaplastic carcinoma (or large cell carcinoma):* The cells vary greatly in shape and size. The parent structure cannot be identified and thus known as anaplastic type. There is presence of sheets of small or large undifferentiated pleomorphic cells.
d. *Small cell carcinoma (or oat cell carcinoma):* These cells have scanty cytoplasm, small hyperchromatic nuclei with a fine chromatin pattern and prominent nucleoli.

Squamous cell carcinoma and small cell carcinoma are strongly associated with smoking.

Answer type (model): A specimen of lung showing a firm, grehish-white mass within—probably a specimen of bronchogenic carcinoma.

II. KIDNEY

1. Acute Glomerulonephritis

Macroscopic

Both the kidneys are involved, slightly enlarged and congested. The capsule is tense but can be removed easily. The cut surface shows pale cortex and congested medulla.

Microscopic

Initially, there is dilatation of glomerular capillaries followed by proliferation of endothelial cells. Thus Bowman's capsule is distended and obliterates the Bowman's space. Capsular space contains serum, fibrin, RBC and WBC.

Tubular cells show cloudy swelling and fatty changes. The lumen of the tubule contains inflammatory exudate. Interstitial tissue shows lymphocytic infiltration.

2. Granular Contracted Kidney

Macroscopic (Fig. 2.7)

Both the kidneys look smaller and pale with a granular surface. Pelvic fat and cortex are thinned out. The final stage of chronic renal failure produces granular contracted kidney and the common aetiology are:

1. Chronic glomerulonephritis.
2. Benign nephrosclerosis.
3. Chronic pyelonephritis.
4. Late stage of tuberculosis of kidney.

The differential diagnosis is done by:

a. *Chronic glomerulonephritis:* The kidneys are small, pale, hard and finely granular. The capsule is adherent and cannot be stripped off easily. The outer surface may have few retention cysts. The cut section shows extreme irregularity and atrophy of cortex. Medulla remains normal. Pelvic fat is increased.

b. *Benign nephrosclerosis:* Same as chronic glomerulonephritis except:
   1. The colour is red.
   2. Coarse granularities.
   3. Retention cysts are more common, and
   4. More contracted.

c. *Chronic pyelonephritis:* The surface is coarse and irregularly granular, capsule is adherent. The cut section reveals involvement of both cortex and medulla.

d. *Late stage of tuberculosis of kidney:* In the early stage, kidney is enlarged but fibrous tissue develops in the late stage, and the kidney becomes small and contracted. The cut section shows presence of tubercle (both in cortex and medulla), tuberculous ulcers, yellow streaks, etc.

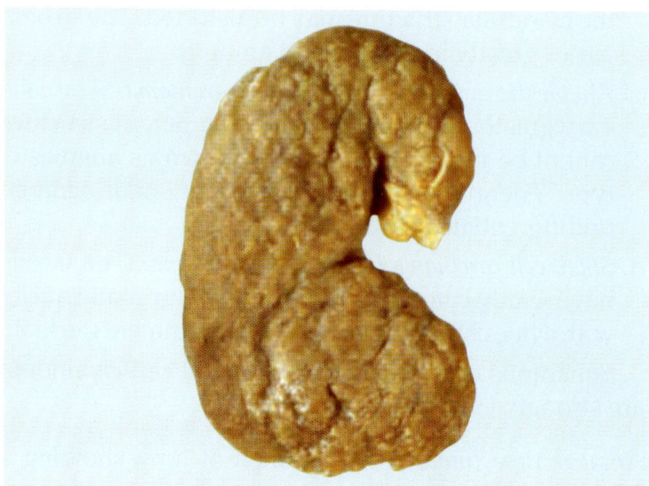

Fig. 2.7: Granular contracted kidney

Microscopic

a. *Chronic glomerulonephritis:* Varying degree of atrophy, hypertrophy and hyalinisation are seen in glomeruli and tubules.

b. *Benign nephrosclerosis:* Smallest vessels show hyaline degeneration (e.g. afferent arterioles). There is sharply defined acidophilic thickening of the sub-intimal tissue (gradually the entire thickness is involved and thus, the lumen is obliterated). The internal elastic lamina splits up into several layers by the process of reduplication. Ultimately, closure of the arterioles ends in hyalinisation of glomeruli.

c. *Chronic pyelonephritis:* The most characteristic feature is peri-glomerular fibrosis. There is round cell infiltration in the interstitium. End-arteritis obliterans may be noted.

d. *Late stage of tuberculosis of kidney:* Classical picture of a tubercle is seen.

3. Large White Kidney

Macroscopic

The kidneys are large in size, smooth, pale (white) and soft. The capsule is tense and thickened but can be stripped off easily.

The different aetiology are:

1. Subacute glomerulonephritis.
2. Amyloidosis.
3. Nephrotic syndrome.
4. Lipoid nephrosis.
5. Diabetic nephrosis (KW syndrome).
6. Toxaemia of pregnancy.
7. Leukaemic infiltrations.
8. Early stages of tuberculosis of kidney.
9. Hydronephrosis.
10. Polycystic kidney.

Microscopic

a. *Subacute glomerulonephritis:* There is proliferation of the parietal layer of the capsular epithelium into the capsular space and is known as 'epithelial crescents'.

b. *Amyloid nephrosis:* Waxy pale amyloid deposits are characteristically seen in glomeruli between the basement membrane, in the wall of arterioles and around the collecting tubules.

c. *Hydronephrosis:* Complete destruction of renal parenchyma is noted. Some glomeruli are normal and some are fibrosed; tubules are atrophied, and the renal parenchyma is replaced by fibrous tissue.

Why large?

Collection of fluid within the kidney (i.e. interstitium) as well as deposition of lipid makes the kidney large.

Why white?

Deposition of lipid and collection of fluid within the interstitial space (blood vessels are compressed) make the kidney pale (white).

4. Flea-bitten Kidney

Macroscopic

The kidney is enlarged and soft; outer surface is smooth with multiple tiny haemorrhagic areas varying from dark red to black in colour, giving the 'flea-bitten' appearance. The cut section shows similar haemorrhagic areas on cortex.

The different aetiology are:

1. Subacute bacterial endocarditis (SBE).
2. Malignant hypertension.
3. Septicaemia.
4. Disseminated intravascular coagulation (DIC).
5. Microangiopathic haemolytic anaemia, e.g. thrombotic throbocytopenic purpura; abruptio placentae or amniotic fluid embolism.
6. Systemic lupus erythematosus (SLE).
7. Rapidly progressive glomerulonephritis (RPGN).

Microscopic

This depends on the underlying aetiology. There is cellular hyperplasia and arteriolar necrosis in the vessels; focal glomerulitis with presence of small 'focal glomerular thrombi'; tubular hyperplasia (compensatory) may be seen.

5. Polycystic Kidney

Macroscopic (Fig. 2.8)

This congenital malformation almost always affects both the kidneys. The kidneys are enlarged, sometimes enormously, and one kidney may be more bigger than the other. There are numerous thin-walled cysts of different sizes present in the kidney (irregular outline) giving the appearance of bunch of grapes. Some of the cysts are white in colour, whereas others are brown (due to haemorrhagic fluid). The cut section shows numerous, irregular cysts of different sizes often filled with greenish-yellow gel; the cut surface lacks normal kidney tissue.

Microscopic

Small cysts lined by tubular epithelium are seen. Surrounding normal kidney tissue is attenuated.

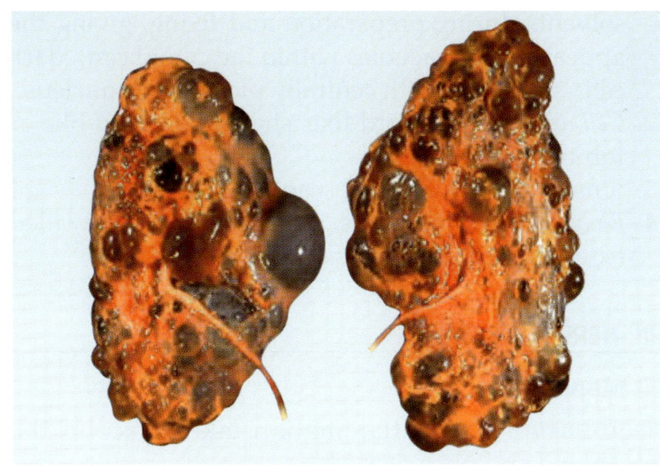

Fig. 2.8: Polycystic kidney

6. Hypernephroma (Renal Cell Carcinoma) (Fig. 2.9)

Macroscopic

The tumour may arise from any one pole of the kidney, commonly the upper one (thus the shape of the kidney is preserved). The mass is usually oval or spherical in shape, and may have lobulations on the surface. The tumour is imperfectly coverd by a capsule made of condensed renal tissue and fibrous tissue; from the capsule, fibrous trabeculae run radially inside the tumour mass, subdividing it into numerous lobules.

The cut section shows characteristic variegated appearance:

1. Healthy parts of the tumour may look golden-yellow in colour (due to deposition of cholesterol and fat), but may be white.
2. The other areas may show fibrosis, necrosis, haemorrhage or cystic changes (containing clear fluid or haemorrhagic fluid; cysts may have red, brown, green or black colour).

Microscopic

Unlike variegated macroscopic appearance, hypernephroma has a characteristic uniform appearance under the microscope.

1. *Cell character:* Anaplastic or foamy cells (most characteristic cells; cytoplasm contain glycogen and lipid materials which are washed out by the fat

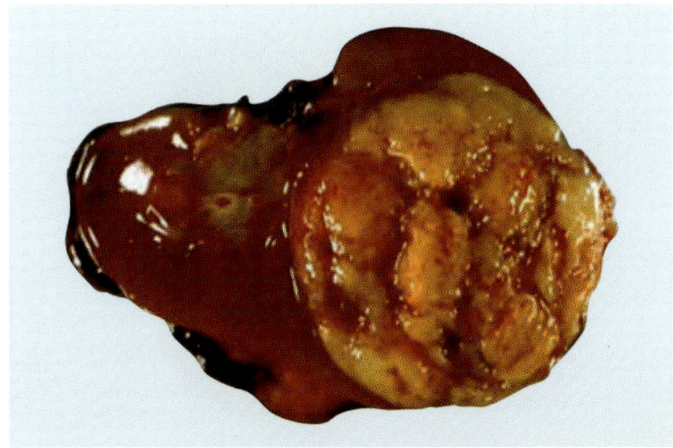

Fig. 2.9: Hypernephroma

solvents during preparation and fixing, giving the appearance of vacuoles within the cytoplasm), dark cells, clear cells with centrally placed dark nucleus.

2. *Cell arrangement:* Cord-like, sheet-like, gland-like or tubular pattern.
3. *Stroma:* Fibrous tissue is scanty.
4. *Blood vessels:* Numerous, immature and thin-walled (so, haemorrhage occurs commonly).

III. NERVOUS SYSTEM

1. Meningitis

Leptomeningitis: Inflammation takes place in the arachnoid and pia mater.

Patchy meningitis: The dura mater is inflamed.

Macroscopic

a. *Pyogenic meningitis:* Purulent exudate extend mainly over the frontal and parietal regions of the brain. Exudate may look green; though thick, it is less thicker than tuberculous meningitis.
b. *Tuberculous meningitis:* Abundant, creamy or gelatinous exudate is seen, mainly over the base of the brain. The exudate is thick and may encase all the structures of the brain. Numerous small tubercles may be found scattered over the brain.

Microscopic

a. *Pyogenic meningitis:* The subarachnoid space is filled with inflammatory exudate consisting mainly of polymorphs, scanty fibrin, RBC and bacteria. The blood vessels are congested.
b. *Tuberculous meningitis:* The inflammatory exudate mainly contains lymphocytes. Tubercles may be seen in various stages of formation.

2. Brain Abscess

Macroscopic (Fig. 2.10)

Any area of brain may be affected depending on the source of infection. A solitary abscess may be formed or multiple small abscesses may be seen in septicaemia. On the surface, an area of congestion is seen with suppuration. Features of cerebral oedema may be present (obliteration of sulci and flattening of gyri). The cut section shows an abscess with loculation of pus. A chronic abscess may have a tough capsule.

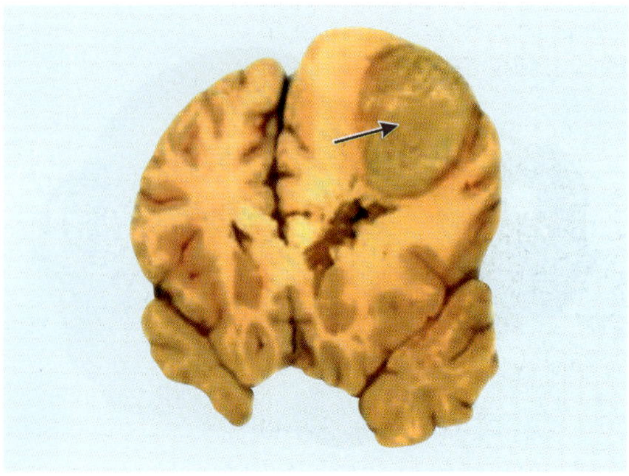

Fig. 2.10: Brain abscess

Microscopic

Area of necrosis with cellular infiltration, mainly polymorphs and macrophages, are seen.

IV. CARDIOVASCULAR SYSTEM

1. Rheumatic Heart Disease

The pathology of rheumatic heart disease is described in three stages, i.e.

a. Stage of exudation, oedema and fibrinoid degeneration of collagen tissues.
b. Stage of proliferation with Aschoff bodies formation, and
c. Stage of healing by fibrosis.

All the three layers of the heart are inflamed, i.e. it is 'pancarditis'.

Macroscopic

a. *Endocarditis* (Fig. 2.11): MacCallum patch or plaque, i.e. a whitish, rough and thickened patch may be seen, particularly on the posterior wall of the left auricle just above the mitral valve. In the valvular endocardium, mitral and aortic valves are commonly affected. Valve cusps become oedematous, thickened and there is formation of Aschoff bodies in the subendothelial connective tissue. In course of time the surface endothelium becomes raw, and platelet and fibrin are deposited there giving rise to minute pale thrombi; ultimately these rheumatic nodules become organised and covered by adjacent endocardium, and is known as 'rheumatic vegetations'. These are very small (size of a pin's head), sessile, warty nodules present a few millimeter away from the margin of the cusps and are arranged in a row. Aschoff bodies are found in chordae tendineae which ultimately becomes thickned, shortened and fibrosed. Valves may be stenosed, especially the mitral and the aortic valve.
b. *Myocarditis:* Aschoff bodies are formed in the left side of the heart mainly (due to more strain). They are mostly found in the left ventricle, base of the interventricular septum and base of the mitral valve. Ultimately myocardial fibrosis and myocardial failure may result.
c. *Pericarditis:* The pericardium loses its shiny appearance and becomes rough. Acute fibrinous inflammation binds the two layers of pericardium, and when separated the rough surfaces show 'bread and butter' appearance. There may be exudative collection in the pericardial sac.

Microscopic

The Aschoff bodies are found around the blood vessels. They are the fundamental units of lesion in rheumatic heart disease, and consist of:

a. Central necrotic area,
b. Surrounded by lymphocytes, plasma cells and occasionally polymorphs,
c. Aschoff cells: Large, multinucleated giant cells containing 5–7 nucleoli, and
d. Proliferation of fibroblasts encircling the above elements.

Anitschkow myocytes: Large vesicular nucleus containing coarse chromatin, and threads of fibrin from the center to the periphery (cardiac cell with 'caterpillar nucleus') may also be seen in myocardium, cardiac valves and coronary vessel wall.

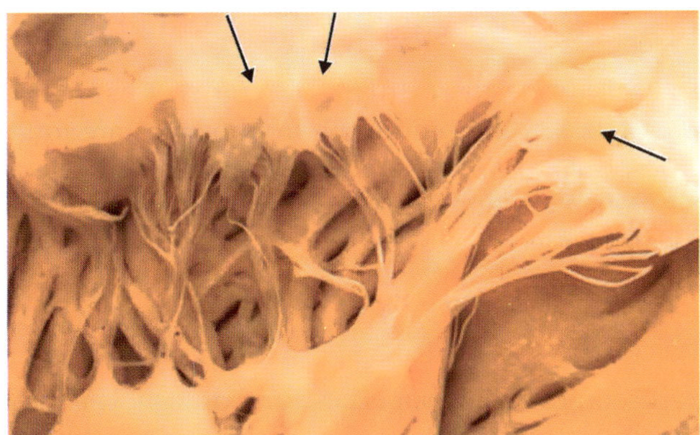

Fig. 2.11: Rheumatic heart disease (endocarditis)

2. Pericarditis

Macroscopic

Commonly fibrinous pericarditis is dealt with. The glossy appearance of pericardium is lost, and it becomes rough. Fibrinous exudate binds, organises and produces adhesions between the two layers of pericardium. If the layers are tried to be separated, they give a 'bread and butter' appearance.

Besides this (fbrinous exudate) serous, sero-fibrinous, haemorrhagic or purulent exudate may be collected within the pericardial sac.

3. Bacterial (Infective) Endocarditis

Macroscopic

Large, friable, polypoid vegetations originate in the line of contact of valve (commonly mitral and aortic) and may spread to involve the whole valve and the mural endocardium. The vegetations get easily detached and produce embolism. The vegetations in subacute bacterial endocarditis are larger than rheumatic vegetations but smaller than that of acute bacterial endocarditis.

Microscopic

The **vegetations** consist of network of platelet and fibrin entangling inflammatory cells, chiefly polymorphs, clumps of bacteria and desquamated endothelial cells.

4. Atherosclerosis of the Aorta

It is a degenerative condition of the arterial wall characterised by deposition of lipid materials in the deepest part of intima of large elastic and muscular arteries.

Macroscopic (**Fig. 2.12**)

Most commonly the abdominal aorta is involved (as a result of maximum trauma and greater hydrostatic presure). Coronary, cerebral, renal, and other visceral vassels as well as big vessels of the limbs may be affected by the process. Depending of the stage, there may be presence of fatty streaks, wax like drops, atheromatous ulcer, thrombi (fibrin and platelet clump), calcification or haemorrhages in the intima.

Microscopic

a. Cytoplasm of intimal smooth muscle fibres accumulates lipid and transforms into foamy cells.
b. The foamy cells die and release their contents; extracellular lipid pool appears. This leads to classical slit-like spaces in cholesterol crystals.
c. Connective tissues of intima overlying the cholesterol deposit becomes thickened: The sclerotic part of atherosclerosis.
d. A mature 'fibro-lipid plaque' consists of a core of extracellular lipid surrounded by smooth muscle cells is formed and is separated from the lumen of the vessel by collagen-rich fibrous tissue. There may be vascularisation under the plaque.
e. Haemorrhage, thrombus formation or calcification may be noted.

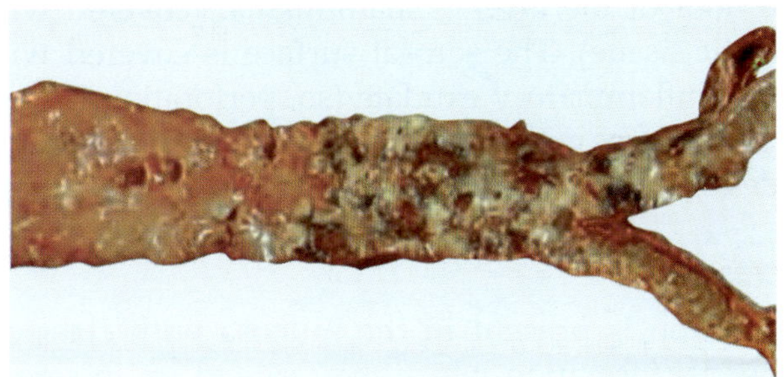

Fig. 2.12: Atherosclerosis of the aorta

5. Syphilitic Aortitis

Macroscopic

The lesion starts at the root of the ascending aorta just distal to the aortic valve, and spreads horizontally around the root of aorta and distally as far as the mouths of the great vessels. Ascending aorta, arch of aorta and rarely the descending thoracic aorta are the sites of involvement due to their rich lymph supply (organisms are carried through lymphatics). It never affects the coronary artery except its opening; never affects the endocardium except the endocardium covering the aortic valve. The aortic valve may be thickned with shortened cusps and widened commissures.

Affected intima may be raised into patches: At first smooth and pearly, later pitted and scarred. Intervening area is wrinkled. It is the fine transverse wrinkles (as a result of stellate scars), which are highly characteristic of syphilis (tree-bark appearance). Atherosclerosis of the aorta often complicates syphilitic aortitis.

Microscopic

There is periaortitis and mesoaortitis with secondary changes in the intima.

Intima shows marked fibrous proliferation, hyalinisation and endarteritis obliterans. Media shows ischaemic necrosis with foci of inflammatory cells. Vasa vasorum shows perivascular infiltration of lymphocytes and plasma cells. There is **gumma** formation, especially around the lymphatic channels and vasa vasorum.

V. INTESTINE

A. Small Intestine

1. Tuberculosis of Intestine

Macroscopic

Classical site is ileocaecal junction but it may extend up to ascending colon or descend up to caecum. Small grey tubercles are seen over the Peyer's patches or lymph follicles opposite the attachment of mesentery. Tubercles undergo caseation necrosis and breaks down into ulcers with ragged and undermined edge. The lie of the ulcer is 'transverse' and thus known as 'girdle ulcer'; when this ulcer heals by fibrosis, it may result in intestinal obstruction (there may be stricture formation). The floor of the ulcer is mammilated (covered with necrotic tissue). The serosal surface is covered with plastic inflammatory exudate (so, perforation is rare) and sometimes with small tubercles. Mensenteric lymph nodes are caseated.

Microscopic

Ulceration is present in the mucosa with classical 'tubercle' formation which may extend up to serous layer. Blood vessels may show endarteritis obliterans.

2. Typhoid Intestine (Enteric Fever)

Macroscopic

Classical site of involvement is terminal ileum and ileocaecal region. There is hypertrophy of the Peyer's patches and solitary lymph follicles opposite the mesenteric attachment with occasional ulcer formation. The ulcer is oval or round, and they grow along the 'longitudinal' axis of the gut (vertical ulcer); Crohn's disease also produces 'longitudinal ulcer'. The edge is raised and smooth, but not undermined. The floor is sieve-like (worm-eaten); the floor is formed by submucous and muscle coat but may extend up to serous coat (so, perforations are likely). Mesenteric lymph nodes are enlarged and congested.

Microscopic

Ulcerated mucosa, hyperplasia of lymph follicles and hypertrophy of Peyer's patches with submucosa infiltrated by mononuclear cells are seen.

B. Large Intestine

1. Amoebic Dysentery Ulcer

Macroscopic

Classically there are two levels of involvement: more commonly the ileocaecal region and less commonly the rectosigmoid region. The shape is oval or round; the margin is undermined and ragged, often formed by the overhanging mucosa (flask-shaped ulcer). The floor is formed by the muscle coat and covered by the necrotic slough (yellow or black). The intervening mucosa seems to be normal. The overlying serous coat may be thickened.

Microscopic

Flask-shaped ulcer formation with absence of *E. histolytica* at the centre; the trophozoites are found at the periphery. Proliferation of endothelial cells of neighbouring blood vessels causing their thrombosis may also be seen.

2. Bacillary Dysentery Ulcer

Macroscopic

The ulcers are mainly superficial and diffuse. The shape is irregular or snail-track, sometimes communicate with the submucous coat. The floor of the ulcer is very shallow and remain on the mucous coat; the margin is sharp. The intervening mucosa is swollen and oedematous. Overlying peritoneum is usually normal

Microscopic

There is absence of mucous membrane; presence of fibrin, RBC, WBC and pus cells over the mucous coat which forms a 'pseudomembrane'. All the layers of intestine are infiltrated with inflammatory cells. The blood vessels are dilated.

VI. LIVER

1. Cirrhosis of Liver

Macroscopic (Fig. 2.13)

The size of the liver is variable (i.e. increased or decreased) depending upon hyperplasia and fibrosis; usually shrunken. The outer surface may have fine nodules (micronodular cirrhosis) giving the liver 'Hob-nail appearance', or have large-irregular nodules (macronodular cirrhosis). The colour of the liver in portal cirrhosis is usually brownish (due to deposition of iron pigment) and it is greenish in biliary cirrhosis. The consistency is very firm (due to fibrosis). The liver gives resistance on cutting and the cut section shows nodules and strands of pale yellow bands of fibrous tissue intercepting the hepatic architecture.

Microscopic

The hepatic lobular architecture is destroyed. Broad bands of fibrous tissue divide and sub-divide a lobule with the result that the position of the central vein is no longer at the center of the lobule. There is presence of necrosis as well as regeneration of new liver cells (irregular in size and arrangement). Round cell infiltration with proliferation of biliary epithelium are seen in the portal canal.

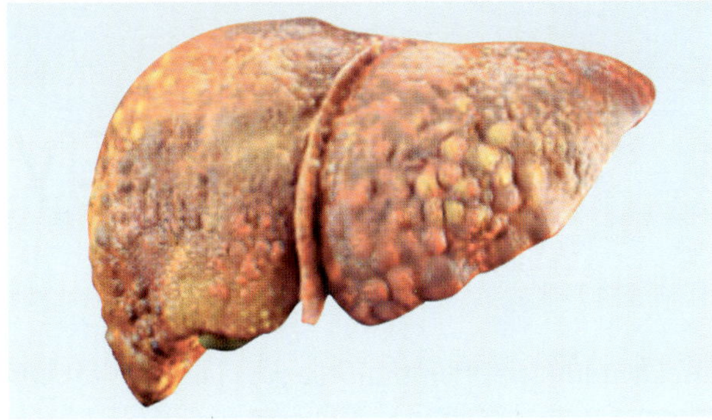

Fig. 2.13: Cirrhosis of liver

2. Amoebic Liver Abscess

Macrocopic (Fig. 2.14)

The liver is enlarged and congested. There is presence of a big abscess, commonly at the postero-superior part of the right lobe. Usually a single abscess (big) is seen which may be surrounded by multiple small abscesses. The cut section would show an abscess filled with chocolate coloured pus, better known as 'anchovy sauce' pus. The content is not true pus but it is an admixture of cytolysed hepatocytes with blood. The wall of the cavity in irregular and ragged.

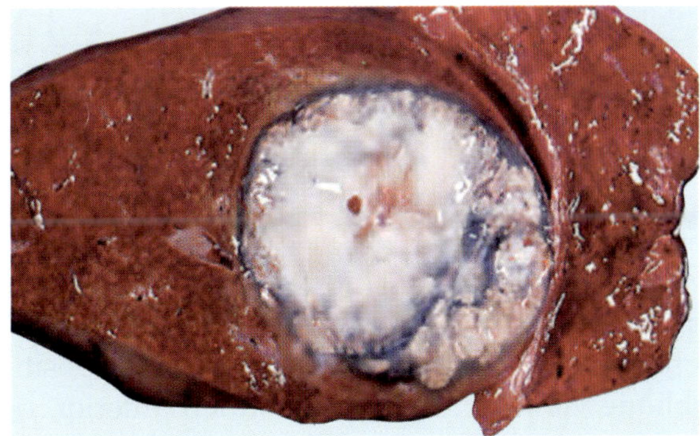

Fig. 2.14: Amoebic liver abscess

3. Pyogenic Liver Abscess

Macroscopic (Fig. 2.15)

The whole of the liver is enlarged. There are multiple, small abscesses (necrosed area) seen scattered throughout the liver. Any lobe of the liver may be affected and the right lobe is affected more than the left lobe. The cut section would reveal yellow-coloured pus coming out from the abscess cavity. The wall of the abscess cavity is usually ragged.

4. Hepato-cellular Carcinoma (Hepatoma)

Macroscopic (Fig. 2.16)

In primary carcinoma of the liver, the enlargement usually occurs irregularly. Commonly, one large tumour

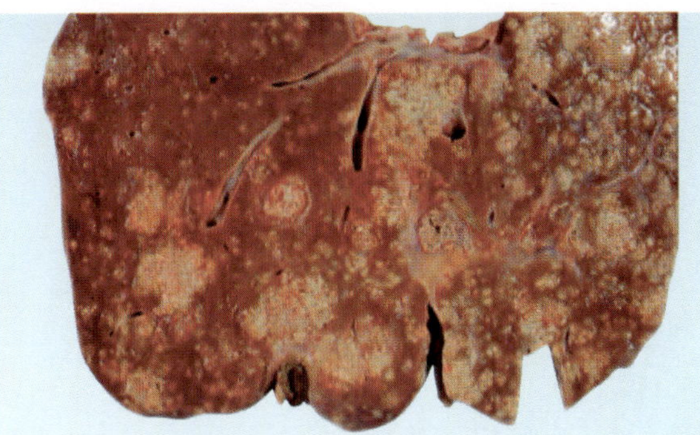

Fig. 2.15: Pyogenic liver abscess

(nodular or diffuse) may be seen with a few small outlying seedling nodules. The intervening portions of the liver is very firm as hepatomas are commonly seen in a patient of cirrhosis of liver. The blood vessels or the bile duct may be involved by extension.

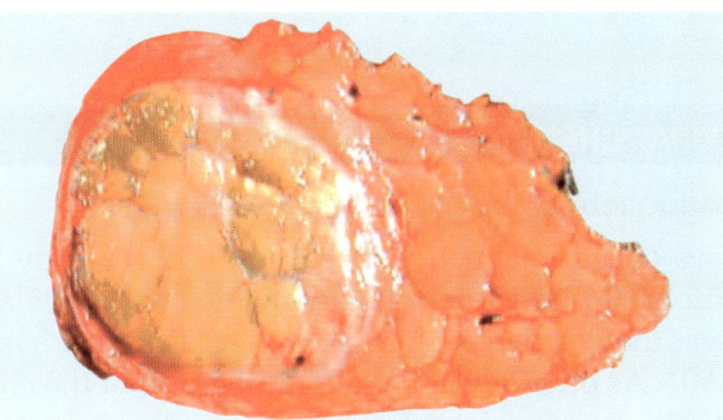

Fig. 2.16: Hepato-cellular carcinoma

5. Secondary Carcinoma of the Liver (Metastases)

Macroscopic (Fig. 2.17)

The liver is enlarged and studded with multiple big nodules. The irregular nodules show depression at the top and is known as 'umbilication' (due to rapid growth of the tumour, there is dimpling as a result of central necrosis). The cut section of a nodule may show area of haemorrhage and necrosis but usually it is greyish-white in colour. There is absence of cirrhotic changes in the intervening areas. 'Umbilication' differentiates secondary carcinoma of liver from nodular liver arising out of post-necrotic cirrhosis or hepato-cellular carcinoma (hepatoma).

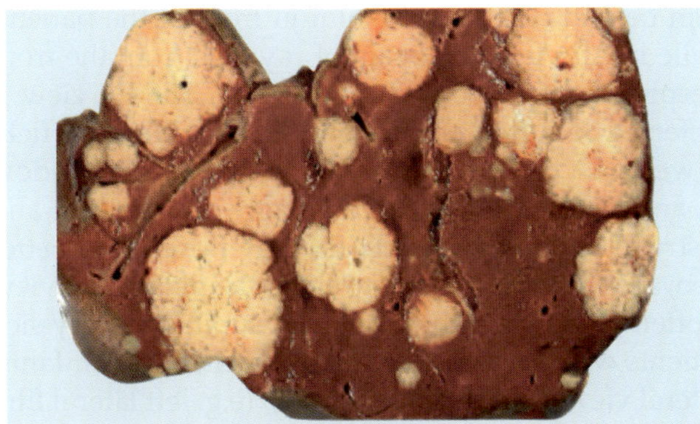

Fig. 2.17: Metastases in liver

Chapter

3

Radiology

"Great discoveries are made accidentally less often than the populace likes to think."

—**William Cecil Dampier** (1867-1952), a British scientist, agriculturist and science historian, referring to the accidental discovery of X-ray by **Wilhelm Roentgen**

[Accidental discoveries: X-ray, penicillin and chloroform]

A. X-RAY CHEST

Introduction

X-rays (electromagnetic rays) were discovered by **Sir Wilhelm Conrad Roentgen** in November 8, 1895 and he was the first person to receive Nobel Prize in Physics in 1901. As on today, the plain radiograph of the chest is still the primary investigation for chest examination.

In the day-to-day practice, postero-anterior and lateral view of the chest are taken to visualise the lung details. Depending upon the direction of the rays from the X-ray tube to the X-ray plate, antero-posterior (AP), postero-anterior (PA) and lateral projections are made in roentgenographic examination.

In the PA view (the standard view for chest), the person should stand erect with the anterior chest closely attached against the X-ray cassette containing the X-ray film, with the hands placed on the waist and the elbows drawn a bit anteriorly. By placing the elbows in a forward direction, the scapulae goes apart and thus they never produce obstruction to the lung fields. The tube-film distance should be about 6 feet or 2 meters, in order to minimise distortion, and magnification (also for radiation protection). In PA view, the beam of ray falls from behind (keeping the film in front of the patient) while in AP view, the beam of ray falls from the front (keeping the film behind the patient). The PA view is preferred because, (a) this view gives a wider lung field as well as a clear picture of bronchovascular shadow (in an AP view, cardiac size is more exaggerated and obstructs part of lung fields) (b) posterior ribs are better seen, and (c) radiation-risk to eyes is negligible. AP view is often ordered (with the patient supine) in very sick patients who are unable to stand or sit, and in infants. Lateral view **(Fig. 3.1A_1 and 3.1A_2)** (e.g. left lateral film is one which is taken with the left side of the patient's chest placed next to the film), recumbent view (X-ray taken in lying down position, usually supine when the patient is unable to stand due to serious illness), decubitus film (right or left lateral decubitus position) or oblique view (i.e. right anterior, left anterior, right posterior, and left posterior oblique) are taken in special situations. Lateral view of the chest is essential for the identification of lobes and segmental details of lung.

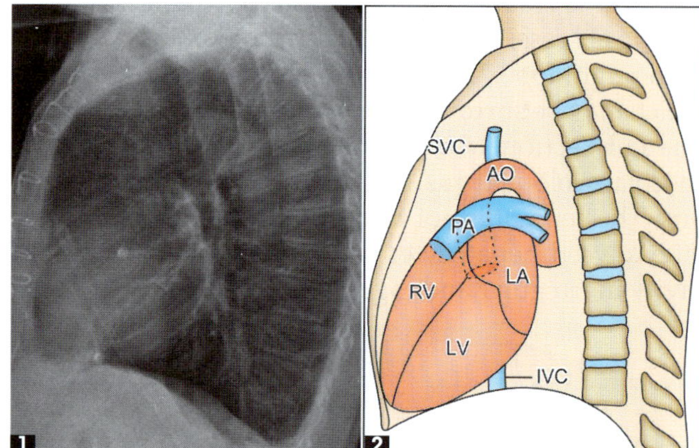

Fig. 3.1A: (1) Chest X-ray—lateral view; (2) Chest X-ray—lateral view (diagrammatic)

Nowadays, digital radiology is the most commonly used modality. **The view of plain films may be:**

1. PA, lateral.
2. AP (patient unable to stand/portable X-ray), decubitus (sub-pulmonary effusion or minimal pleural effusion), supine or recumbent, oblique (for retrocardiac area) view.
3. End-expiratory (to detect small pneumothorax).
4. Lordotic—apical (for better visualisation of apex), penetrated (for enlarged left atrium and aorta).
5. Portable/mobile X-ray.

An ideal chest X-ray film should have:

1. *Proper exposure (i.e. dose of radiation):* In general, it is desirable that the upper four thoracic vertebrae (not

all vertebrae) be just barely discernible through the cardiomediastinal shadow with adequate exposure. **Overexposure** makes the lung fields more black with a clear view of vertebral bodies; **underexposure** makes the lung fields hazy while the thoracic vertebrae are not visible. In overpenetrated films, one may overlook low density lesions. Ideally films should be of medium contrast. Exposure may be adequate, under- or overexposed.

2. *Proper labelling by radiology technician:* The technician puts 'R' (right) or 'L' (left) in the upper comer of the X-ray plate for side determination. He should also label the plate properly with name of the patient and date of exposure. The physician should read the label at the beginning, otherwise a case of dextrocardia may be missed.
3. *Proper centering:* The clavicles should be at the same level and the inner ends of the clavicles should be equidistant from the midline, i.e. from the spinous process of the vertebral column (or, the gap in the sternoclavicular articulation should be the same on both sides).

- In an ideal PA view of chest, clavicle should lie over the posterior end of 3rd rib to clearly visualise the apex of the lungs—the 'normal angulation'.

The cartilagenous rings of **trachea** are not visible though the air within trachea may be seen as a dark column (black). Normally, the trachea is centrally placed or slightly deviated to the right.

The scapulae should not project over the lung fields. It should be remembered that approximately 75% of the lung fields are seen in routine PA view of the chest (25% lung fields are obstructed by clavicles, ribs, cardiovascular shadow and subdiaphragmatic tissue).

A routine chest X-ray should be always taken in full inspiration except in a case of suspected small or hair-line pneumothorax. PA view of chest taken in expiration makes the cardiac size enlarged and lung bases hazy. While taking an X-ray, the patient should be unclothed, long hairs should be pinned up. Radio-opaque materials e.g. jewelleries should be removed. For lateral view, the patient's arms are folded and extended above the head.

The X-ray plate should be examined in a 'view-box', usually from a distance of 2 feet. The plate should be correctly mounted in the view-box. The **side determination** (maintaining the anatomical position) is done by the following methods:

1. Label put by the radiology technician (L or R).
2. Apex of the heart should be on the left side.
3. Fundal gas shadow should be on the left side.
4. Right dome of the diaphragm is placed at a higher level than the left.
5. Aortic knuckle should be on the left side.

In a case of rotation of viscera (dextrocardia with or without situs inversus), the above formula does not serve the purpose and one has to depend only on radiographer's labelling.

The normal chest X-ray should be assessed or described in the following order:

1. View or X-ray projection (PA, lateral, oblique).
2. Exposure or penetration.
3. Centralisation.
4. Skeletal structures (thoracic cage).
5. Lung fields including blood vessels and pleura.
6. Cardiovascular silhouette.
7. Mediastinum (including position of the trachea and cardiac apex).
8. Costophrenic and cardiophrenic angle.
9. Diaphragm.
10. Soft tissue abnormalities.
11. Final diagnosis or conclusion.

Each part is described below in a nutshell:

1. *View*
2. *Exposure*
3. *Centralisation*

} Described above

4. *Skeletal structures (i.e. vertebrae, ribs, sternum, scapulae, clavicles):* In full inspiration, 10 posterior and 6 anterior ribs should be visible. Ribs slant down postero-anteriorly. Actually the thoracic bony cage (rib cage, thoracic spines, clavicles and bones of the shoulder girdle) is looked for:
   a. Kyphosis, scoliosis, straight back, or paravertebral pathology (e.g. cold abscess).
   b. Any distortion of size or shape of the chest, i.e. symmetrical or not.
   c. Crowding (e.g. collapse or fibrosis of the lung) or widely spaced (e.g. emphysema) ribs.
   d. Absence of clavicle (e.g. aleidocranial dysostosis) or erosion of clavicle (e.g. bronchogenic carcinoma or multiple myeloma).
   e. Rib erosion (e.g. multiple myeloma, bronchogenic carcinoma, hyperparathyroidism) or rib notching (e.g. coarctation of aorta), fracture or healed fracture in ribs.
   f. Presence of cervical rib, bifid rib, resected rib, absent rib or hemivertebra.

- Soft tissues are breast shadows, axillae and supraclavicular areas.

5. *Lung fields including blood vessels and pleura:* Normally lung fields are translucent and look reticular too (due to bronchovascular markings). One has to look for radio-opaque shadows or hypertranslucency in the lung shadows. The X-ray appearance of the lung fields and the normal bronchovascular tree depends on the degree of aeration and vascular filling at the time of exposure, the size of the bronchi, and other associated anatomic and physiologic factors.

   The vascular shadows (looks white linear) in the lung are casted by the branches of pulmonary artery. Pulmonary veins (often seen in upper lobes) produce low-density shadow. Branches of pulmonary artery (form major bulk of hilar density) and veins are accompanied by a corresponding branch of the bronchus. The alveoli, pleura, interstitium and lymphatics produce a very low-density shadow which are rarely identified in the X-ray film. Increase in the white linear shadows (i.e. **bronchovascular markings** radiating from the hilar region to the periphery) may be seen in:

a. *Accentuated pulmonary arteries:* Left-to-right shunt in ASD, VSD and PDA.
b. *Distension of pulmonary veins:* In the left-sided heart failure (i.e. left ventricular or left atrial failure).
c. *Accentuation of bronchial pattern:* Seen in chronic bronchitis, bronchiectasis.
d. *Prominence of lymphatic vessels:* Commonly seen in bronchogenic carcinoma.
e. *Thickened alveolar septum:* Seen in pneumoconiosis, pulmonary fibrosis (interstitial lung disease).

In a normal person, the **'hilar shadows'** (the lung roots) are made up of pulmonary arteries, pulmonary veins, bronchi, hilar lymph glands, lymphatics and connective tissue components. Left hilum is slightly higher in position (0.5–2.0 cm) than the right, and both the hila have concave borders with equal density. For the purpose of radiological description, **lung fields are divided by two horizontal lines into three zones,** i.e. upper, middle and lower zones. The 'upper line' passes horizontally through the inferior borders of the anterior ends of the second costal cartilages; similarly the 'lower line' passes horizontally through the inferior borders of the anterior ends of the fourth costal cartilages. The upper zone is restricted above the upper horizontal line, the mid-zone lies in between upper and lower horizontal lines, and the lower zone extends from lower horizontal line to the bases of lungs. Zones in the X-ray plate do not correspond with the lobes of the lung. Each zone is examined symmetrically on two sides and an area of abnormality is meticulously compared with the corresponding area on the other side.

The normal pleural structures are seldom visible. The pleura may be visible, if thickened or calcified.

- Bronchovascular markings become less prominent in pulmonary stenosis and pericardial effusion.

6. *Cardiovascular silhouette:* The cardiothoracic ratio (CTR) is expressed as a percentage of the ratio between the maximum transverse diameter of the heart and the maximum internal diameter of the chest (thorax). In health, the transverse diameter of the heart is usually equal to half the internal diameter of the chest or just less, i.e. CTR 0.5:1 or it is just <0.5 : 1; cardiac enlargement is suspected if the CTR is >0.57 : 1 or the transverse diameter of the heart is >16 cm (though often varies with age, sex, build and nutrition). In a PA view of the chest, 2/3rd of the cardiac shadow lies on the left and 1/3rd on the right from the midline.

The CTR is a simple method to estimate cardiac enlargement. The CTR is estimated in a better way by the following measurements. First, draw a vertical line over the spinous process in the midline to divide the heart into two halves. Now, maximum extension of the heart to the right of midline (X) and maximum extension of heart to the left of midline (Y) is measured. Next, maximum internal diameter (ID) of the thorax is measured as the maximum measurement of the thorax to the inside of the ribs, at the lowermost part of the PA view of chest.

Finally, the CTR is calculated as $\frac{X+Y}{ID}$; X + Y is equivalent to maximum transverse diameter of the heart (Fig. 3.1B).

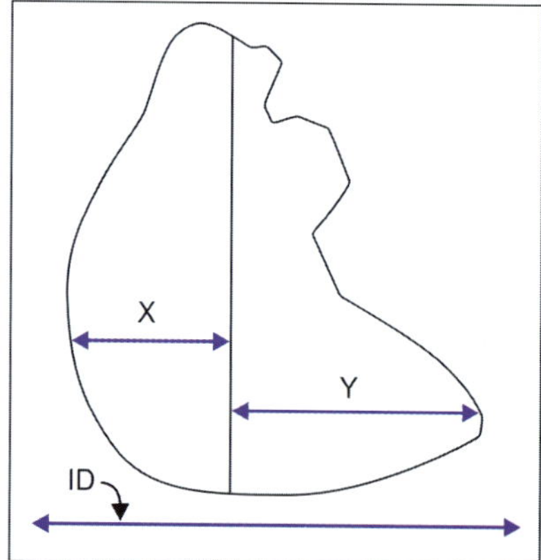

Fig. 3.1B: Diagramatic representation of maximum transverse diameter of the heart

- **Borders of cardiac silhouette in PA view of chest:**
  a. Right border (from above downwards):
    1. Superior vena cava (sometimes, ascending arch of the aorta takes part): The upper straight portion.
    2. Outer border of the right atrium (sometimes, inferior vena cava may be visible just right to the right atrium): The lower curved portion.
  b. Left border (from above downwards):
    1. Aortic knuckle: A convexity (at the level of 2nd ICS).
    2. Pulmonary trunk (conus) or left pulmonary artery: A straight line or a concavity (known as 'pulmonary bay'; at the level of 3rd ICS).
    3. Left atrial appendages: The short straight portion.
    4. Outer border of the left ventricle: The convexity in the lower part, ending at the apex.
- Inferior border of heart is contiguous with the diaphragm and is not visible. In the PA view of chest, right ventricle does not form any border, rather in lateral view it forms most of the anterior heart border.

Changes in the Cardiac Size, Shape and Position

a. *Prominent aortic knuckle:* Old age (i.e. unfolding of the aorta and atherosclerosis), aortic aneurysm, post-stenotic dilatation and aortitis.
b. *Concavity of the pulmonary trunk becomes convex:* Pulmonary hypertension, left-to-right shunt in the heart, i.e. ASD, VSD, PDA, and idiopathic dilatation of pulmonary artery.

c. *Absent pulmonary artery shadow:* Pulmonary stenosis or pulmonary atresia.
d. *Enlargement of cardiac size:* Enlarged chambers of heart, pericardial effusion, cardiomyopathy. Enlargement in transverse diameter indicates RVH, and increase in oblique diameter features LVH.
e. *Right atrial enlargement:* Enlargement of the right border of the heart (a bulge is seen in PA view).
f. *Left atrial enlargement:*
   i. Straightening of the left border of the heart (the base of the pulmonary bay).
   ii. Prominence of the left atrial appendages in the left border of the heart.
   iii. Double contour of the right border of the heart (the outer and upper border is due to LA, and the inner and lower border is due to RA enlargement)—as seen in mitral stenosis.
   iv. Upwards displacement of left main bronchus, and it becomes horizontal; widening of angle of carina.
   v. Posterior displacement of barium-filled oesophagus in right anterior oblique view.

❍ Atrial enlargement (right or left) is often better seen in the lateral view as a posterior bulge.

g. *Right ventricular enlargement:*
   i. PA view: Shifting of the apex to the left (i.e. outward enlargement only) with 'upturned' apex and increase in the transverse diameter of the heart with boot-shaped configuration.
   ii. Lateral view: Obliteration of retrosternal air space from below upwards.
h. *Left ventricular enlargement:*
   i. Increase in the oblique diameter of the heart.
   ii. Shifting of the apex outwards (to the left) and downwards.

7. *Mediastinum:* In a normal chest X-ray, trachea (the black airy tube) remains central or slightly towards the right, and evenly calibred. The mediastinal borders are made of right heart, ascending aorta, superior vena cava, aortic knuckle, descending aorta and the left heart. Mediastimum is central and cardiac borders are clearly seen. The thymus, pleural reflections and fibrofatty tissue may or may not be visible. Observe, whether the mediastinum is widened or not. Positions of the cardiac apex (outwards, or out and downwards) and the trachea indirectly indicate shifting of the mediastinum. Is there any shadow 'behind the heart'?
8. *Costophrenic and cardiophrenic angle:*
   a. Costophrenic angle (the angle between the diaphragm and the rib): In a PA view of the chest, costophrenic angles should be clearly visible. Normally, it is sharp and acute in angle. In pleural effusion or empyema thoracis, this angle is obliterated first.
   b. Cardiophrenic angle (the angle between the diaphragm and the cardiac broder): In health, the right-sided angle is acute or near about right angle. In pericardial effusion, the right-sided angle becomes more acute (Rotch's sign). The left-sided angle cannot be distinctly seen owing to the presence of epicardial pad of fat (especially in elderly fatty people) and thus it is of no importance radiologically.
9. *Diaphragm:* The right and left dome of the diaphragm are convex upwards and sharp in outline. The right dome is placed high-up (0.5–2.5 cm in erect posture) than the left dome. In the midclavicular line, the upper limit of the right dome should be between 6th and 7th intercostal space anteriorly and 10th intercostal space posteriorly. Fundal gas shadow is seen below the left diaphragm.
   a. *Elevated diaphragm:* Collapse or fibrosis of the lung (basal), ascites, pregnancy, diaphragmatic palsy, abdominal mass, amoebic liver abscess (right dome).
   b. *Depressed or flattened dome:* Emphysema (bilateral), pneumothorax (unilateral).
   c. *Localised bulge or tenting:* Amoebic liver abscess, subdiaphragmatic abscess, pleural tumour.
10. *Soft tissue abnormalities (including root of neck):* Soft tissues of the chest wall (wart, angioma, neurofibroma), upper abdomen, neck (calcified lymph nodes) and shoulder may be visible in chest X-ray film. Costal cartilage calcification has no clinical significance. Breast and nipple shadows in female (partially obstructs lung bases), sternomastoid shadows (especially in male) or gas shadows (subcutaneous or surgical emphysema) should be especially looked for. Artefacts (errors in film handling by technician may give rise to white linear shadows or hair balls, buttons may cast rounded shadows, especially in females) should be carefully identified. Check for any foreign body like endotracheal tube, Ryle's tube, ECG leads, chest drain, sternotomy sutures and clips, or pacemaker.
11. *Conclusion:* A normal chest X-ray should be described in the following way (Fig. 3.1C): **This is a PA view of the chest with adequate exposure, proper centering and without any apparent bony abnormality. The trachea is centrally placed and the lung fields are clear with normal bronchovascular markings; cardiovascular silhouette is within normal limit with normal cardiothoracic ratio. The mediastinum, costophrenic and cardiophrenic angles, domes of the diaphragm and soft tissues show no abnormality.**

Clinical Wisdom

For cardiological check-up, following views are necessary: 1. PA, 2. Lateral, 3. Oblique (right and left anterior oblique views with barium swallow film of oesophagus).

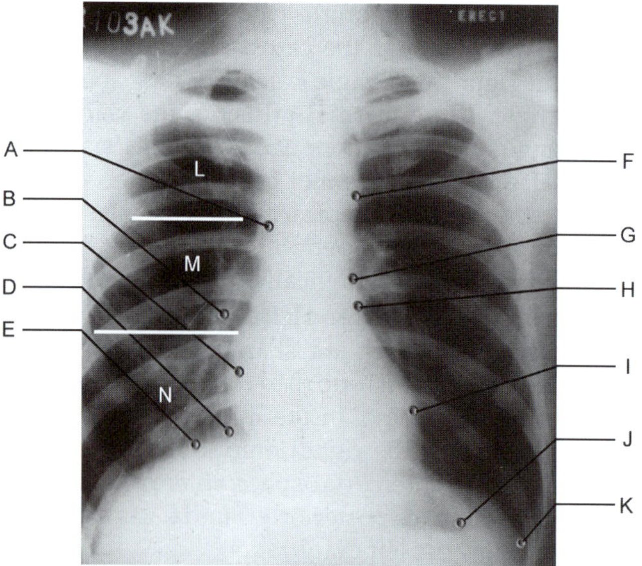

Fig. 3.1C: PA view of the chest X-ray in a normal adult. A: Superior vena cava; B: Bronchovascular marking; C: Right atrium; D: Cardiophrenic angle (right); E: Dome of diaphragm (right); F: Aortic knuckle; G: Main pulmonary artery; H: Left atrial appendages; I: Left ventricle; J: Fundal gas shadow; K: Costophrenic angle (left); L,M,N: Respectively upper zone, mid-zone and lower zone of the lung

- While describing an X-ray plate, always try to maintain the frame of words described in conclusion, along with the abnormalities seen. While describing individual X-ray plates in the following pages, particularly the abnormalities have been highlighted.
- **Always search for the following, in an apparently normal looking chest X-ray:**
  1. Small apical pneumothorax.
  2. Very small collection of pleural fluid.
  3. Fluid level (e.g. hiatus hernia) or air-fluid level (e.g. achalasia) behind the cardiac shadow.
  4. Rib notching, rib erosion, rib fracture, or whiteness of ribs (osteopetrosis).
  5. Gas shadow under the diaphragm (right side).
  6. Deviation of the trachea.
  7. Paratracheal lymph node enlargement.
  8. Cervical ribs (additional rib/ribs arising from the C_7 vetebra).
  9. Mastectomy.
  10. Right middle lobe collapse with loss of clear outline of right cardiac border.
  11. Soft tissue shadows: subcutaneous emphysema (looks black), axillary lymph node swelling.
- The different images seen in chest radiograph as difference in **densities** from least dense (black) to most dense (white) are:
  a. Gas (air present in the lungs).
  b. Fat (soft tissue, epicardial pad of fat).
  c. Water (density same as heart).
  d. Bone (maximum density among the tissues).
  e. Metal (any metallic foreign body, pacemaker).

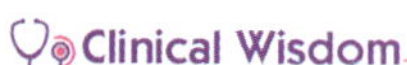

Inspiratory versus expiratory film: Normally, chest X-ray is taken in full inspiration. *In a good inspiratory film:* 6 anterior ribs and 10 posterior ribs are visible.

In expiratory film: Cardiac shadow seems larger. As the lung volume is reduced, a small pneumothorax is easily visualised.

- **Digital chest X-ray** is clean-cut, accurate, more bright and thus revolutionary.
- **Ultrasonography of chest** is indicated in:
  1. To differentiate pleural thickening from pleural fluid.
  2. To diagnose solid or cystic nature of a superficial lesion.
  3. To examine diaphragmatic movement (e.g. in diaphragmatic paralysis).
- **CT scan of chest** is indicated in:
  1. Abnormal or doubtful shadow in chest X-ray.
  2. Staging of bronchogenic carcinoma.
  3. Widening of mediastinum.
  4. Hilar abnormality.
  5. Interstitial lung disease, bronchiectasis.
  6. Abnormalities in pleura.
  7. Embolism in pulmonary artery.
  8. Lesions in the chest wall.

Different imaging modalities in clinical medicine:

Many imaging methods are now available, which are used with consideration of nature of clinical problem, urgency, availability and cost. They are:

1. Screening.
2. Conventional and digital radiography (most commonly used) (Fig. 3.1D).
3. Tomography.

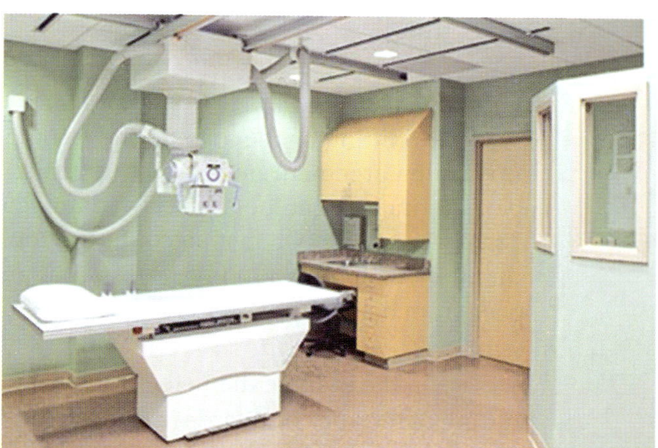

Fig. 3.1D: Conventional X-ray room

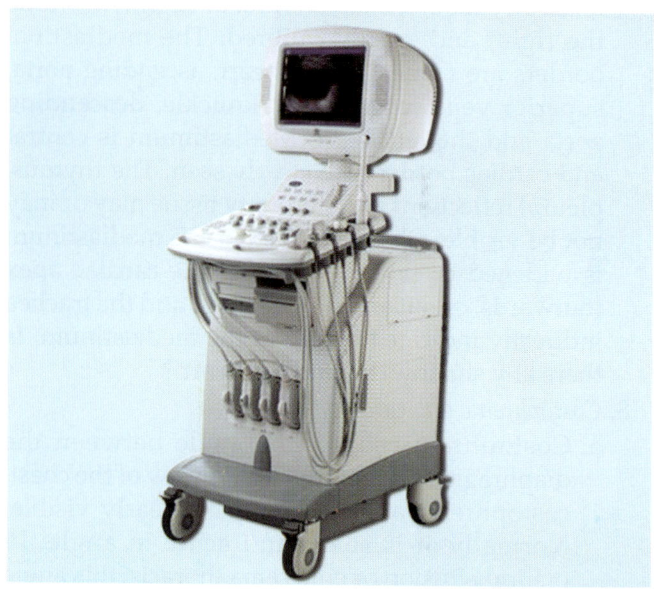

Fig. 3.1E: USG machine

4. Fluoroscopy (e.g. to see diaphragmatic movements).
5. Contrast studies (e.g. barlum study, contrast CT/MRI of brain or spinal cord, coronary angiography).
6. USG (ultrasonography) (Fig. 3.1E).
7. CT (computed tomography) scan (Fig. 3.1F).
8. MRI (magnetic resonance imaging) scan (Fig. 3.1G).
9. PET (positron emission tomography) scan (Fig. 3.1H).
10. SPECT (single-photon emission computed tomography) scan.

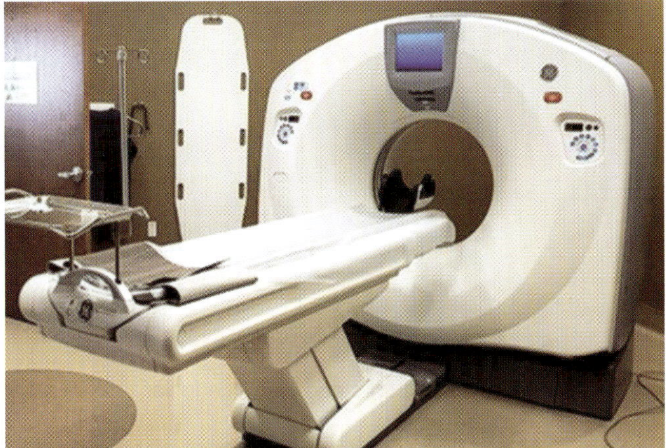

Fig. 3.1F: CT scan machine

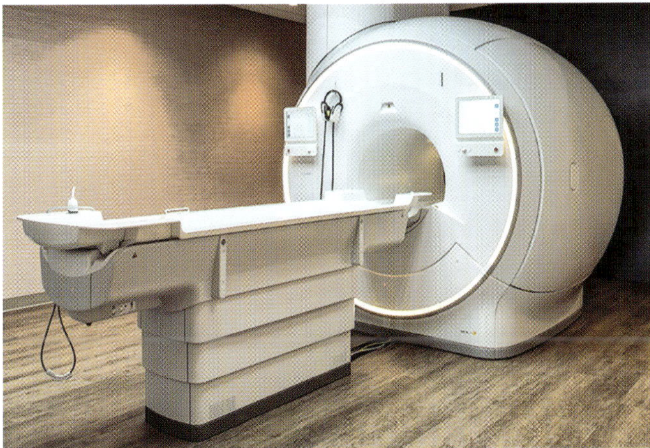

Fig. 3.1G: MRI machine

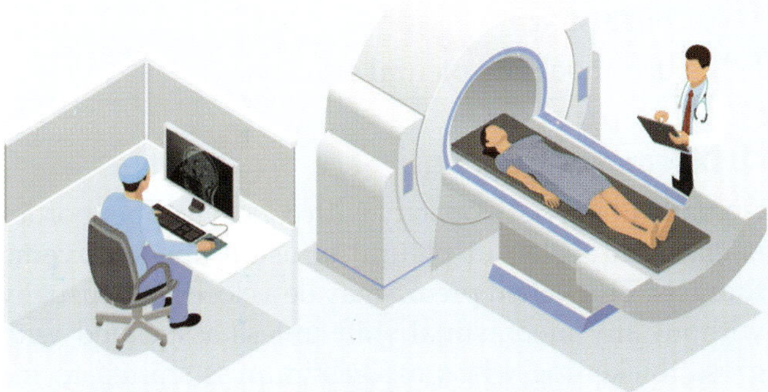

Fig. 3.1H: PET scan room

CONSOLIDATION OF THE LUNG (Fig. 3.2)

Q. Description:

This is a PA view of the chest showing a sharply-defined triangular uniformly homogeneous opacity involving

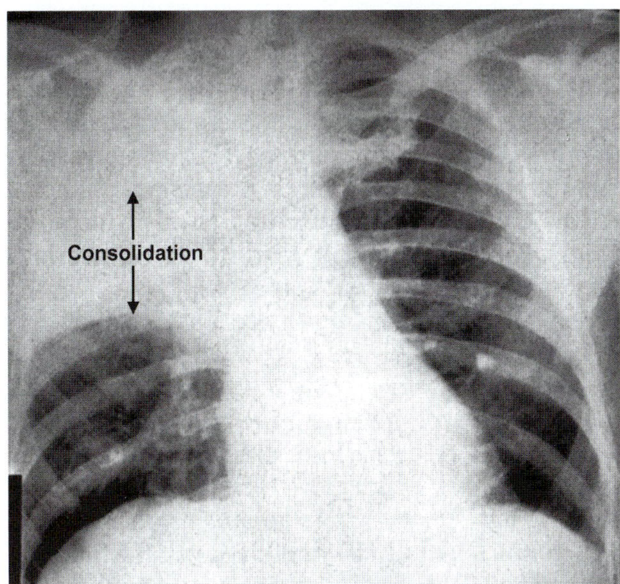

Fig. 3.2: Consolidation of the right lung

the right upper and mid-zone. Trachea and apex beat are normal in position. Both the costophrenic angles are clear.

Other points: Within normal limit.

- Air bronchogram is not clearly seen here. There is no loss of lung volume.

 *Conclusion*

Consolidation of the right lung.

- **Pneumonia or consolidation** is the exudative solidification of lung parenchyma.

Q. Which lobe of right lung is involved?

It needs a lateral X-ray film to diagnose. It is expected that right upper lobe has been affected.

Q. Differential diagnosis:

1. Collapse of the lung (mediastinum moves to the diseased side, absent air bronchogram).
2. Bronchogenic carcinoma (pleural reaction, i.e. pleural effusion is commonly seen, absence of 'air bronchogram' and there may be presence of rib erosion).
3. Pulmonary tuberculosis (classically sharply-defined consolidation is rare, pleural reaction is more common).
4. Pulmonary infarction (may be a possibility because in pulmonary infarction wedge-shaped, homogeneous, poorly-defined opacity is produced, attached against pleura; thus blunting of costophrenic angle is commonly seen here).

Q. What is air bronchogram?

Bronchus contains air and the air is not visible separately in a normal chest X-ray. But in consolidation of the lung (pneumonia), the air within the bronchus casts linear translucency (black) over the background of homogeneous opacity (e.g. consolidation, which looks white). These are commonly seen as scattered linear translucencies rather than continuous branching structures. Air bronchogram reflects that an opacity is intrapulmonary. **It is seen in consolidation,** pulmonary oedema, alveolar cell carcinoma and hyaline membrane disease. It needs a good quality of X-ray film and the observer should have an eagle's eye.

Q. 'Pulmonary opacities' in chest X-ray:

They are usually classified as: alveolar or interstitial.

- *Alveolar (acinar):* Alveoli are filled-up with fluid, blood or cells. They produce ill-defined, non-segmental small shadows which may give rise to larger shadows after merging. Air bronchogram is characteristic. Common example is consolidation of the lung.
- *Interstitial:* They produce reticular, reticulonodular or ground glass opacity as a result of thickening of perivascular interstitial tissue. The lesions may be small (e.g. miliary) or large. Common example is fibrosing alveolitis.

Q. What is 'silhouette sign'?

When two structures of same radiologic density are in same plane, then the interface between the two is obliterated, and the lack of interface is known as silhouette sign (i.e. loss of demarcation between pulmonary shadow and neighbouring structures). For example, right heart border is obliterated by right middle lobe lesion (consolidation or collapse), and left heart border is obliterated by lesion in lingular lobe.

Q. Outstanding feature in the X-ray film

The is no shifting of mediastinum.

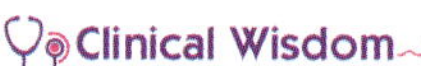

Bronchopneumonia gives rise to heterogenously scattered patchy opacities without air bronchogram.

PLEURAL EFFUSION (Fig. 3.3A and B)

Q. Description:

This is a PA view of the chest showing a triangular homogeneous dense opacity (opacity decreases from below upwards) on the left chest with a curved upper border which is 'concave' medially and upwards, and extends towards the axilla. Left costophrenic angle is obliterated while the right angle is clear. The cardiac shadow and trachea (lower part) have shifted slightly towards the right. Lung fields are apparently normal.

Other points: Within normal limit.

- In **pleural effusion,** serous fluid collects in between two layers of pleura, i.e. visceral and parietal pleura.
- There is absence of air bronchogram in pleural effusion. If the curved upper border of fluid seems convex, think of 'loculated' pleural effusion.

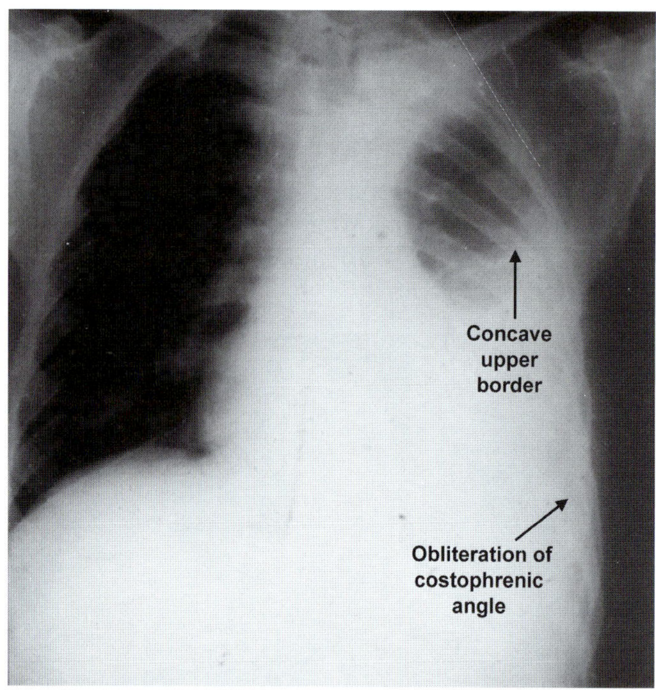

Fig. 3.3A: Left-sided pleural effusion

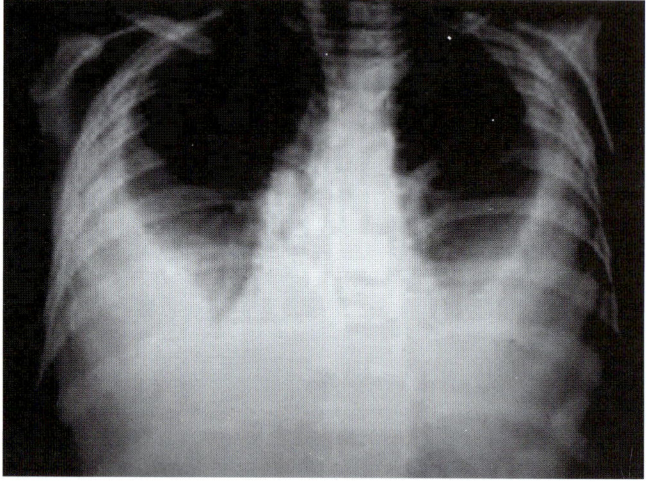

Fig. 3.3B: Bilateral pleural effusion

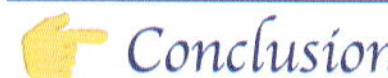

Left-sided moderate pleural effusion.

Q. Differential diagnosis:

Actually this type of opacity with concave upper border is classically seen in pleural effusion and **empyema thoracis**. **Thickened pleura** may be a close D/D (usually without any mediastinal shift unless associated with gross thickening when mediastinum is shifted to the same side; ribs may be visible within the opacity, i.e. opacity is not truely dense; upper margin is fading and not concave). **Bronchogenic carcinoma** or **consolidation** (with parapneumonic effusion) may be present underneath the effusion. **Fibrosis** or **collapse of the lung** (if considered in the D/D) produces mediastinal shifting to the diseased side.

Q. Hemithorax opacity without any mediastinal shift:

1. Consolidation of the lung.
2. Malignant pleural effusion (due to associated absorption collapse of the lung).
3. Mesothelioma of the pleura.
4. Fibrothorax (i.e. grossly thickened pleura).

Q. Blunt costophrenic angle without any fluid collection (spurious):

1. Breast shadow in females.
2. X-ray taken in expiration.
3. Basal pneumonia in the elderly.
4. Thickened pleura.

Q. Minimal collection for radiological detection:

At least 300 mL fluid is required (earliest clinical detection requires 500 mL fluid).

Clinical Wisdom

Normally, a small amount of pleural fluid (i.e. 5–15 mL) is produced from capillaries in parietal pleura at a rate of 0.01 mL/kg/hour which is removed by lymphatics in parietal pleura.

Q. Earliest site of fluid collection in X-ray film (PA view):

Small amount of fluid <50 mL is not detected on PA view of chest X-ray. However, small effusions (e.g. 100 mL) are diagnosed earlier on lateral film where the fluid is collected in most dependent recess of pleura, the posterior costophrenic angle. A more collection (approximately 300 mL) produces obliteration of lateral costophrenic angle in PA view of chest radiograph.

Q. Why the upper margin of fluid goes towards axilla in chest X-ray?

Actually it is a radiological illusion. A horizontal section of hemithorax at the level of the upper margin of fluid shows that there is same amount of fluid present anteriorly, posteriorly and laterally. But it is a fact that X-ray beam traverse more fluid laterally than they do centrally because of the peculiar shape of hemithorax. So, we see the curved upper margin going towards axilla in X-ray picture.

Some clinicians opine that it is due to capillary suction between two layers of pleura, which draws the fluid up.

Q. How to diagnose small pleural effusion?

1. X-ray in lateral decubitus position.
2. USG of the chest.

Q. X-ray picture mimicking pleural effusion but 'dry tap' after needling reasons behind?

1. Thickened pleura.
2. Empyema thoracis (wide-bore needle required).
3. A mass lesion.

Q. Bilateral pleural effusion–possibilities (Fig. 3.3B):

1. Rheumatoid arthritis.
2. Systemic lupus erythematosus (SLE).
3. Lymphomas and leukaemias.
4. Bilateral tuberculous effusion (rare).
5. Pulmonary infarction.
6. Multiple pleural metastases.

- Remember, hydrothorax is usually bilateral.

Q. How malignant pleural effusion is suspected?

1. A convex bulge may be seen above the concave fluid level.
2. Collapse (absorption) of the lung may be associated with (in any part of either lung).
3. Trachea may be shifted to the same side (due to associated absorption collapse).
4. Elevated hemidiaphragm may indicate diaphragmatic palsy.
5. Prominence of hilar or parahilar shadow; erosion of ribs may be seen.
6. Recurrent, rapid collection of fluid.

- In this situation, first aspirate the fluid and again take a film.
- USG and CT scan of thorax differentiate easily a mass from loculated pleural effusion or pleural thickening.

PNEUMOTHORAX (Fig. 3.4)

Q. Description:

This is a PA view of the chest which reveals increased translucency on the right side of the chest with absence

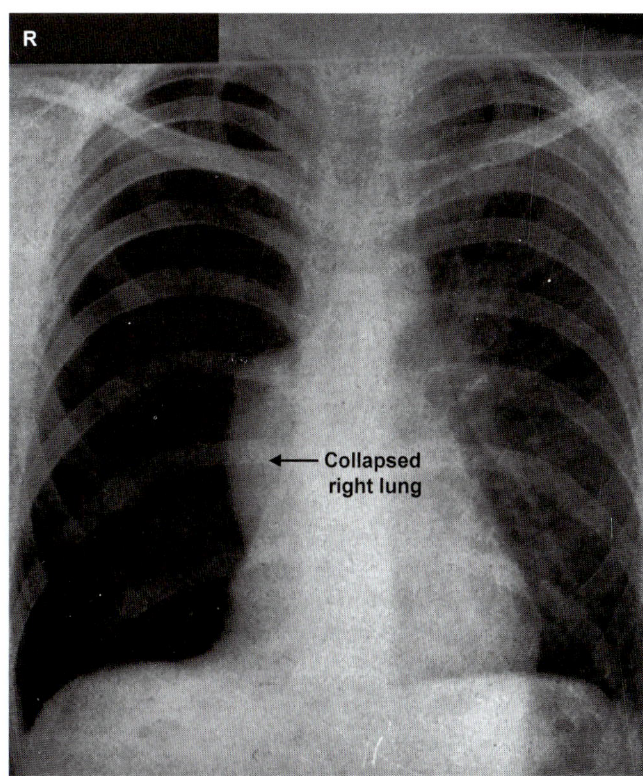

Fig. 3.4: Pneumothorax of right side

of bronchovascular markings. A sharply defined homogeneous opacity is seen lateral to right cardiac border which indicates the collapsed right lung. Both the costophrenic angles are, more or less, clear. Cardiac apex and tracheal shadow are not shifted in the X-ray film probably because of improper centering of the patient (usually shifts to opposite side, i.e. to the left). The left lung field is clear and normal.

Other points: Within normal limit.

- There is absence of bronchovascular markings beyond the collapsed lung border.
- In pneumothorax, these is abnormal collection of air within the pleural cavity.

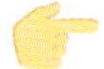 Conclusion

Right-sided pneumothorax.

- In a suspected case of pneumothorax, X-ray film is taken in erect posture while breath to hold in expiration.

Q. Types of pneumothorax:

a. Artificial,
b. Traumatic, and
c. Spontaneous
(i) Closed (ii) Open, and (ii) Valvular (tension).

- Recent classification of spontaneous pneumothorax: Primary (no known lung disease), and secondary types.
- To diagnose the type of pneumothorax, H/o onset and progress of symptoms are the two most important determinants.

Q. Why tension pneumothorax is lethal to the patients?

Marked mediastinal shift → decreased venous return → diminished cardiac output
\+
Severely compromised ventilation → arterial hypoxaemia
↓
Death may result, unless tackled immediately. It is a medical emergency to the internist.

Q. Unilateral hypertranslucency in chest X-ray film (D/D):

1. Pneumothorax (large).
2. Bulla.
3. Lung cyst.
4. Eventration of the left dome of the diaphragm.
5. Partial bronchial obstruction (unilateral): Obstructive emphysema.
6. Compensatory emphysema (secondary to post-lobectomy).
7. Contralateral thickened pleura (produces apparent increased translucency).
8. Mastectomy, congenital absence or atrophy (e.g. poliomyelitis) of pectoral muscle, Poland syndrome (absence of unilateral chest wall muscles).
9. Ball valve endobronchial obstruction.
10. Pulmonary thromboembolism.
11. Poor technique (e.g. rotation), scoliosis.

- In pneumothorax, always search for stigmata of tuberculosis in the other lung. Also look for signs of tube drainage and surgical emphysema (i.e. collection of air in the soft tissue).
- Sudden onset of unilateral pleuritic chest pain and dyspnoea are two chief complaints in pneumothorax.

HYDROPNEUMOTHORAX (Fig. 3.5)

Description:

This is a PA view of the chest (taken in erect posture) which shows a horizontal fluid level on right chest. There is increased translucency above the horizontal level which is lacking in lung markings ('pneumo' component) and a homogeneous opacity is seen below the horizontal level ('hydro' component). The homogeneous opacity ('hydro' component) is uniform, and medially it has merged with the cardiac silhouette. Trachea and cardiac shadows are shifted towards the left side. The left-sided costophrenic angle and the left lung show no apparent abnormality.

Other points: Within normal limit.

 Conclusion

Right-sided hydropneumothorax.

- *The X-ray picture of hydropneumothorax should always be taken in erect posture.*

Q. Can you localise the collapsed right lung?

No. It is usually hidden within the fluid and is not visible in the X-ray.

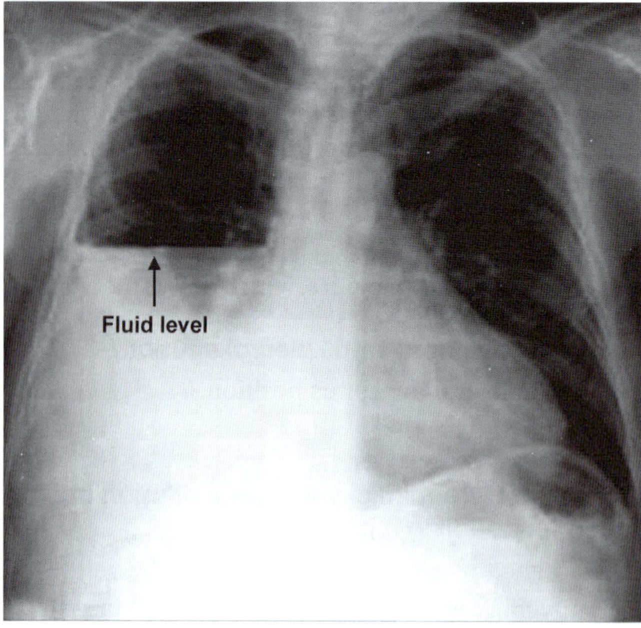

Fig. 3.5: Hydropneumothorax of right side

Q. Cardinal features of hydropneumothorax:

1. Shitting dullness.
2. Succussion splash, and
3. Horizontal fluid level (upper limit of dullness is horizontal).

Q. Differential diagnosis:

1. Haemopneumothorax or pyopneumothorax.
2. Infected lung cyst.
3. Very big lung abscess.

- Multiple air-fluid levels in lung suggest multiple lung abscess or loculated hydropneumothorax.

EMPHYSEMA (Fig. 3.6)

Q. Description:

This is a PA view of the chest which shows hypertranslucency, (i.e. dark lung fields indicating hyperinflation) of both the lung fields, wide intercostal spaces with horizontal ribs, low-flat diaphragm, narrow vertical heart (tear-drop heart or tubular heart), large and prominent hilar shadows with diminished peripheral vascular pattern. Few 'bullae' are seen as rounded areas of increased translucency with thin hair-line shadow forming the walls. There is no mediastinal shift.

Other points: Within normal limit.

- **Emphysema** is the permanent overinflation of air spaces in lung distal to terminal respiratory bronchioles as well as destruction of alveolar septae.
- HRCT of the chest is presently the definitive test to diagnose emphysema.

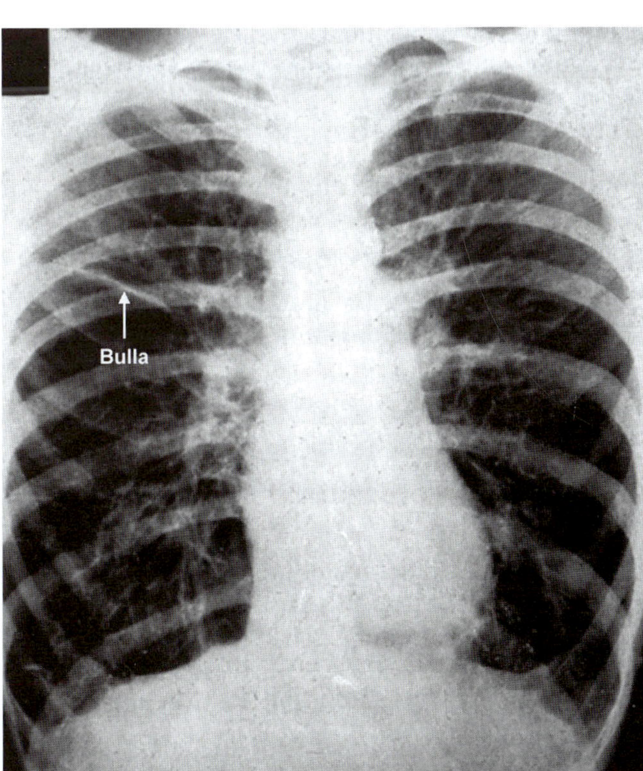

Fig. 3.6: Emphysema

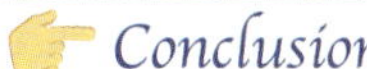

Conclusion

Bullous emphysema.

Q. Bilateral hypertranslucency in chest X-ray film (D/D):

1. Emphysema.
2. Bilateral pneumothorax.
3. Hyperinflated lungs.
4. Multiple bullae.
5. Bronchial asthma.
6. Overexposed (overpenetrated) film.
7. Fallot's tetralogy with pulmonary atresia, Ebstein's anomaly.

- **Bullae** are thin-walled (<1 mm in thickness) air spaces more than one centimeter in diameter, produced by rupture of alveolar walls. Bullae are usually situated subpleurally, and may be single or multiple, large or small. Rupture of bullae gives rise to pneumothorax.
- **Petite heart** (tubular heart, chicken heart or tear-drop heart), i.e. vertical, long and tubular heart is found in PA view of chest X-ray in emphysema, Addison's disease, anorexia nervosa, panhypopituitarism and constrictive pericarditis. The CTR is <25%.

BRONCHIECTASIS (Fig. 3.7)

Q. Description:

This is a PA view of the chest which shows multiple ring shadows at both lower zones (left > right). Areas of haziness or fibrosis is seen at places (bases). There is a big bulla seen in the right apex: Right costophrenic angle is blunt. There is no mediastinal shift.

Other points: Within normal limit.

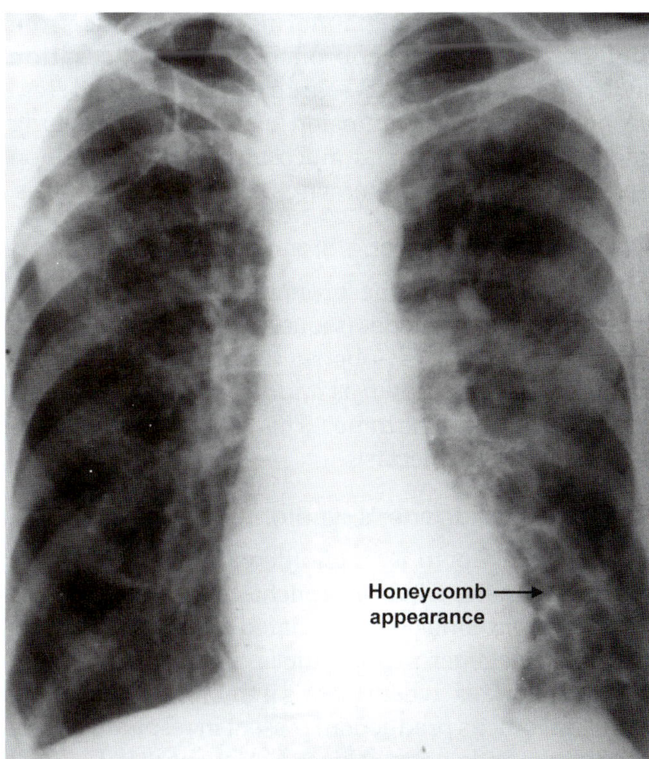

Fig. 3.7: Bronchiectasis

- Dilated bronchi give rise to 'tram line shadows' (linear streaks) or 'ring shadows', while dilated air-filled bronchi may produce 'gloved finger shadows'.
- **Bronchiectasis** is a chronic necrotizing infection of the bronchi and bronchioles which leads to abnormal and permanent dilatation of the airways.

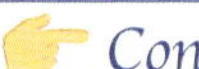 *Conclusion*

Bronchiectasis (bilateral and basal).

- Commonest site of bronchiectasis is left lower lobe and lingula.

Q. How a bronchiectasis patient presents?

The common presentation is cough with profuse (and often foetid) expectoration of sputum, usually more marked in the morning after waking from sleep. The patient may have haemoptysis and breathlessness. Features due to secondary infection may be associated with.

On examination, there is clubbing and coarse crepitations which are mostly found on the back of the chest (i.e. base of lung), and may reduce or disappear after coughing.

Q. What is bronchiectasis sicca (dry bronchiectasis)?

It is also known as dry bronchiectasis. Here, apices of lungs are affected (e.g. post-tuberculous bronchiectasis) in contrast to bases, and the patient will have minimum or no sputum production (i.e. dry cough as a result of easy drainage of sputum). Haemoptysis may be the only symptom.

Q. What is pseudobronchiectasis?

It is a bronchographic abnormality resulting from atelectasis and tracheobronchitis with ulceration in bronchial mucosa which mimic cylindrical bronchiectasis. Re-expansion of the collapsed lung and healing of bronchial mucosa make the condition reversible and thus it is known as pseudobronchiectasis.

Q. Describe middle lobe bronchiectasis:

When the middle lobe bronchus is obstructed by tuberculous lymph nodes (sequel to primary pulmonary tuberculosis), a post-obstructive bronchiectasis is formed, which is known as middle lobe bronchiectasis or 'middle lobe syndrome'. This is a variety of post-obstructive bronchiectasis.

Q. What is Kartagener's syndrome?

This is also known as immotile cilia syndrome. The syndrome is the triad of bronchiectasis, dextrocardia and recurrent sinusitis, associated with infertility (in males). Kartagener's syndrome is a variety of 'primary ciliary dyskinesia' where there is immotility of cilia (with abnormal mucus production) present in respiratory tract epithelium and sperm. Manes Kartagener (1897–1975) was a Swiss physician.

Q. Pathological types of bronchiectasis:

1. *Cylindrical (tubular) bronchiectasis:* Uniform dilatation of bronchi.
2. *Varicose bronchiectasis:* Beaded pattern of dilated bronchi.
3. *Cystic bronchiectasis:* Ballooned or saccular dilatation.

This classification (Reid's classification) is based on gross histological appearance.

- Haemoptysis in bronchiectasis is due to → hypertrophy of bronchial wall → friable mucosa → sloughing out of mucosa → opening of capillaries → bleeding.

Q. Outline of management of bronchiectasis:

1. Antibiotics (long-term azithromycin has an immunomodulatory effect) for infection control.
2. Autogenic (self-) drainage and postural drainage—A position is adopted where the lobe to be drained remains uppermost. This is to be continued for 20 minutes, once or twice daily, in empty stomach. Gentle purcussion over the front and back of the chest with cupped hands helps dislodgement of sputum (chest physiotherapy). Postural drainage should be assisted by deep breathing exercises.
3. Bronchodilators, mucolytics as and when necessary. Inhaled or oral corticosteroid may be helpful.
4. Bronchoscopic aspiration of inspissated sputum is rarely needed.
5. Surgery: Lobectomy in localised and unilateral lesion in young adults (<40 years) who are unresponsive to medical treatment; also in recurrent haemoptysis/pneumonias. Heart-lung transplantation is performed in bilateral extensive disease.
6. Pulmonary rehabiliation.
7. General: Nutritious diet, correction of anaemia.

- *Complications:* Recurrent pneumonia, pleurisy, pleural effusion, lung abscess, brain abscess, cor pulmonale, respiratory failure, amyloidosis.

Q. How to confirm your diagnosis?

Diagnosis can only be made with certainty by bronchography (old procedure) or high-resolution CT (HRCT) scan of thorax (definitive and preferred investigation). HRCT shows both the extent and distribution of bronchiectasis.

Q. Causes of 'honeycombing' or 'honeycomb lung' (D/D):

X-ray picture in honeycombing shows multiple air containing cyst-like shadows or ring shadows measuring 0.5–2 cm in diameter (mimicking bunch of grapes). This shadows are best visualised on high-resolution CT scan (HRCT) of chest and are found in:

1. Bronchiectasis.
2. Fibrosing alveolitis, systemic sclerosis, SLE, rheumatoid arthritis.

3. Cystic fibrosis, tuberous sclerosis, histiocytosis X, pneumoconiosis, asbestosis, sarcoidosis.
4. Extrinsic allergic alveolitis.
5. After use of drugs like busulphan, nitrofurantoin, bleomycin or melphalan.

Q. Why the right costophrenic angle is blunt?

It may be due to mild pleural reaction or developed as a result of small collection of fluid.

Q. 'Three-layer sputum test' in bronchiectasis:

When the copious and foetid sputum from a bronchiectatic patient is collected in a conical glass, it separates into three layers arbitrarily if allowed to stand for sometime and the layers are:

- Upper layer (serous layer) contain's froth (watery),
- Middle layer (mucoid layer) contain's liquid or thick sputum,
- Lower layer (purulent layer) contain's heavier particles, e.g. epithelial debris, masses of bacteria, clumps of pus cells, foul-smelling Dettrich's plugs, blood clots.

Q. Bedside diagnosis of bronchiectasis:

Read the section on 'Fibrosis or collapse of the lung' from 'Bedside Clinics in Medicine, Part I'.

LUNG ABSCESS (Fig. 3.8)

Q. Description:

This is a PA view of the chest showing a big cavity occupying the left-sided mid- and lower zones with thick, rough and shaggy inner wall. The cavity is circular, the lower homogeneous opacity with a horizontal level indicates fluid inside the cavity, and the hypertranslucency (devoid of lung markings) above the fluid level indicates air within the cavity. Rest of the lung fields are clear. Trachea and cardiac apex are in normal position.

Other points: Within normal limit.

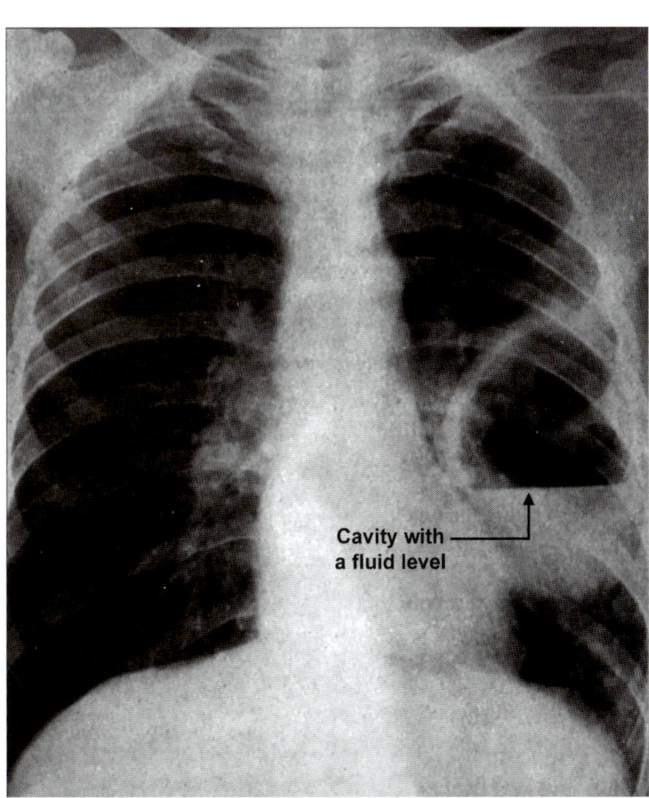

Fig. 3.8: Left-sided lung abscess

- Air-fluid level is the hallmark of lung abscess.
- **Lung abscess** is localised parenchymal destruction due to suppuration within the lung.

 *Conclusion*

Left-sided solitary lung abscess.

Q. Differential diagnosis:

Differentiate between the causes of 'horizontal fluid level' seen in the chest X-ray plate. They are:

1. Lung abscess (infiammation associated with necrosis of lung tissue).
2. Hydropneumothorax, haemopneumothorax or pyopneumothorax—Loculated variety.
3. Cardiospasm or achalasia cardia.
4. Diaphragmatic hernia (obstructed).
5. Infected lung cyst.
6. Carcinoma of the oesophagus.
7. Hydropneumopericardium (rare).

Q. Predisposing factors and bedside diagnosis of lung abscess:

a. Predisposing factors:

1. Alcoholism.
2. Old age.
3. Diabetes mellitus.
4. H/o convulsions.
5. H/o general anaesthesia.
6. Malnutrition or immunocompromised patients (e.g. corticosteroid therapy, AIDS).
7. Oral or pharyngeal sepsis, sinusitis, drowning, following bronchial obstruction, tracheo-oesophageal fistula, bulbar palsy, unconscious patients, achalasia cardia—predisposes aspiration of infected material.
8. Cystic fibrosis (thick, viscid sputum production).
9. Inadequately treated pneumonia, septic emboli, pulmonary infarction, infection of lung cyst.
10. Pulmonary tuberculosis (an important cause of lung abscess).

b. Specific infection by: *Streptococcus pneumoniae*, *Staphylococcus aureus*, *Klebsiella pneumoniae*, different fungi, etc.

c. Obstruction by: Bronchogenic carcinoma, foreign body, bronchial adenoma or enlarged lymph node.

d. Spread: ('local' from liver abscess or subphrenic abscess; 'haematogenous' from septicaemia, pelvic abscess).

e. Bedside diagnosis (clinical features):

I. *Symptoms:*

i. Anorexia, malaise, weakness, loss of weight and symptom of toxaemia; the onset may be insidious, acute or chronic.
ii. Fever: Intermittent, may be hectic; profuse sweating (often nocturnal).
iii. Cough with profuse, foetid, purulent and often blood-tinged sputum.
iv. Pleuritic chest pain or deep-seated chest discomfort.
v. Haemoptysis.

II. *Signs:*

i. Fever; may look toxic.
ii. Halitosis.
iii. Pallor (i.e. anaemia).
iv. Clubbing (develops rapidly).
v. Examination of the chest may be normal or may include signs of consolidation, i.e. no shifting of mediastinum, woody dullness on percussion, bronchial breath sound (cavernous or amphoric), pleural rub, coarse crepitations (often post-tussive crepitations) with increased vocal resonance. Sometimes, feature of empyema thoracis may be found.

- Frank signs of cavity are rarely found. Clubbing and pallor are present in chronic cases.
- Usually features of consolidation, rarely features of cavitation, and combined features of both are sometimes found in large abscess.

Q. Possible causes of 'multiple' lung abscess:

1. Aspiration of infected material.
2. Infection by *Staphylococcus aureus*, *Klebsiella* and fungus.
3. Amoebic liver abscess ruptured into lung.

Q. Causes of cavitary lesion in lung:

Infection [tuberculosis, *Klebsiella*, staphylococcal (lung abscess)], cavitating bronchogenic carcinoma, cystic lung disease, cystic bronchiectasis, hydatid cyst, bulla, Wegener's granulomatosis, pulmonary sequestration, rheumatoid nodule, preumatocele, and traumatic.

Q. Complications:

1. Massive haemoptysis.
2. Acute dry pleurisy.
3. Empyema thoracis.
4. Pneumothorax or pyopneumothorax.
5. Metastatic cerebral abscess.
6. Pyaemia.
7. Aspergillosis (fungus ball).
8. Trapped lung.
9. Bronchopleural fistula.
10. Amyloidosis (rare)—in chronic cases.

Q. Differential diagnosis of cavity containing air or fluid:

1. *Cavity with shaggy walls:* Lung abscess, bronchogenic carcinoma, tuberculous cavity (empty).
2. *Cavity with thin walls:* Tuberculous cavity (caseous), lung cyst, bullae, mycotic cavitation.
3. *Very small cavity with much thicker wall:* Bronchogenic carcinoma.

Q. Differential diagnosis of intracavitary mass lesion in chest X-ray:

1. Aspergilloma or mycetoma (the opacity or 'fungus ball' shifts with change of posture).
2. Cavitating carcinoma of lung.
3. Blood clot.

Q. What is 'pseudocavity'?

Cavity: Liquefaction necrosis within the lung (may remain empty or filled with secretion) surrounded by a wall whose thickness is >1 mm and is usually communicating with a patent bronchus.

Pseudocavity: Radiological appearance mimicking pulmonary cavity as a result of summation shadows of ribs, vessels, fibrotic bands, calcification or artefacts.

Clinical Wisdom

Bronchiectasis mimicks lung abscess clinically. In bronchiectasis, like lung abscess, there are profuse and foetid sputum production with clubbing, and presence of crepitations. To differentiate, in bronchiectasis the patient has no fever, is non-toxic and predominantly there are basal crepitations.

- In lung abscess, for areas of lung involvement in most of the times, read page 55.

Clinical Wisdom

Lung abscess is treated by appropriate antibiotics assisted by chest physiotherapy and postural drainage.

HOMOGENEOUS OPACITY OF HEMITHORAX (Fig. 3.9)

Q. Description:

This is a PA view of the chest which shows homogeneous opacity of the whole of the left chest. Left costophrenic angle is obliterated and the mediastinum has shifted to the right side. The right lung apparently shows no abnormality.

Other points: Within normal limit.

Conclusion

Homogeneous opacity of left hemithorax. The causes of unilateral dense homogeneous opacity are:

1. Massive pleural effusion.
2. Empyema thoracis.
3. Collapse of the lung (whole lung) or dense pulmonary fibrosis.

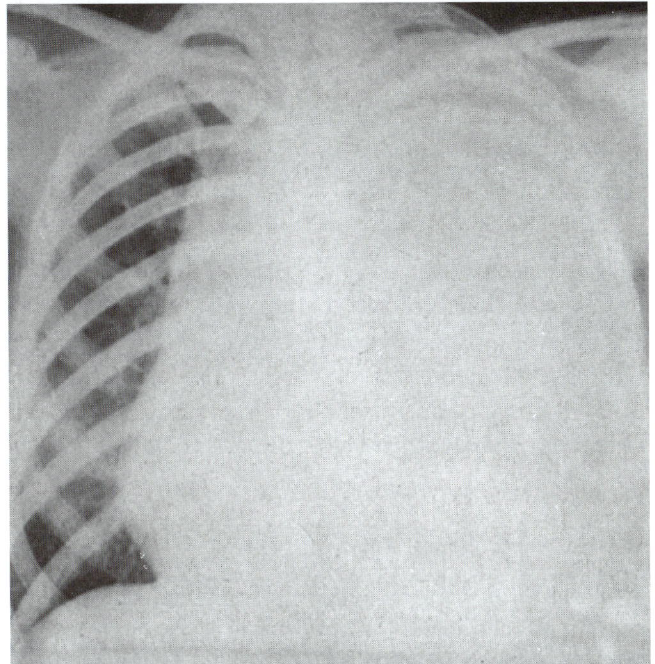

Fig. 3.9: Homogeneous opacity of left hemithorax

4. Consolidation (massive).
5. Thickened pleura.
6. Pleural mesothelioma or large pulmonary growth.
7. Agenesis of the lung.
8. Pneumonectomy (associated with crowding of ribs and resected ribs).
9. Destroyed lung (e.g. from chronic inflammation and fibrosis).
10. Technical (rotation scoliosis).

As there is mediastinal shifting towards the opposite side, No 1 and 2 are the most probable possibilities here.

Causes of **bilateral opaque hemithorax** are ARDS, bilateral pleural effusion, extensive bilateral consolidation and hyaline membrane disease.

Q. Shifting of trachea and cardiac shadow in all (see question above):

1. Massive pleural effusion or empyema thoracis: Opposite side.
2. Collapse or fibrosis of the lung: Same side.
3. Consolidation: No shifting.
4. Thickened pleura: Same side (in gross thickening).
5. Pleural mesothelioma or large pulmonary growth: Usually no shifting.
6. Agenesis of lung, pneumonectomy and destroyed lung: Same side with compensatory emphysema of the other lung.

COLLAPSE OF THE LUNG (Fig. 3.10)

Q. Description:

This is a PA view of the chest showing an opacity which is rather homogeneous and involving almost whole of

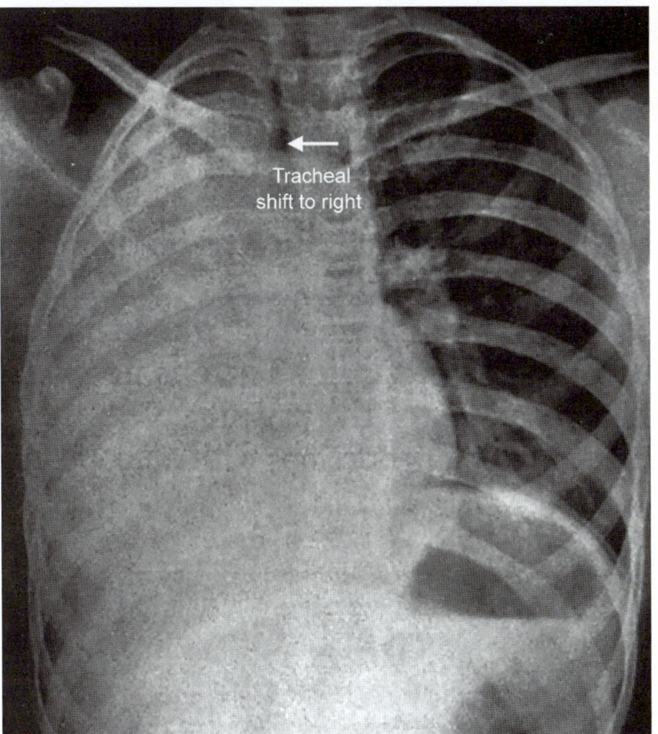

Fig. 3.10: Collapse of the right lung

the right lung. The trachea and cardiac apex have shifted towards the right side. Neither elevation of the right dome of diaphragm nor compensatory emphysema of the left lung is noted. Crowding of the ribs are seen on the right side with shrunken hemithorax.

Other points: Within normal limit.

Conclusion

Collapse (absorption) of the right lung.

- To diagnose collapse of the lung, both PA and lateral films are necessary.

Q. What is collapse of the lung?

Collapse of the lung is the reduction in lung volume due to absorption of alveolar air (absorption collapse) or resulting from expulsion of air from the alveoli (compression collapse).

Q. Types of collapse:

1. Absorption or active collapse, e.g. mucus plug, foreign body, bronchogenic carcinoma.
2. Compression or passive collapse, e.g. pleural effusion, pneumothorax, hydropneumothorax.

[3. Infarction collapse, e.g. pulmonary thromboembolism.]

Q. Clinical features of collapse:

1. *Absorption or active collapse:* Read 'Bedside Clinics in Medicine, Part I'.
2. *Compression or passive collapse:* Features of pleural effusion, pneumothorax or hydropneumothorax are clinically manifested.

Q. Differential diagnosis:

Same as 'homogeneous opacity of one hemithorax' described earlier.

FIBROSIS OF THE LUNG (Fig. 3.11)

Q. Description:

This is a PA view of the chest showing non-homogenous haziness, predominantly in the upper zone of the left lung with shifting of trachea and cardiac apex towards the left side. Crowding of the ribs at the left upper chest is seen. Left hemithorax is smaller than the right one. Both the costophrenic angles are clear Diaphragmatic contours are normal. Other points: Within normal limit.

- In chest X-ray of fibrosis of the lung one should also search for fibrous bands, pulled-up hilum and tenting of diaphragm which are absent here.

 *Conclusion*

Fibrosis involving upper zone of the left lung.

Q. Types and clinical features of fibrosis:

Read 'Bedside Clinics in Medicine, Part I'.

Q. Differential diagnosis of such localised haziness:

1. Fibrosis of the lung.
2. Pulmonary tuberculosis (primary).
3. Resolving bacterial pneumonia.
4. Thickened pleura.
5. Localised bronchiectasis (usually basal).
6. Alveolar cell carcinoma.

Q. Causes of fibrosis of the lung of cardiac origin:

1. Mitral stenosis, and
2. Pulmonary infarction (multiple).

Q. Basic clinical differentiation between fibrosis and collapse:

A. Fibrosis of the lung:

a. Onset is chronic.
b. Chest wall is retracted on the affected side.
c. Crowding of the ribs and drooping of the shoulder on the affected side.
d. Clubbing may be present. Breath sound is diminished but never absent. Fine crepitations may be heard.

B. Collapse of the lung:

a. Onset is acute.
b. Chest wall is flattened on the affected side.
c. Crowding of the ribs and drooping of the shoulder may be evident, if the collapse is prolonged.
d. Clubbing is absent. Breath sound is absent if a major bronchus is obstructed; usually no added sound.

- Fibrosis: Opacity is non-homogeneous; collapse: Opacity is homogeneous.
- In chest X-ray, features of collapse are more or less same as fibrosis but is of lesser in degree.

TUBERCULOUS INFILTRATIONS (Fig. 3.12)

Q. Description:

This is a PA view of the chest which reveals multiple wooly opacities involving both the lung fields, giving the

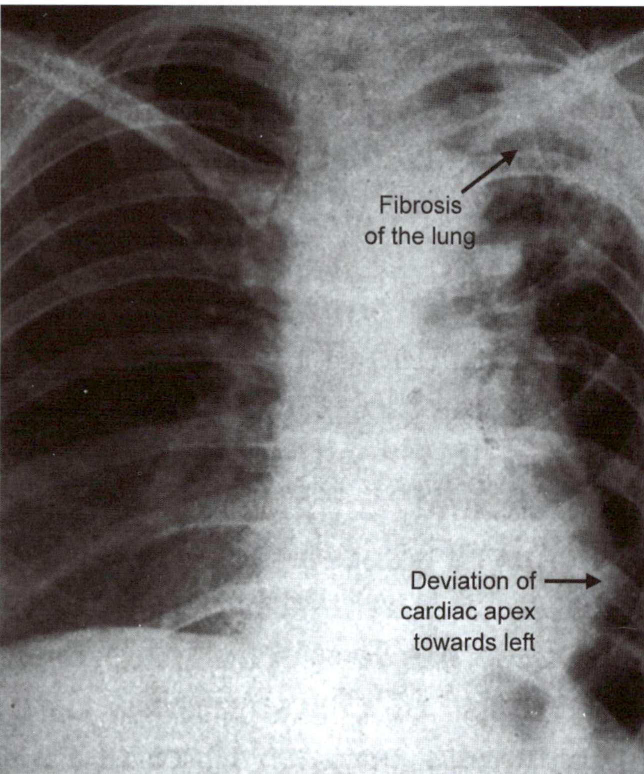

Fig. 3.11: Fibrosis of the left upper lobe

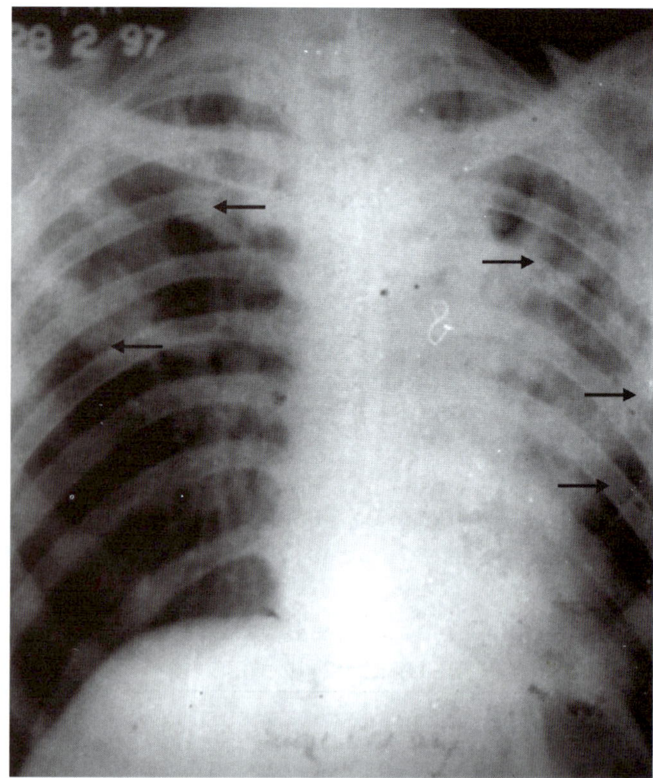

Fig. 3.12: Tuberculous infiltrations

X-ray film a 'moth-eaten appearance'. The costophrenic angles are clear. No mediastinal shift is seen.

Other points: Within normal limit.

Conclusion

Pulmonary tuberculosis (possibly post-primary type).

Q. Differential diagnosis of such an X-ray picture:

1. Pulmonary tuberculosis.
2. Resolving bacterial pneumonia.
3. Alveolar cell carcinoma.
4. Pulmonary oedema.
5. Fungal disease of the lung.
6. Pulmonary haemorrhage.

Q. Different radiological findings in pulmonary tuberculosis:

1. Wooly opacites or soft fluffy shadows (exudative phase).
2. Uni- or bilateral apical infiltrations.
3. Dense nodular shadow (proliferative phase).
4. Miliary mottlings.
5. Cavities (bilateral or multiple).
6. Fibrocaseous lesion.
7. Reticulonodular (if interstitium is involved).
8. Calcification (healed disease).
9. Tuberculoma (round or oval solitary shadow).
10. Bronchiectasis, especially affecting the upper zones.

- Involvement of pleura and pericardium is excluded.
- In adults, pulmonary component and in children, the glandular component is more prominent.

Clinical Wisdom

Active tuberculosis—1–4, cavities (thin-walled).
Healed tuberculosis— 6, 8, cavities (thick-walled).

Q. Features of tuberculous 'activity' in a patient:

1. Presence of AFB in sputum (i.e. sputum +ve cases), certainly indicates activity.
2. Patients having tuberculous toxaemia, i.e. evening rise of temperature, night sweats, anorexia, malaise, cough or loss of body weight are in favour of activity.
3. Crepitations heard after coughing (post-tussive crepitations) are often diagnostic of tuberculous cavity, and indicates activity.
4. A high ESR may be an indicator of activity.
5. Radiological features of activity are:
   a. Presence of a cavity.
   b. Soft shadows, even if very small.
   c. In case of extensive shadow, activity is likely.
   d. Progression of shadows in spite of treatment (in serial chest X-rays).

- Surest sign of activity: Sputumn positivity for AFB in direct smear examination.

Clinical Wisdom

A strongly +ve Mantoux test (e.g. induration >30 mm) may be quite compatible with activity.

Q. Types of pulmonary tuberculosis:

A. Parenchymatous:

a. Primary
b. Progressive primary
c. Post-primary
d. Miliary
e. 'Cryptic' miliary

B. Respiratory tract or airway infection:

a. Laryngitis
b. Bronchitis

C. Pleural:

a. Pleurisy
b. Pleural effusion
c. Pneumothorax
d. Hydropneumothorax

Q. What is 'primary complex'?

The subpleural tuberculous focus in the lung, hilar lymphadenopathy and interconnecting lymphatics constitute the primary complex (Ghon's complex).

Q. Can you describe the fate of a primary complex?

1. Commonly resolves within weeks or months.
2. Fibrosis/calcification/scar or cavity (reactivation) seen in chest X-ray.
3. In young children and immuno-compromised host—progressive primary disease or miliary tuberculosis may supervene.

Q. Enumerate different tuberculous foci in various organs:

1. Pulmonary:
   a. Subpleural: Ghon's focus.
   b. Deep apical: Ashman's focus.
   c. Subpleural focus in the upper lobe: Simon's focus.
2. Cerebral: Rich's focus.
3. Hepatic: Simmond's focus.
4. Blood vessels: Wigard's focus (present within tunica intima).
5. Besides these, there are primary lymph node, splenic, renal and intestinal focus.

Q. How post-primary tuberculosis develops?

It may arise by:

1. Direct progression of a primary tuberculosis.
2. Reactivation of a (dormant) primary lesion.
3. Haematogenous spread to lungs.
4. Exogenous re-infection.

Q. Factors implicated in reactivation of latent tuberculosis/re-infection of tuberculosis:

1. HIV infection (involves lower lobes of lung: Cavitation is rare).

2. Diabetes mellitus.
3. Immunosuppressive therapy including corticosteroids, antimetabolites, biologics in rheumatological diseases (e.g. infliximab).
4. Severe undernutrition.
5. End-stage chronic renal failure (CRF).
6. Malignancy.
7. Old age (Ageing).
8. Silicosis.

- Tuberculosis commonly affects the upper zone of lung but with associated immunodeficiency, lower and mid-zones may be involved.

Q. Complications of pulmonary tuberculosis:

Haemoptysis, pneumothorax, pleural effusion, hydropneumothorax, empyema thoracis, bronchiectasis, bronchopleural fistula, fibrosis of the lung, aspergilloma (in lung cavity), cor pulmonale, spread of tuberculosis to other organs, scar carcinoma of the lung, laryngitis, intestinal tuberculosis (from swallowed sputum), Poncet's polyarthritis and amyloidosis

Q. What is extrapulmonary tuberculosis (EPTB)?

These are isolated sites affected by *M. tuberculosis*, other than the lung. In reactivation tuberculosis, pulmonary disease is 55% and EPTB is 45%. The commonly affected extrapulmonary sites are lymph nodes (with non-healing sinuses over skin), pleural, gastrointestinal, pericardial, genitourinary (including kidney), nervous system (brain and meninges), skeletal system (osteomyelitis, caries spine, cold abscess), miliary tuberculosis (extrapulmonary), adrenal gland (Addison's disease), skin (lupus vulgaris), and eye (phlyctenular keratoconjunctivitis, choroiditis, iritis); there may be disseminated tuberculosis.

Q. Common causes of apical shadows (infiltrates) in chest X-ray:

1. Tuberculosis.
2. Aspergillosis.
3. Pancoast's tumour.
4. Bullae.
5. Pneumothorax.
6. Ankylosing spondylitis (i.e. upper lobe fibrosis).
7. Nocardiasis, actinomycosis, *Klebsiella pneumoniae* infection, silicosis.
8. Artefacts (hair balls or sternomastoid shadow).
9. Pleural cap (irregular crescentic, commonly left-sided, may represent old pleural thickening, incidence 7%).

Q. Haemoptysis in post-primary tuberculosis:

Mechanisms responsible:

1. Tuberculous pneumonitis: Bronchiolar ulceration and necrosis of adjacent vessels.
2. Rupture of Rasmussen's aneurysm (aneurysmally dilated pulmonary artery in a cavity).
3. Invasion of blood vessels by active tuberculous granulation tissue.
4. Oozing from the wall of an active cavitary lesion.

- Haemoptysis may result from aspergillosis in tuberculous cavity; lately, post-tuberculous bronchiectasis or scar carcinoma may lead to haemoptysis.

Q. How do you like to investigate a suspected case of pulmonary tuberculosis?

1. *Routine blood examination:* Hb, TC, DC, ESR (anaemia, mild elevation of lymphocytes and high ESR may be found).
2. *X-ray chest:* PA view, apical lordotic view to visualise the apex in a better way.
3. *Mantoux test:* Negative reaction usually rules out tuberculosis but a positive reaction (induration ≥10 mm) is observed in the presence of tuberculosis whether it is healed or active. It is often said that a +++ reaction (induration>30 mm, which may ulcerate) or a positive reaction below 3 years of age (non-BCG-vaccinated) indicates towards active tuberculosis.
4. Sputum examination for AFB (acid-fast bacilli) for consecutive 2 days (as per RNTCP), or detection of AFB in gastric aspirate or gastric lavage in children, or search for AFB from laryngeal swab, bronchoalveolar lavage in selected cases—confirms the diagnosis.
5. Biopsy of the cervical lymph nodes, and examination of pleural fluid in selected cases.
6. Culture of sputum for *M. tuberculosis* in Lowenstein-Jensen media (or Middlebrook agar); result usually comes within 8–12 weeks.
7. Newer diagnostic techniques (costly and not routinely practised):
   a. ELISA (IgG or IgM)—not much useful as the bacilli contains complex antigenic structure; having high specificity (97%) with low sensitivity (65%). The result is not dependent on tuberculin test or BCG-vaccination status.
   b. Adenosine deaminase activity (ADA)—in CSF, pleural, pericardial or ascitic fluid.
   c. Detection of tuberculostearic acid.
   d. Polymerase chain reaction (PCR) for tuberculosis from sputum, pleural fluid, CSF or blood—to detect mycobacterial DNA.
   e. Radiolabelled DNA and RNA probes, specific for different mycobacterial species, identify organisms in culture—nucleic acid amplification assay.
   f. 'Bactec' test—radioisometric blood culture; result within 7 days.
   g. Cartridge-based nucleic acid amplification test (CB-NAAT) is known as GeneXpert test, which is helpful in early diagnosis of tuberculosis (usually done from sputum).
   h. QuantiFERON-TB Gold test—requires a whole blood sample and the result is available within 24 hours, and is also known as 'interferon-gamma

release assays (IGRAs)'. This test detects latent as well as active disease.

MILIARY MOTTLINGS (Fig. 3.13)

Q. Description:

This is a PA view of the chest which shows small discrete nodules or miliary opacities (spotted or mottled appearance) of the size of 1–2 mm diameter, involving all the zones of both the lungs. There is no mediastinal shifting. Both the costophrenic angles are clear.

A dense homogeneous opacity is seen in left apex which may be encysted pleural effusion, benign tumour of lung or a soft tissue shadow.

Other points: Within normal limit.

Conclusion

The probable differential diagnosis of **'miliary mottlings'** in chest X-ray are:

1. Acute millary tuberculosis (generalised, uniform size, smaller shadows, usually hilar lymph nodes are not affected, and common in children; upper zones are always involved).
2. Tropical eosinophilia (usually involves the mid- and lower zones, non-uniform, larger shadows with hilar lymph nodes involvement, persons of any age are affected).
3. Miliary carcinomatosis (rare, slightly larger shadows of secondary deposits; may be the primary source in breast, bronchus, kidney or thyroid).
4. Pneumoconiosis (size 3–5 mm coal-miners commonly).
5. Acute extrinsic allergic alveolitis (often more pronounced in upper zones).
6. Acute lymphangitis carcinomatosa [a form of metastatic carcinoma where the pulmonary lymphatics are invaded and are often blocked by malignant cells; 2–3 mm nodules with thickening of pulmonary septa (Kerley's A and B lines); may be the primary source in bronchus, stomach, breast, colon or prostate].
7. Pulmonary haemosiderosis (smaller but dense shadows).
8. Sarcoidosis (larger shadows, spare apices but hilar lymph nodes may be enlarged).
9. Fungal diseases like histoplasmosis, coccidioidomycosis.
10. Miscellaneous: Collagen vascular diseases, post-chickenpox bronchopneumonia, mycoplasma pneumonia, mitral stenosis (having pulmonary haemosiderosis from recurrent haemoptysis), aspiration of blood or vomitus, multiple pulmonary infarction, Loeffler's syndrome, hyaline membrane disease, alveolar microlithiasis, Langerhans cell histiocytosis, after lipoidal bronchography, artefacts like multiple skin warts or neurofibromatosis.

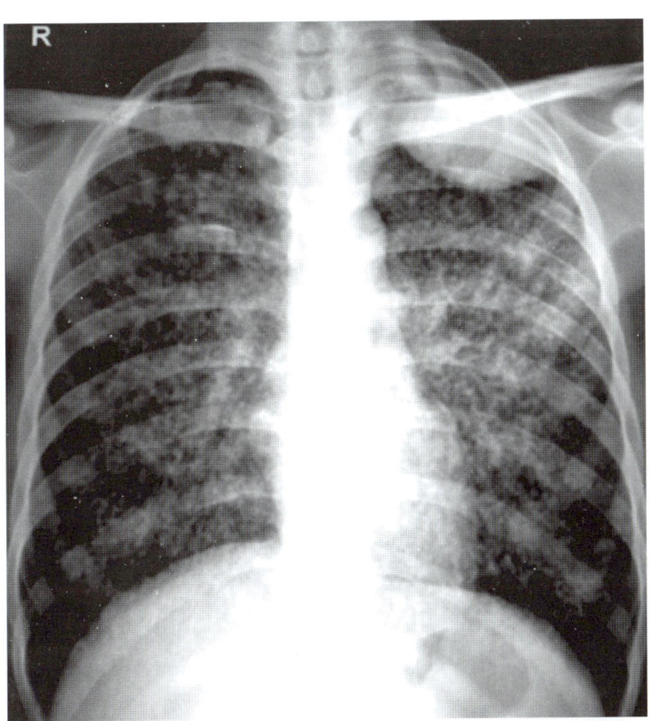

Fig. 3.13: Miliary mottlings

- Early lesions of 'miliary mottlings' are often better visualised in over-penetrated PA view of the chest with viewing the X-ray plate by putting a bright light behind. The nodular shadows of miliary mottlings are detected earlier in CT scan than plain radiograph.

Q. Clinical features of acute miliary tuberculosis:

Read 'Bedside Clinics in Medicine. Part I'.

- The 1–2 mm miliary opacities mimic millet seeds and it is why these type of shadows are known as 'miliary mottlings'.

Q. 'Calcification' seen in the chest X-ray:

a. *Parenchymal (lung):* Tuberculosis (commonest), histoplasmosis, hamartomas (popcorn calcification), silicosis (egg-shell calcification), post-chickenpox bronchopneumonia, tumour (usually benign), alveolar microlithiasis, haemosiderosis from recurrent haemoptysis, lung abscess.
b. *Pleural:* Tuberculosis, asbestosis, empyema thoracis.
c. *Cardiac:* Aortic arch (ring shaped), pericardial (constrictive pericarditis), calcification of heart valves (e.g. mitral and aortic), prosthetic valve, ventricular aneurysm (oval calcification), calcification of coronary arteries, left atrial myxoma with thrombi.
d. *Mediastinal (hilar):* Lymphadenopathy from tuberculosis or sarcoidosis, teratodermold, silicosis.
e. *Chest wall:* Costal cartilage calcification, cervical or axillary lymph nodes, nipple in females, phleboliths, Guinea worm in soft tissue, artefact.

MEDIASTINAL WIDENING (Fig. 3.14)

Q. Description:

This is a PA view of the chest which shows few circumscribed, tiny, coin-like shadows involving the

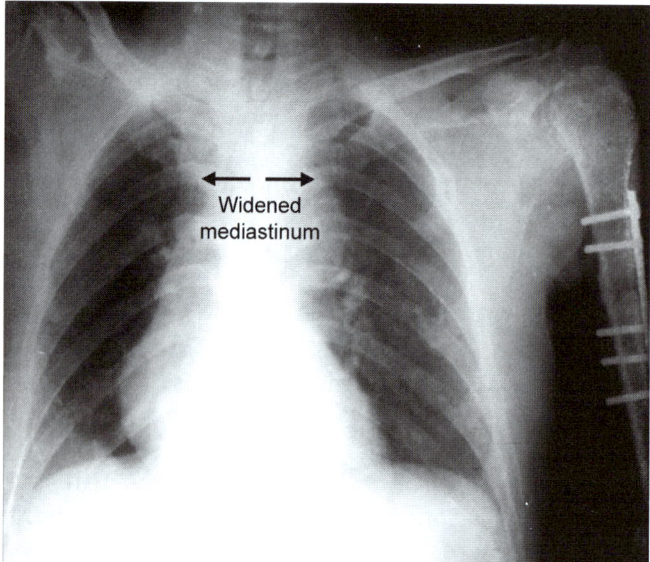

Fig. 3.14: Mediastinal widening

left lung field with gross mediastinal widening. The left hilum is heavy. Both the costophrenic angles are clear and there is absence of mediastinal shifting. Diaphragms are normal in position with normal contour. The left humerus shows fracture, treated by nailing and plating.

Other points: Within normal limit.

Conclusion

Apparently it is a case of bronchogenic carcinoma with pathological fracture of left humerus.

Q. Differential diagnosis of 'coin lesion' (or solitary nodule) in the lung:

1. Bronchogenic carcinoma.
2. Bronchial adenoma.
3. Metastatic nodules (secondary infiltrations).
4. Hamartomas.
5. Granuloma (tuberculosis, fungal infection, e.g. histoplasmosis, eosinophilic granuloma, Wegener's granulomatosis).
6. Cyst (congenital, hydatid, dermoid, polycystic disease), lipoma, fibroma.
7. Miscellaneous: Arteriovenous fistula, tuberculoma, interlobar effusion, mesothelioma of pleura, pulmonary infarction, fat embolism, lung abscess, localised pneumonia, rheumatoid nodule, intrapulmonary lymph nodes, bronchopulmonary sequestration.

- ***Coin lesion:*** Coin-shaped round lesion (usually of 1–5 cm) with well-circumscribed margin which is completely surrounded by normal aerated lung, and without associated lung, pleural or mediastinal pathology. It may or may not be associated with calcification.

Solitary pulmonary nodule: Spherical, <3 cm in diameter, intrapulmonary, roentgenographic density (granuloma, carcinoma, metastasis).

Mass lesion: Lesions >3 cm in size, and are often malignant (carcinoma, metastasis, hamartoma).

Cannonball shadow: Well circumscribed, large, round shadows mimicking cannonballs, and are commonly due to metastases from extra-thoracic malignancy (e.g. hypernephroma or carcinoma of breast, thyroid, etc.).

Features of malignant pulmonary nodule in chest X-ray:
1. Size >3 cm.
2. Irregular border.
3. Lack of calcification.

Plus, age >40 years with history of smoking (past or present).

Q. Differential diagnosis of mediastinal widening:

1. Lymph node enlargement as a result of bronchogenic carcinoma (primary or secondary), lymphoma, tuberculosis, sarcoidosis, fungal infection of the lung.
2. *Mediastinal mass:*
   a. *Anterior and middle mediastinum:* Teratodermoid, thymoma, lymphoma, metastatic carcinoma, aortic aneurysm, bronchogenic cyst, pericardial cyst.
   b. *Superior mediastinum:* Thymoma, retrosternal thyroid, metastatic carcinoma, aortic aneurysm, Zenker's diverticulum, dermoid cyst, tumours of parathyroid.
   c. *Posterior mediastinum:* Neurogenic tumour (neurofibroma), lymphoma, aortic aneurysm, achalasia cardia, hiatus hernia, paravertebral abscess, pharyngo-oesophageal pouch.

- Bronchogenic carcinoma and lymphoma are common causes of mediastinal widening in clinical practice.

Q. Causes of hilar enlargement (or lymphadenopathy):

A. Bilateral:

1. Expiratory film.
2. Sarcoidosis.
3. Lymphoma, bronchogenic carcinoma.
4. Tuberculosis, histoplasmosis.
5. Increased pulmonary flow due to septal defects in heart.
6. Pulmonary hypertension.
7. Silicosis.
8. Lymphangitis carcinomatosa.

B. Unilateral:

1. Rotation, scoliosis.
2. Bronchogenic carcinoma.
3. Sarcoidosis.
4. Lymphoma.
5. Tuberculosis.
6. Pulmonary artery aneurysm.
7. Pericardial cyst or tumour.
8. Secondaries in lung.
9. Pulmonary thromboembolism.

- 'Displaced hilar shadows' are found in post-tubercular fibrosis (upper lobe) with pulled-up hilum, or in lobar or segmental collapse of the lung.

Q. Differential diagnosis of elevation of diaphragm:

a. *Unilateral:* Phrenic nerve paralysis, amoebic liver abscess, basal pulmonary infarction, subphrenic abscess, basal collapse or fibrosis, sub-pulmonary pleural effusion, eventration of the diaphragm, splenic cyst, scoliosis, massive hepatomegaly or splenomegaly.

b. *Bilateral:* Poor inspiration, obesity, ascites, abdominal distension, pregnancy, huge mass in the abdomen, hepatosplenomegaly, fibrosing alveolitis, bilateral phrenic nerve paralysis, bilateral basal collapse, pneumoperitoneum, restrictive lung disease.

- ***Diaphragmatic hump:*** This is a localised elevation on the medial aspect of right dome of diaphragm. The hump is smooth and convex upwards, and is usually a normal finding.
- ***Tenting of diaphragm:*** The diaphragm may be pulled upwards losing its smooth upward convex contour by basal pleurisy. Here, the elevation of diaphragm is abrupt and 'tent-like'.
- ***Flat diaphragm:*** Perpendicular height of diaphragm is <2.5 cm from base, i.e. in emphysema.

Q. Types of bronchogenic carcinoma:

a. Non-small cell carcinoma (80%):
   1. Squamous or epidermoid carcinoma (35%)
   2. Adenocarcinoma (including bronchioloalveolar) (30%)
   3. Large cell carcinoma (also known as anaplastic carcinoma) 15%

b. Small-cell carcinoma or oat cell carcinoma (20%).

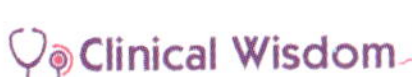

Clinical Wisdom

This is the pattern of bronchogenic carcinoma in UK. In USA, the incidence of adenocarcinoma is a bit higher replacing squamous cell carcinoma (as in India).

Q. Clinical findings expected in this patient:

Features of 'superior mediastinal syndrome' may be present.

PULMONARY OEDEMA (Fig. 3.15)

Q. Description:

This is a PA view of the chest which shows "bat's wing" or "butterfly" appearance of confluent shadows which extends from the hilum to the mid- and upper zones. These bilateral pulmonary clouding (perihilar opacities) escapes the peripheral and basal zones. Cardiac silhouette is enlarged. Costophrenic angles are clear and there is no mediastinal shifting.

Other points: Within normal limit.

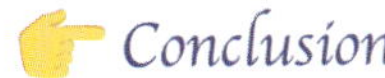

Conclusion

Pulmonary oedema.

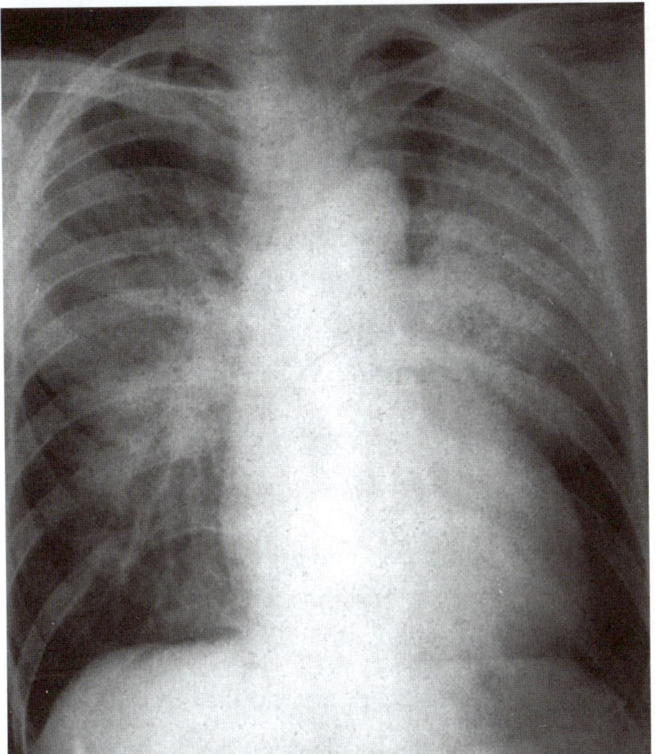

Fig. 3.15: Pulmonary oedema

Q. Differential diagnosis (of widespread alveolar opacities):

1. Pneumonia.
2. Acute lung injury or ARDS.
3. Alveolar cell carcinoma.
4. Uraemic pneumonitis.
5. Intra-alveolar haemorrhage.
6. Fat emboli.
7. Metastasis by haematogenous route.
8. Fungal disease of lung.

- One has to differentiate pulmonary oedema from pulmonary infection. Pulmonary oedema is acute in onset, usually bilateral and rapidly resolves with treatment, while the patient is afebrile.
- In CT scan of thorax, pulmonary oedema gives a 'ground-glass opacity'.

Q. Different causes of pulmonary oedema:

a. *Cardiogenic:* Left-sided heart failure (i.e. left ventricular or left atrial failure), acute myocardial infarction, cardiac dysrrhythmias, pulmonary thromboembolism.

b. *Non-cardiogenic:* Drowning, inhalation of toxins, Gram-ve septicaemia, fluid overload, insecticide poisoning, narcotic overdose, haemorrhagic pancreatitis, falciparum malaria, high altitude.

Q. Causes of unilateral pulmonary oedema:

1. Too much aspiration of pleural fluid (ipsilateral pulmonary oedema).

2. Bursting of lung abscess open within the lung (ipsilateral).
3. Aspiration of foreign body (ipsilateral).

Q. X-ray shows pulmonary oedema without any cardiac enlargement:

1. Mitral stenosis (producing left atrial failure).
2. Constrictive pericarditis, and
3. Causes of non-cardiogenic pulmonary oedema.

Q. 'Pressure changes in left atrium' in evolution of pulmonary oedema:

1. *Normal left atrial pressure:* 2–10 mm of Hg.
2. *Prominence of upper lobar pulmonary veins in X-ray:* 12 mm of Hg.
3. *Interstitial oedema:* >15 mm of Hg.
4. *Kerley's B lines in chest X-ray:* >20 mm of Hg.
5. *Pulmonary oedema:* >25 mm of Hg.

Q. Evolution of radiographic features in pulmonary oedema:

a. *Interestitial oedema:* As the left atrial pressure rises >20 mm of Hg (i.e. pulmonary venous pressure increases), normally invisible interstitial septa becomes visible as a result of interstitial oedema (Kerley's B and A lines).
b. *Alveolar (pulmonary) oedema:* When the left atrial pressure is >25 mm of Hg, fluid collects within the alveoli giving rise to parahilar "bat's-wing" or "butterfly" shadow in chest X-ray.

THORACIC NEOPLASM (Fig. 3.16)

Q. Description:

This is a skiagram of the chest, PA view which shows a dense homogeneous opacity (with sharp margin) occupying the left upper and mid-zone. There is absence of 'air bronchogram'. Mediastinal widening, mediastinal shifting, obliteration of the costophrenic angles (though not clearly seen), elevation of diaphragm are absent. There is absence of any rib destruction. Radiographer's signal (L for left) is wrongly given.

Other points: Within normal limit.

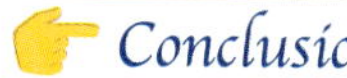
Conclusion

Apparently it is a case of pulmonary neoplasm.

Q. Differential diagnosis of such a lesion in X-ray:

1. Bronchogenic carcinoma.
2. Pneumonia.
3. Lung cyst.
4. Aortic aneurysm.
5. Granuloma.
6. Artefact.

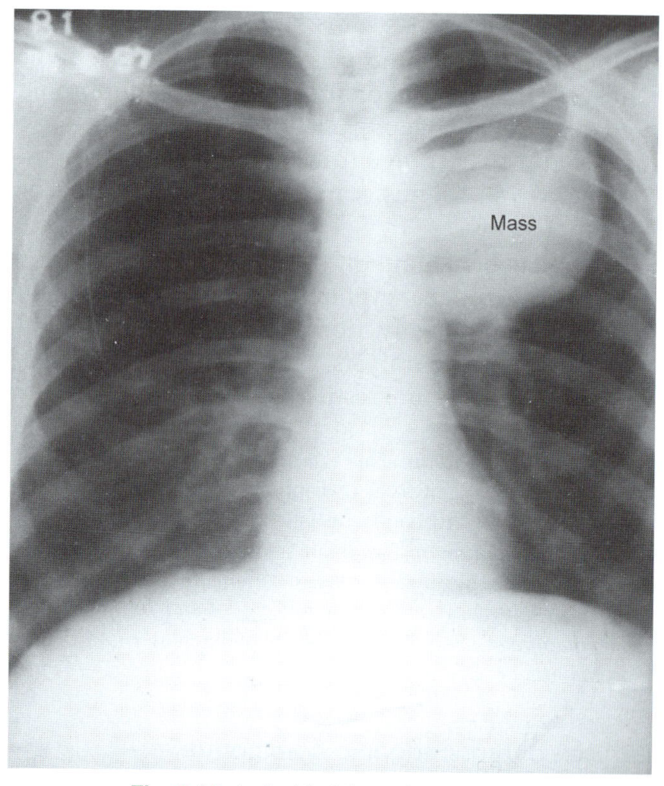

Fig. 3.16: Left-sided thoracic neoplasm

Q. Common symptoms in bronchogenic carcinoma:

1. *Non-specific systemic symptoms:* Anorexia, weakness, loss of weight, nausea and vomiting, pyrexia.
2. *Pulmonary symptoms:* Cough, haemoptysis, chest pain, breathlessness.
3. *Metastatic symptoms:* Jaundice, neuralgic pain over the extremities, haematuria, convulsions, pathological fracture, SVC syndrome (dysphagia, dyspnoea, hoarseness of voice), lymphoedema of chest and upper extremity with severe breathlessness, spinal cord compression with paraplegia.
4. ***Paraneoplastic syndrome*** (not related to metastasis):
   a. *Systemic:* Anorexia, loss of weight, cachexia, lassitude.
   b. *Endocrine:* Cushing's syndrome, hyperparathyroidism, carcinoid syndrome, syndrome of inappropriate ADH secretion (SIADH), hypoglycaemia.
   c. *Neuromuscular:* Peripheral neuropathy, myasthenic syndrome (Lambert-Eaton syndrome), myopathy, polymyositis, cortical degeneration, subacute cerebellar degeneration, encephalomyelopathy.
   d. *Haematological:* Normoblastic anaemia, granulocytosis, leucoerythroblastosis, polycythemia, haemolytic anaemia, thrombocytopenia, disseminated intravascular coagulation (DIC).
   e. *Cutaneous:* Dermatomyositis, acanthosis nigricans, pruritus, herpes zoster.
   f. *Bones and connective tissue:* Clubbing, hypertrophic pulmonary osteoarthropathy (HPOA) and pachydermoperiostitis.

g. *Vascular:* Migratory thrombophlebitis, marantic endocarditis, gangrene.
h. *Renal:* Nephrotic syndrome, glomerulonephritis.
i. *Miscellaneous:* Gynaecomastia.

- Paraneoplastic syndrome is seen when a hormone with biologic activity is secreted by the tumour.

Q. Mention special features of Pancoast tumour (or superior pulmonary sulcus tumour syndrome):

It is an apical bronchogenic carcinoma usually of non-small cell variety. It rapidly infiltrates brachial plexus, sympathetic trunk, pleura, pericardium and ribs, which gives rise to:
1. Severe shoulder and upper extremity pain.
2. Wasting and weakness of ipsilateral hand.
3. Horner's syndrome
4. Hoarseness of voice and bovine cough (by pressure over recurrent laryngeal nerve).

Q. Rib erosion and rib notching:

a. *Rib erosion:* There is destruction of ribs; ribs may look moth-eaten. It is found in bronchogenic carcinoma, multiple myeloma, histiocytosis X disease.
b. *Rib notching:* Notching of the ribs may be present in the upper border, lower border or randomly. It is found in coarctation of aorta (lower border of 3rd to 8th rib), hyperparathyroidism (random), chronic SVC and IVC obstruction, subclavian artery obstruction, arteriovenous fistula, neurofibromatosis (upper border), enlarged nerve, Fallot's tetralogy, pulmonary stenosis, after Blalock-Taussig shunt operation done in Fallot's tetralogy.

- Rib notching of coarctation of aorta in chest X-ray is known as Dock's sign, and is due to collaterals.
- Bilateral rib notching is congenital, or found in coarctation of aorta and neurofibromatosis.

Q. Different radiological features of bronchogenic carcinoma in chest X-ray:

1. Solitary, dense, well-circumscribed pulmonary opacity; sometimes a cavity within.
2. Dense, irregular hilar opacity with peripheral extension.
3. Localised emphysema (an early feature), atelectasis involving a segment, lobe, or the whole lung.
4. Mediastinal widening, rib erosion, elevated hemi-diaphragm (phrenic nerve palsy), pleural effusion may be seen.
5. Linear streaks radiating from hilum, or miliary mottlings developing as a result of lymphangitis carcinomatosa.
6. Hilar and mediastinal lymphadenopathy.

- In a suspected X-ray of thoracic neoplasm, always search for rib erosion, pleural effusion and diaphragmatic palsy. 18F-FDG-PET (fluorodeoxyglucose positron emission tomography) scan distinguishes benign and malignant lesion, as cancer cells take up FDG very quickly.

Q. Different investigations done to diagnose bronchogenic carcinoma:

1. Chest X-ray and HRCT scan of chest.
2. Sputum examination for cytology (e.g. malignant cells).
3. Pleural fluid examination, if pleural effusion develops.
4. Biopsy of scalene node.
5. Bronchoscopy.
6. Lung biopsy.
7. FDG-PET scan.

Q. 'Pseudotumour' (mimicking neoplasm in lung) in chest X-ray:

1. Paravertebral cold abscess.
2. Scoliosis.
3. Aortic aneurysm.
4. Achalasia cardia.
5. Extramedullary haematopoiesis in chronic haemolytic anaemia (e.g. thalassaemia).

B. X-RAY CHEST—HEART

MITRAL STENOSIS (Fig. 3.17)

Q. Description:

This is a PA view of the chest which shows **'mitralisation' of heart**, or straightening of the left border of heart and is due to (from above downwards),

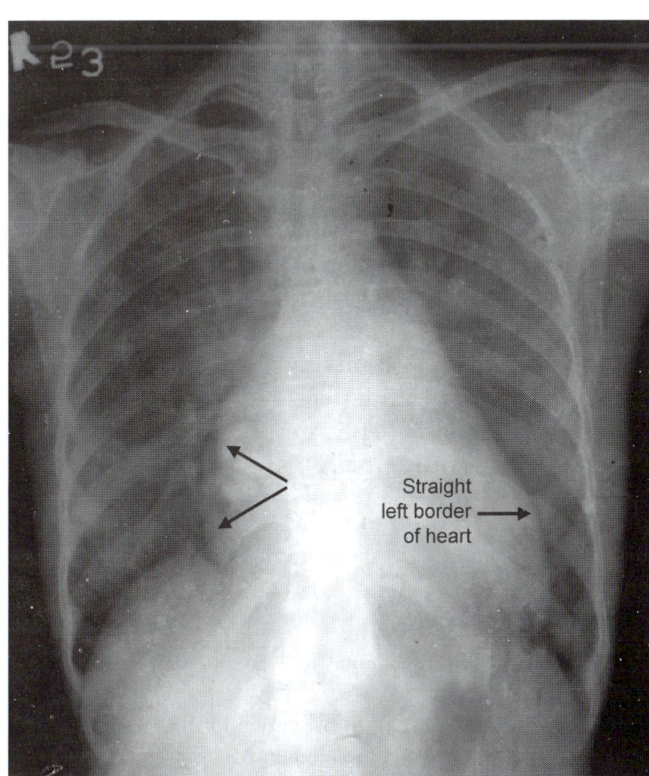

Fig. 3.17: Mitral stenosis

Radiology

a. Small aortic knuckle (due to low cardiac output),
b. Conspicuous convexity due to dilated pulmonary artery (due to pulmonary hypertension),
c. Convexity produced due to prominent left atrial appendages, and
d. Normal left border of left ventricle.

Double contour of the right border of heart or double-density sign (the upper and outer border is due to LA, and the lower and inner border is due to RA enlargement) is present here (shown by arrows).

The cardiac size shows enlargement in transverse diameter (RVH). Dilated pulmonary arteries at hilum with peripheral pruning is seen (evidence of pulmonary hypertension). Upper lobar pulmonary veins are dilated (or upper lobe diversion).

Kerley's B line, fan-shaped opacity at hilum (pulmonary oedema), mitral valve calcification, features of haemosiderosis are not evident here.

Other points: Within normal limit.

- The apex of the heart in the X-ray plate seems to be downwards as well as outwards (RVH + LVH). As MS does not produce LVH, think of other causes associated with MS (see the question below), i.e. this X-ray plate probably does not belong to a case of isolated MS.
- The D/D of this X-ray picture is ASD or left atrial myxoma.

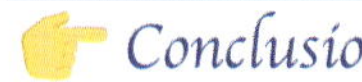

Mitral stenosis with features of pulmonary hypertension.

Q. What are "Kerley's—A, B and C" lines?

a. *Kerley's A lines:* Ragged, unbranched lines which spread out from hilum into the mid- and upper zones.
b. *Kerley's B lines:* Fine, dense, 1–2 cm in length, non-branching horizontal lines at the base of the lung (near costophrenic angles).
c. *Kerley's C lines:* Fine, interlacing lines and are seen in the central and parahilar region.

A, B and C lines are also known as 'septal lines'. These white lines represent 'dilated lymphatics and distended interlobular septa'. B line is most commonly seen. They occur most often in pulmonary oedema as a result of chronic pulmonary venous hypertension. Kerley's B line has a relation with left atrial pressure (B-lines are invariably present if LA pressure goes above 20 mm of Hg). These lines are actually found in left-sided heart failure.

- Kerley's **A** line stands for apex, **B** line for base and **C** line for central region of the lung.
- Kerley's B lines are found in:
  a. Pulmonary venous hypertension, e.g. LVF, left atrial failure from MS.
  b. Dilated lymphatics due to lymphatic obstruction, e.g. lymphangitis carcinomatosa, pneumoconiosis.
- PJ Kerley (1900–1979) was a British radiologist.

Q. Radiological features of raised left atrial pressure:

1. Prominence of hilar pulmonary vascular shadows.
2. Dilated upper lobar pulmonary veins.
3. Kerley's B lines, and
4. Interstitial pattern of pulmonary shadow—either diffuse haziness or "bat's-wing" appearance of acute pulmonary oedema.

Q. Radiological evidences of pulmonary arterial hypertension:

Causes:

1. Left-to-right shunt (ASD, VSD, PDA).
2. Long standing left-sided heart disease (MS).
3. COPD or other chronic pulmonary diseases (e.g. interstitial lung disease).

Radiological features:

1. Bulging pulmonary arteries at hilum (parahilar prominence).
2. Peripheral 'pruning' (peripherally pulmonary arteries taper sharply).
3. Disappearance of Kerley's B lines.

- Enlarged pulmonary artery (>16 mm) in chest X-ray is due to left-to-right shunt (e.g. ASD, VSD, PDA), pulmonary hypertension and poststenotic dilatation of pulmonary stenosis.

Q. Radiological evidences of pulmonary venous hypertension:

Pulmonary venous hypertension is due to backward pressure passed on from left heart chambers to the pulmonary veins.

Causes:

1. Left-sided heart failure (LAF/LVF), i.e. mitral or aortic valve disease, IHD, cardiomyopathy, left atrial myxoma.
2. Chronic cor pulmonale.
3. Pulmonary thromboembolism.
4. Pulmonary venous obstruction (veno-occlusive disease).

Radiological features: Prominent vascular markings as a result of venous congestion in lung (upper lobe vessels become prominent initially followed by parahilar congestion) → followed by features of raised left atrial pressure, i.e. development of Kerley's B lines and pulmonary oedema (see above).

Q. X-ray shows 'mitralisation', but the apex is down and out—possibilities:

Always try to determine to position of the cardiac apex by counting intercostal spaces (whether outwards, or downwards as well as outwards) in all chest X-ray (PA view).

Isolated MS with pulmonary hypertension and RVH will have outward apex. As MS (evidenced by mitralisation) does not produce LVH, other causes of LVH should be considered to be associated with MS if the apex goes downwards and outwards (Fig. 3.17). So the likely possibilities are:

MS associated with:

1. MI, AI, AS.
2. Systemic hypertension.
3. Ischaemic heart disease.
4. Severe anaemia.
5. Cardiomyopathy.
6. Thyrotoxicosis.

Q. A patient of MS becomes symptomatic suddenly or within few days—possibilities:

A patient of MS may develop heart failure in conditions like:

1. Left atrial failure and pulmonary oedema.
2. Development of tachyarrhythmias, e.g. atrial fibrillation.
3. Sudden embolic manifestations (e.g. pulmonary embolism).
4. Physical (unaccustomed exercise) and emotional stress.
5. Severe anaemia, intercurrent illness (e.g. infection), development of thyrotoxicosis.
6. Pregnancy.
7. Attacks of active rheumatic carditis.
8. Excess intake of salt, poor compliance with therapy.

- In MS, a chest X-ray done in right anterior oblique (RAO) view with barium-filled oesophagus may reveal the backward curving of oesophagus (sickling of oesophagus) as a result of left atrial enlargement.
- Double contour of the right border of heart may also be found in isolated mitral regurgitation.

PERICARDIAL EFFUSION (Fig. 3.18)

Q. Description:

This is a PA view of the chest which shows grossly enlarged (globular) cardiac silhouette with a 'water-bottle configuration' or 'pear-shaped heart'. The cardiothoracic ratio is increased. The cardiac land-marks (indentations) on the borders of the heart (i.e. ups and downs, or convexity-concavity) are obliterated (i.e. stencil-cut outline). Right cardiophrenic angle is more acute (*Rotch's sign*). The lung fields are oligaemic. Both the costophrenic angles are apparently clear.

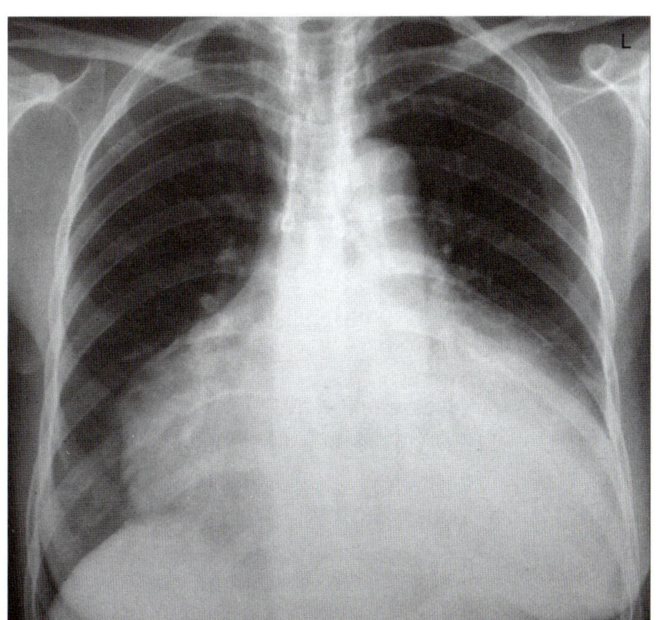

Fig. 3.18: Pericardial effusion

Other points: Within normal limit.

- In pericardial effusion, fluid collects in-between visceral and parietal pericardium.

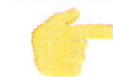 *Conclusion*

Pericardial effusion.

Q. Causes of pulmonary oligaemia and plethora:

A. Pulmonary oligaemia (i.e. reduction in pulmonary blood flow or vascularity):

a. *Radiological features:* Bronchovascular markings are less conspicuous and lung vessels are of diminished calibre.

b. *Causes:* Fallot's tetralogy, truncus arteriosus, severe pulmonary stenosis, pulmonary atresia, pulmonary thromboembolism, pericardial effusion, right-to-left shunt.

B. Pulmonary plethora (i.e. increased pulmonary perfusion or vascularity):

a. *Radiological features:* Dilated vessels are seen throughout the lung fields (from hilum to periphery) due to increased pulmonary blood flow [With the onset of pulmonary hypertension, plethora disappears and the peripheral 1/3rd of lung will have less arterial markings ('pruning' or 'pruned tree appearance')].

b. *Causes:* MS, MI, AS, AI, left ventricular failure, left-to-right shunt (ASD, VSD, PDA).

- ASD is an important cause of pulmonary plethora in clinical practice.

Q. How much pericardial fluid is required to show enlarged cardiac silhouette in chest X-ray?

It is approximately 250 mL.

Q. Minimum amount of fluid required to diagnose pericardial effusion by echocardiography:

Echocardiography can detect pericardial effusion as small as 15 mL.

Q. Common causes and clinical features of pericardial effusion:

Read 'Bedside Clinics in Medicine, Part I'.

- In a patient of pericardial effusion, if the X-ray is taken in Trendelenberg's position, there is widening of superior mediastinal shadow.

Q. Possible aetiology of combined pleural plus pericardial effusions!

1. Tuberculosis/viral.
2. Hydrothorax (e.g. CCF, cirrhosis of liver).
3. Lymphoma or acute leukaemias.
4. Collagen vascular diseases (e.g. SLE).
5. Polyserositis.
6. Septicaemia.
7. Neoplastic or post-irradiation.
8. Familial Mediterranean fever (FMF).
9. Dressler's syndrome (post-myocardial infarction syndrome).

- **Polyserositis** or Concato's disease: Inflammation of several serous membranes (i.e. pleura, pericardium and/or peritoneum) at the same time, and may be due to tuberculosis, SLE, malignancy, asbestosis, drug-induced or idiopathic.

ENLARGED CARDIAC SHADOW (Fig. 3.19A)

Q. Description:

This is a PA view of the chest which shows grossly enlarged cardiac shadow with increased cardiothoracic ratio. The indentations on the borders of the heart are retained. Bronchovascular markings and right cardiophrenic angle are within normal limit. The right costophrenic angle is blunt. The lung fields look normal (i.e. not oligaemic).

Other points: Within normal limit.

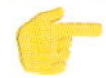 *Conclusion*

Cardiomegaly, apparently due to cardiomyopathy.

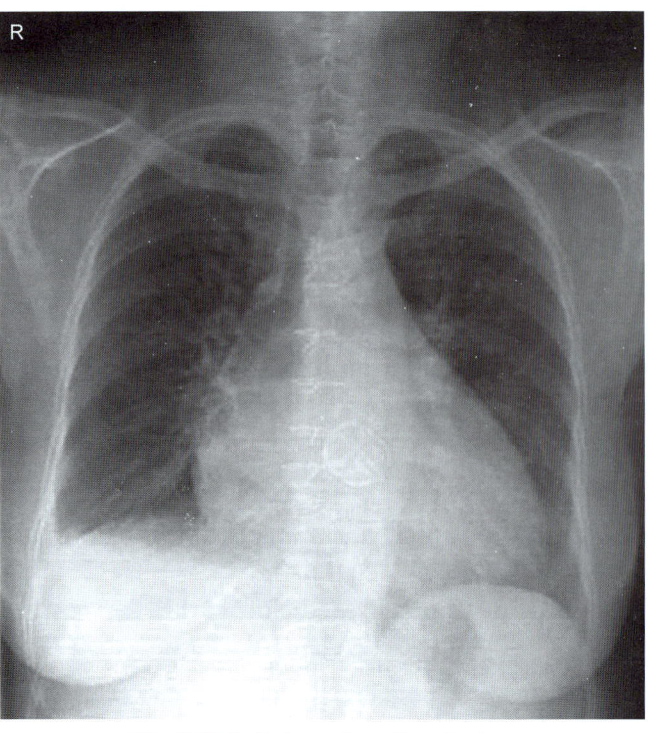

Fig. 3.19A: Enlarged cardiac shadow

Q. Enlarged cardiac shadow (cardiomegaly) in radiology:

1. Cardiomyopathy (indentations at cardiac borders are retained, absence of pulmonary oligaemia, right cardiophrenic angle remains acute, i.e. normal).
2. Pericardial effusion (indentations at cardiac borders are lost and cardiac enlargement is generalised, pulmonary oligaemia, more acute right cardiophrenic angle).
3. Enlargement of heart chambers (commonly from multiple valvular heart disease):
   a. Enlargement in transverse diameter with a boot-shaped configuration—RVH.
   b. Enlargement in oblique diameter—LVH.
   c. Double contour of the right border—LAH.
   d. Extension of the right atrial border with increased convexity—RAH.

- Read the causes of chamber enlargement of heart from 'Bedside Clinics in Medicine, Part I'.

4. Advanced congestive cardiac failure [upper lobar veins are prominent, evidence of Kerley's B line, phantom tumour (interlobar effusion) or even hydrothorax may be present].
5. Atrial septal defect (↑CTR, RVH, prominent pulmonary artery with pulmonary plethora).
6. Ebstein's anomaly (↑ CTR with big right atrium).
7. Left ventricular aneurysm (a distinct bulge is seen from the wall of the left ventricle).
8. Chest X-rays taken in full expiration or lying down position, patients with high diaphragm, or with cardiac pad of fat, or with skeletal deformity (e.g. depressed sternum, scoliosis) may give a false impression of cardiomegaly (spurious).

- In chest X-ray reporting, it is better to say chamber enlargement (e.g. left or right ventricle) while in ECG interpretation, chamber hypertrophy is a better terminology.

Clinical Wisdom

In clinical practice, common causes of gross cardiomegaly (wall-to-wall heart) are:

1. Pericardial effusion.
2. Cardiomyopathy (dilated).
3. Valvular heart diseases present singly or in combination, e.g. AI, MI, MS with MI, etc.
4. Systemic hypertension.
5. Ischaemic heart disease.
6. Congenital heart disease (ASD, VSD, Ebstein's anomaly).

Q. What is cardiomyopathy?

These are diseases primarily involving the myocardium in the absence of congenital, rheumatic, hypertensive, coronary arterial, thyrotoxic or pericardial abnormalities, and is present with cardiac enlargement.

Q. Clinical classification of cardiomyopathy:

a. *Dilated or congestive (commonest):* LVH and/or RVH, CCF, arrhythmias, embolism, systolic dysfunction.
b. *Restrictive (rare):* Restriction of LV and/or RV filling, abnormal diastolic function.
c. *Hypertrophic (rare):* Disproportionate LVH. Massive hypertrophy of interventricular septum. Double kicking apex, diastolic dysfunction.

- Features of restrictive variety mimic constrictive pericarditis.
- Arrhythmogenic cardiomyopathy: There is progressive dystrophy of right ventricular muscle, often familial, leading to ventricular arrhythmias and sudden cardiac death (SCD).
- Left ventricular non-compaction cardiomyopathy—a disease of endomyocardial trabeculations with LV dysfunction, malignant arrhythmias and thromboembolic epidoses. It is a cogenital condition.

Q. Management of cardiomyopathy:

a. *Dilated:* Management of heart failure, alcohol withdrawal, cardiac transplantation.
b. *Restrictive:* Diuretics, excision of the fibrotic endocardium, cardiac transplantation.
c. *Hypertrophic:* Beta blockers, dual chamber pacing, surgery of hypertrophied septum.

- Cardiac transplantation in human was first performed by Christiaan Barnard, a South African cardiac surgeon, in 1967.

DEXTROCARDIA (Fig. 3.19B)

Q. How to diagnose dextrocardia in PA view of chest?

A. Isolated dextrocardia (i.e. without situs inversus):

1. The cardiac apex is in right hemithorax. Major portions of heart is on right side.
2. See the radiographer's labelling of 'R' on the side of the apex.
3. The left diaphragm is higher than the right diaphragm (heart pushes the right diaphragm).
4. Fundal gas shadow is on the left side.
5. Trachea is central (so, dextroversion is absent, i.e. push-pull effects of lung is not present here).
6. Liver, spleen and stomach are in normal position

B. Dextrocardia with situs inversus (i.e. rotation of abdominal or thoracic organs to opposite side):

1. All remain same except the fundal gas shadow remains on the right side (Fig. 3.19B).
2. Liver lies on the left, and spleen and stomach on the right side.

Q. Does peripheral blood smear help to diagnose dextrocardia?

Dextrocardia may be associated with asplenia, and thus peripheral smear shows nucleated RBCs, Howell-Jolly bodies and Heinz bodies.

Q. Conditions associated with dextrocardia:

1. Kartagener's syndrome.
2. Heterotaxy syndrome in children.
3. Asplenia or hyposplenia.

C. STRAIGHT X-RAY OF THE ABDOMEN

GAS UNDER THE DIAPHRAGM (Fig. 3.20A and B)

Q. Description:

This is a straight (plain) X-ray of the abdomen (taken in erect posture) which shows semilunar gas shadow

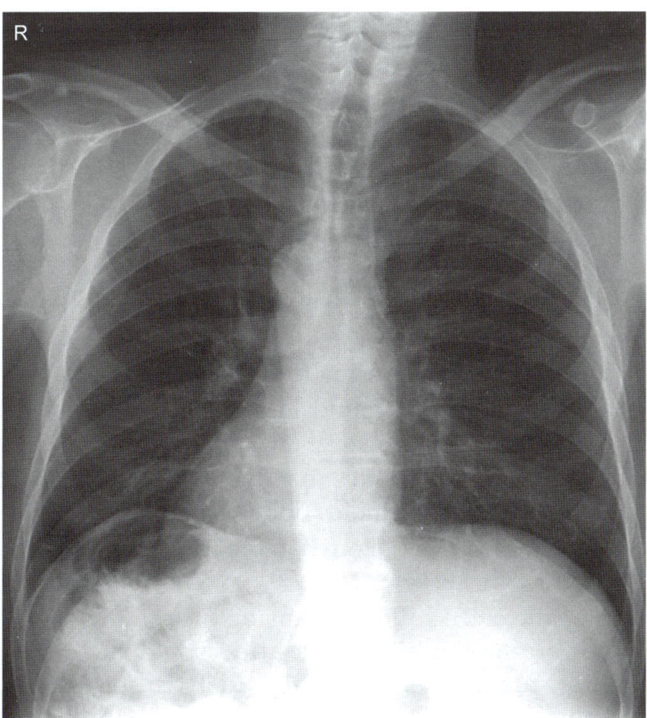

Fig. 3.19B: Dextrocardia

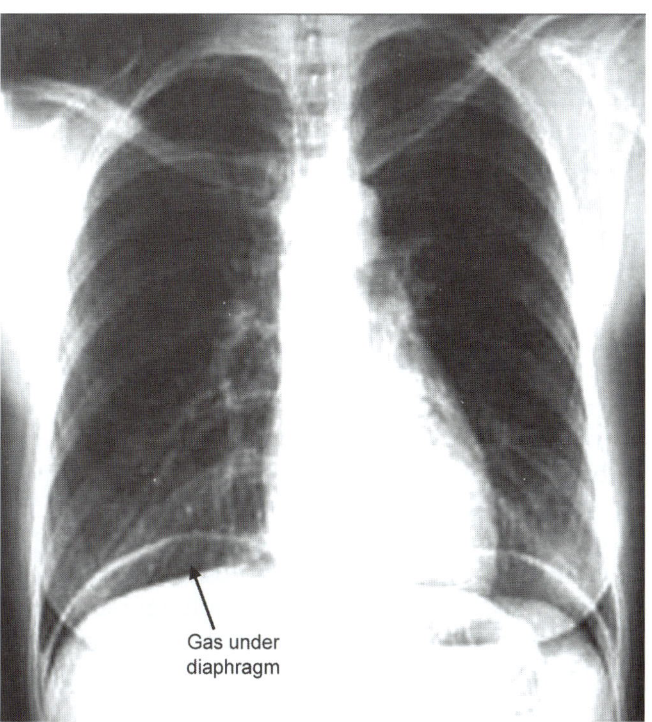

Fig. 3.20A: Gas under the diaphragm

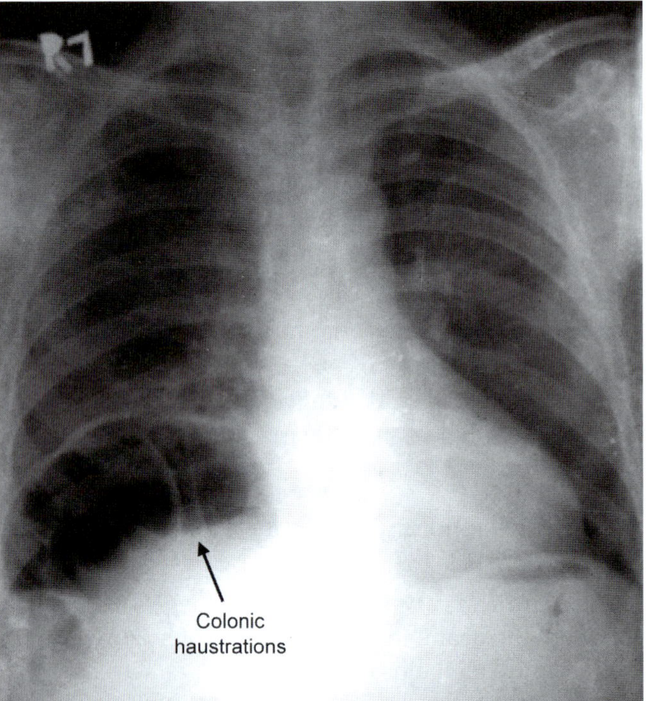

Fig. 3.20B: Chilaiditi's syndrome

under the right dome of diaphragm. Normal fundal gas shadow is seen under the left dome of diaphragm.

Psoas shadow, feature of bowel obstruction, calculus or any sign of calcification is absent. Lung bases are normal with clear costophrenic angles (Fig. 3.20A).

- Never say PA or AP view of the abdomen though it is the antero-posterior erect view.

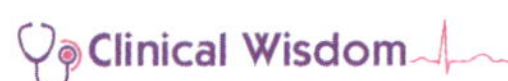

Clinical Wisdom

Conventional gastrointestinal radiology includes:
- Straight X-ray of the abdomen (suspected perforation, renal or biliary colic, intestinal obstruction, or foreign body ingestion).
- Barium study.

Conclusion

This X-ray film strongly suggests perforation of hollow viscus, most probably it is acute perforation of a peptic ulcer. The other possibilities are:

1. Peritonitis by gas forming organism.
2. Subdiaphragmatic abscess (right) by gas forming organism.
3. Following (CO_2 is the most commonly used gas for creating 'pneumoperitoneum'):
   a. Tubal insuffiation test (Rubin's test).
   b. Abdominal surgery.
   c. Laparoscopy.
   d. Peritoneal dialysis.
4. Chilaiditi's syndrome, i.e. interposition of transverse colon between the liver and the diaphragm simulating pneumoperitoneum (colonic haustrations are seen). This is a normal finding (anatomical variation) as well as a transient phenomenon (Fig. 3.20B) though the patient may have pain abdomen.

Q. Clinically, how to suspect the presence of gas under the diaphragm?

Percussion of the liver is done from above downwards along right MCL. Loss of liver dullness clinches the above diagnosis in a patient with acute abdomen.

Q. What is *Helicobacter pylori*?

Human are the only important source of *H. pylori*, which is now regarded as an important pathogen. These are spiral, curved or comma-shaped, microaerophilic, Gram–ve and Giemsa+ve multiflagellated, urease-producing, highly motile organism measuring 3–5 μm in length, which colonises the stomach in the deep portion of mucous gel layer that coats mucosa and also in the surface epithelial cells. They adhere to gastric epithelium but never invade. *H. pylori* is responsible for 80% patients developing gastric ulcer, 95–100% cases of duodenal ulcer and 50% cases of non-ulcer dyspepsia. Gastric acid cannot destroy the bacteria. It spreads from person to person by faecal-oral or oral-oral route.

Q. How to eradicate *Helicobacter pylori*?

Eradication of *H. pylori* is not an easy matter. *H. pylori* has been implicated in gastroduodenal ulceration: It is considered a carcinogen and as such plays a role in the development of gastric adenocarcinoma and mucosa-associated lymphoid tissue (MALT) lymphoma, and thus it should be eradicated at its earliest. Newer regimens consist of a proton-pump inhibitor (PPI) and 2–3 antimicrobial agents used for 7–14 days. There are many drug schedules but the accepted regimens are described in Table 3.1.

Q. Causes of pneumoperitoneum (i.e. abnormal presence of air or gas in the peritoneal cavity):

Pneumoperitoneum is seen as dark, crescentic air shadows below the diaphragms, and is found in:

1. Perforation of a hollow viscus.
2. After laparotomy or laparoscopic surgery.
3. Post-peritoneal dialysis.
4. Post-tubal insufflation test.

Q. 'Calcification' seen in the straight X-ray of abdomen:

1. Fecoliths (i.e. a stone made of very hard feces).
2. Phleboliths (small, round, local calcification within a vein).
3. Calcified lymph nodes (e.g. tuberculosis), calcified aorta, calcified dermoid/fibroid/foetus.
4. Calculi in organs like renal, biliary, pancreatic and splenic.
5. Hepatic calcification: Haemangioma, tuberculosis, hepatoma, calcified hydatid cyst, brucellosis, histoplasmosis; bladder wall (tuberculosis, schistosomiasis); uterus (fibroid); vas deferens (diabetes).

Table 3.1: Eradication regimen of *H. pylori* (concept from Harrison's Principles of Internal Medicine)

Regimen	Drug combinations
Regimen 1 (7–14 days)	Omeprazole (20 mg BDAC) + Clarithromycin (500) mg BDS) + Metronidazole (500 mg BDS)
Regimen 2 (7–14 days)	Omeprazole (20 mg BDAC) + Clarithromycin (500 mg BDS) + Amoxicillin (1g BDS)
Regimen 3 (14 days)	Omeprazole (20 mg BDAC) + Bismuth subsalicylate (2 tab QDAC) + Tetracycline (500 mg QDS) plus metronidazole (500 mg TDS)
Regimen 4 Sequential (5 days + 5 days)	Omeprazole (20 mg BDAC) + Amoxicillin (1g BDS) Omeprazole (20 mg BDAC) + Clarithromycin (500 mg BDS) + Tinidazole (500 mg BDS)
Regimen 5 (14 days)	Omeprazole (20 mg BDAC) + Amoxicillin (1g BDS) + Clarithromycin (500 mg BDS) plus Tinidazole (500 mg BDS)
Regimen 6 (10 days)	Omeprazole (20 mg BDAC) + Amoxicillin (1g BDS) + Levofloxacin (500 mg BDS)

- Regimen 1and 2 are 'Tripple therapy' (i.e. **first-line therapy**). Bismuth subsalicylate 1 tab = 262 mg. There is a high incidence of resistance to clarithromycin and metronidazole in some population. Levofloxacin or bismuth-based quadruple therapy is **second-line therapy**.
- 'Rescue therapy' **(third-line therapy)**—when standard regimens fail ciprofloxacin/levofloxacin, furazolidone and rifabutin are used as tripple therapy.

6. Miscellaneous: Chronic pancreatitis, Addison's disease, calcification of abdominal wall (e.g. cysticercosis), soft tissue (Guinea worm).

D. BARIUM STUDY

The GI tract can be viewed and studied, if it is filled with some radio-opaque material like barium. For barium studies of the GI tract, the patient swallows radio-opaque barium sulfate. The radiologist carefully observes the passage of barium on a fluorescent screen/TV monitor with an image intensifier and takes X-ray films for permanent recording. For the study of oesophagus, **barium swallow** X-ray is required (for stricture, oesophageal varices, achalasia cardia, carcinoma, hiatus hernia); for stomach and duodenum **(barium meal X-ray)**; and for small intestine (e.g. narrowing, dilatation, diverticula, flocculation of barium in malabsorption, narrowing of ileocaecal valve) barium meal X-ray are taken sequentially after few minutes of swallow **(barium follow-through)**. **Barium enema** (barium suspension introduced per rectum) is used for diagnosis of large intestinal (e.g. ulcerative colitis) and rectal diseases. Small bowel enema or **enteroclysis** (for small intestine) is nowadays done frequently in selective cases.

For better visualisation in barium enema study, when barium and air both are used, it is known as 'double contrast' study.

Water-soluble Gastrografin is particularly indicated when viscous barium sulphate (not water-soluble) may be potentially dangerous in conditions like suspected intestinal obstruction, haemorrhage or perforation.

DUODENAL ULCER (Fig. 3.21)

Q. Description:

This is a barium meal X-ray of stomach and duodenum which shows deformity of the duodenal cap. The outline of stomach is within normal limit. It is seen that barium has passed into the small intestine.

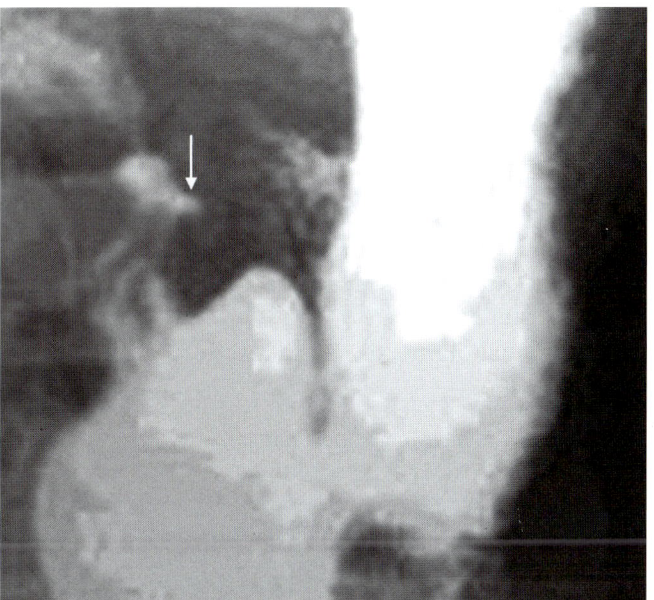

Fig. 3.21: Duodenal ulcer

- 'Duodenal cap' is the very first part of duodenum seen by X-ray or fluoroscopy.

Conclusion

Duodenal ulcer.

- Deformity of the duodenal cap is due to an ulcer crater, oedema, muscular spasm, fibrosis or their combination.

Q. Enumerate the deformities of duodenal cap:

One of the deformities is known as clover leaf or trefoil deformity.

Q. How do you diagnose *Helicobacter pylori*?

1. *Histology* by gastric mucosal biopsy (gold-standard for diagnosis; the morphology of the organism has

been discussed in X-ray picture of 'Gas under the diaphragm'. The biopsy tissue is stained by:

a. Haematoxylin and eosin.
b. Special stain (modified Giemsa, Warthin-Starry, Gram's stain).
c. Immunohistochemistry (endonuclease analysis).

2. *Biopsy culture:* Most specific but may not be very sensitive.
3. *Serology (ELISA):* Detects IgG antibody to *H. pylori*, and are reasonably sensitive (90%) as well as specific (83%). Detection of IgG antibody in saliva may also be done.
4. *Rapid urease test:* Biopsy tissue is put into urea-containing broth (*Chlamydia*-like organism or CLO test; also known as helicochek test: urea-containing broth is broken down to NH_3, if urease is produced by *H. pylori* and the colour of the broth is changed to red in a positive test).
5. *Carbon-urea (13_C or 14_C) breath test:* Most consistently accurate test; useful for screening test to detect *H. pylori*, and also to follow-up after treatment. It is often cosidered as the gold standard test for diagnosis of *H. pylori*.
6. *Stool antigen test for H. pylori (HpSA):* A new promising test, where sensitivity and specificity is >95%.
7. *Saliva test:* An immunochromatographic assay of unique antibodies in saliva for detection of oral infection.
8. *Emerging:* Polymerase chain reaction (PCR).

- *H. pylori* was discovered by Barry Marshall and Robin Warren in 1982, who received Nobel Prize in 2005.
- Invasive tests—1, 2, 4; non-invasive tests—3, 5, 6, 7, 8.

Q. What is non-ulcer dyspepsia (NUD)?

It is a chronic dyspepsia without any organic disease where the patient complains of abdominal pain or upper abdominal discomfort. The patient is usually a young (<40 years) female who presents with nausea, abdominal fullness, bloating with early satiety. Anxiety may be prominent. The abdomen is inappropriately tender on palpation and there is no history of weight loss. Though NUD is a functional disorder, gallstones, pregnancy or malignancy should always be ruled out by appropriate investigations. Reassurance, prokinetics, PPI or H_2RA, anti-*H. pylori* therapy, low dose amitriptyline may be of some help.

GASTRIC ULCER (Fig. 3.22)

Q. Description:

This is a barium meal X-ray of stomach which shows an ulcer crater (niche) on the lesser curvature of the stomach (the small projection, marked by an arrow) and an indentation or indrawing (notch) on the greater curvature opposite to the ulcer crater due to spasm of the circular muscle fibres locally (not clearly seen in the

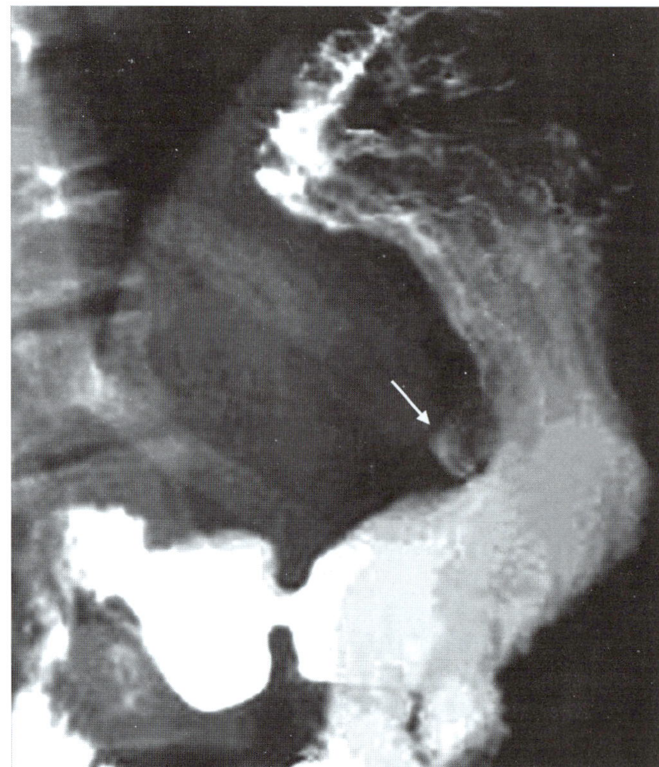

Fig. 3.22: Gastric ulcer

X-ray plate). There is no filling defect seen within the stomach. Duodenal cap is not clearly visualised. Barium has passed into the duodenum and small intestine. Bony and soft tissue structures show no apparent abnormality.

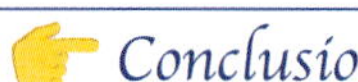 *Conclusion*

Benign gastric ulcer **(Table 3.2)**.

Q. Possible aetiology of 'stress ulcers' and erosions in stomach:

1. NSAID (e.g. aspirin) or corticosteroid-induced.
2. Head injury or increased intracranial tension (Cushing's ulcer), burn (Curling's ulcer), severe sepsis, shock and severe trauma.

OESOPHAGEAL CARCINOMA (Fig. 3.23A and B)

Q. Description:

This is a barium swallow (oblique view) X-ray of oesophagus showing persistent irregular filling defect or a persistently stenotic segment. Proximal dilated part of oesophagus is seen here. Classical 'rat-tail' like deformity of lower part of oesophagus is evident. Bony structure shows no apparent abnormality. The dye (radio-opaque barium sulfate) has passed into the stomach.

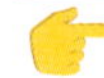 *Conclusion*

Carcinoma of the oesophagus (involving middle and lower third).

Table 3.2: Differentiation between benign and malignant ulcer in stomach

Benign ulcer	Malignant ulcer
1. Projects beyond the margin of lesser curvature	1. Remains within the margin of lesser curvature
2. Deep	2. Shallow
3. Sharply marginated, round	3 Irregular in shape
4. Rugae converge towards ulcer	4. Rugae are interrupted
5. Smooth ulcer 'collar'	5. Absence of ulcer 'collar'
6. Hampton's line (linear radiolucent line at the base of projection in lesser curvature) is present	6. Hampton's line is absent
7. No adjacent nodules or masses	7. Adjacent wall is rigid or nodular
8. Heals completely	8. Complete healing is rare

- Larger ulcers (>3 cm) are likely to be malignant. Ulcers in lesser curvature are usually benign whereas greater curvature ulcers are likely to be malignant.
- Carcinoma of the stomach may occur in gastric ulcer but not in duodenal ulcer.

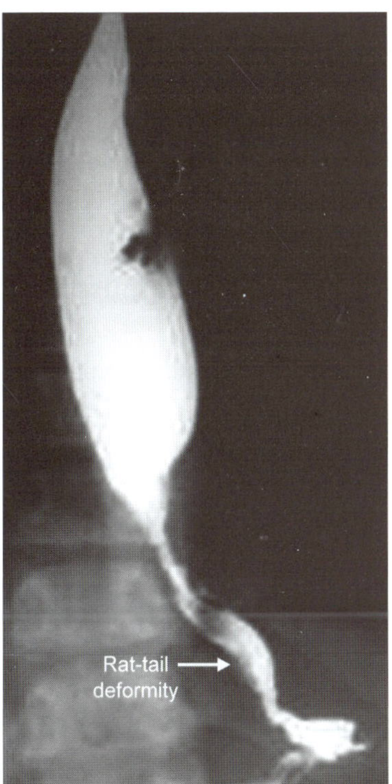

Fig. 3.23A: Oesophageal carcinoma

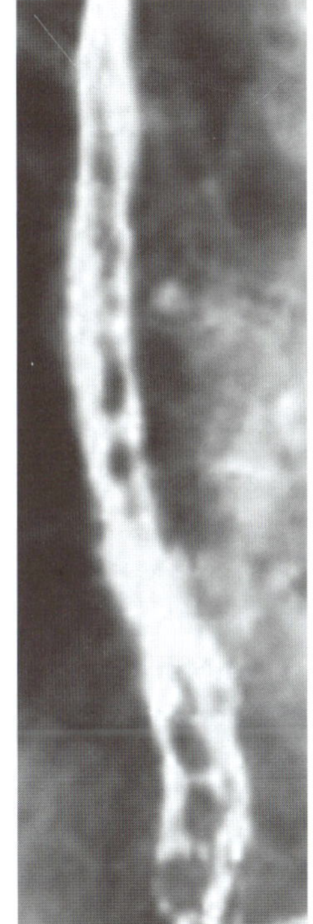

Fig. 3.23B: Oesophageal varices

Q. How to confirm the diagnosis?

By endoscopic biopsy and cytology.

Q. Irregular filling defect of oesophagus in barium swallow:

1. Carcinoma of the oesophagus (rat-tail deformity)
2. Oesophageal varices.
3. Multiple stricture following strong acid or alkali poisoning.
4. Leiomyoma of the oesophagus.
5. Diffuse oesophageal spasm (corkscrew oesophagus).
6. *Candida* (monilial) oesophagitis.

Q. Describe the barium swallow picture of oesophageal varices (Fig. 3.23B):

Multiple filling defects give a picture of 'moth-eaten' or 'worm-eaten' appearance of the oesophagus and the irregularity is maximum near the lower end. The varices (indicate portal hypertension) formed by anastomosing channels of portal and systemic veins produce those serpiginous filling defects in the regular contour of oesophagus. Oesophageal varices also need endoscopic confirmation and grading.

CARDIOSPASM (Fig. 3.24)

Q. Description:

This is a barium swallow X-ray of oesophagus which shows smooth and symmetrical beak-like narrowing of

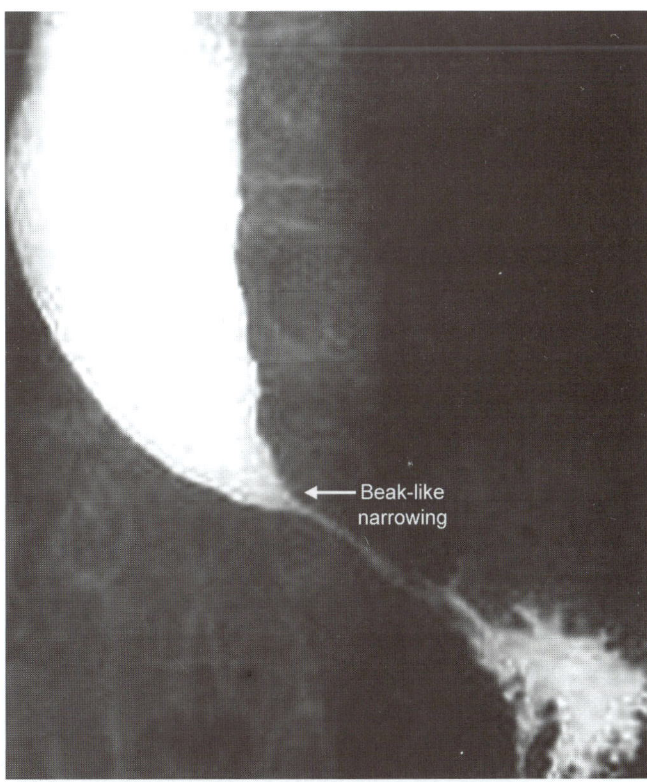

Fig. 3.24: Cardiospasm (achalasia cardia)

the terminal part of oesophagus (bird's beak appearance) with funnel-like gross dilatation of the proximal part. There is absence of fundal gas shadow. Air-fluid level within dilated oesophagus (oftern evident) is not seen here. Bony and soft tissue structures show no apparent abnormality.

 *Conclusion*

Cardiospasm or achalasia cardia.

Q. D/D with carcinoma of the oesophagus:

a. *Cardiospasm:* Outline is smooth, central narrowing of lumen, beak-like narrowing and non-rigid affected area (fluoroscopy), absent fundal gas shadow.
b. *Carcinoma of the oesophagus:* Outline is irregular, eccentric narrowing of lumen, irregular narrowing and rigid affected area (fluoroscopy); fundal gas shadow is visible.

Q. Symptoms at presentation:

Usually a middle-aged patient presents with:

1. *Dysphagia:* Difficulty in swalloing (first with solids, then both with solids and liquids).
2. Retrosternal chest pain (vigorous achalasia).
3. Regurgitation (effortless apperance of gastric contents in mouth).
4. Cough due to recurrent pulmonary aspiration.
5. Sense of fullness or a gurgling sound while taking meal.
6. Loss of weight.

Q. Different causes of cardiospasm:

a. *Primary or idiopathic:* Congenital defect of smooth muscle innervation [reduction in myenteric neurones which is related to abnormal nitric oxide synthesis within the lower oesophageal sphincter (LES)].
b. *Secondary:* Infiltrating gastric carcinoma, lymphoma, irradiation, Chagas disease, toxins and drugs (chronic narcotic use).

Q. Investigations commonly done:

1. *PA view of the chest:* Midline opacity with horizontal fluid level may be seen in upright posture; absence of fundal gas shadow.
2. *Barium swallow of oesophagus:* Described above.
3. *Oesophagoscopy:* Endoscopy may reveal inflammation and ulceration; oesophagus is dilated. On gentle pressure, the instrument can be pushed into the stomach (may not be possible in oesophageal carcinoma). Endoscopy is very helpful in excluding secondary causes, especially gastric carcinoma (biopsy is taken, if necessary). Proper cleansing of oesophagus is necessary before endoscopy.
4. *Oesophageal manometry:* Elevated resting lower oesophageal sphincter (LES) pressure; absence of swallow-induced relaxation of LES; simultaneous-onset contractions replace primary peristaltic waves; injection of mecholyl (cholinergic drug) raises the baseline oesophageal pressure instead of lowering it.
5. *CT scan:* To exclude distal oesophageal carcinoma.

Q. Line of management:

Basically the treatment is palliative:

1. Calcium channel blockers like nifedipine, or isosorbide dinitrate sublingually, or sildenafil is tried initially; soft foods, sedatives, anticholinergic drugs are not very helpful. Mild cases may not require treatment.
2. Hydrostatic or pneumatic balloon dilatation: One or more dilatations may be required.
3. Endoscope-aided injection of botulinum toxin into the LES may induce temporary clinical remission.
4. *Heller's cardiomyotomy operation:* Risk of development of reflux oesophagitis and peptic stricture of oesophagus are there. In this operation, the circular muscle layer is incised. Anti-reflux procedure (fundoplication) may also be done laparoscopically. Per oral endoscopic myotomy, a novel technique, which incises the LES is tried.
5. Oesophageal resection with colonic interposition may be done.

Q. Common causes of motor (neuromuscular) dysphagia:

1. Motor neurone disease: Leading to bulbar palsy.
2. Pseudobulbar palsy
3. Myasthenia gravis.
4. Polymyositis or dermatomyositis.
5. Myopathy (i.e. oculopharyngeal).
6. Myotonic dystrophy.
7. Stroke or CVA.
8. Multiple sclerosis.

Q. 'Opacity' seen within cardiac opacity in a PA view of chest X-ray—reasons behind:

1. Aortic aneurysm.
2. Paravertebral abscess (e.g. cold abscess).
3. Any soft tissue mass (e.g. mediastinal mass).
4. Extramedullary haematopoiesis (e.g. thalassaemia).
5. Achalasia cardia.

- In achalasia, there is impaired relaxation of lower oesophageal sphincter (LES) and oesophageal aperistalsis. Achalasia cardia has an increased incidence of developing squamous cell carcinoma of the oesophagus after few years.

PYLORIC STENOSIS (Fig. 3.25)

Q. Description:

This is a barium meal X-ray (of stomach) which shows grossly distended stomach (with excessive fasting contents). An obstruction is seen near the pylorus though the dye has passed into the duodenum. Bony and soft tissue structures show no apparent abnormality.

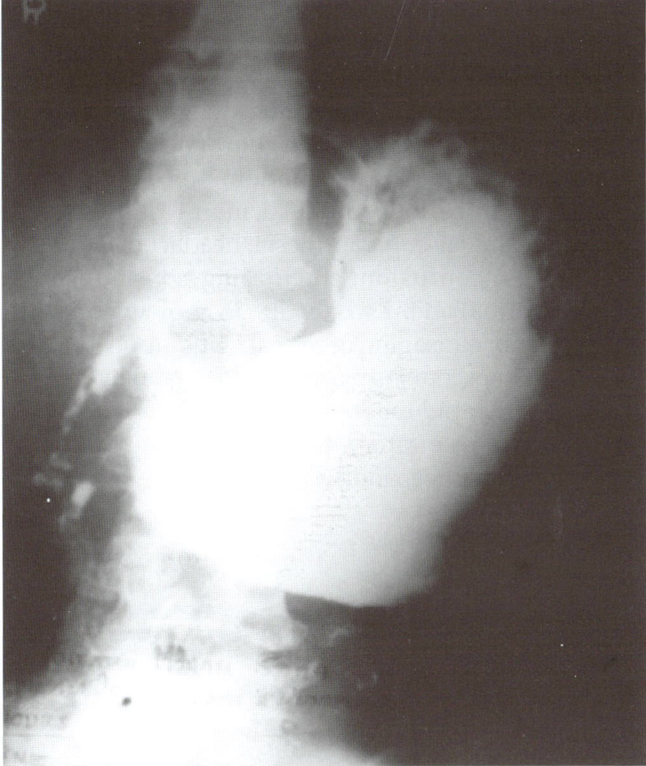

Fig. 3.25: Pyloric stenosis

Conclusion

Gastric outlet obstruction, most probably pyloric stenosis.

Q. Confirmation of diagnosis:

a. Failure of the stomach to evacuate the barium meal even after 6 hours.
b. Upper GI endoscopy.

Q. Differential diagnosis:

a. *Gastric outlet obstruction:* Other than pyloric stenosis (resulting from duodenal cicatrisation as a complication of chronic duodenal ulcer) they are carcinoma of the pylorus, oedema of the pylorus, adult hypertrophic pyloric stenosis, hypertrophic gastritis, bezoars (trichobezoars or phytobezoars) and congenital hypertrophic pyloric stenosis (infants).
b. *Non-obstructive gastric dilatation:* Gastroparesis diabeticorum (from diabetes mellitus), postpartum and postoperative gastric dilatation, drugs (clonidine, tricyclic antidepressants, e.g. amitriptyline), scleroderma, dermatomyositis or polymyositis, myotonia dystrophica. In this category, radioisotopic gastric emptying study often confirms the diagnosis.

Q. Important bedside signs in pyloric stenosis:

1. Diffuse swelling present in the upper abdomen.
2. Visible peristalsis traversing from left-to-right hypochondrium.
3. Positive succussion splash.
4. Positive ausculto-percussion test.

Q. Thickened mucosal fold of small intestine in barium follow-through:

1. Lymphoma.
2. Zollinger-Ellison syndrome.
3. Intestinal lymphangiectasia.
4. Amyloidosis.
5. Paraproteinaemia.

E. X-RAY OF SKULL

MULTIPLE MYELOMA (Fig. 3.26)

Q. Description:

This is a lateral view of the skull which shows multiple small, rounded, 'punched-out' areas (radiolucent osteolytic lesions) of different sizes. The margin of the radiolucent areas are sharply defined and are not surrounded by zone of osteosclerosis.

Orbital fossa, sinuses, pituitary fossa are within normal limit. No intracerebral calcification is noted.

Conclusion

Probably, it is the skull X-ray of multiple myeloma.

Q. Single or multiple 'osteolytic lesion' in skull:

1. Mutiple myeloma (classical rounded 'punched-out' areas without surrounding osteosclerosis).
2. Metastatic carcinoma from bronchus, thyroid, breast or kidney (osteoblastic reaction, i.e. osteosclerosis is seen at the margin of osteolytic lesions).
3. Hyperparathyroidism (spotty decalcification).
4. Paget's disease in active phase (moth-eaten appearance).
5. Histiocytosis X disease (big mappy area of radiolucency or 'geographical skull').

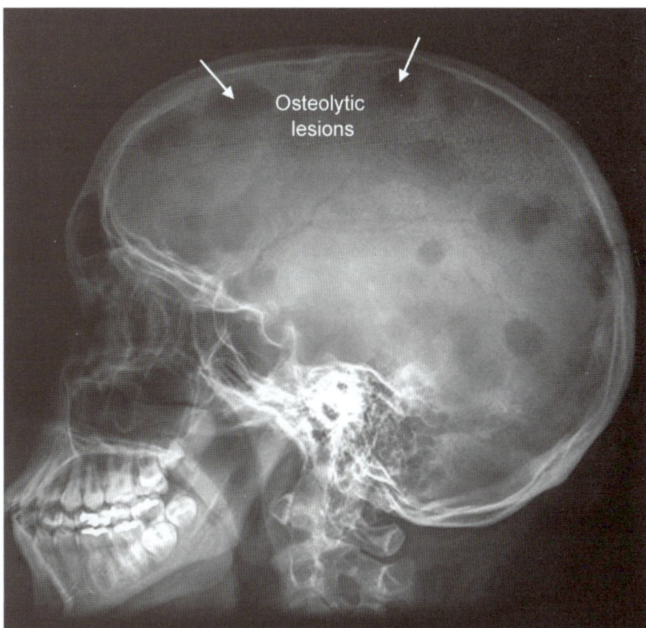

Fig. 3.26: Multiple myeloma

6. Leukaemic or lymphomatous deposits (small to large).
7. Burr-hole (Iatrogenic).
8. Sarcoidosis (small to large).
9. *Miscellaneous:* Big diploic foramen, silver-beaten appearance of raised intracranial tension (children), congenital venous lakes, haemangioma of the vault, fibrous dysplasia, arachnoid granulations.

- Mandible may be affected in multiple myeloma, which is usually not a feature of metastatic carcinoma.
- Radionuclide scan is taken up by secondaries but not by osteolytic lesions of multiple myeloma.

Q. Radiographic examination in multiple myeloma:

1. *Skull:* Multiple punched-out osteolytic lesions.
2. *Spine:* Collapse of one or more vertebrae, and osteoporosis; spinal deformity.
3. *Chest:* Punched-out lesions in ribs (i.e. rib erosion), clavicle and sternum; drumstick expansion of anterior end of ribs and there may be pathological fracture in ribs.
4. *Pelvis:* Multiple punched-out osteolytic lesions; osteoporosis.
5. *Kidney:* Nephrocalcinosis.

Q. Features noted in examination of any X-ray of skull:

X-ray of skull is viewed as follows:

1. Calvarium and base (e.g. physiological radiolucencies like sutures, vascular imprints; or fracture; or sinuses, fontanelles).
2. Sella turcica (shape, size, erosion of posterior clinoid process, mineralisation, etc.).
3. Calcification.

Q. Presentation of multiple myeloma:

It is a 'plasma cell neoplasm', and other related plasma cell disorders are Waldenstrom's macroglobulinaemia, benign monoclonal gammopathy, heavy chain diseases and primary amyloidosis. These are monoclonal neoplasms which are developed from common progenitors in the B-lymphocyte lineage, and are also known as paraproteinaemias, dysproteinaemias, plasma cell disorders or monoclonal gammopathies. The patient of multiple myeloma is classically a male one, in-between 60 and 70 years of age who presents with:

1. Bone pain (most common symptom)—especially in the spine (60%).
2. Severe weakness with wasting.
3. Low-grade pyrexia.
4. Pre-syncope, syncope, vertigo, breathlessness as a result of severe anaemia.
5. Paraplegia (with plasmacytoma or localised myeloma).
6. Renal failure [hypercalcaemia, tubular damage due to excretion of light chains (Bence Jones proteinuria), hyperuricaemia, amyloid deposits, recurrent infections and infiltrations of the kidney by myeloma cells are the contributory factors].
7. Joint pain.
8. **Hyperviscosity syndrome** due to aggregation of IgM paraproteins (bleeding from gum or nose, thrombotic episodes, Raynaud's phenomenon, congestive heart failure, neurological manifestations like fatigue, malaise, paraesthesia, headache, faintness, tinnitus, confusion, fluctuating consciousness, mild impairment to abrupt loss of vision with 'boxcar or sausaging of retinal veins' appearance in ophthalmoscopy)— plasmapheresis (and hydration) may give rapid relief.
9. Recurrent respiratory tract infections.
10. Amyloidosis (secondary).

Q. Low-trauma fractures occur in:

1. Severe osteoporosis.
2. Metastatic bone disease.
3. Multiple myeloma.
4. Fragility fracture (e.g. osteomyelitis).

Q. Causes of diffuse and widespread bone pain:

1. Osteomalacia and rickets.
2. Widespread secondary bony metastases.
3. Multiple myeloma.
4. Osteoporosis with fracture (osteoporosis *per se* is painless).
5. Leukaemias (e.g. CML).

Q. M-band or M-component on electrophoretic strip—causes behind:

1. Plasma cell neoplasms/disorders (mentioned above).
2. CML, CLL, lymphomas, breast carcinoma.
3. *Non-neoplastic conditions:* Cirrhosis of liver, rheumatoid arthritis, sarcoidosis, myasthenia gravis.

Q. What is 'paraprotein'?

Normal immunoglobulins are polyclonal but in multiple myeloma, plasma cells produce immunoglobulin of a single heavy and light chain, a 'monoclonal protein', which is known as paraprotein, and appears on electrophoretic strip as a clear-cut band (M-band). These paraproteins are responsible for hyperviscosity, renal damage and amyloidosis (rare).

Q. Confirmation of diagnosis in multiple myeloma

Presence of at least two of the following confirms the diagnosis:

1. Monoclonal immunoglobulin, or light chains in blood or urine (by protein electrophoresis).
2. Bone marrow infiltration with malignant plasma cells (by bone marrow biopsy).
3. Osteolytic bone lesions (by radiology).

- Very high ESR (stormy ESR) and increased rouleaux formation make the pathologist suspicious.

Table 3.3: Biochemical features of common bone diseases

Diseases	Calcium	Phosphate	Alkaline phosphatase
Osteoporosis	N	N	N
Osteomalacia or rickets	↓ or N	↓ or N	↑
Hyperparathyroidism (primary)	↑	↓	N
Hypoparathyroidism	↓	↑	N
Secondary deposits	↑	N	↑
Multiple myeloma	↑	N	N
Paget's disease	N	N	↑↑
Chronic renal failure	↓ or N	↑ or N	N (↑ in osteodystrophy)

- Alkaline phosphatase is increased in hyperparathyroidism with significant bone involvement, and in multiple myeloma with healing fracture of bones (as osteoblastic activity tries to repair fracture).

- Plasma alkaline phosphatase level remains normal unless there is a fracture (**Table 3.3**).

Q. What is Bence Jones protein (BJP)?

The clone which produces increased amount of intact monoclonal immunoglobulin, also synthesizes and secretes excess of free light chains that **appear in the urine** as monoclonal light chains, and are known as Bence Jones protein (by Bradshaw test). Bence Jones proteinuria may also be found in primary amyloidosis, Waldenstrom's macroglobulinaemia and lymphoma. BJP is found in 50–80% patients of multiple myeloma.

- BJP was described by the English physician Henry Bence Jones in 1847.

Q. Possible causes of 'osteosclerotic lesion' (bone turns absolutely whitish):

1. Fluorosis (i.e. overexposure of fluoride).
2. Secondary deposits from carcinoma of prostate (commonly), and rarely from breast, intestine or bronchus.
3. Hodgkin's disease (ivory vertebra).
4. Marble bone disease (osteopetrosis or Albers-Schönberg disease).
5. Vitamin A or D toxicity (i.e., hypervitaminosis).
6. Diffuse idiopathic skeletal hyperostosis (Forestier's disease or DISH).
7. Jaw in Paget's disease.
8. Meningioma gives rise to sclerotic lesion in skull.
9. Renal osteodystrophy.
10. Neuroblastoma, medulloblastoma, mastocytosis.
11. Osteopoikilosis.
12. Pycnodysostosis.

Q. How to recognise 'osteoporosis'?

X-ray is not sensitive enough in this regard and radiological changes in bony structures are revealed when 30% of the bone is lost. Bone in osteoporosis usually shows diminished density, thinning of cortex, loss of horizontal trabeculae with prominent vertical trabeculae, loss of height of vertebra with biconcave vertebra, and anterior vertebral wedging resulting in kyphosis (Dowager's hump or widow's stoop).

Osteopenia and osteoporosis are diagnosed by measuring bone mineral density (BMD) with the preferred technology of dual energy X-ray absorptiometry (DEXA), and the preferred sites are lumbar spine and hip.

T-score in BMD may be above –1.0 (normal), lie between –1.0 and –2.5 (osteopenia), falls to –2.5 or below (osteoporosis).

THALASSAEMIA (Fig. 3.27)

Q. Description:

This is a lateral view of the skull which shows widening of diploic space (i.e. separation of two tables), cortical thinning with faint outer table. The bony trabeculae are arranged perpendicular to the inner table giving rise to 'hair on end' appearance (indicated by arrows).

Orbital fossa, sinuses, pituitary fossa are within normal limit. No intracerebral calcification is noted.

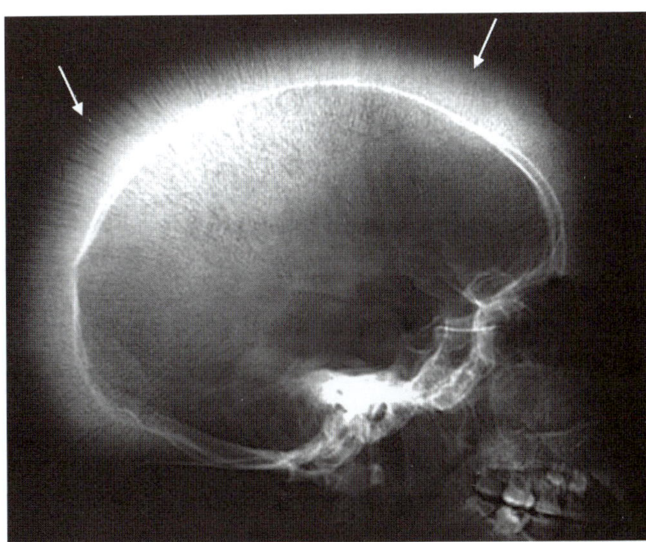

Fig. 3.27: Thalassaemia

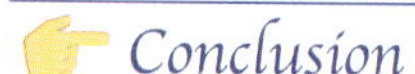

Conclusion

Chronic haemolytic anaemia, most probably thalassaemia major (commonest cause).

Q. Radiological features of small bones of hand in thalassaemia:

1. Wide medullary cavity with coarse trabeculae and thinned out cortex (mosaic-patterns).
2. Phalanges may loose their biconcave shape and ultimately become rectangular or biconvex.

[3.Long bones may also give rise to mosaic pattern].

Q. Does thalassaemia minor produce these skeletal changes?

Usually skeletal changes are absent in thalassaemia minor.

Q. What are the other possible radiological changes in skull?

1. Obliteration of paranasal air sinuses.
2. Slight prominence of frontal and maxillary bones.
3. Dental malposition.

- Very rarely, 'hair on end' appearance in skull X-ray is seen in severe iron deficiency anaemia and cyanotic congenital heart diseases.
- Chest X-ray may show extramedullary haematopoiesis in ribs, and cardiomegaly. Vertebrae may reveal osteoporosis and compression fracture.

MISCELLANEOUS SKULL X-RAYS

1. Raised intracranial tension

a. Silver-beaten appearance (in children).
b. Sutural diastasis or separation (in children).
c. Erosion of posterior clinoid process.
d. Deepened sella turcica.
e. Enlargement of internal auditory meatus.

2. Acromegaly

a. Thickened skull vault.
b. Enlarged sella turcica (i.e. pituitary fossa) with a double floor.
c. Large frontal and maxillary sinuses, large mastoid air cells.
d. Prognathism (prominent lower jaw).

3. Hyperparathyroidism

Spotty decalcification of skull (salt and pepper appearance—Pepper pot skull).

4. Paget's disease

a. Increase in size of the skull.
b. Marked thickening of cortical bone.
c. Hazy opaque mottled appearance (moth-eaten appearance).

5. Intracranial calcification (on plain films)

A. Physiological:

a. Pineal body.
b. Choroid plexus.
c. Falx cerebri.
d. Petroclinoid ligament.
e. Habenula.

B. Pathological:

a. *Primary tumours:* They are glioma, meningioma, craniopharyngioma. Basal ganglia may show calcification in hypoparathyroidism. Cerebral metastases do not give rise to calcification.
b. *Vascular malformations:* Arteriovenous malformations, Sturge-Weber disease ('railroad track' or curvilinear calcification), cerebral aneurysm, old subdural haematoma, atherosclerotic arteries.
c. Multiple small discrete calcifications are produced by tuberous sclerosis, hypoparathyroidism.
d. *Infection:* Tuberculoma, cysticercosis, toxoplasmosis (congenital), rubella, cytomegalovirus infection, hydatid cyst and old cerebral abscesses.

F. X-RAY OF HANDS

SCURVY (Fig. 3.28)

Q. Description:

This is an AP view of lower part of the thigh, knee joint, leg and foot of both sides which reveals:

1. Pencilling of cortex of epiphysis or signet ring appearance of epiphysis (Wimberger's ring sign).
2. Increased density and widening at ends of tibia and fibula seen as white line (white line of Frankel).
3. Transverse band of radiolucency (black line) in the metaphysis, adjacent to white line of Frankel ('scurvy line' or Trummerfeld zone)—Specific sign of scurvy.

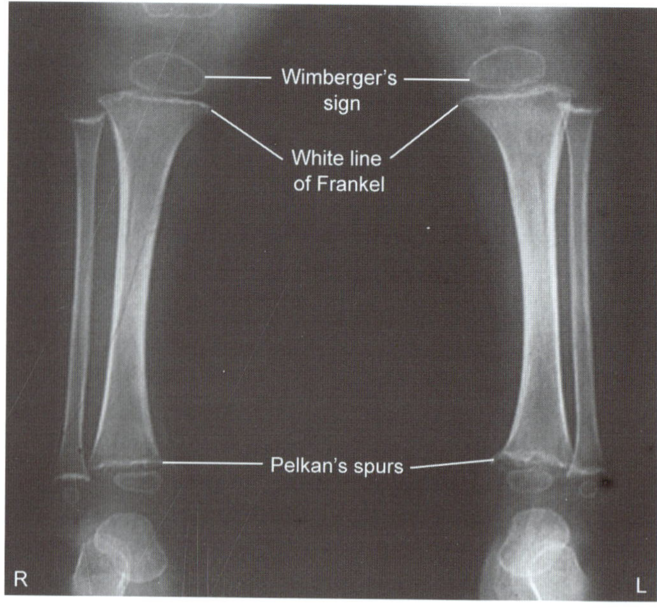

Fig. 3.28: Scurvy

4. Ground-glass appearance of the shaft of diaphysis (uniform demineralisation).
5. Angular lateral bony spurs of marginal fractures in the junction of diaphysis and metaphysis (Pelkan's sign).
6. Elevation of periosteum (as a result of subperiosteal haematoma which may rarely calcified).

- No. 3 and 6 are not seen here.

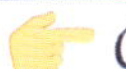
Conclusion

It is the radiological features of scurvy.

Q. Why the white line and black line are formed?

a. White line of Frankel reflects impaired growth and continued deposition of calcium phosphate.
b. Scurvy line (black line) reflects failure of primary ossification.

- **Vitamin C deficiency (scurvy)** creates a condition where there is diminished production and maintenance of intracellular ground substance.

Q. Differential diagnosis:

1. Traumatised child syndrome (absence of demineralisation of bone).
2. Heavy metal poisoning, e.g. lead poisoning (no osteopenia, and absence of zone of translucency).

Q. Clinical features of infantile scurvy:

Usually it is seen in between 6 and 18 months of age.

1. Fretful, listless and anorectic child who cries on being handled.
2. Reluctance to move the painful limbs (pseudoparalysis).
3. Symptoms due to haemorrhage:
   a. *Subperiosteal:* 'Frog position' with thighs flexed as well as abducted, and knees flexed.
   b. Bleeding from gum, gum is swollen and spongy too.
   c. *Bleeding into skin, mucous membrane; orbit:* Petechiae, or proptosis.
   d. *Beading of ribs as a result of posterior displacement of sternum:* Scorbutic rosary (angular and sharp in contrast to rachitic rosary which in semicircular and dome-shaped); painful.
   e. Haematochezia, haematuria and intracranial haemorrhages are rarely seen.
4. Low grade pyrexia, pallor (anaemia) and extreme weakness.

- In adults, there is spongy-swollen-bleeding gums, perifollicular haemorrhages and hyperkeratotic papules, petechiae, ecchymoses, splinter haemorrhages, deformed 'cork-screw' hair projecting from hair follicle, poor wound healing, and muscle and joint haemorrhages.
- Manifestations of scurvy in gums are not seen in edentulous (teethless) persons.

Q. Dose of vitamin C in scurvy:

250 mg of vitamin C should be given 3 times daily orally and encouraged to eat fresh fruits and vegetables.

- Recommended daily intake of ascorbic acid for children and adults are respectively 25 mg and 90 mg.

Q. Dietary sources of vitamin C:

Fresh citrus fruits and vegetables are good sources. Amla, guava, orange, lemon, tomato, drumstick leaves, amaranth, papaya, cabbage, cauliflower are rich in ascorbic acid. Breast milk contains adequate amount of vitamin C.

RICKETS (Fig. 3.29)

Q. Description:

This skiagram shows AP view of lower parts of the forearm, wrist joint and part of the hand of both sides which reveal cupping, widening and fraying (saucer deformity) of the lower end of radius and ulna. There is generalised demineralisation of bones (osteopenia) present. The epiphysis appears indistinct and lacks a bony cortical margin. Broadening of the wrist (soft tissue shadow) is seen. There is increased distance between the distal end of radius-ulna and metacarpal bones because of non-calcification of rachitic metaphysis.

Other radiological features not present in Fig. 3.29 are, cortical spurs from metaphysis growing towards displaced epiphysis (produces deformity), and greenstick fracture with bending and deformities.

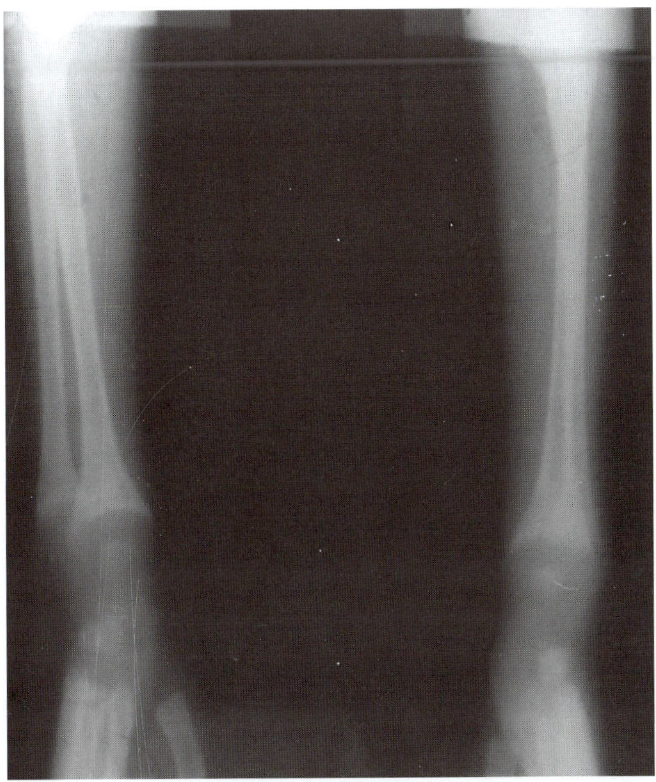

Fig. 3.29: Rickets

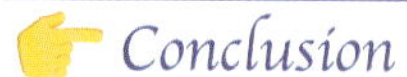

Rickets (vitamin D deficiency in the growing child before the fusion of epiphysis).

Q. Radiological features of X-ray skull in rickets:

1. Delayed closure of anterior fontanelle.
2. Small islands of unossified area.
3. Frontal and parietal bossing.
4. Quadrate skull.
5. Widening of sutures.
6. Late appearance of temporary teeth.

Q. Differential diagnosis:

One cannot differentiate among different causes of rickets by seeing the X-ray plate only. The X-ray plate of rickets (cupping and fraying) may be confused with metaphyseal dysostosis and hypophosphatasia.

Q. Radiological signs of 'healing' rickets:

1. The radiological density is increased and roughness is diminished.
2. Epiphyseal cartilage becomes horizontal.
3. Horizontal "Harrison's line" are seen in the lower end of diaphysis (initialy near the epiphysis).

Q. Causes of rickets:

1. *Deficiency of vitamin D:* Dietary deficiency, deficient endogenous synthesis (e.g. inadequate exposure to sunlight).
2. *Gastrointestinal disturbances:* Malabsorption, e.g. cystic fibrosis, Crohn's disease, gastrectomy, hepatic disorders, chronic pancreatic insufficiency.
3. *Disturbances of vitamin D metabolism:* Hereditary and acquired (use of anticonvulsants, e.g. phenytoin sodium or chronic renal failure).
4. *Renal disorders:*
   a. Renal tubular acidosis.
   b. Fanconi's syndrome.
   c. Familial hypophosphataemic rickets.
5. *Primary defect in mineralisation of bone:*
   a. Hypophosphatasia (deficiency of alkaline phosphatase).
   b. Treatment by fluoride.
6. Prolonged lactation and frequent pregnancies.
7. *Non-renal acidosis:*
   a. Ureterosigmoidostomy.
   b. Chronic acetazolamide or ammonium chloride intake.
8. Conditions with rapid bone formation, e.g. osteopetrosis or marble bone disease.

Q. What is Looser's zone (pseudofracture)?

These zones are specific of **osteomalacia** (vitamin D deficiency in adults when epiphyseal growth plates have closed) which resemble 'fracture lines'. Actually, these are 1–3 mm wide, translucent bands of decalcification lying at right angle to cortex. The classical sites are axillary borders of scapulae, ribs, lower ends of radius and ulna, ischiopubic rami, and medial border of femoral neck. These lines are formed as a result of pulsations of nutrient arteries over the soft bones as a result of deficient vitamin D.

MISCELLANEOUS HAND X-RAYS

1. Rheumatoid arthritis

a. Periarticular osteopenia.
b. Loss of articular cartilage (↓ of joint space).
c. Periarticular bone erosions.
d. Subluxation of the joints (or ankylosis).
e. Marked osteoporosis may be evident.
f. Varying degree of deformities.

- In the hand, mainly the PIP and MCP joints are affected.

2. Osteoarthritis

a. Arthritis of the thumb, i.e. involvement of 1st carpometacarpal joint (the joint space is ↓).
b. Hard bony nodules are seen over the dorsal aspect of DIP (Heberden's node) and PIP (Bouchard's node). Angular deformities of distal digits. DIP joints are mostly affected.

3. Chronic haemolytic anaemia

Read radiology of 'Thalassaemia' (*see* page 98).

4. Acromegaly

a. The hand is large (enlargement of soft tissue).
b. Tufting of terminal phalanges, i.e. 'arrow-head appearance'.
c. Widening of MCP joints spaces due to overgrowth of articular cartilage.
d. Thickening of the sesamoid bones in hand.
e. Chondrocalcinosis or pseudogout (rare).

5. Resorption of terminal phalanges

Subperiosteal bone resorption in terminal phalanx is characteristic of:

a. Scleroderma (may have soft tissue calification).
b. Leprosy.
c. Hyperparathyroidism (rarely may reveal arterial calcification).
d. Acromegaly.

- The fingers may mimick clubbing (known as pseudoclubbing).

6. Gout

a. Soft tissue swelling (due to underlying arthritis): Periarticular.
b. Typical well-defined punched-out erosion with an overhanging edge over the joints (Martel's sign).
c. Tophi: Large soft tissue lumps (due to deposits of monosodium urate crystals) are seen; may show calcification.

Short Description of Fig. 3.30 to Fig. 3.33:

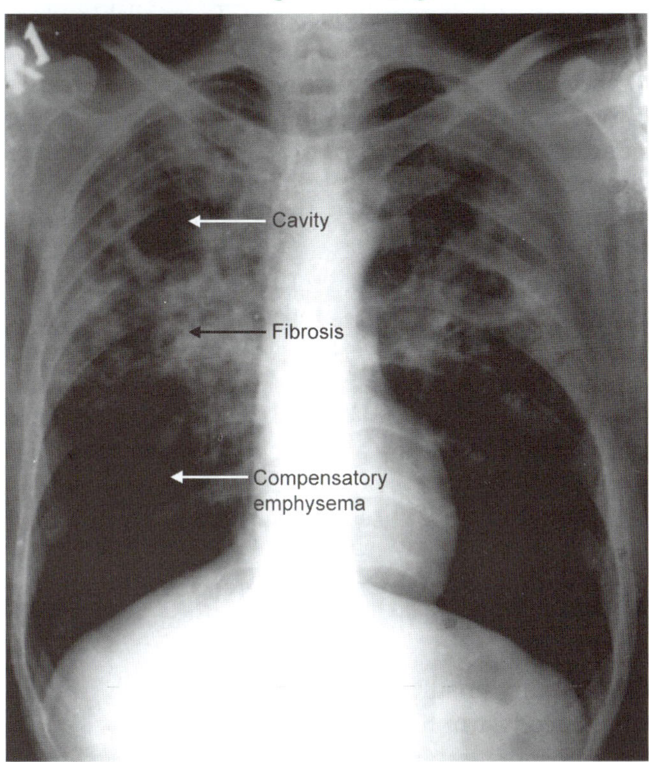

Fig. 3.30: This is a sklagram of the chest, PA view which shows bilateral upper and mid-zonal fibrosis (right > left) with cavity formations. Lower zones of the lungs reveal evidence of compensatory emphysema. The costophrenic angles are clear. **Impression:** Fibro-cavitary lesion of the lung probably resulting from tuberculosis

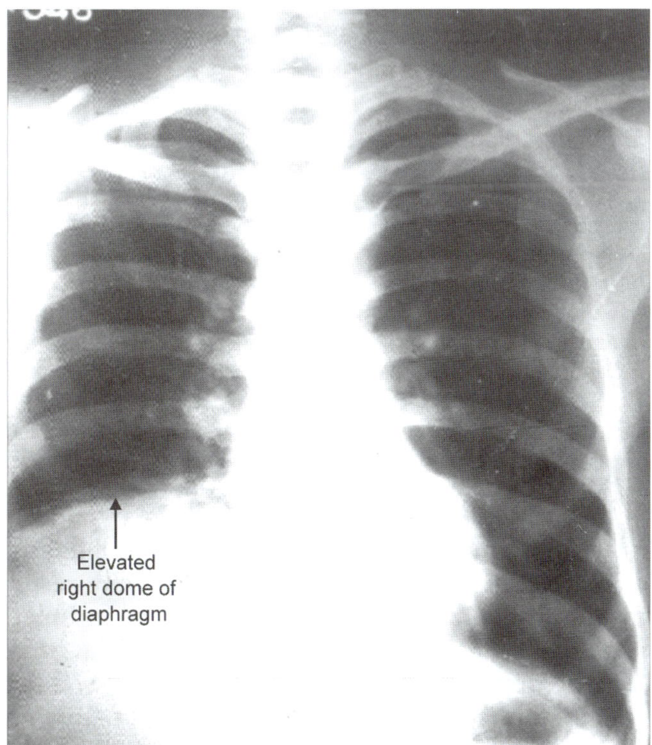

Fig. 3.31: The X-ray plate reveals skiagram of the chest, PA view demonstrating elevated right dome of diaphragm. The pulmonary parenchyma, costophrenic angles, cardiac silhouette and mediastinum are with in normal limit. **Impression:** Elevated right dome of diaphragm (the possibilities are mentioned in page 83)

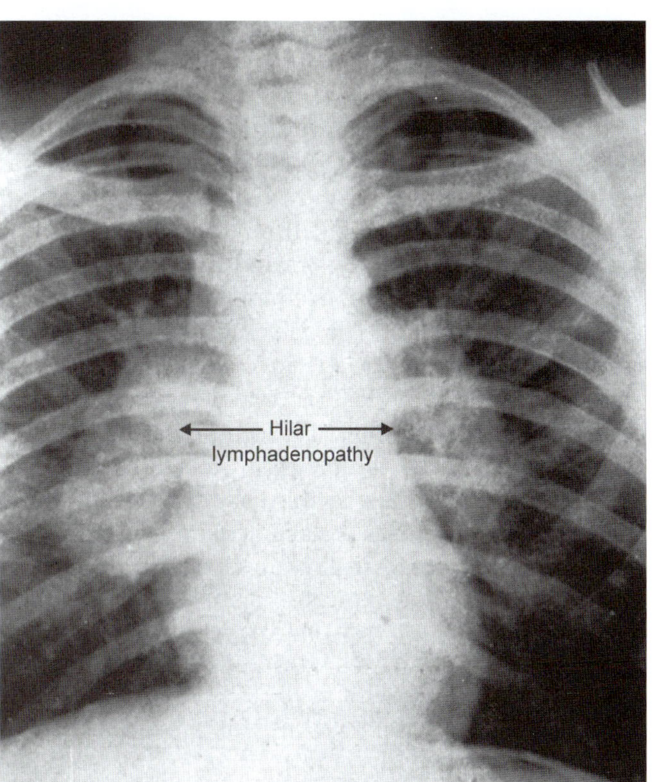

Fig. 3.32: This is a PA view of the chest which shows bilateral hilar lymphadenopathy. The pulmonary parenchyma, costophrenic angles, cardiac silhouette and mediastinum are within normal limit. **Impression:** Sarcoidosis (read 'hilar enlargement' from page 82)

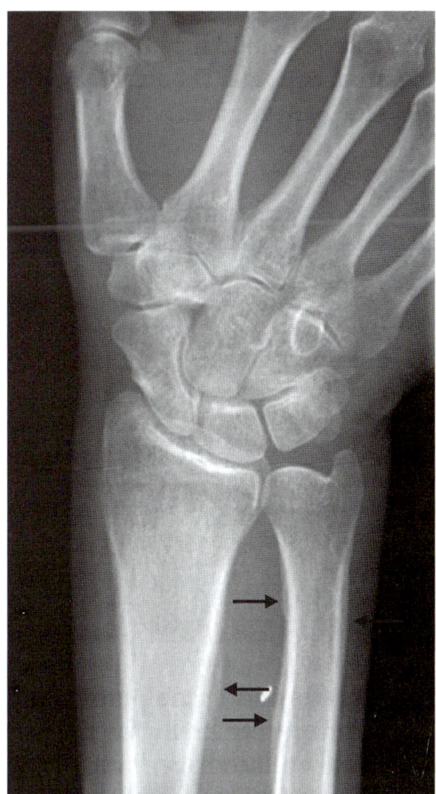

Fig. 3.33: This is AP view of lower part of radius and ulna, carpals, metacarpals and phalanges of right hand featuring 'subperiosteal new bone formation' at lower end of both radius and ulna. **Impression:** Hypertrophic osteoarthropathy (i.e. Grade IV clubbing; differential diagnosis closely resembles thyroid acropachy)

G. SYNOPSIS OF COMPUTED TOMOGRAPHY (CT) AND MAGNETIC RESONANCE IMAGING (MRI) SCAN

The advent of X-ray computed tomography (CT) in the year 1972 was a major milestone, since it has revolutionised the ability to visualize the inside of a patient's body. In 1979, the Nobel Prize for the Invention of CT scan was shared by **Sir Godfrey N Hounsfield**, a British engineer and **Allan M Cormack**, an American physicist. The CT came in 1970s, magnetic resonance imaging (MRI) in 1980s, and positron emission tomography (PET) and single-photon emission computed tomography (SPECT) thereafter in 1990. CT scan is a special radiological procedure that uses attenuation characters of the tissue to X-ray beam. CT scanning provides a very sensitive method for evaluating suspected lesions in the central nervous system.

The parallel and thinly collimated X-ray beam traverse synchronously across a slice of brain tissue between 2 mm and 13 mm thick; the X-irradiation is computer processed and a value (Hounsfield number) is given to its density scale [e.g. air (black) = –1000 units, water (less black than air) = 0, and bone (white) = +1000]. The difference in density (i.e. X-ray attenuation) makes it possible to differentiate between extravasated blood, cerebral oedema, space-occupying lesion (SOL) or infarction **(Table 3.4)**. Contrast enhancement by intravenous iodinated contrast media helps to diagnose lesions with increased blood supply (e.g. angioma, some SOL) and cerebral oedema. The irradiation involved in CT and MRI scan is negligible.

Table 3.4: Attenuation values of different tissues

Tissue	Hounsfield units
Air	–1000
Fat	up to –100
Water	0
Fluid	0–20
Soft tissue	20–100
White matter	30–35
Grey matter	35–45
Acute haemorrhage	55–75
Calcification	90–200
Bone	+1000

CT scan of brain and spinal cord demonstrates cerebral haemorrhage, cerebral infarction, intracranial SOL, subarachnoid haemorrhage, 'mass effect' by lateral shifting of midline structures, hydrocephalus, subdural and epidural haematoma, calcification within a lesion, cerebral atrophy, fracture of skull or vertebra, spinal tumours (CT-myelography), etc.

Contrast-enhanced CT scan (by using contrast agents like iothalamate meglumine/iopamidol/iodixanol) are used to visualise the blood flow to an organ or tissue. Nowadays, 64-slice multidetector CT is available which can detect several images at the same time.

In *MRI scan*, protons are imaged with radiofrequency waves, and T_1, T_2 and other sequence-weighted high-quality images are recorded. T_1-weighted sequence accentuates fat-containing substances, whereas T_2-weighted sequence accentuates water-containing substances. The magnetic strength of MRI is measured in Tesla (one Tesla is equal to 10000 gauss). One of the advantages of MRI scan is that it involves no ionising radiation, and the other is that it distinguishes between white and grey matter in the brain and spinal cord. The intravenous contrast used in MRI scan contains gadolinium. Following are the situations where MRI is especially useful for evaluation:

1. Demyelinating disease (e.g. plaques of multiple sclerosis).
2. Posterior fossa tumours (e.g. cerebellum) or vascular lesions, or disorders of cranio-vertebral junction.
3. Dementia.
4. Pituitary imaging.
5. Leucodystrophies.
6. MR angiography for arteriovenous malformations, aneurysm or arterial stenosis.
7. Myelopathy (spinal cord, spinal canal and nerve roots are imaged clearly), e.g. prolapsed intervertebral disc, syringomyelia, vascular malformations.
8. Imaging musculo-skeletal soft tissue diseases, in rheumatological disorder (e.g. to detect sacroiliitis in ankylosing spondylitis), tumours or injuries, e.g. shoulder or knee pain.
9. AIDS-associated diseases of brain.
10. Visual disturbances—For imaging beyond retina.

- MRI scan is very helpful in detecting hypothalamic and cranial nerve lesions, white matter lesion and lesion in brainstem. Types of MRI sequences are: T_1, T_2, Flair (fluid-attenuated inversion recovery, preferred in demyelinating diseases), DWI (diffusion-weighted images, preferred to detect early infarcts) and ADC (apparent diffusion coefficient). **PC Lautebur**, an American chemist and **P Mansfield**, an English physicist received Nobel Prize jointly in 2003 for their discoveries concerning development of MRI, while R Damadian was first inventor of MR scanning.

CT and MRI scan are very safe except the contrast-related systemic reactions experienced by a minority of patients. Contrasts used in CT scan may result in anaphylactoid reactions or contrast-induced nephropathy; gadolinium used in MRI as contrast may lead to 'nephrogenic systemic fibrosis' (mimicking scleroderma) in patients with chronic renal failure on haemodialysis. MRI is costlier than CT scan and is more time-consuming. The common **contraindications of MRI scan** are:

1. Patients having pacemaker.
2. Bullet injury (bullets inside the body) or intraocular foreign body.

3. Cochlear implant and deep brain stimulators.
4. Along with splint and traction,
5. Tattoed eye-liner, and
6. Any ferro-magnetic metal clip (e.g. clipping cerebral aneurysm) present within the body. Claustrophobia is a relative contraindication (an open-gantry MRI is helpful for claustrophobic, obese and pediatric patients).

CT scan of thorax gives an excellent anatomic details of hilum, pulmonary parenchyma and pleura. Coventionally thick slices (10 mm) are taken. High-resolution computed tomography (HRCT) produces thinner slices (1.5 mm). HRCT helps in diagnosis of bronchiectasis, insterstitial lung disease, infiltrative diseases of lung, pulmonary neoplasms, asbestos-related pleural plaques, and planning for radiotherapy.

CT scan of abdomen delineates liver, spleen, gallbladder, kidney, aorta, stomach (barium-filled), pancreas, adrenal gland and spine (vertebra). It is helpful in diagnosis of pancreatic diseases, hepatic neoplasms, malignant deposits, ascites, assessment of vascularity of tumour and tumour staging.

In *pregnancy*, CT scan is better avoided but MRI is believed to be safe for the fetus (as there is no radiation exposure).

A *PET (position emission tomography) scan* uses radiation to show activity within the human body on a cellular level. Other than the anatomical configuration, PET scan demonstrates its functions too. The biologically active tracer molecule used in PET scan is FDG (fluorodeoxyglucose), an analogue of glucose. **EJ Hoffman** along with **MM Ter-Pogossian** and **ME Phelps** invented PET scan, which is widely used by 1990s. It is helpful in oncology (e.g. to search for metastases), certain diffuse brain disease (e.g. dementia), and to map normal brain and cardiac function.

In the examination, mount the CT-plate correctly in the view-box (by seeing the patient's name and other write-up) and say: it is the CT scan plate of brain showing different cut sections .... and there is a big hyperdense shadow in right parieto-temporal region .....; the final dignosis is ....; try to comment on skull bone (e.g. any fracture), ventricles (e.g. full with blood or 'cupping' seen), midline shift, brain parenchyma (e.g. cerebral oedema), etc.

The CT and MRI scan plates are described below:

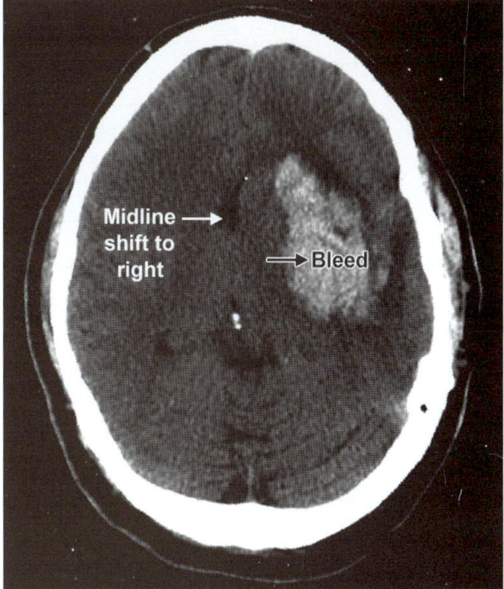

Fig. 3.34: This is a CT scan of brain which reveals a big hyperdense lesion due to **intracerebral bleed/haematoma** (white) in left cerebral hemisphere with perilesional cerebral oedema (black). Mass effect with midline shift to the right is noted. Normal intracerebral calcification is seen in the midline. The skull bone is intact

Clinical Wisdom

The patient will have right-sided complete hemiplegia. It is a patient of **cerebral haemorrhage**.

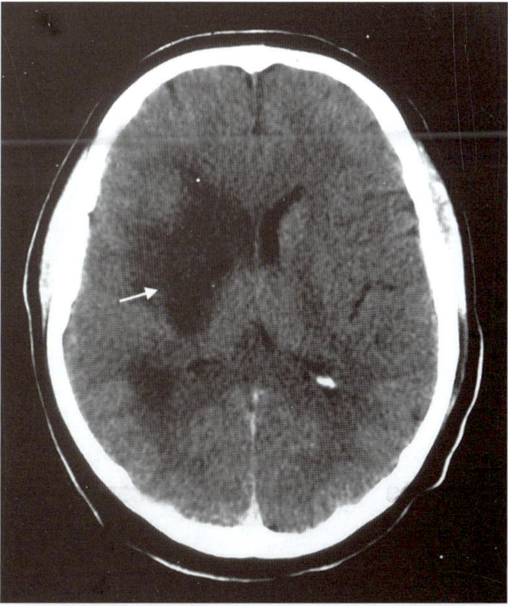

Fig. 3.35: This is a CT scan of brain showing paraventricular triangular hypodense lesion (looks black as shown by arrow) of **cerebral infarction** on the right hemisphere. Choroid plexus calcification is seen in the left side

Clinical Wisdom

The patient will have left-sided complete hemiplegia, and is due to cerebral thrombosis, cerebral embolism or vasculitis (rare).

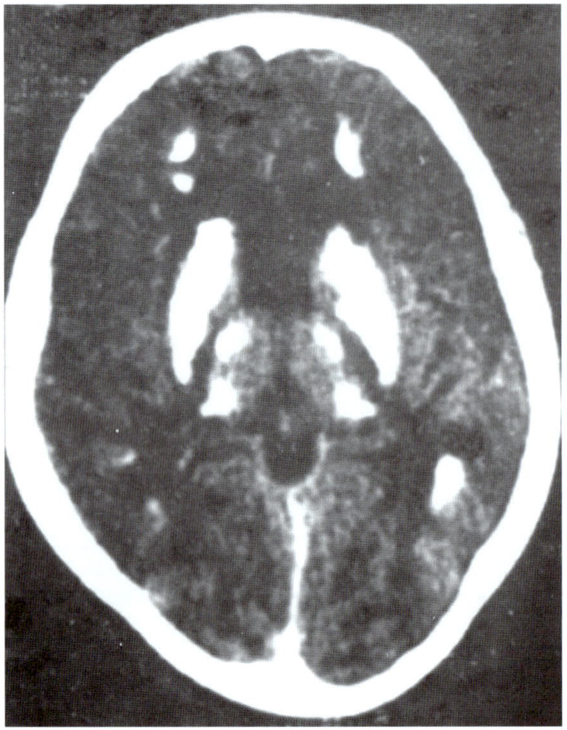

Fig. 3.36: This is a CT scan of brain which shows bilateral **basal ganglia calcification** (white). Calcification in other parts of brain is also seen

Clinical Wisdom

The common causes of basal ganglia calcification are idiopathic (commonest), familial, hypoparathyroidism, pseudo-hypoparathyroidism, carbon monoxide poisoning (attempted hanging), neurodegenerative disorder (Fahr's syndrome), and toxoplasmosis (congenital).

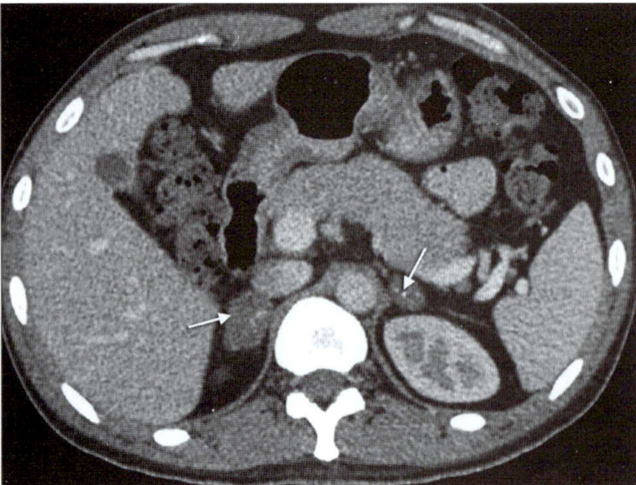

Fig. 3.37: The CT scan of abdomen demonstrates liver, spleen, aorta, stomach and spine. **Bilateral adrenal (suprarenal) masses** are seen as pointed by arrows

Clinical Wisdom

This is a CT scan picture of adrenal histoplasmosis. The usual mode of presentation is Addison's disease (i.e. hypofunction of adrenal cortex).

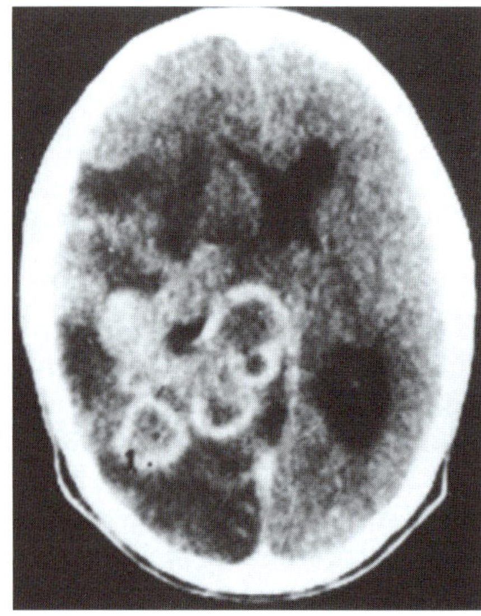

Fig. 3.38 Contrast-enhanced CT scan of brain (CECT) showing multiple isodense masses with ring enhancement in the right periventricular region with enlargement of ventricles. This is a patient with **tuberculoma** in brain

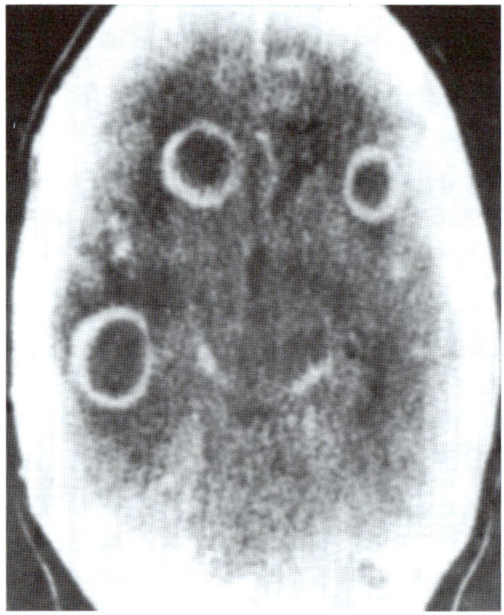

Fig. 3.39: CECT scan of brain reveals multiple large 'ring lesions'. This is a case of **multiple cerebral abscesses** in the white matter

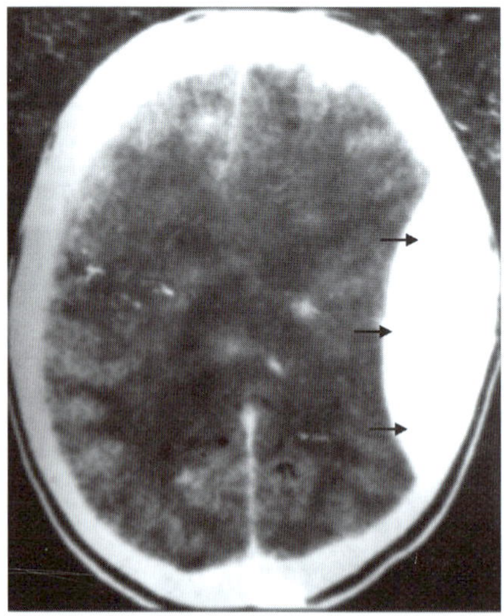

Fig. 3.40: The non-contrast-enhanced CT scan of brain showing a peripheral high-density 'biconvex' blood collection. This patient suffers from subacute **epidural haematoma**

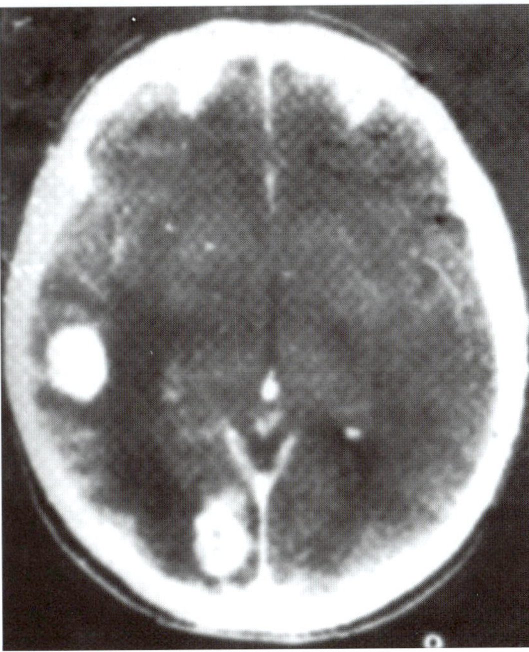

Fig. 3.41: CECT scan of brain shows two hyperdense masses in the right posterior temporal and occipital lobes. The lesions enhance homogeneously. Perilesional cerebral oedema and a slight midline shift to the left is seen. This is a patient of **cerebral metastases** from carcinoma of colon

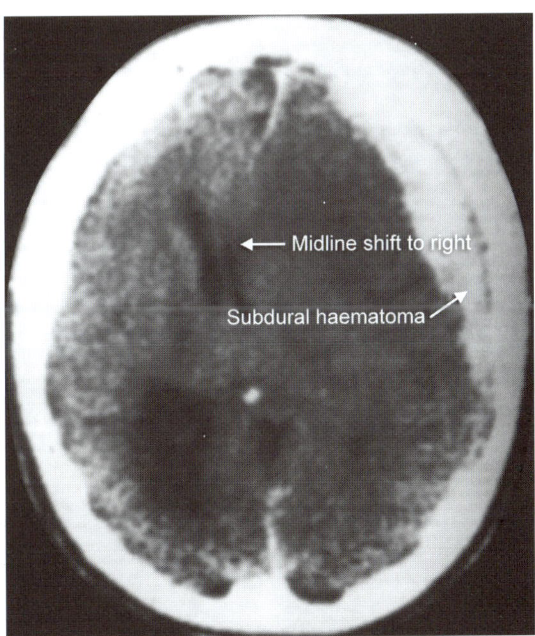

Fig. 3.42: This is an axial non-contrast-enhanced CT scan of brain showing a peripheral high density extracerebral collection within the subdural space which compresses the left cerebral hemisphere; there is a midline shift. This is a patient of acute **subdural haematoma**

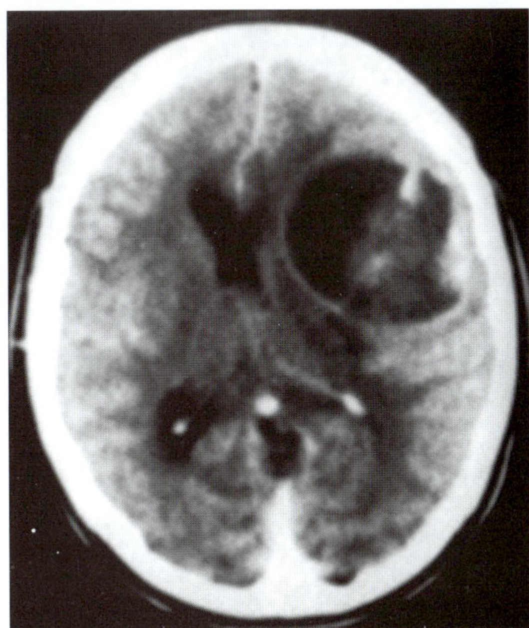

Fig. 3.43: CECT scan of brain demonstrates a well-marginated cyst with central mass in the left cerebral hemisphere; there is midline shift towards right. This is a case of **intracerebral tumour** (astrocytoma)

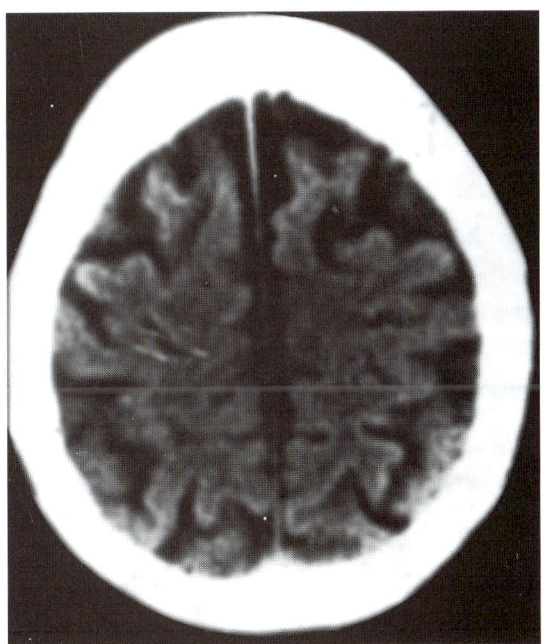

Fig. 3.44: Axial CT sections of brain shows enlargement of cortical sulci over the convexities. This is the CT scan brain of a 83-years old man having **cerebral (cortical) atrophy**

- CT scan feature of meningitis is 'diffuse meningeal enhancement'.
- **'Ring lesions'** (single or multiple: outer white ring with inner black shadow as shown in Fig. 3.39) in brain is seen in:
  1. Tuberculoma.
  2. Neurocysticercosis.
  3. Brain abscess.
  4. Cerebral metastasis.
  5. Venous infarcts.
  6. Others: Fungal infection, glioma, demyelinating disorders, toxoplasma, resolving haematoma, CNS lymphoma, radiation necrosis, etc.

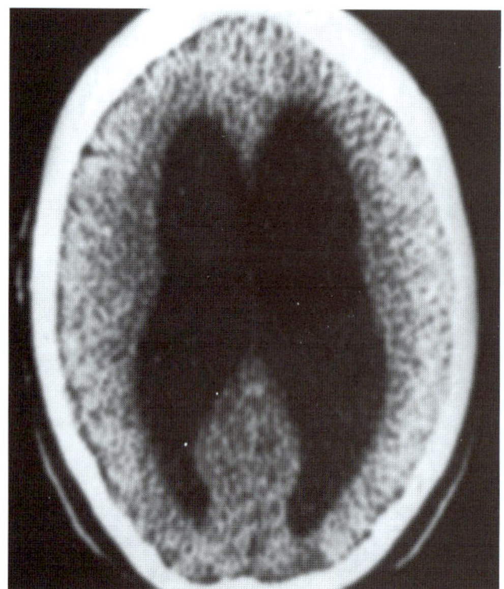

Fig. 3.45: This is a CT scan of brain showing symmetrical enlargement (dilatation) of the entire ventricular system. The patient is suffering from communicating **hydrocephalus**

- In CT scan: White shadow means hyperdense lesion and black shadow means hypodense lesion.
- In MRI **(Fig. 3.46)**: (a) T_1-weighted image: The signal characteristics of CSF, grey matter and white matter are hypointense, grey and white respectively. (b) In T_2-weighted image: They are hyperintense, white and grey respectively.

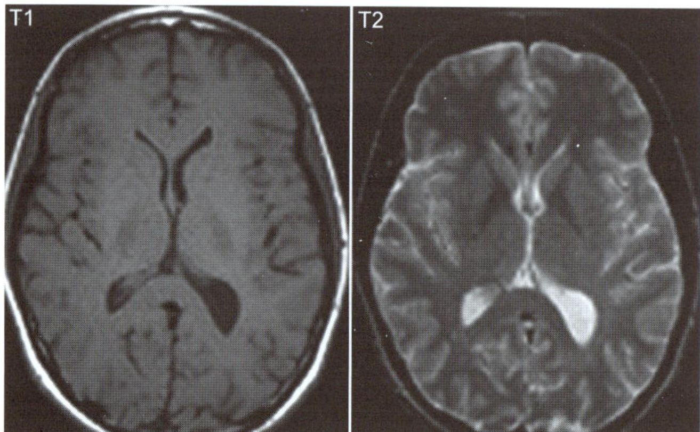

Fig. 3.46: MRI of brain—T_1 and T_2-weighted images

Clinical Wisdom

One has to remember that imaging modalities of choice during pregnancy are ultrasound and MRI. In disorders of musculoskeletal system, investigation of choice is MRI.

Chapter 4

Electrocardiography

"Ups and downs in life are very important to keep us going, because a straight line even in an ECG means we are not alive."

—**Ratan Naval Tata** (born on 28/12/1937),
an Indian businessman, investor, leader, philanthropist and former Chairman of Tata sons

Introduction and Basic Principles (fundamentals) of ECG

The graphic recording of the electrical activity generated by the heart is known as electrocardiogram or ECG. The ECG is recorded by applying electrodes to different parts of the body (wrists, ankles and chest wall) and connecting those electrodes to an electrocardiographic apparatus. It is inexpensive, easily accessible, simple to interpret, and provides wealth of information about cardiac status of the patient. 'Pattern recognition' of ECG in different diseases are important for a beginner.

The specially prepared ECG thermal paper (usually light pink or blue in colour) is made of small and large squares (Fig. 4.1A). Five small squares make one large square. The horizontal and vertical lines are present at 1 mm interval. Heavier lines of large squares are present in every 5 mm. Time is measured along the horizontal lines; **one small square (1 mm) is equal to 0.04 second in duration**, and one large square (5 mm) is equal to 0.2 second (i.e. 0.04 × 5). Voltage is measured along the vertical lines and is expressed in mm, and **10 mm is equal to 1 mV** (i.e. the usual calibration in ECG is a 1 mV signal that produces a 10 mm deflection). The **ECG paper moves at a speed of 25 mm/second**, i.e. 1500 mm/minute, i.e. 1500 small squares (so called, 300 large squares) are covered in 1 minute and thus to *calculate the heart rate*, one should divide 1500 by the number of small squares present in between two heart beats (R-R interval).

Any deflection above the **baseline (isoelectric line)** is known as positive deflection and that below the baseline is regarded as negative deflection.

A normal heart has P, Q, R, S, T and U waves (>5 mm) in ECG. Small waves of <5 mm in height are designated by small letters (q, r, s) (Fig. 4.1B).

P wave	Normally upright and signifies atrial depolarisation; precedes the QRS complex.
Q wave	The initial negative deflection that precedes R wave.
R wave	The first positive deflection of the QRS complex, i.e. ventricular depolarisation.
S wave	The negative deflection of QRS complex that follows R wave.
T wave	Normally upright and signifies ventricular repolarisation; follows S wave.

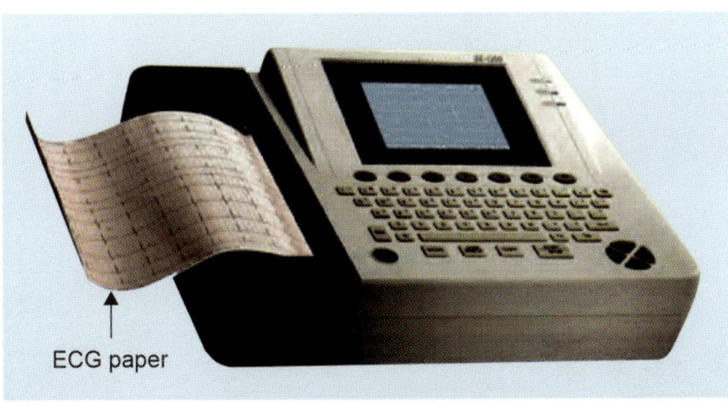

Fig. 4.1A: Portable ECG machine

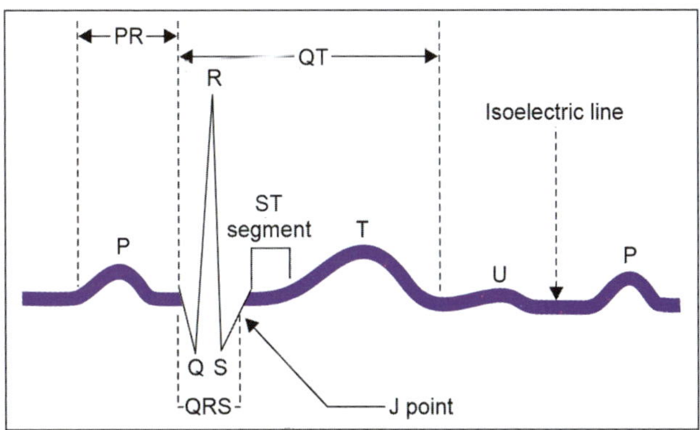

Fig. 4.1B: ECG complexes, segments and intervals

U wave	The small positive deflection that follows T wave and is probably due to slow repolarisation of interventricular (Purkinje) conduction system.
R-R interval	Distance between two successive R waves. It helps in counting the heart rate, i.e. R-R interval 15 mm = heart rate 100/minute (1500/15), and R-R interval 25 mm = heart rate 60/minute (1500/25).
P-R interval	It is the time taken for an impulse to traverse from the SA node to the ventricles. This is the period of conduction pause at AV node. It is measured from the beginning of the P wave to the onset of the QRS complex (more accurately P-Q interval) and is normally in the range of 0.12–0.20 second (i.e. 3–5 small squares in duration). P-R interval must be correlated with the heart rate (short with tachycardia and prolonged with bradycardia).
Q-T interval	It is the time taken for the total ventricular events (i.e. depolarisation as well as repolarisation) and is measured from the beginning of the Q wave to the end of the T wave. The normal Q-T interval is usually 0.35–0.44 second.

Uses of ECG in Clinical Practice

1. Hypertrophy of cardiac chambers, myocardial ischaemia or infarction, arrhythmias, different heart blocks, pericardial diseases.
2. Effects of drugs and electrolytes on the heart.
3. Evaluation of efficacy of angioplasty or by-pass surgery.
4. Holter monitoring and stress ECG.
5. Perioperative anaesthesia monitoring.
6. Screening tool in a sports physical examination.

Leads in Surface ECG

Conventionally, **12-leads ECG** (six limb leads and six precordial leads) are used in day-to-day practice (I, II, III, aVR, aVL, aVF, V_{1-6}). The right leg electrode and the lead act as a ground wire.

6 limb leads

- Bipolar standard limb leads: Lead I, Lead II, Lead III
- Unipolar (augmented) limb leads: aVR, aVL, aVF

6 precordial leads

- Unipolar precordial or chest leads: V_1, V_2, V_3, V_4, V_5, V_6

The unipolar (augmented) limb leads aVR, aVL and aVF record electrical activity of heart from right arm, left arm and left leg, respectively.

Lead I, II, III, aVR, aVL, aVF reflect electrical activity of heart in the frontal plane while lead V_1 to V_6 reflect the same in the horizontal plane. Each standard lead measures the potential differences in voltage between two extremity electrodes: lead I = left arm–right arm, lead II = left leg–right arm, and lead III = left leg–left arm voltages.

Besides these leads, oesophageal leads (E) are there to record magnified atrial complexes and to explore the posterior surface of left ventricle (introduced through nasal catheter). Unipolar intracardiac leads (recorded from right atrium or right ventricle) may be used for clarification of different types of arrhythmias.

Though in routine screening of ECG '12-leads' are employed, in following progress of arrhythmia a **'long lead II'** or V_1 is needed, or it is wise to explore higher (e.g. $3V_{1-9}$) and more lateral areas of precordium (e.g. V_{3R}, V_{4R}) in a doubtful case of acute myocardial infarction. The common precordial positions of the chest leads are (Fig. 4.1C):

V_1	4th intercostal space (ICS) at the right sternal border
V_2	4th ICS at the left sternal border
V_3	Equidistant from V_2 and V_4 leads
V_4	5th ICS in the left MCL (midclavicular line). All the subsequent leads (V_{5-9}) are placed in the same horizontal plane (i.e. in left 5th ICS) as V_4
V_5	Anterior axillary line (left)
V_6	Midaxillary line (left)
V_7	Posterior axillary line (left)
V_8	Posterior scapular line (left)
V_9	Left border of the spine
V_{3R-9R}	Taken on the right chest in the same location as left-sided leads V_{3-9}; V_{2R} is therefore same as V_1
$3V_{1-9}$	Taken one intercostal space higher than V_{1-9}; these are 3rd intercostal space leads. Similarly 2nd ICS and 6th ICS leads will be respectively $2V_{1-9}$ and $6V_{1-9}$
VE	Taken over ensiform cartilage

- ECG is also known as EKG. Lead aVR is oriented to the cavity of the heart and thus deflections of P-QRST are normally negative in this lead. Here, lead described after V_6 are additional leads and are not used routinely.

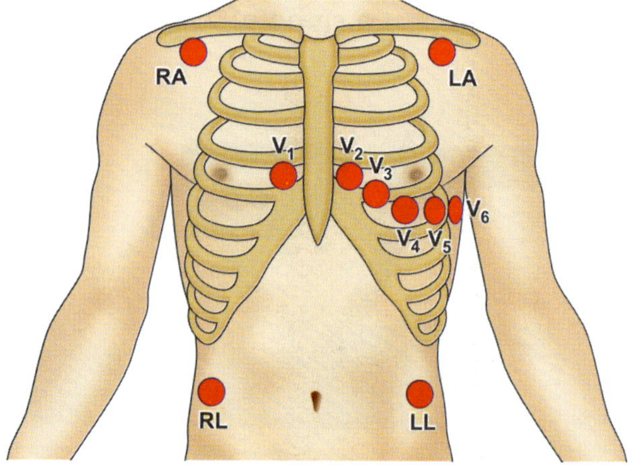

Fig. 4.1C: ECG leads placement

Axis Deviation

A 'hexaxial reference system' using standard leads and unipolar limb leads (the most popular and easy method for axis determination), deduced from **'Einthoven triangle'** reflects the mean QRS vector as follows **(Fig. 4.2)**:

- Normal axis lies between –30° and +100°
- Left axis deviation between –30° and –90°
- Right axis deviation between +100° and ±180
- Indeterminate axis (or extreme right axis deviation) between –90° and ±180°

- Axis lying between 0° and –30° is often known as mild left axis deviation.
- **Willem Einthoven** (1860–1927) of Netherlands was awarded Nobel Prize in 1924 for discovery of the mechanism of ECG.

Determination of Axis

The upper half of the horizontal line in the hexaxial system is negative and the lower half is positive. The positive pole of lead I is considered as 0° and the negative pole of lead I as ±180°; the positive pole of aVF is designated as +90° and the negative pole of aVF as –90°. The QRS complexes (positive or negative deflection) is marked or plotted in lead I and aVF accordingly, and the axis is determined accurately **(lead I and aVF are perpendicular to each other, and are routinely used to calculate the axis in clinical practice)**. One may consider lead II and aVL (perpendicular to each other), or lead III and aVR (perpendicular to each other) for axis calculation. Actually, the net positive or net negative QRS deflection in lead I and lead aVF is calculated (by subtracting the smaller deflection above or below the isoelectric line, from the larger deflection) and finally plotted for axis determination. One example is given below for better understanding **(Fig. 4.3)**:

Causes of Left Axis Deviation

1. Left ventricular hypertrophy (LVH).
2. Left bundle branch block.
3. Left anterior hemiblock.
4. W-P-W syndrome.

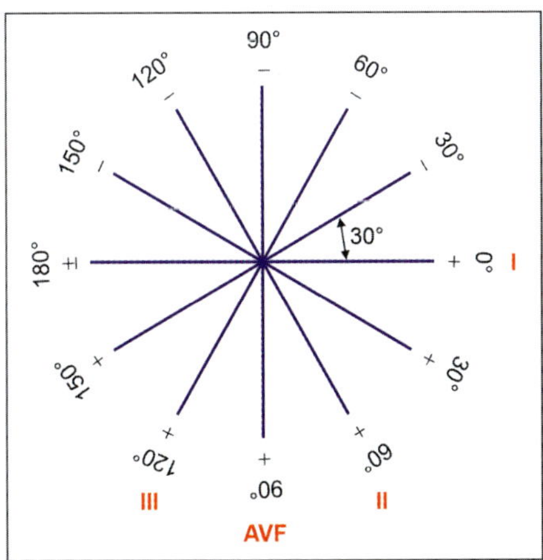

Fig. 4.2: Hexaxial reference system

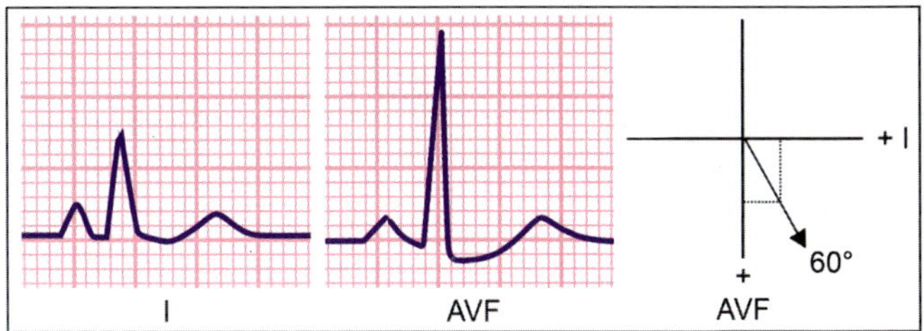

Fig. 4.3: Axis determination. The QRS axis is approximately +60°

5. Hyperkalaemia.
6. Endocardial cushion defect, e.g. ostium primum type ASD.
7. Hypertrophic cardiomyopathy.
8. Mechanical shifts, e.g. expiration, obesity, high diaphragm resulting from pregnancy, ascites, abdominal tumours; elderly subjects.

Causes of Right Axis Deviation

1. Right ventricular hypertrophy (RVH), right ventricular strain.
2. Right bundle branch block.
3. Left posterior hemiblock.
4. Normal variation; infants.
5. During inspiration; thin built adults.
6. Dextrocardia.
7. Emphysema and cor pulmonale.
8. Ostium secundum type ASD, Fallot's tetralogy.

Causes of Indeterminate Axis

1. Dextrocardia.
2. Hyperkalemia.
3. Severe emphysema.
4. Transposition of leads.
5. Ventricular pacing.
6. Ventricular tachycardia.

Position of the Heart

As anatomical rotation is rare, rotation of the heart refers to rotation of the electrical forces. Rotation of the heart may occur on either the antero-posterior axis (i.e. frontal plane) or the oblique axis (i.e. horizontal plane).

Rotation on the antero-posterior axis or **lie of the heart** is diagnosed by axis deviation:

a. Horizontal (–30°): aVL shows major upward deflection while aVF shows major downward deflection of QRS complex.
b. Semihorizontal (0°).
c. Intermediate (+30°): Both aVL and aVF show major upward deflection (it is the normal position of heart).
d. Semivertical (+60°), and
e. Vertical (+90°): aVF shows major upward deflection and aVL shows major downward deflection.

Rotation (electrical) on the oblique axis is diagnosed by the precordial leads:

a. Clockwise rotation: Persisting S waves in V_5 and V_6 (i.e. rS complexes in V_5 and V_6).

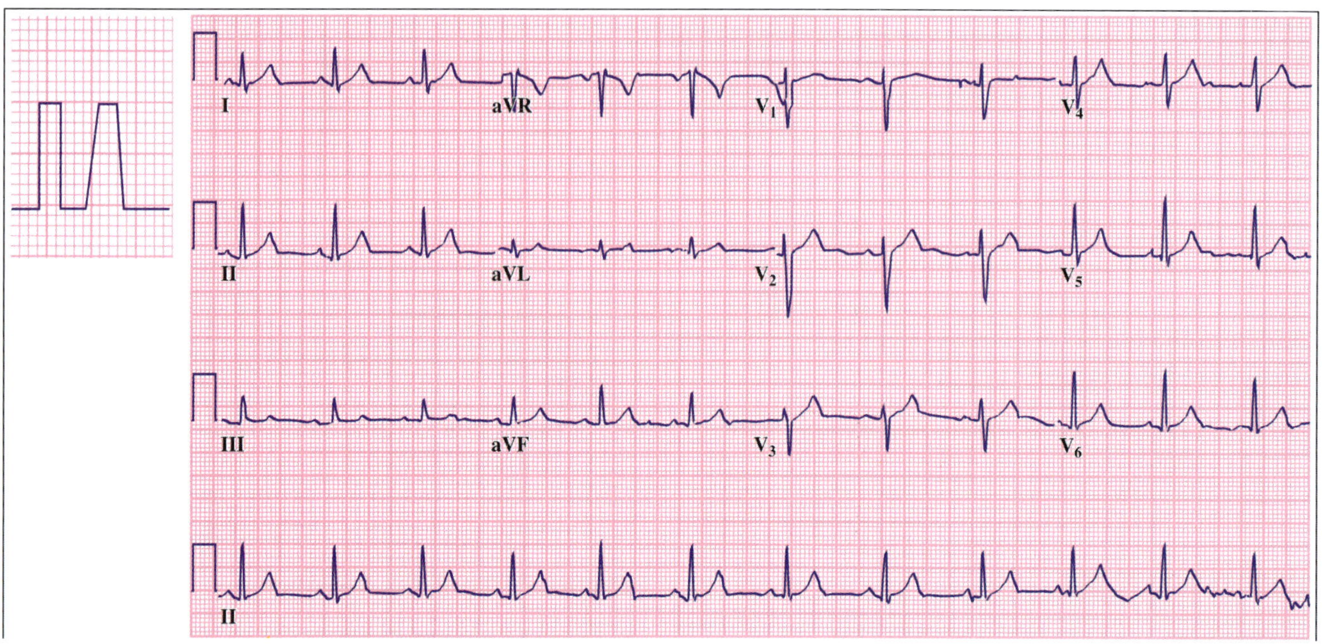

Fig. 4.4A: Normal electrocardiogram with long lead II (lowermost strip)

b. Anti-clockwise rotation: Appearance of left ventricular complexes as early as V_2 (i.e. qR complexes in V_2, V_3).

- Clockwise or anti-clockwise rotation is considered when the heart is viewed through the diaphragm.
- **The normal position is intermediate.** Normally, there is no clockwise or anti-clockwise rotation.

Technique of Reading or Reporting ECG (Fig. 4.4A and B)

1. Standardisation
2. Voltage
3. Heart rate
4. Rhythm
5. Axis
6. Lie and rotation
7. P wave
8. P-R interval
9. QRS complex and duration
10. ST segment
11. T wave
12. U wave
13. Q-T interval
14. Final diagnosis or conclusion

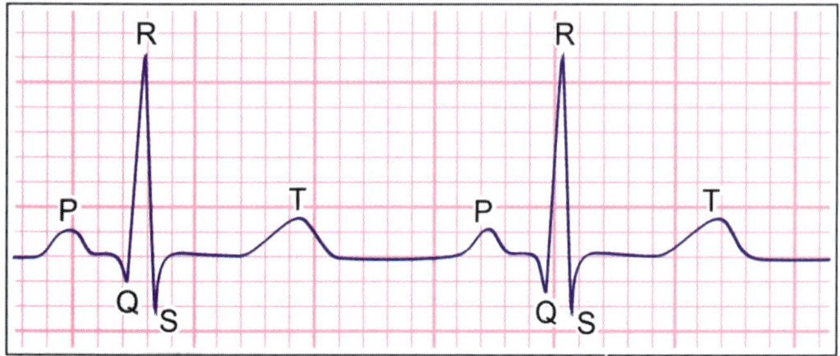

Fig. 4.4B: Normal ECG graph illustration

- In arrhythmia, study of 'long strip' of lead II is necessary (rhythm strip).
- **In the examination**, hold the ECG strip correctly (put your left hand over lead I and right hand over V_6; some small printing from ECG paper manufacturer will help you to select the upper and lower borders of ECG strip) and read the ECG in this way: 'it is the 12-lead strip of electrocardiogram showing normal standardisation......... voltage .... heart rate .... rhythm .... axis, ...and the final diagnosis is ....'.

DIFFERENT WAVES, COMPLEXES AND INTERVALS

P Wave

P wave signifies atrial activity (depolarisation) where the early part of P wave represents right atrial activity and the terminal part represents left atrial activity. Conventionally, the positive deflection is upward and the negative deflection is downwards. This is best visualised in lead II and V_1, and normally it is upright in lead I, II, aVF and V_{3-6}. P wave is inverted in aVR and frequently in V_1. Normally it does not exceed 2.5 mm in height and 0.12 second in duration (i.e. horizontally).

The abnormalities are:

1. Wide and notched (also known as **P-mitrale** (Fig. 4.5A); as mitral valve disease is a common cause of this abnormality): Indicates left atrial hypertrophy. Notching is considered significant when the distance between two peaks exceeds 0.04 second.
2. Tall and peaked (also known as **P-pulmonale** (Fig. 4.5B); as severe pulmonary disease is a common cause of this abnormality): Indicates right atrial hypertrophy when the height of P wave is greater than 2.5 mm.
3. Absent: In atrial fibrillation, nodal rhythm, SA block and sometimes in hyperkalaemia.

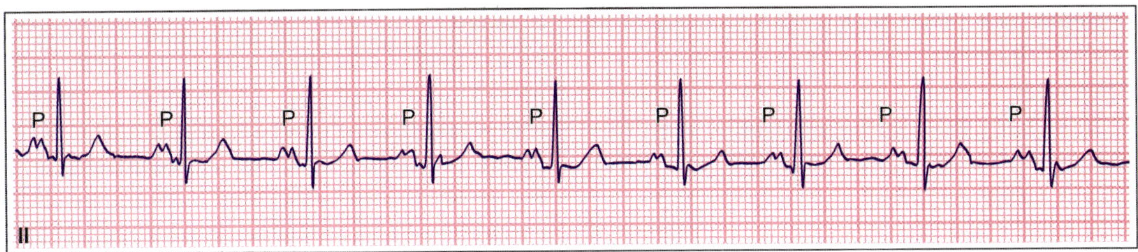

Fig. 4.5A: P-mitrale

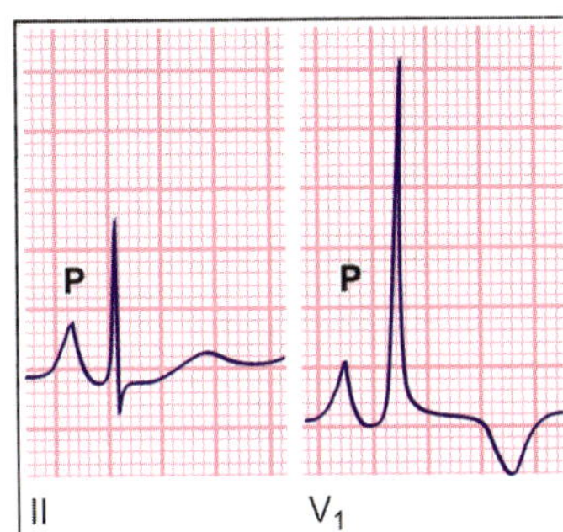

Fig. 4.5B: P-pulmonale

4. Inverted (in lead I): In wrong electrode placement by the technician, dextrocardia or possibly due to retrograde atrial activation (e.g. nodal rhythm).
5. Diphasic or biphasic P wave: The P wave in V_1 may be normally biphasic with a shallow, terminal negative component. If the terminal negative component is prominent, it indicates left atrial hypertrophy.
6. Himalayan P wave (height >5 mm): In Ebstein's anomaly, tricuspid atresia, restrictive cardiomyopathy, COPD.
7. Deformed: In atrial fibrillation, P waves are replaced by numerous small, rapid, irregular fibrillation (f) waves. In atrial flutter, P waves are replaced by flutter (F) waves which give the baseline a corrugated or saw-toothed appearance.

Summary:

Right atrial enlargement	P-pulmonale in lead II and lead V_1
Left atrial enlargement	P-mitrale in lead II, and or diphasic P wave with prominent negative terminal component in lead V_1

- Common **causes of atrial hypertrophy/enlargement** are: Mitral or tricuspid stenosis, secondary to LVH (develops left atrial enlargement) or RVH (develops right atrial enlargement), secondary to pulmonary hypertension or cor pulmonale, mitral incompetence, left atrial myxoma, etc.

QRS Complex

This complex comprises of Q, R and S waves, and is produced as a result of total ventricular muscle depolarisation (i.e. septal activation). QRS complex is upright (i.e. upward deflection >downward deflection) in most of the leads except in aVR.

a. ***Q wave:*** It is the negative deflection that precedes R wave. It signifies depolarisation of the ventricular septum from left to right side.
b. ***R wave:*** It is the first positive deflection of QRS complex. It signifies depolarisation of the ventricles. Initially, the anteroseptal portion is depolarised followed by the major muscle mass of ventricles.
c. ***S wave:*** It is the negative deflection of QRS complex that follows R wave. It denotes depolarisation of the posterobasal part of the left ventricle, pulmonary conus and the superiormost part of the ventricular septum.

In standard leads, R wave is dominant. In V_1, the r wave is small with a big S wave; gradually from V_1 to V_6, R wave increases (absent R wave progression is seen in anterior wall AMI) and S wave decreases in height. The height of QRS complex also depends on the position of the heart and the degree of abnormality.

- An entirely negative deflection without an R wave is known as QS deflection.

Voltage Criteria of QRS Complex

a. ***Low voltage* (Fig. 4.6)*:*** When the QRS complex is <5 mm (i.e. 5 small squares) in limb leads visiting Lead I, II, III, aVR, aVL and aVF, and <10 mm (i.e. 10 small squares) in precordial leads visiting V_1 to V_6, it is designated as low voltage. The common causes are:
   1. Incorrect standardisation by the technician.
   2. Obesity or thick chest wall.
   3. Emphysema.
   4. Pericardial effusion or chronic constrictive pericarditis; myocarditis.

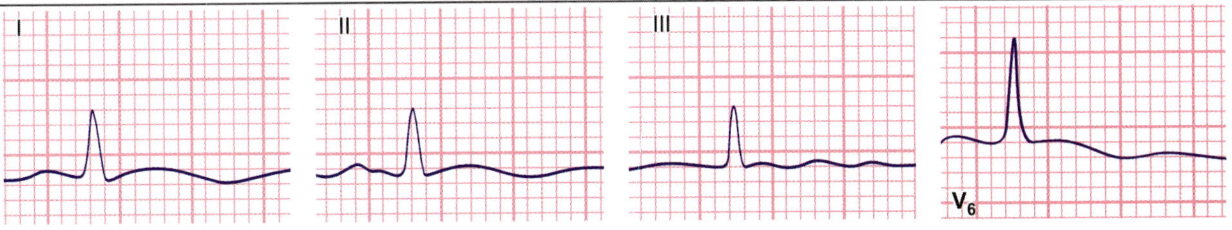

Fig. 4.6: Low voltage in a case of myxoedema

5. Myxoedema.
6. Panhypopituitarism.
7. Hypothermia.

b. ***High voltage:*** Tall QRS complexes usually signifies ventricular hypertrophy (criteria for LVH and RVH are described afterwards).

T Wave

It is a dome-shaped wave with two asymmetrical limbs, and is produced as a result of ventricular repolarisation; it follows QRS complex. It is normally upright (i.e. T wave is in the same direction as the main QRS complex), except in leads III, aVR, V_1 and V_2.

The abnormalities are:

1. ***Tall peaked T wave*** (>10 mm in height) (Fig. 4.7): In hyperkalaemia, acute subendocardial ischaemia or infarction, hyperacute myocardial infarction, often in true posterior wall myocardial infarction.
2. ***Low or inverted T wave*** (Fig. 4.8): Indicates coronary heart disease or myocardial ischaemia, ventricular 'strain' pattern, constrictive pericarditis, hypokalaemia, CVA (subarachnoid haemorrhage). In myocardial infarction, two limbs of the T wave may be symmetrical.
3. ***Flat T wave:*** In thick chest wall, emphysema, myocardial ischaemia, myocarditis, pericardial effusion, myxoedema and hypokalaemia.

- Following the T wave there is a brief 'isoelectric period' of 0.04 sec.
- Inverted T wave is usually accompanied by ST segment depression, and as a whole this is known as **ST-T changes**.

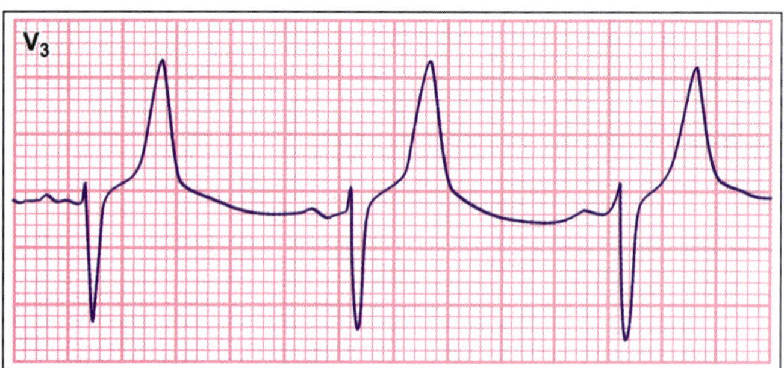

Fig. 4.7: Tall T wave

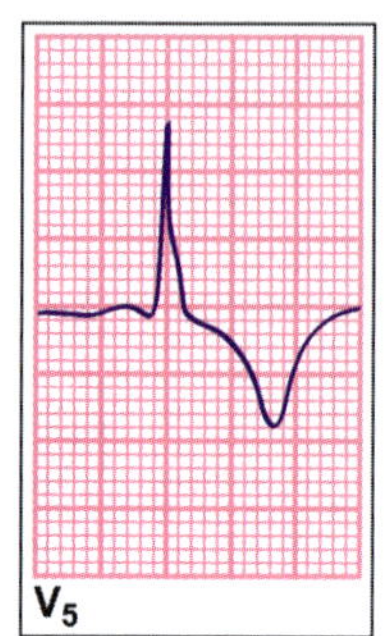

Fig. 4.8: Inverted T wave

U Wave

It is usually a small positive deflection which comes after T wave and precedes the P wave of the next cycle. It is possibly produced as a result of slow repolarisation of the Purkinje fibres, the interventricular septum and the papillary muscles. Many a time, the U wave is not evident in ECG. It is usually best seen in lead V_2 to V_4.

The abnormalities are:

1. Prominent U wave (almost resembling T wave) (Fig. 4.9): In hypokalaemia (commonest cause), thyrotoxicosis, exposure to quinidine or amiodarone.
2. Inverted U wave (i.e. U wave which is opposite in direction to the T wave): In coronary heart disease (acute myocardial infarction), hypertensive heart disease, acute pulmonary thromboembolism, intracerebral haemorrhage.

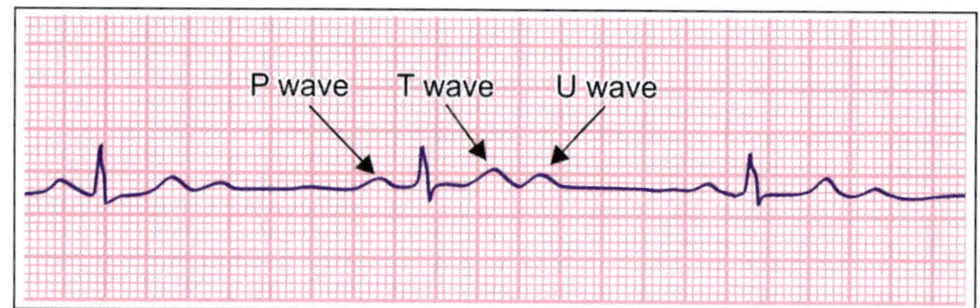

Fig. 4.9: U wave in hypokalaemia. Bradycardia is evident

ST Segment

The ST segment measurement is taken from the end of the QRS complex to the beginning of the T wave. Though normally it is 'isoelectric', it may vary from –0.5 mm (depressed) to +1 mm (elevated) in precordial leads (if ST segment is deviated more than the normal variation, the deviation is considered significant). The diagnosis of depressed or elevated ST segment is evaluated in comparison to the **T-P segment** (i.e. the base line between the termination of the T wave and the begenning of the P wave of the next cycle). The point where the QRS complex ends and the ST segment begins is known as **'J point'**, which is an important point for evaluation of ST segment deviation. ST segment represents the time interval between ventricular depolarisation and repolarisation.

The abnormalities are:

1. ***Elevated (with convexity upwards)***: In acute myocardial infarction (Fig. 4.10), coronary spasm, LV aneurysm.

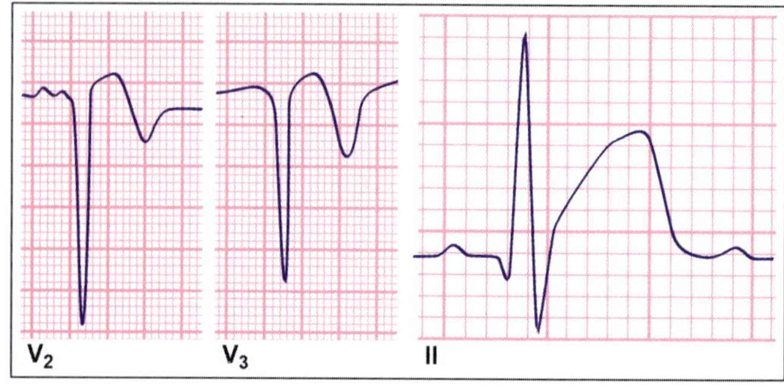

Fig. 4.10: Acute myocardial infarction with ST elevation (convexity upwards)

2. *Elevated (with concavity upwards):* In acute pericarditis (Fig. 4.11).
3. *Depressed (oblique, plane or sagging)* (Figs 4.12 and 4.13): In coronary artery disease (angina pectoris).
4. *Depressed with mirror-image of a 'correction mark':* In digitalis effect (Fig. 4.14).
5. *Depressed with upward convexity:* In strain pattern of ventricular hypertrophy (Fig. 4.15).

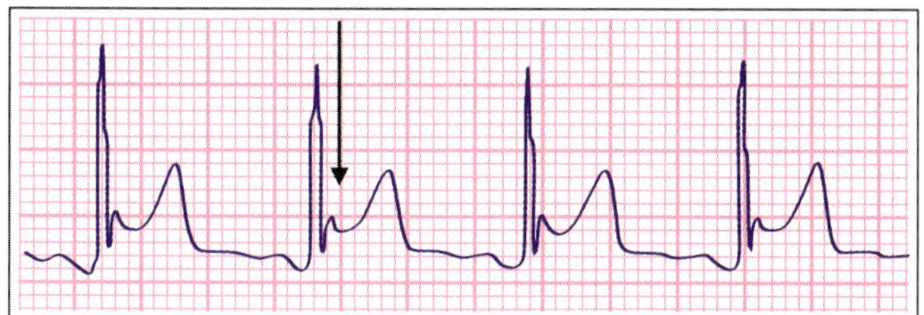

Fig. 4.11: Acute pericarditis with ST elevation (concavity upwards)

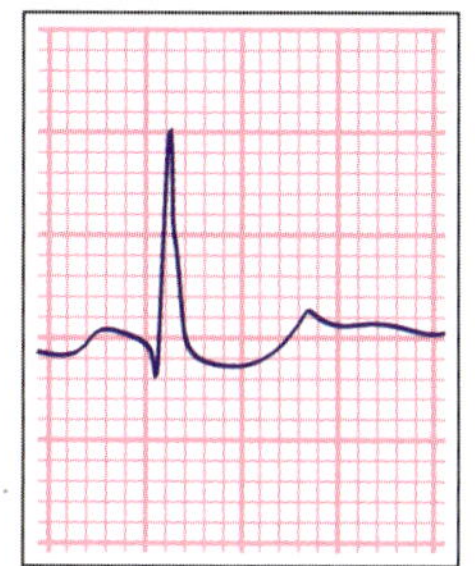

Fig. 4.12: Sagging depression

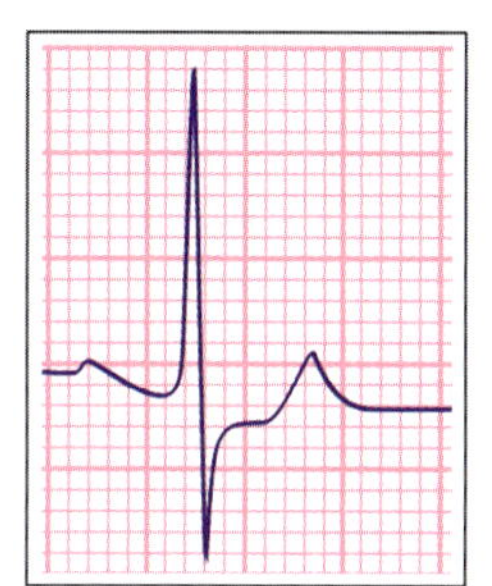

Fig. 4.13: Plane depression

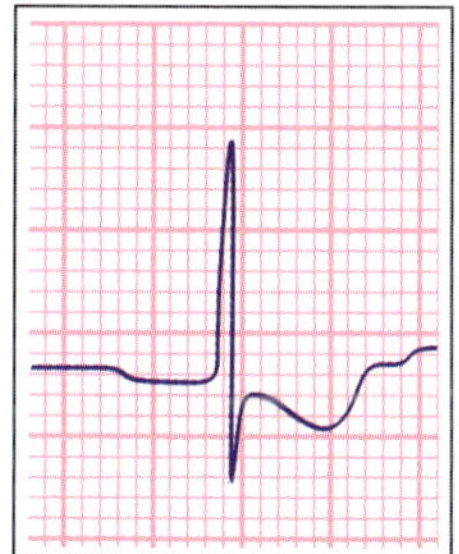

Fig. 4.14: Digitalis effect

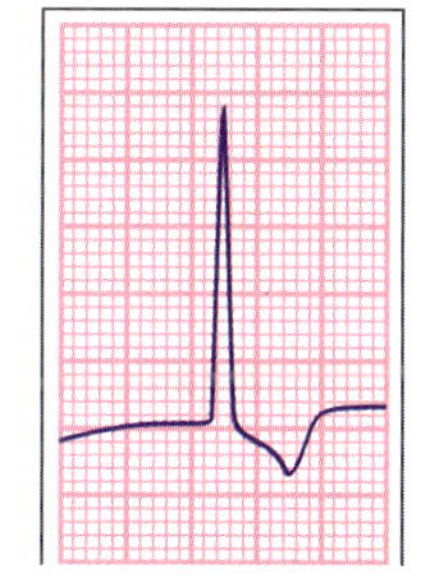

Fig. 4.15: Strain pattern

ST Segment Deviation

a. ST elevation

1. Acute myocardial infarction.
2. Prinzmetal's angina.
3. Acute pericarditis.
4. Ventricular aneurysm.
5. Hyperkalaemia.
6. Pulmonary thromboembolism.

b. ST depression

1. Angina pectoris.
2. Acute subendocardial infarction.
3. Myocarditis, posterior MI.
4. Ventricular hypertrophy with strain.
5. Digitalis effect.
6. CVA.

P-P and R-R Interval

The P-P interval is the distance between two successive P waves, and the R-R interval is the distance between two successive R waves. In sinus rhythm, the P-P and R-R intervals are same in duration. In heart blocks, some of the P waves are conducted while some are blocked and thus the P-P interval is different from R-R interval. Atrial rate is reflected in P-P interval and so the ventricular rate in R-R interval.

Calculation of Heart Rate (Fig. 4.16)

If the **rhythm is regular**, count the small squares present between two consecutive P waves or R waves, and then divide 1500 by that number. For example, if the R-R or P-P interval becomes 20 small squares (i.e. 20 mm), the heart rate with be 1500 ÷ 20 = 75/minute. In a case of complete heart block, the R-R interval (not the P-P interval) will help in calculation of heart rate (i.e. ventricular rate).

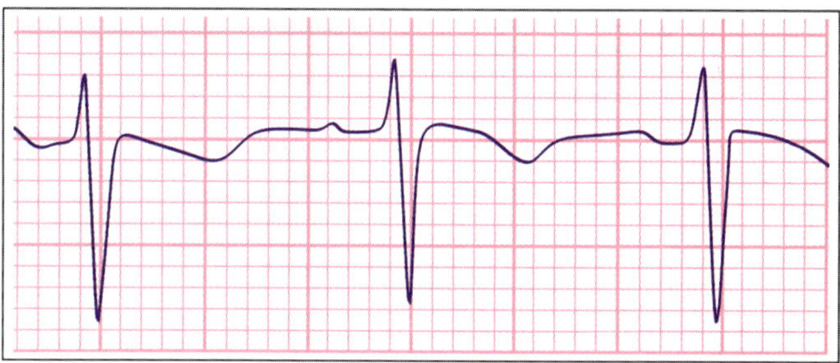

Fig. 4.16: Patient with heart rate 100/minute (1500/15)

If the **rhythm is irregular**, select consecutive 20 large squares (i.e. 0.2 × 20 = 4 seconds) in long strip of lead II, and count the number of R waves (or QRS complex) present in the time span of 4 seconds. Multiply the number of R waves by 15 to get the number of beats/minute or heart rate. This is practised in a case of atrial fibrillation.

P-R Interval

It is measured from the beginning of the P wave to the beginning of the QRS complex. The normal P-R interval is 0.12–0.20 second; the duration decreases with increase in heart rate and *vice versa* in decrease in heart rate. It is an indirect measurement of the time interval between atrial and ventricular depolarisation, and reflects intra-atrial, AV nodal and His-Purkinje conduction.

Clinical correlation: P-R interval determines the intensity of first heart wound (S_1). S_1 is loud if P-R interval is short, and S_1 becomes muffled in prolonged P-R interval.

The abnormalities are:

1. *Increased P-R interval* (>0.20 second; synonymous with 1° heart block) (Fig. 4.17): In acute rheumatic fever (i.e. Duckett Jones minor criteria), ischaemic heart disease, after digitalis or β-blocker therapy, myxoedema, hypothermia, ASD and as rare normal variation.

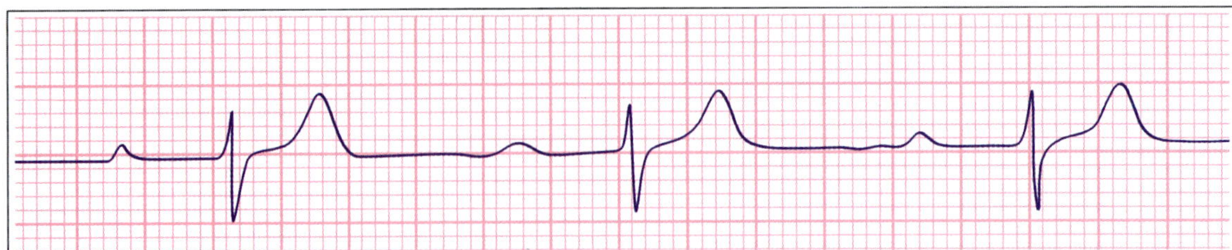

Fig. 4.17: Increased P-R interval. Heart rate is also slow, i.e. 50/minute

2. ***Shortened P-R interval*** (<0.12 second) **(Fig. 4.18)**: Tachycardia, in different pre-excitation syndrome like Wolff-Parkinson-White (W-P-W) syndrome; AV nodal rhythm, low atrial rhythm.

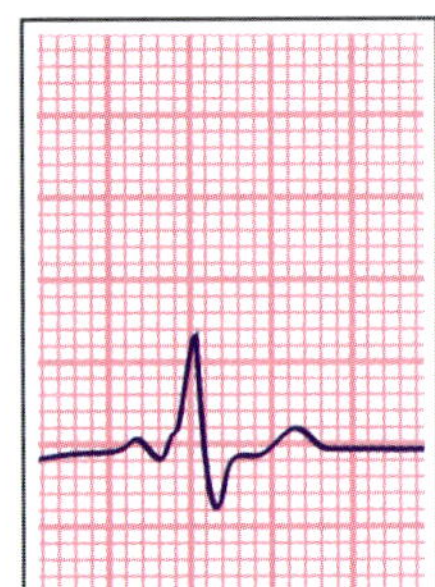

Fig. 4.18: Shortened P-R interval

3. Progressive prolongation of P-R interval is found in Wenckebach 2° heart block.
4. Variable P-R intervals are found in wandering atrial pacemaker or multifocal atrial tachycardia.

QRS Interval

It measures the total ventricular depolarisation time. The QRS interval is measured from the beginning of the Q wave (or, consider R wave if no Q wave is visible) to the termination of the S wave. The upper limit of normal QRS interval is 0.10 second.

If the QRS interval goes above 0.12 second, bundle branch block or intraventricular conduction defect is considered.

Prolongation of the QRS interval ≥0.12 second = Complete bundle branch block, and if the QRS interval is <0.12 second = Incomplete bundle branch block.

- *Intrinsicoid deflection or ventricular activation time (VAT)* is the time taken for an impulse to traverse the myocardium from its endocardial to epicardial surface. Measurement is taken from the beginning of the Q wave to the peak of the R wave. The VAT should not exceed 0.03 second in V_{1-2} (i.e. RV) and 0.04 second in V_{5-6} (i.e. LV).

Q-T Interval

It is measured from the beginning of the Q wave to the end of the T wave. It measures the total duration of ventricular systole. The Q-T interval should be corrected (Q-Tc) as it changes with the heart rate. Though Q-T interval varies from 0.35 to 0.44 second, the Q-Tc (corrected Q-T interval in response to different heart rate) should be:

$$\text{Q-Tc} = \frac{\text{Q-T interval (in second)}}{\sqrt{\text{R-R interval (in second)}}}$$

This is *Bazett's formula* (rate related) and according to this formula, Q-Tc is ≤0.44 second. The abnormalities are:

1. ***Prolonged Q-T interval*** (>0.44 second) **(Fig. 4.19)**: Hypocalcaemia, hypokalaemia, acute rheumatic carditis, acute myocardial infarction, myocarditis of any aetiology, quinidine or procainamide therapy, CVA (i.e. increased intracranial tension), hypothermia and congestive cardiac failure.
2. ***Shortened Q-T interval*** (<0.35 second): Hypercalcaemia, digitalis therapy, vagal stimulation and hyperthermia.

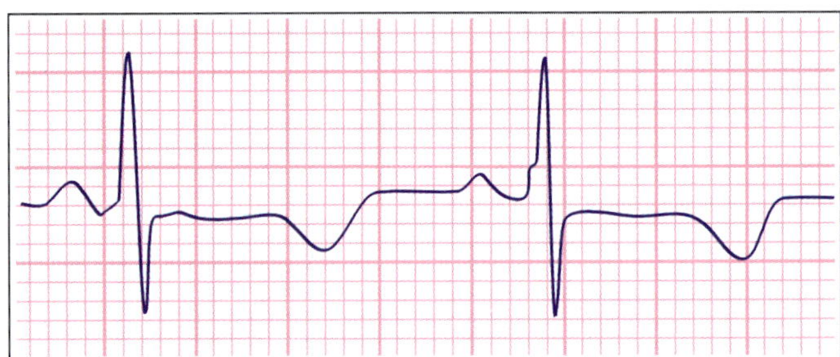

Fig. 4.19: Prolonged Q-T interval

Rhythm

Often a glance to the ECG recording is enough to say whether the rhythm is regular or irregular.

1. ***Regular (sinus rhythm)*** **(Fig. 4.4A)**: Sino-atrial, A-V nodal or idioventricular; the normal rhythm is regular.
2. ***Irregular (arrhythmia or dysrhythmia)***: Whether any definite pattern is present (i.e. beats grouped in pairs or every fourth beat is dropped) or not (i.e. totally irregular or with erratic irregularity like atrial fibrillation).

Measure the R-R or P-P interval and compare with corresponding two R or P waves.

Avoidance of Technical Difficulties before Recording

To avoid poor technical records, follow these instructions:

1. Patient should be explained the procedure to allay anxiety. Patient should be totally relaxed. A comfortable bed is necessary. Shivering or tremor should be avoided.
2. Good contact between the skin and the electrode is a must. Electrolyte jelly should be rubbed properly in the skin.

3. The ECG machine should be properly grounded to avoid AC interference.
4. Remove all electronic or magnetic equipments, or metal from the patient's body.
5. Enquire about presence of pacemaker.
6. Correct standardisaton (*see* below).

Standardisation

Normal coventional standardisation (calibration) is 1 mV which will produce an upward deflection of 10 mm (Fig. 4.20). Incorrect standardisation will lead to faulty interpretation as a result of incorrect voltage of the complexes (e.g. overstandardisation will unnecesarily diagnose ventricular hypertrophy and understandardisation will incorrectly diagnose a normal person as hypothyroid). Furthermore, the stylus of the ECG machine should have a correct pressure on the recording edge; otherwise the recording stylus will not move properly. Half standardisation is done in case of very high voltage (e.g. ventricular hypertrophy) and double standardisation is done in very low voltage (e.g. myxoedema).

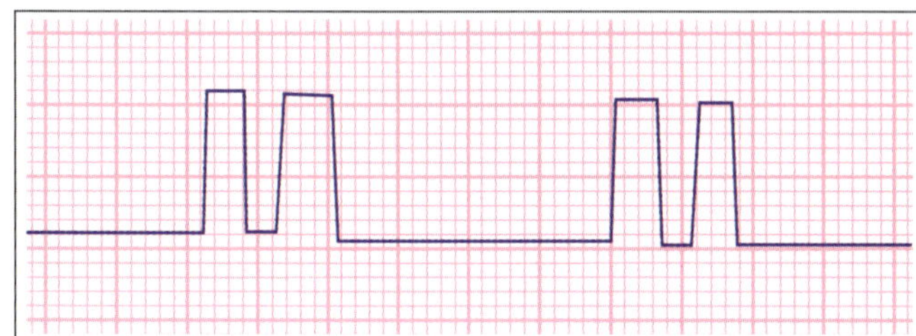

Fig. 4.20: Correct standardisation (calibration of 10 mm = 1 mV)

Effect of Deep Respiration on ECG

Deep inspiration makes the heart more vertical with clockwise rotation, and in deep expiration heart becomes more horizontal with anti-clockwise rotation. Often in lead III, a small q wave appears which disappears on taking deep inspiration (i.e. lead III R should be a routine procedure in the standard ECG tracing; R stands for respiration).

Exercise (Stress) Electrocardiography

Since the resting ECG is normal in 25–40% of patients with angina, stress (exercise) ECG is used to assess the cardiac response to exercise. The ECG is recorded while the patient walks or runs on a motorized treadmill **(TMT or treadmill test)** or bicycle ergometer, which follows the 'Bruce protocol'. Exercise can result in relative myocardial ischaemia as it increases myocardial demand on coronary blood supply.

In stress ECG testing, the limb leads are placed on shoulders and hips instead of wrists and ankles. The common indications are diagnosis and evaluation of angina, to assess the outcome of coronary angioplasty and to assess the prognosis following AMI. Patient's symptoms are assessed and BP is recorded during the test. If the patient complains of anginal pain, BP falls or fails to rise, or there is ST depression of >1 mm—the test is declared 'positive'. Subsequently, the patient is advised for coronary angiography to establish coronary arterial disease.

A. HYPERTROPHY PATTERNS (Chamber Enlargement)

'Hypertrophy' refers to an actual increase in muscle mass (pressure overload), commonly resulting from systemic hypertension (↑ LV) and aortic stenosis (↑ LV). 'Enlargement' is due to dilatation of heart chamber due to stretching of cardiac muscles (volume overload), commonly as a result of valvular heart diseases, e.g. aortic regurgitation (LV enlargement), or mitral stenosis/regurgitation (LA enlargement); hypertrophy and enlargement may co-exist.

Atrial Hypertrophy

Read the P wave in details (described earlier): P-mitrale and P-pulmonale.

Ventricular Hypertrophy

1. Left Ventricular Hypertrophy (LVH) (Fig. 4.21)

Criteria for diagnosis:

a. *Voltage criteria:* There is tall R waves in V_5 and V_6, lead I and aVL; deep S waves in V_1 and V_2; R in V_5 or V_6 is >27 mm; a sum of S in V_1 + R in V_5 or V_6 is >35 mm (Sokolow-Lyon criteria), and
b. R in AVL is >11 mm.
c. Horizontal heart with frontal plane QRS axis <–30° and anti-clockwise rotation.
d. The intrinsicoid deflection in V_{5-6} >0.04 second, i.e. VAT is increased.
e. Strain pattern (Fig. 4.15): Depressed and convex upwards ST segment with inverted T wave in lead I, aVL, V_5 and V_6.

- Left axis deviation is not an invariable accompaniment of LVH and if the axis is > –30°, think of associated left anterior hemiblock. Remember, lead V_5 represents the left ventricular forces.
- Nowadays, **Romhilt and Estes point scoring system** is probably the best formula to diagnose LVH.
- There may be associated P-mitrale.

2. Right Ventricular Hypertrophy (RVH) (Fig. 4.22)

Criteria for diagnosis:

a. *Voltage criteria:* R wave is greater than S wave in V_1 or V_{3R}, i.e. R : S = >1; usually a tall R wave >5 small squares in V_1 is suggestive of RVH.
b. A sum of R in V_1 + S in V_6 is >10 mm.
c. Persistent deep S wave in V_5 and V_6.
d. Normal axis or usually with right axis deviation (> +100°).
e. Vertical heart with clockwise rotation.
f. Intrinsicoid deflection in V_1 or V_{3R} is over 0.03 second, i.e. VAT is increased.

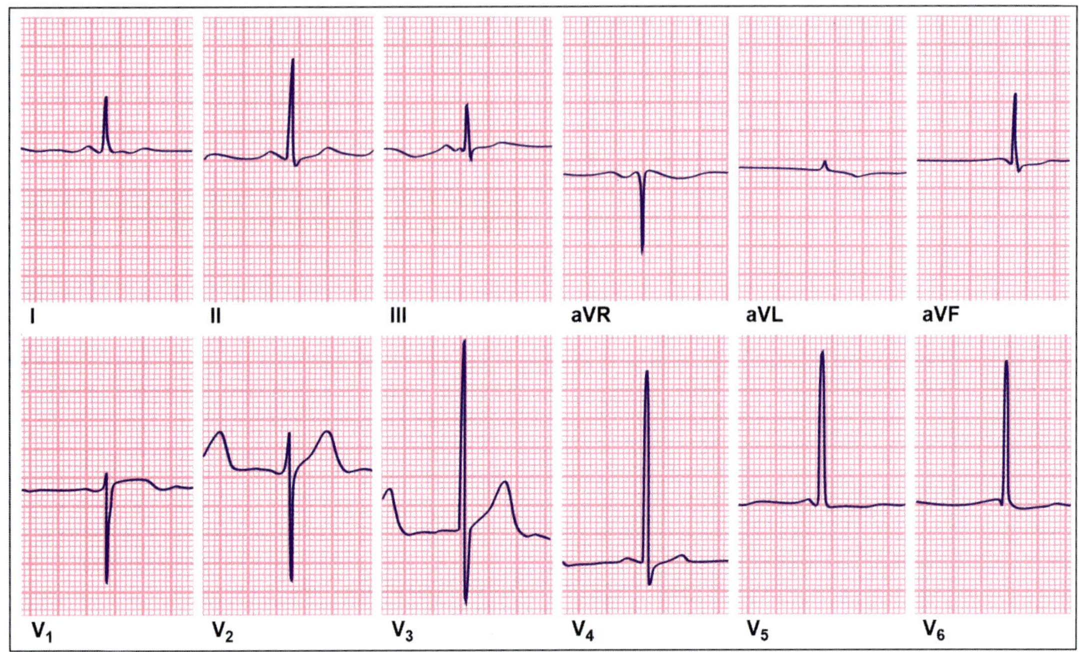

Fig. 4.21: Left ventricular hypertrophy

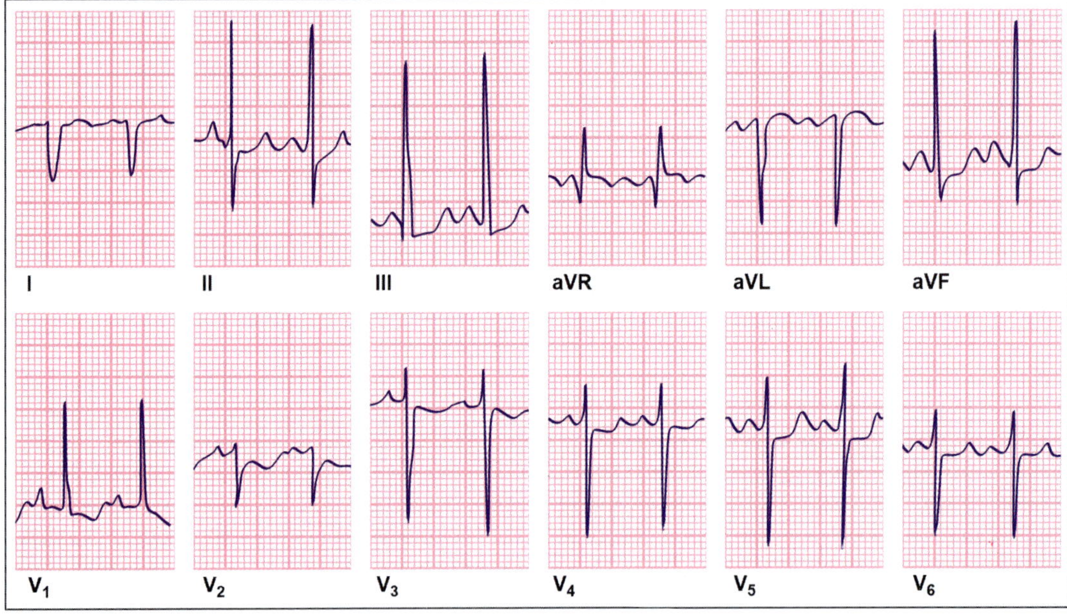

Fig. 4.22: Right ventricular hypertrophy with strain

g. Strain pattern (Fig. 4.15): Depressed and convex upwards ST segment with inverted T wave in right ventricular leads (V_1, aVR, V_{3R}).

- There may be associated P-pulmonale. Remember, lead V_1 represents the right ventricular forces.

3. Combined Left and Right Ventricular Hypertrophy

It is difficult to diagnose because very often the features of RVH are obscured by those of LVH. The most reliable criteria are the features of LVH in precordial leads associated with an axis deviation > +90° (signifies RVH); features of RVH with left axis deviation (signifies LVH) also point towards biventricular hypertrophy.

- **Katz-Wachtel phenomenon:** Large amplitude equiphasic RS complexes in mid-precordial leads (V_2 to V_5) are seen in biventricular hypertrophy (commonly in VSD).

4. Chronic Cor Pulmonale (Fig. 4.23)

a. P-pulmonale in lead II, III and aVF.
b. Vertical heart with clockwise rotation; there may be right axis deviation due to RVH.
c. Features of RVH.
d. Low voltage due to the presence of emphysema.
e. Right bundle branch block (rsR′-pattern in V_1).
f. ‘S_1, S_2, S_3 syndrome’ (producing S wave in standard leads I, II and III) as a result of emphysema.

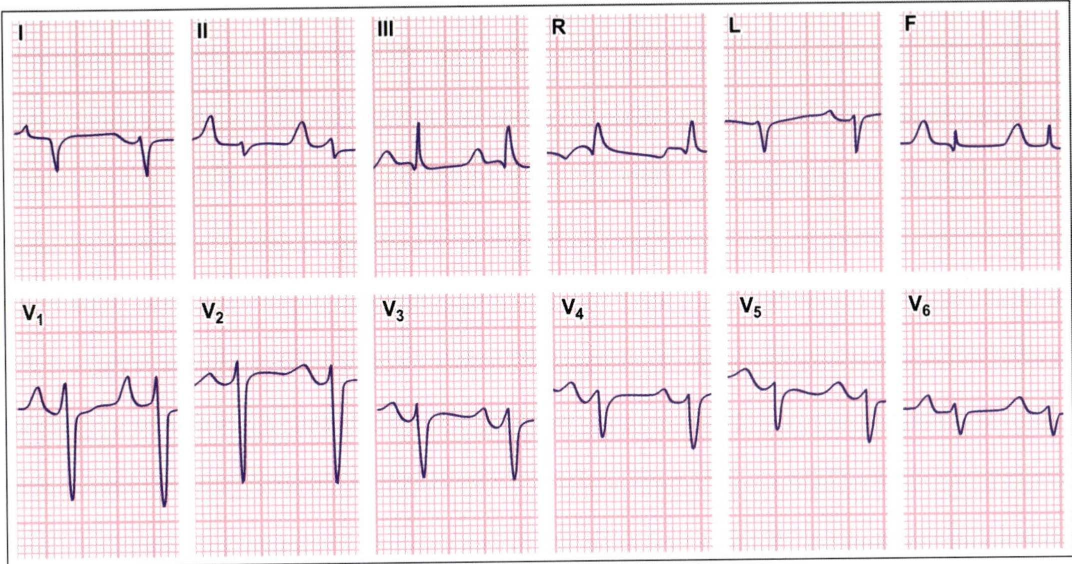

Fig. 4.23: Chronic cor pulmonale

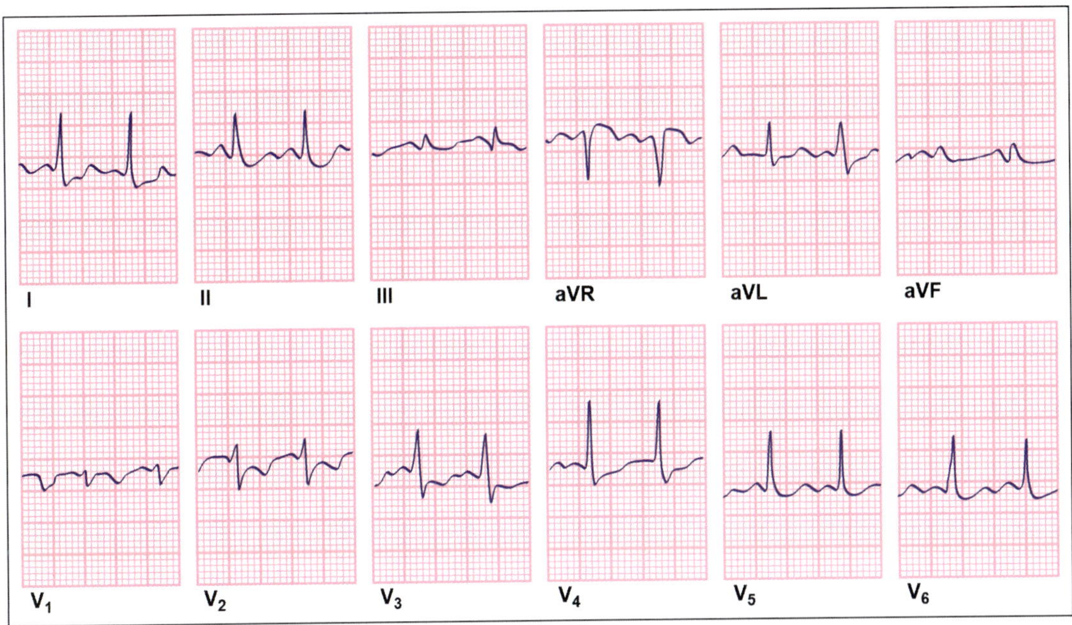

Fig. 4.24: Acute pulmonary thromboembolism

- The S_1, S_2, S_3 syndrome constitutes supportive evidence of RVH.

5. Acute Cor Pulmonale (Acute Pulmonary Thromboembolism) (Fig. 4.24)

a. Sinus tachycardia.
b. RVH with strain pattern.
c. Right axis deviation.
d. Right bundle branch block.
e. P-pulmonale.
f. 'S_1, Q_3, T_3 pattern', i.e. prominent S wave in lead I, prominent Q wave in lead III and inverted T wave in lead III (a reflection of right heart strain).

- Read the causes of atrial and ventricular hypertrophy from 'Bedside Clinics in Medicine, Part I'.

B. MYOCARDIAL ISCHAEMIA AND INFARCTION

Myocardial Ischaemia (Angina Pectoris)

Criteria: ST depression or T wave inversion, or both in standard leads, extremity leads and precordial leads. The ST depression may be of plane, oblique or sagging depression (Fig. 4.25).

- ST depression in angina pectoris (or Heberden's angina) usually indicates transient subendocardial ischaemia (Fig. 4.26). In Prinzmetal's angina, there is ST elevation seen as a result of transient subepicardial injury.

Myocardial Infarction

Three zones, i.e. ischaemia-injury-necrosis sequence in myocardial infarction is reflected in ECG. The ECG tracing (fully evolved phase) is the summation of,

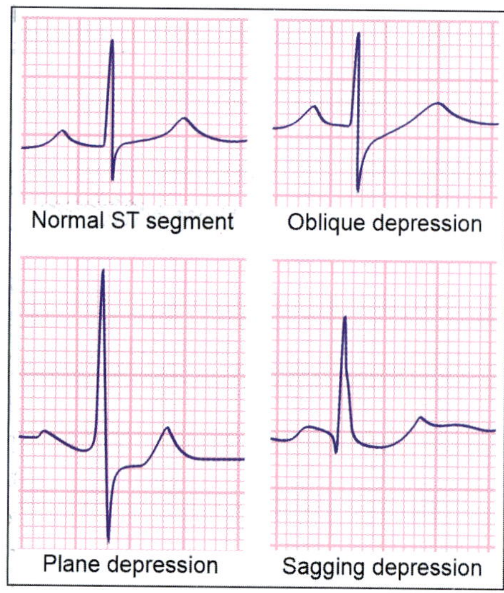

Fig. 4.25: Normal and abnormal ST segment

Table 4.1: Ventricular surfaces and leads reflecting ischaemia/ infarction

Surfaces (left ventricle)	Lead orientation
1. Anterior	V_{1-6}
2. Anteroseptal	V_{1-4}
3. Anterolateral	I, aVL, V_{4-6}
4. Extensive anterior wall	I, aVL, V_{1-6}
5. High lateral	I, aVL
6. Apical	V_{5-6}
7. Inferior	II, III, aVF
8. Posterior	No direct lead specification. 'Mirror-image' changes (ST depression and tall R) are seen in V_{1-3}
Surfaces (left ventricle)	**Lead orientation**
Right ventricle	aVR, V_1 and right-sided precordial leads, especially V_{4R}

1. *Myocardial injury:* ST elevation with convexity upwards.
2. *Myocardial necrosis:* Wide and deep Q wave.
3. *Myocardial ischaemia:* T inversion; T wave is peaked and both the limbs are symmetrical (arrowhead T wave).

- Acute myocardial infarction (AMI) is diagnosed on ECG by infarction pattern (presence of Q wave, ST elevation and T wave inversion), seen in more than two consequtive leads (Fig. 4.27); the infarction pattern observed in different leads determines the site (e.g. anterior, lateral, inferior) (Table 4.1).

Pathological Q Wave in Myocardial Infarction

1. Wide: >0.04 second in duration.
2. Deep: Usually >4 mm in depth.
3. Usually >1/4 th of R wave (in height) with substantial loss in the height of ensuing R wave.
4. Pathological Q waves are usually present in several leads, e.g. in inferior wall infarction, it is present in lead II, III and aVF.

The process of infarction progresses through three phases:

a. *Early 'hyperacute' phase* (within a few hours of the onset: Fig. 4.28):
   1. Slope-elevation of the ST segment with
   2. Wide and tall T wave.
b. *Fully evolved phase* (usually within 24 hours of the onset: Fig. 4.27):
   1. Pathological Q wave.
   2. Coved and elevated ST segment.
   3. Symmetrically inverted T wave.
c. *Phase of resolution or old infarction:*
   1. Pathological Q wave.
   2. ST segment and T wave may be normal, equivocal or point towards coronary insufficiency.

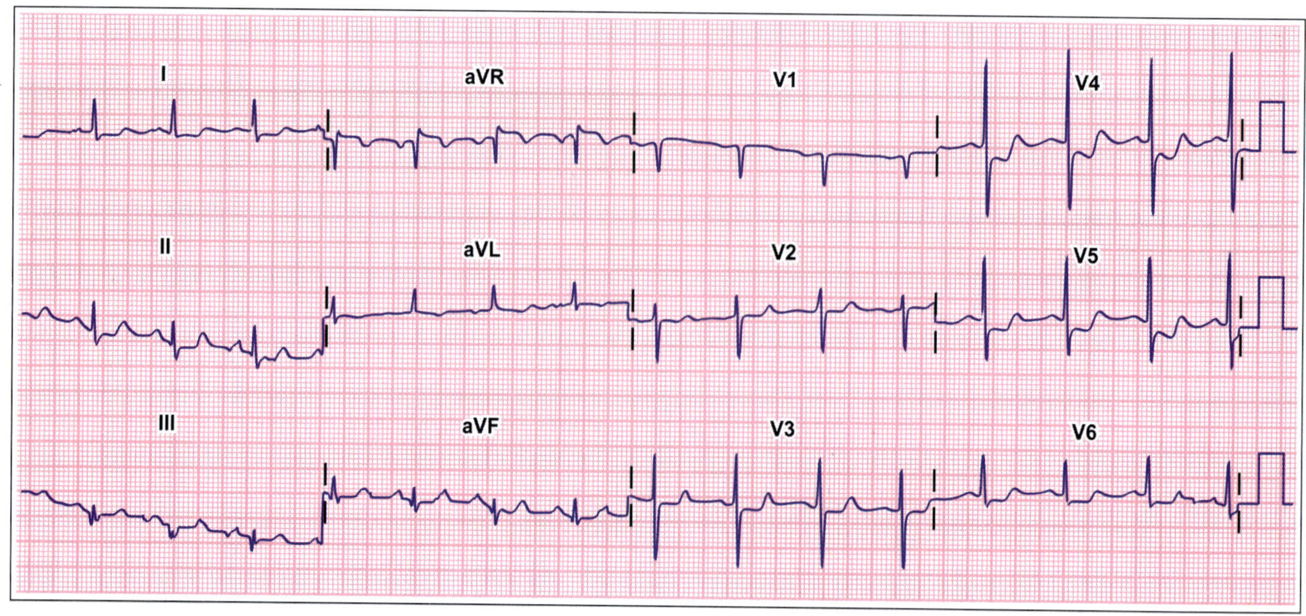

Fig. 4.26: Angina pectoris (coronary insufficiency). Anterolateral ischaemia is present

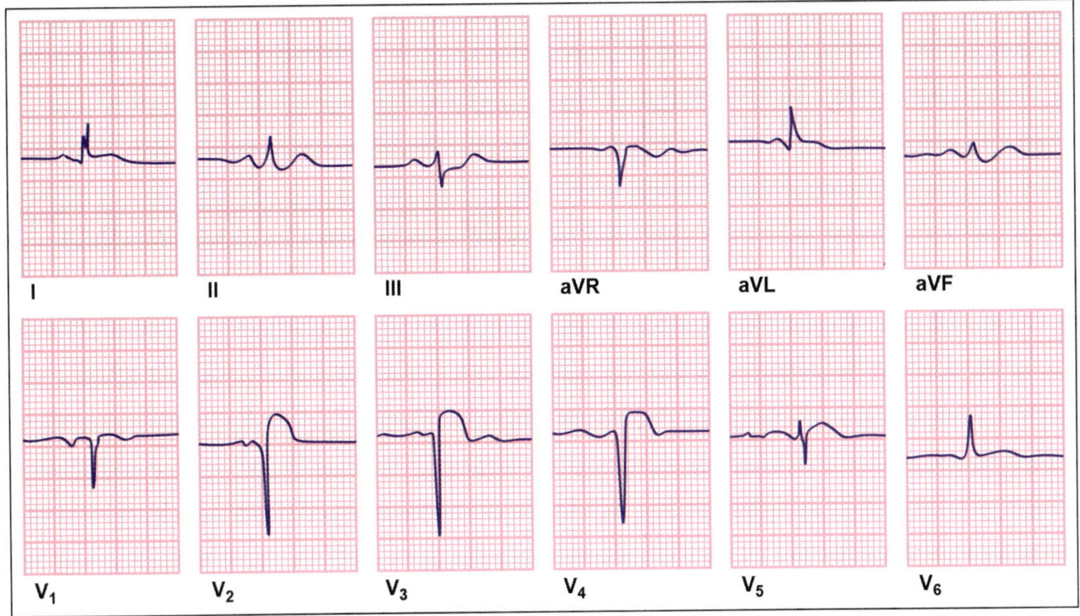

Fig. 4.27: Acute anterior wall myocardial infarction (extensive)—fully evolved phase

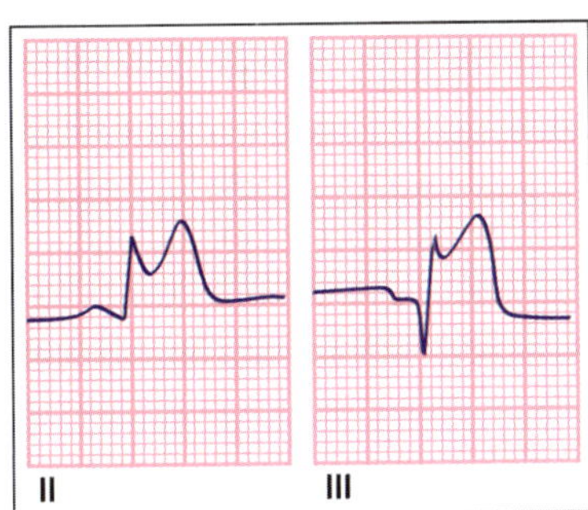

Fig. 4.28: Hyperacute phase of AMI

Table 4.2: Indicator leads and reciprocal leads in AMI

Indicator leads of AMI	Reciprocal leads
Anterior: I, aVL, V_{1-6}	II, III, aVF
Inferior: II, III, aVF	I, aVL and some precordial leads
Lateral: I, aVL, V_{5-6}	V_1, V_{3R}

- The reciprocal leads will show ST depression in case of acute myocardial infarction (AMI) **(Table 4.2)**.
- The above features give an idea of transmural (full thickness) infarction. Subendocardial (partial thickness) infarction is a bit different in acute coronary syndrome (ACS) patients, so that ECG shows deep symmetrical T wave inversion and loss of height of R waves facing the infarction (there is neither Q wave nor ST elevation)—non-ST-elevation myocardial infarction (NSTEMI).
- In high antero-lateral infarction, third intercostal space leads are recorded. Remember, QS complexes may normally be seen in V_{1-2} (in clockwise rotation) and in AVF (in horizontal heart). Persistence of ST segment elevation for a period of months or years after AMI indicates development of ventricular aneurysm.

Clinical Wisdom

Pathological Q wave, isoelectric ST segment and symmetrically inverted T wave are found in **'AMI of some duration'** (e.g. after 3–5 days).

C. DISORDERS OF RHYTHM

Sinus Rhythm

The rate and rhythm of the normal heart are controlled by the SA node which is again influenced by the vagus nerve. When the impulse is produced by the SA node, it is known as *sinus rhythm* which is the normal rhythm of the heart **(Fig. 4.29)**. The average heart rate is 60–100 beats/minute. If vagal tone increases, the heart rate is decreased and in decrease in vagal tone, there is accentuation of the heart rate.

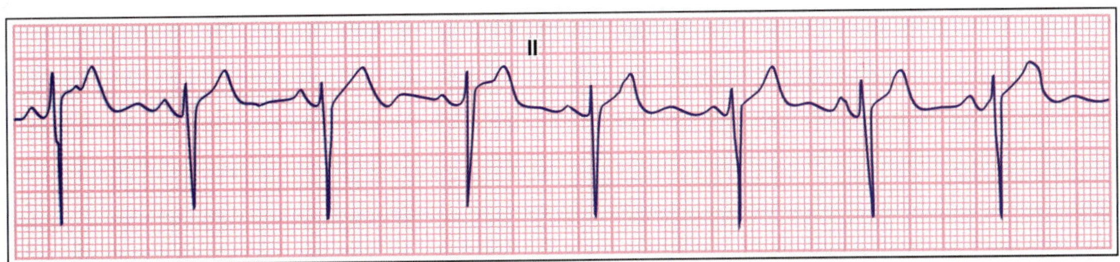

Fig. 4.29: Sinus rhythm

Sinus Arrhythmia

Heart rate increases with inspiration and decreases with expiration in sinus arrhythmia (i.e. alternate tachycardia and bradycardia associated with phases of normal respiration) **(Fig. 4.30)**. It is due to variation in vagal tone. This physiological phenomenon is commonly seen in children than in adults and is often associated with sinus bradycardia. Sinus arrhythmia is accentuated by vagotonic produres like carotid sinus massage, and is abolished by vagolytic procedures like exercise. The ECG tracing is diagnosed by gradual lengthening and gradual shortening of R-R interval in a normal ECG with normal P-QRST complexes.

Sinus Tachycardia

It is a regular sinus rhythm with SA node discharging in excess of 100 times/minute (usually 100–160 times/minute) **(Fig. 4.31)**. Common causes are adrenergic stimulation, strenuous exercise, emotion, anxiety, excitement, congestive cardiac failure, severe anaemia, thyrotoxicosis, shock, pain, pyrexia, myocarditis, acute haemorrhage, pregnancy, atropinisation and administration of drugs like nifedipine. The ECG tracing is diagnosed by R-R interval less than 15 small squares with normal P-QRST complexes.

Sinus Bradycardia

It is a regular sinus rhythm with SA node discharging in less than 60 times/minute **(Fig. 4.32)**. Common causes are vagal stimulation, athletes, deep sleep, fright, myxoedema, obstructive jaundice, increased intracranial tension, vasovagal attacks, sick sinus syndrome, heart blocks, hypersensitive carotid sinus, hypothermia, administration of drugs like propranolol and digitalis. The ECG tracing is diagnosed by R-R interval more than 25 small squares with normal P-QRST complexes.

SUPRAVENTRICULAR RHYTHM DISTURBANCES

Tachyarrhythmias are classified into two groups:

a. *Supraventricular:* Focus originating from atria or AV node.
b. *Ventricular:* Focus lies in ventricles.

Supraventricular Premature Beats (SVPB) or Extrasystoles

The ectopic impulse is due to premature discharge either from the atrium or the AV node.

Features

1. As the atrial ectopic beat (P′) occurs prematurely, it comes earlier than the anticipated sinus P wave.
2. The P′ wave may be upright, inverted or diphasic; it may be pointed or notched, i.e. P′ wave is bizarre.
3. The P′ wave is usually followed by a normal QRST complex (an ectopic P′ wave may be blocked and thus it may not be followed by a QRST complex). The QRS complex is of normal duration and same morphology.
4. The 'compensatory pause' is incomplete, i.e. the sum total of the R-R intervals of the normal beat before and after the ectopic beat is less than double of the normal R-R interval, i.e. A-B interval is <B-C interval in **Fig. 4.33**.

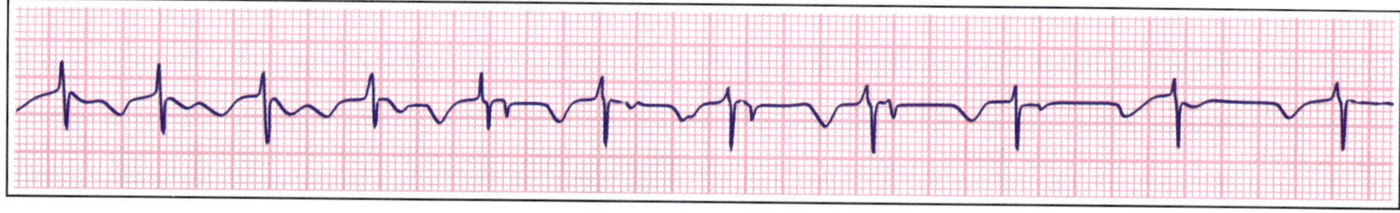

Fig. 4.30: Sinus arrhythmia

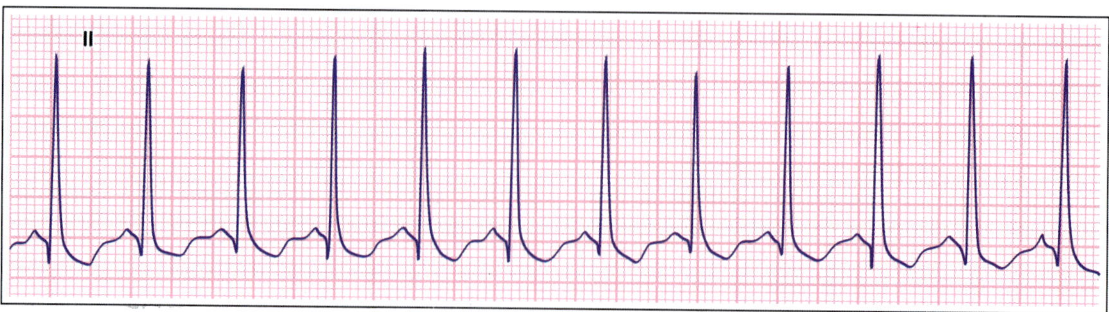

Fig. 4.31: Sinus tachycardia. Heart rate is 135/minute

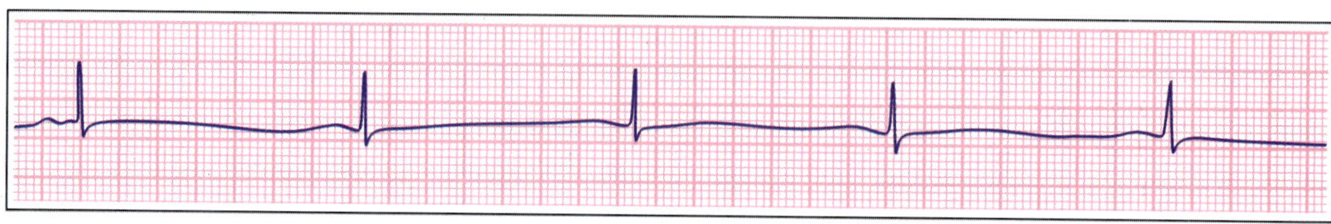

Fig. 4.32: Sinus bradycardia. Heart rate is 42/minute

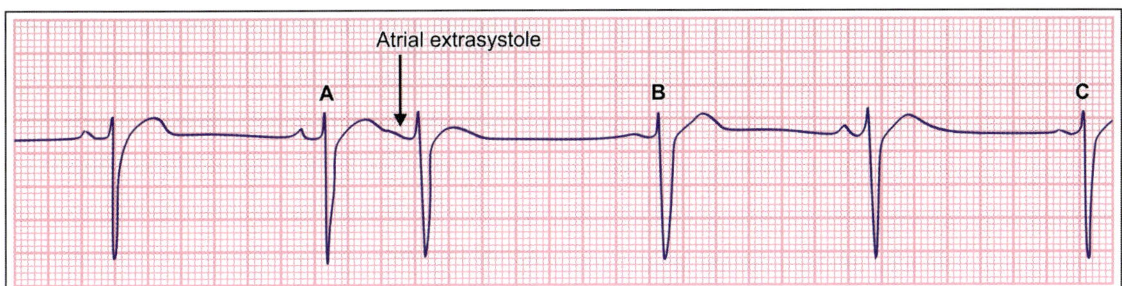

Fig. 4.33: Atrial extrasystole

Aetiology

1. Overindulgence of tea, coffee, cigarettes, alcohol.
2. Anxiety, dyspepsia.
3. Rheumatic, ischaemic, hypertensive, thyrotoxic, diphtheritic and cardiomyopathic heart diseases.
4. Drugs: Digitalis, emetine, thyroxine, adrenaline.
5. Hypoxia: Severe anaemia, shock.
6. During cardiac surgery.

- Two to four SVPB may result from smoking, insomnia, overindulgence of coffee or alcohol, and very often regarded as normal.

Symptoms pertaining to extrasystoles: Symptoms, if present are due to,

a. Extrasystoles or ectopics: Palpitations, extra beat.
b. As a result of compensatory pause: Vertigo, syncope, stoppage of heart, chest pain.
c. As a result of forceful contraction after the pause: Palpitations or thumping sensation.

Paroxysmal Supraventricular Tachycardia (PSVT)

PSVT is best thought of as a 'run of rapidly repeated premature beats' of sudden onset, usually three or more consecutive rapidly occuring SVPBs which continue for several hours or days; it may have sudden termination. PSVT is characterised by a regular rhythm at a rate of 160–220/minute.

As PSVT resembles a continuous run of SVPB, each P′ wave is followed by a ventricular QRS complex. PSVT is principally due to AV nodal re-entry mechanism often exaggerated by using a concealed extranodal pathway.

PSVT is also known as paroxysmal atrial tachycardia (PAT).

Features (Fig. 4.34)

1. Abnormal P′ wave preceding QRS complex.
2. Rapid (160–220/minute), regular and normal QRS (narrow) complex.
3. ST segment depression with T wave inversion may be seen.

Usually there is 1 : 1 AV conduction. Sometimes, there is AV block of varying degree, usually 2 : 1 (paroxysmal atrial tachycardia with block). The P′-R interval is often prolonged in PSVT and the P′ wave may be buried in the preceding QRS complex (i.e. no P′ wave seen), mimicking junctional (nodal) tachycardia (Table 4.3).

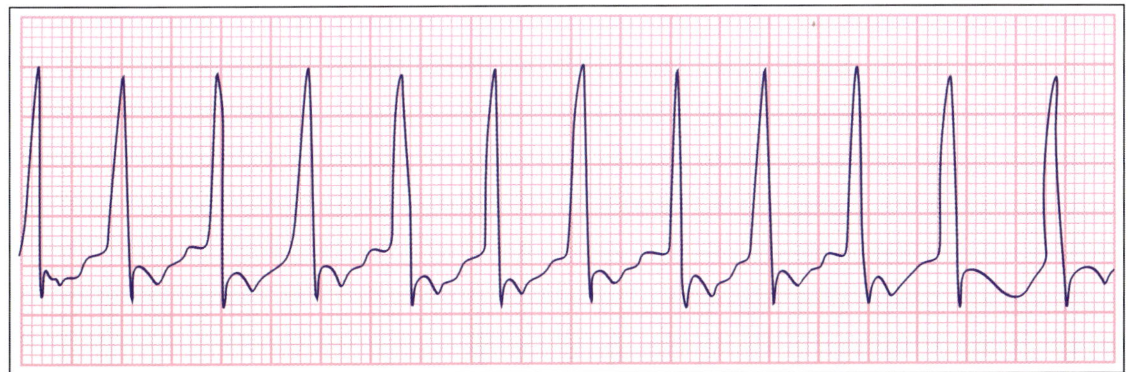

Fig. 4.34: Paroxysmal supraventricular tachycardia (PSVT)

Table 4.3: Differentiation between sinus tachycardia and PAT

Features	Sinus tachycardia	PAT
1. Heart rate	100–160/min	160–220/min
2. Onset and termination	Both are 'gradual'	Both are 'abrupt' or 'sudden'
3. P waves	Normal sinus P waves	Totally different from sinus P waves
4. Regularity	A bit irregular (during breathing)	Regular and no alteration with breathing
5. Effect of carotid massage	Gradual slowing of heart rate	Sudden reversal to normalcy

Significance of PSVT

Aetiologies are same as SVPB (sometimes PSVT may be seen in association with ASD, Ebstein's anomaly, W-P-W syndrome, sick sinus syndrome or floppy mitral valve syndrome). If PSVT continues for a long time, cardiac failure may be precipitated. *Management* is done by carotid sinus massage or with the help of other vagotonic procedures, and administration of drugs like verapramil, adenosine, beta-blockers (e.g. esmolol); lastly cardioversion with synchronized DC shock (100–500 J) may be applied.

Atrial Fibrillation

The excitation and recovery of the atria are totally disorganised and chaotic in atrial fibrillation. The atrial rate is usually 350–600/minute and varying degrees of AV block always exist in an untreated patient. The ventricular rate is usually 100–150/minute.

Features (Fig. 4.35)

1. Atrial deflections are irregular and chaotic, and thus results in a ragged baseline. The P waves are replaced by fibrillatory waves or 'f' waves which are rapid, small and irregular waves.
2. **Irregularly irregular ventricular rhythm.**
3. Normal QRS complexes, sometimes varying in amplitude.

Aetiology

1. *Heart diseases:* Rheumatic (commonly MS), ischaemic, hypertensive, thyrotoxic, diphtheritic and cardiomyopathic.
2. Myocarditis, pericarditis.
3. Drugs: Digitalis, emetine, adrenaline.
4. 'Lone' atrial fibrillation: In elderly persons without any demonstrable organic heart disease.
5. Constrictive pericarditis, ASD, W-P-W syndrome, cor pulmonale, pulmonary thromboembolism.
6. Sinoatrial disease (sick sinus syndrome).
7. Following cardiothoracic surgery.

Atrial Flutter

It is the rapid as well as regular contraction of atria at a rate of approximately 220–350/minute. The ventricular rate is usually regular, being 1/2 to 1/4th of the atrial rate (as AV block is always associated with). Constantly changing AV block makes the ventricular rate irregular. The P' waves of atrial flutter have a 'saw-toothed' appearance and are known as flutter (F) waves (usually in lead II and III).

Features (Fig. 4.36A)

1. 'Saw-toothed' or undulating baseline with 'F' waves (flutter waves) replacing P waves. Usually atrial rate is 220–350/ minute and the ventricular rate is 1/2 to 1/4th of the atrial rate.
2. **Regular ventricular rhythm** unless associated with changing AV block.
3. Normal QRS complexes in a ratio of 2:1 to 8:1.

Aetiology

Same as atrial fibrillation.

Atrial Flutter-Fibrillation

Sometimes, a mixture of atrial flutter with atrial fibrillation is seen and the precise differentiation between them is often very difficult. This is known as flutter-fibrillation (Fig. 4.36B).

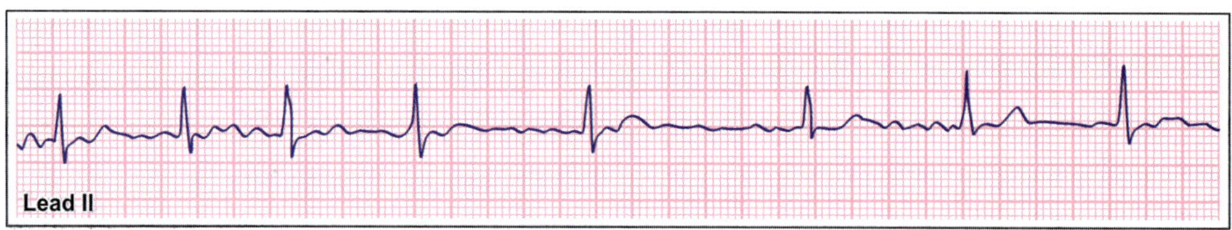

Fig. 4.35: Atrial fibrillation

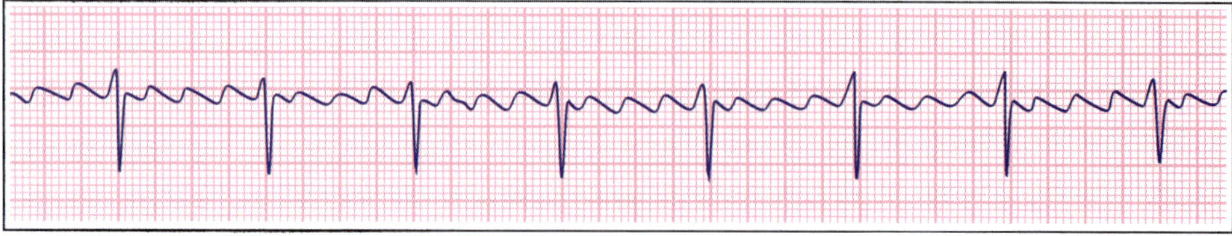

Fig. 4.36A: Atrial flutter

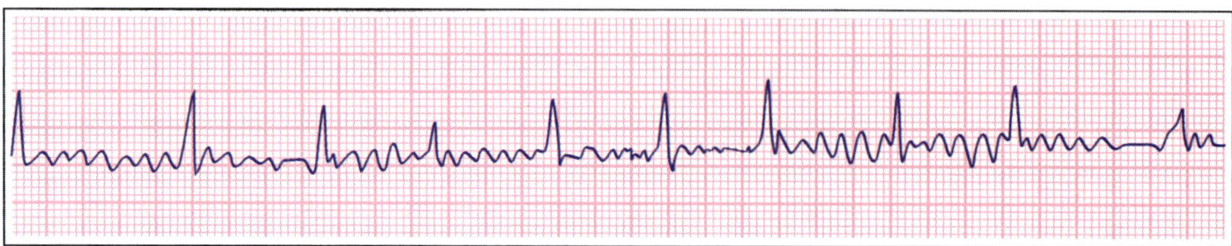

Fig. 4.36B: Atrial flutter-fibrillation

- Fibrillation and flutter waves are best seen in lead II and V_1.
- 'Holiday heart syndrome' is the development of supraventricular tachycardia (SVT), most commonly atrial fibrillation and flutter, following an acute alcoholic binge usually on holidays. These are transient episodes.

VENTRICULAR RHYTHM DISTURBANCES

Ventricular Premature Beats (VPB) or Extrasystoles

The VPB arises from an ectopic focus in any portion of the ventricular myocardium.

Features (Fig. 4.37)

1. The ectopic beat appears prematurely.
2. P' wave is usually hidden in the QRS complex or a retrograde P' wave (usually inverted) may follow the QRS complex.
3. Bizarre, wide and tall QRS complex. The ST segment and T wave are usually displaced in the opposite direction of the major QRS complex.
4. The 'compensatory pause' is complete, i.e. the sum total of the R-R intervals of the normal beat preceding and following a VPB is equal to double of the normal R-R interval.

- Ventricular ectopics or VPBs may be monomorphic (same pattern) or polymorphic (different patterns). They may form 'couplet' (a pair of successive VPBs) or 'bigeminal rhythm' (an ectopic beat alternating with a sinus beat).

Aetiology

Same as SVPB.

- VPB are commonly seen in 24 hours ECG tacing or following acute myocardial infarction.

Significance of VPB

SVPB frequently occurs in normal individuals. Diagnosis of organic heart disease should not be made solely on the ECG criteria of SVPB. Very often atrial extrasystoles occur secondary to emotional disturbances, after consumtion of tea, coffee, tobacco and alcohol.

Though **VPB** may occasionally be found in normal individuals, **it is always significant** if associated with:

1. Bigeminal rhythm (Fig. 4.38).
2. In an individual with organic heart disease, especially myocardial disease.
3. If the VPB are multifocal.
4. If the VPB occur frequently, i.e. in 'crops'.
5. If the VPB are present >5 times/minute.
6. If precipitated by exercise.
7. If occurs in persons >40 years of age.
8. Presence of 'R on T phenomenon' (such an ectopic beat is prone to initiate repetitive discharge, i.e. ventricular tachycardia or fibrillation may be precipitated).

Clinical Wisdom 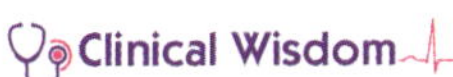

In contrast to SVPB (often found in normal individuals), VPB usually indicates some cardiac disease.

Ventricular Tachycardia (Paroxysmal)

When a series of three or more consecutive VPBs occur for few beats or continue for several hours or days, it is known as ventricular tachycardia (VT). Usually VT has a 'regular rhythm' with a heart rate of 140–220/minute.

Features (Fig. 4.39)

1. Premature, bizarre, tall and wide QRS complexes recorded in rapid succession.
2. The P wave bears no relationship with the QRS complexes (AV dissociation).

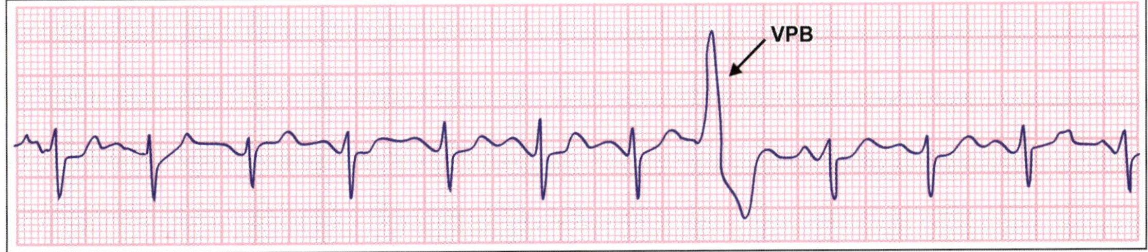

Fig. 4.37: Ventricular extrasystole

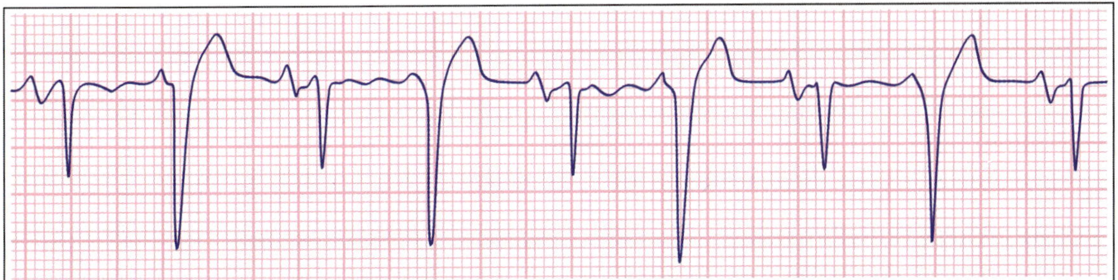

Fig. 4.38: Bigeminal rhythm produced by alternate VPB

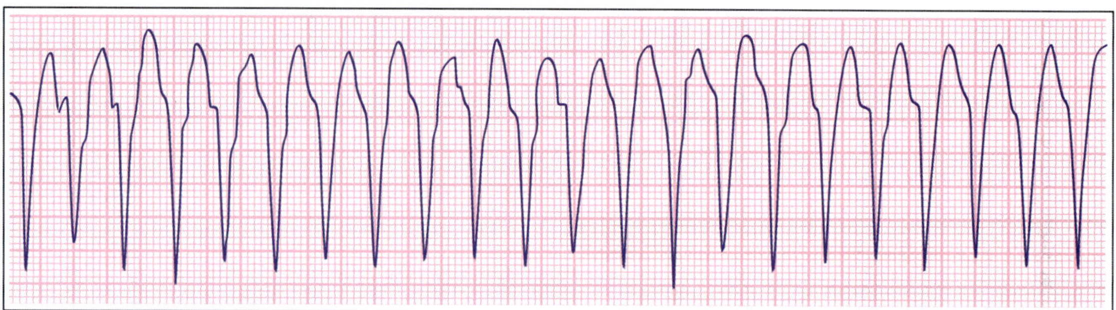

Fig. 4.39: Ventricular tachycardia

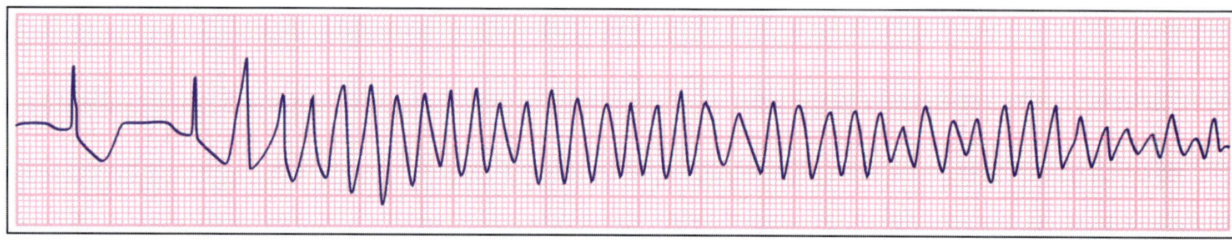

Fig. 4.40: Ventricular fibrillation

3. Presence of **capture beats** (the normal sinus conducted beat occurring during the run of VT) and **fusion beats** (a blending complex beat which is in between normal sinus beat and ventricular ectopic beat) (Table 4.4).
4. Concordant precordial leads (i.e. V_{1-6}): All the complexes are either upwards or downwards.

Aetiology

Same as SVPB (commonly due to IHD, cardiomyopathy, valvular heart disease, thyrotoxicosis, floppy mitral valve syndrome, myocarditis, hypoxia, acidosis, digitalis and hypokalaemia). VT is commonly associated with recent myocardial infarction. It is regarded as a very serious arrhythmia. If not treated properly, VT may degenerate into VF.

- **Torsades de Pointes** is a form of VT manifested by episodes of alternating electrical polarity with the changing QRS amplitude twisting around an isoelectric baseline (hence the name); the rhythm usually starts with a VPB and is preceded by prolongation of Q-T inverval. Certain drugs (e.g. quinidine, procainamide) and electrolyte imbalance ($\downarrow Ca^{++}$, $\downarrow K^{+}$) may precipitate the situation. It is a twisting form of polymorphic ventricular tachycardia. Usually the attacks are self-limiting but may lead to VF.

Ventricular Fibrillation (VF)

VF is a chaotic and incoordinated activity of the heart, which results in totally irregular, bizarre and deformed deflections of the QRS complex of varying height, width and shape (Fig. 4.40). This is a fatal and terminal condition where the peripheral pulses are not palpable and the heart beat is inaudible. Fibrillating ventricles can not effectively pump out blood in the circulation. The treatment is immediate electrical defibrillation.

Aetiology (for ventricular arrhythmias)

1. Ischaemic heart disease, especially acute myocardial infarction.
2. Myocarditis, cardiomyopathy (e.g. dilated, hypertrophic), valvular heart disease.
3. Digitalis, adrenaline or quinidine toxicity, especially if associated with hypokalaemia.
4. Electrical shock (accidental).
5. Hypoxia, especially induced by cardiac surgery; acidosis.
6. Hypothermia.
7. Electrolyte imbalance (high or low K^{+}, low Ca^{++} or Mg^{++}).
8. Cardiac surgery or catheterisation.

Significance

It is considered as the most *serious and catastrophic arrhythmia*, and the prognosis is extremely poor.

Ventricular Flutter

This results from a very rapid and regular ectopic ventricular discharge associated with grossly abnormal intraventricular conduction, and is manifested by bizarre and wide configuration of the QRS complex where the QRS complex is fused with T wave mimicking continuous 'hairpin curves' or 'sine-like wave' form (Fig. 4.41).

Aetiology

Same as VF.

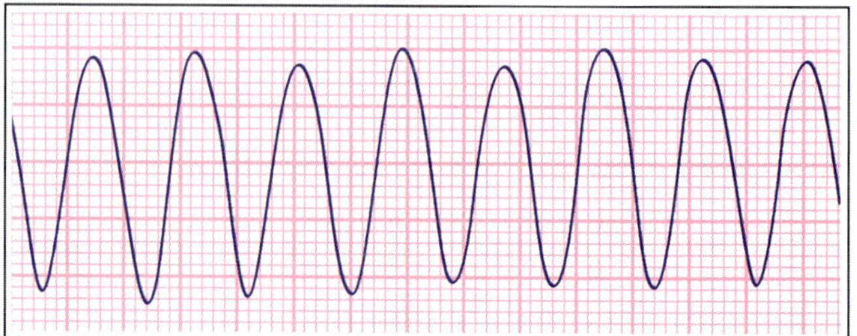

Fig. 4.41: Ventricular flutter

Table 4.4: Differentiation between SVT and VT

Features	SVT with aberrant conduction	VT
1. P wave	A premature P′ wave may precede QRS	QRS complex not preceded by P′ wave
2. Duration of QRS complex >0.14 second	Absent	May be present
3. R-R interval	Perfectly regular and constant	Slightly irregular and not absolutely constant
4. Carotid sinus massage	May be reverted to normal	No effect
5. Left axis deviation	Usually absent	Usually presnt
6. AV dissociation	Not present	Present
7. Capture and fusion beats	Absent	A characteristic feature

- Junctional (nodal) rhythm: When AV node acts as a pacemaker instead of SA node, it is called nodal rhythm (40–60 beats/min). In **junctional premature beats**, the P′ wave is inverted as atria are activated retrogradely, and may precede or blend with or follow the QRS complex; QRS morphology is like sinus rhythm. In **junctional tachycardia**, there is enhanced automaticity of AV node pacemaker with retrograde P′ waves.
- Complete absence of electrical activity of heart is called **ventricular asystole** (i.e. cardiac standstill or cardiac arrest), when there is absence of ventricular complexes in ECG (shows flat line) for seconds to minutes. Clinically, this can not be differentiated from ventricular fibrillation unless ECG monitoring is done.
- Clinically, VT is associated with varying intensity of S_1 and irregular cannon waves in neck vein.
- A patient suspected to suffer from rhythm disturbances should undergo (a) 12-lead ECG, (b) Holter monitoring, and (c) Exercise ECG.

D. INTRAVENTRICULAR CONDUCTION DEFECTS

Pacemaker Tissues and Conducting System of the Heart (Fig. 4.42A)

Certain tissues in the heart responsible for initiation and propagation (i.e. conduction) of the heart beat, are known as 'pacemaker tissues'. They are:

1. *Sinoatrial (SA) node:* It lies in the right atrium at the junction of superior vena cava and right atrial appendages. SA node originates impulses at a rate of 60–100 beats/min (average 72 beats/min) which traverses through three internodal atrial pathways towards atrioventricular (AV) node. **SA node is the natural pacemaker of the heart** and generates **sinus rhythm**.
2. *Atrioventricular (AV) node:* It is located posteriorly on the right side of the interatrial septum. When SA node fails, AV node may generate impulse at the rate of 40–60 beats/min **(nodal rhythm)**.
3. *Bundle of His:* It originates from AV node and divides into right (acting as a single fascicle) and left (left anterior and left posterior fascicles) branches. The right and left bundle branch runs along the right and left side of the ventricular septum, respectively. 'Fascicular block' or 'bundle branch block' results from their delay in conduction.
4. *Purkinje fibres:* They penetrate the ventricular wall after taking origin from terminal divisions of right and left branches of the bundle of His. When SA or AV node fails, the Purkinje cells of the ventricular muscle may beat at the rate of 30-40 beats/min (average 36 beats/min), which is known as **idioventricular rhythm**.

Clinical Wisdom

The cells of AV node, bundle of His and Purkinje fibres also have potential pacemaking properties (back-up pacemaker).

Classification

1. *Unilateral bundle branch block:* Right or left; complete or incomplete.
2. *Peripheral left ventricular conduction defect:* Left anterior fascicular/hemiblock (LAHB) or left posterior fascicular/hemiblock (LPHB), septal block.
3. *Bilateral bundle branch block or bifascicular block:* Right bundle branch block with LAHB or LPHB, alternating RBBB and LBBB, RBBB or LBBB with prolonged AV conduction.
4. Trifascicular block.

I. Right Bundle Branch Block (RBBB)

RBBB is a *fairly common ECG finding* and does not necessarily indicate any organic heart disease.

- Incomplete: QRS interval <0.12 second.
- Complete: QRS interval ≥0.12 second.

Features (Fig. 4.42B)

1. rSR′ or rsR′ pattern or 'M-shaped' complexes in $V_{1–2}$ (also in aVR and V_{3R}); absent q waves in these leads.
2. Wide and slurred S waves in lead I and $V_{5–6}$.
3. ST depression and T wave inversion in $V_{1–3}$.
4. QRS interval is equal, more, or less than 0.12 second (in $V_{1–2}$).
5. Right axis deviation.
6. VAT (intrinsicoid deflection) is prolonged.

Aetiology

1. Normal variant.
2. Right ventricular hypertrophy.
3. Emphysema of lung.

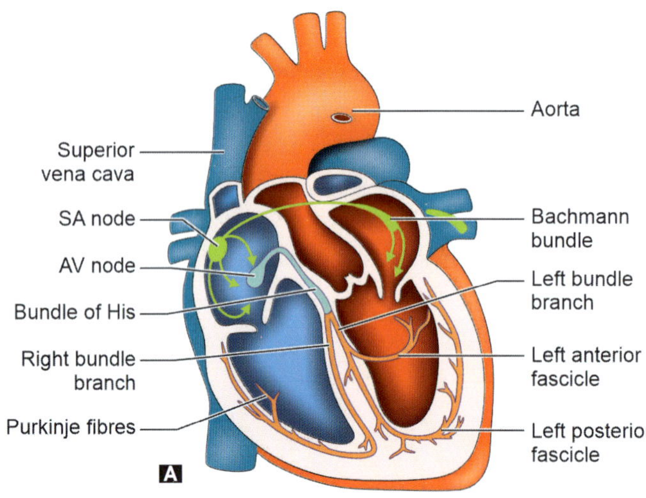

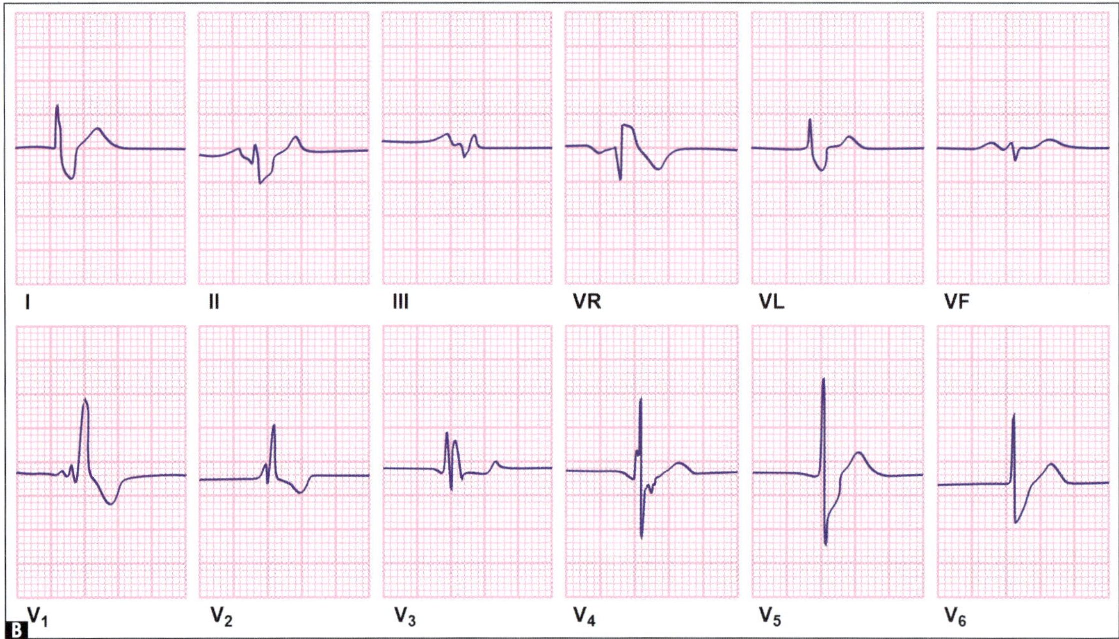

Fig. 4.42A and B: (A) Cardiac conduction system; (B) Right bundle branch block (incomplete)

4. ASD (ostium primum type).
5. Ischaemic heart disease.
6. Myocarditis from any cause.
7. Hypertensive heart disease.
8. Acute pulmonary thromboembolism.
9. Cardiomyopathy.
10. Idiopathic.

Clinical Correlation

In RBBB, there is wide and variable splitting of second heart sound (S_2).

II. Left Bundle Branch Block (LBBB)

Complete LBBB *indicates organic heart disease,* and is commonly associated with ischaemic and hypertensive heart diseases. Prognostically it is worse then RBBB.

Complete or incomplete: Criteria of duration in timing are same as RBBB.

Features (Fig. 4.43)

1. rsR′ or RsR′ pattern or 'M-shaped' complexes in leads V_{4-6}, I and aVL; absent q waves in these leads.
2. Dominant S wave in V_1, and dominant R wave in leads I, aVL.
3. ST depression with T wave inversion in lead I and V_{4-6}.
4. QRS interval is equal, more, or less than 0.12 second (in V_{5-6}).
5. Usually associated with left axis deviation.
6. VAT (intrinsicoid deflection) is prolonged.

Aetiology

1. Ischaemic heart disease.
2. Left ventricular enlargement due to any cause (especially from systemic hypertension).
3. Cardiomyopathy.
4. Myocarditis due to any case.
5. Drugs like quinidine or procainamide.
6. Aortic valve disease, e.g. aortic stenosis.
7. Idiopathic fibrosis.

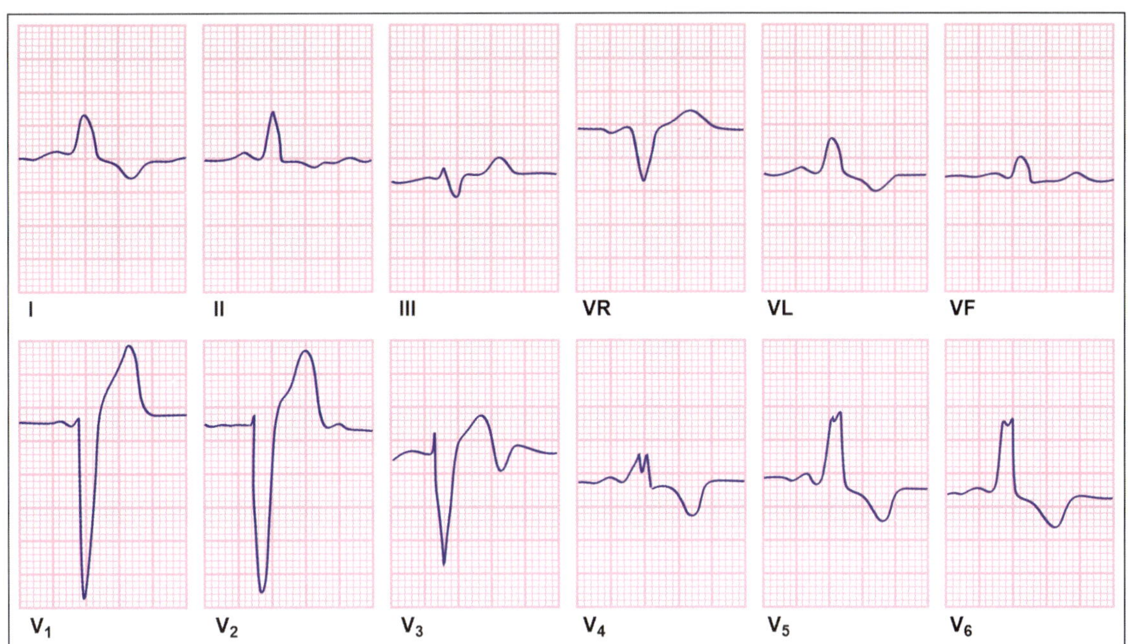

Fig. 4.43: Left bundle branch block (complete)

- The presence of q waves in lead I and V_{5-6} always negate the diagnosis of LBBB or indicates associated acute myocardial infarction (AMI).
- In the presence of AMI, LBBB can not be diagnosed properly.

Peripheral left ventricular conduction defect is divided into:

a. Left Anterior Fascicular Block (also known as left anterior hemiblock or LAHB)

Features

1. Left axis deviation (at least –45°).
2. Narrow QRS complex, qR in lead I, aVL and V_{5-6}; rS in lead II, III, aVF.

b. Left Posterior Fascicular Block (also known as left posterior hemiblock or LPHB)

Features

1. Axis of +100° or greater, i.e. right axis deviation.
2. Narrow QRS complex, and qR in lead II, III, aVF; rS in lead I, aVL and V_{5-6}.
3. 'S_1, Q_3, T_3 pattern' may be seen (like acute pulmonary thromboembolism).

c. Left Septal Block

Feature: Absent q wave in V_{5-6}.

III. Bilateral Bundle Branch Block or 'Bifascicular Block'

The possible combinations are:

- RBBB with LAHB (Fig. 4.44): Features of RBBB plus left axis deviation (commonest),
- RBBB with LPHB: Features of RBBB plus right axis deviation, or
- LBBB (both anterior and posterior fascicles are blocked): LBBB is regarded as a bifascicular block.

IV. Trifascicular Block

When the three fascicles (right bundle, left anterior fascicle and left posterior fascicle) are blocked, it is known as trifascicular block.

Features

1. Features of RBBB.
2. Left axis deviation (indicating left anterior fascicular block).

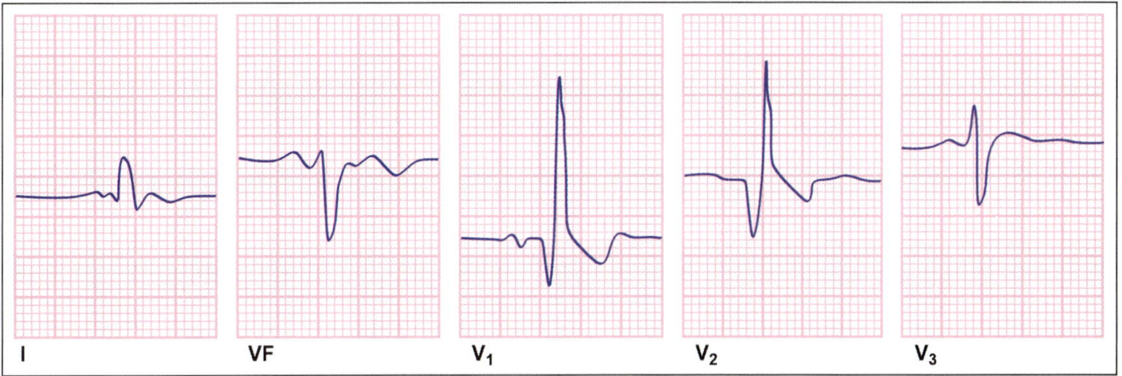

Fig. 4.44: Bifascicular block (RBBB wih LAHB)

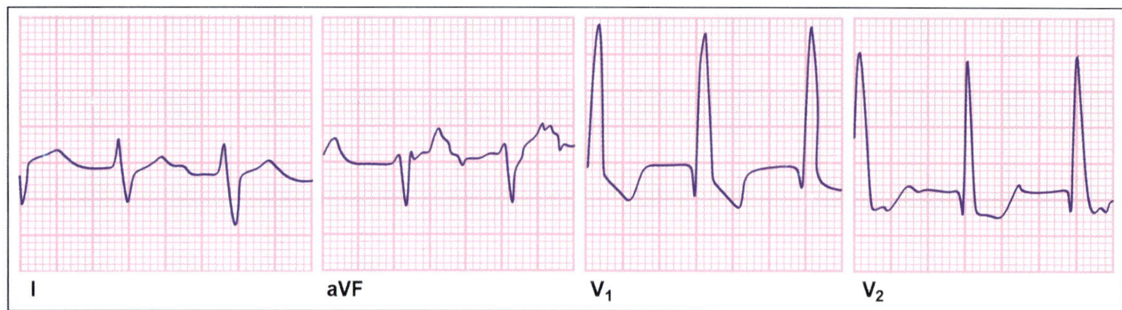

Fig. 4.45: Trifascicular block

3. Prolonged P-R interval (indicating first degree AV block, or may be represented by left posterior fascicular block).

- Fig. 4.45 fulfils all 3 points mentioned above.
- Bifascicular and trifascicular block should undergo pacemaker implantation if associated with syncope, which is not attributable to other causes.

E. ATRIOVENTRICULAR (AV) CONDUCTION DEFECTS

AV block is the disturbance in the conduction of normal sinus impulse through the AV node, the bundle of His, or the intraventricular conduction system.

Classification

A. *Incomplete:*
   a. First degree (1°)
   b. Second degree (2°)
      i. Mobitz type I or Wenckebach phenomenon
      ii. Mobitz type II

B. ***Complete,*** i.e. third degree (3°) heart block

I. 1° Heart Block (Fig. 4.46)

There is disturbance in conduction between the SA node and the AV node, and results in the prolongation of the P-R interval above the upper limit of normal (0.20 second). The rhythm is regular with constant P-P and R-R interval. Atrial rate: ventricular rate = 1:1.

Aetiology

1. Idiopathic, i.e. in the absence of organic heart disease.
2. Acute rheumatic fever (myocarditis).
3. Any acute infectious disease (mainly viral) or inflammatory (SLE, MCTD, rheumatoid arthritis).
4. Digitalis, quinidine or propranolol-induced.
5. Ischaemic heart disease.
6. Congenital heart diseases: ASD or Ebstein 's anomaly.
7. Hyperkalaemia.

Clinical suspicion: If the S_1 becomes muffled in the presence of tachycardia, 1° heart block is thought of. There is *no dropped beat* in peripheral pulse in 1° heart block.

II. 2° Heart Block

From time to time, some atrial impulses are allowed to pass and some are not allowed to pass through the AV node. So the atria contract but as all the contractions do not reach the ventricle, there is **missing beats** in the pulse. This block may be temporary or permanent. Following are the types of 2° heart block:

a. Mobitz Type I or Wenckebach Phenomenon (Fig. 4.47A)

The P-R interval 'progressively increases' till one beat is completely blocked and thus that P wave is not followed by QRS complex. This is more benign and commoner type than Mobitz type II block. This type is commonly associated as transitory change with acute inferior wall myocardial infarction, digitalis toxicity, or following cardiac surgery. Here, the disease lies proximal to the bundle of His. Temporary pacing may be necessary.

The basic rhythm is sinus with a constant P-P interval. The conduction ratio varies, e.g. 5:4, 4:3, etc.

b. Mobitz Type II (Fig. 4.47B)

The ventricle periodically fails to respond to the atrial contraction in Mobitz type II block. Here, P-R interval remains either normal or prolonged but is always 'fixed'; and ultimately misses one beat (progressive prolongation of P-R interval like Wenckebach phenomenon is absent

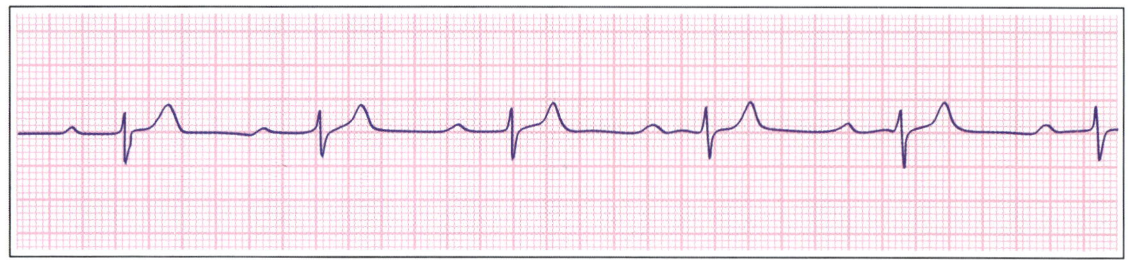

Fig. 4.46: First degree heart block. P-R interval is 0.32 second (incidentally, there is bradycardia)

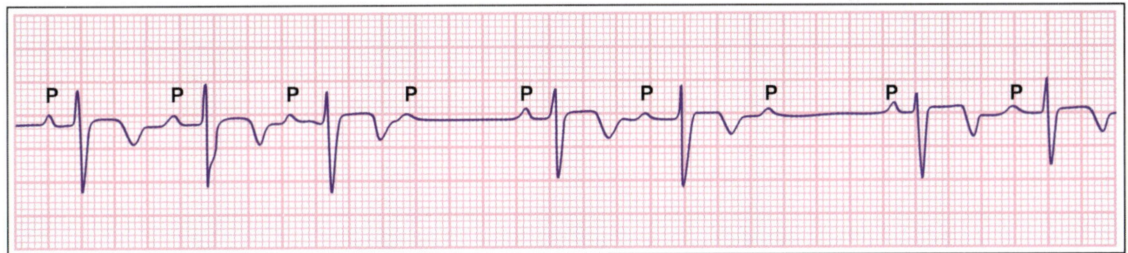

Fig. 4.47A: Second degree heart block (Wenckebach type)

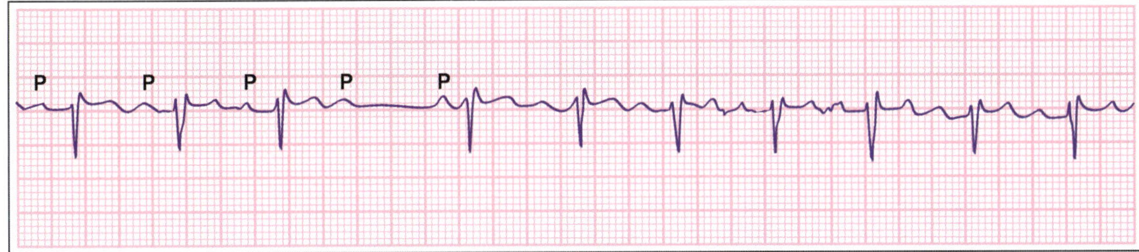

Fig. 4.47B: Second degree heart block (Mobitz type II)

here). This type is commonly associated with acute inferior wall myocardial infarction. Here, the block lies below the bundle of His and prognostically worse than Mobitz type I block. This rhythm often progresses to 3° heart block.

The basic rhythm is sinus with constant P-P and P-R intervals. The conduction ratio may be fixed (4:3, 2:1) or variable. This type of block usually needs pacing.

c. 2° Constant (advanced) Heart Block (2:1 or 3:1 type) (Fig. 4.48)

- There is a fixed AV relationship in constant 2° block. In 3:2 block, there are 3-P waves (atrial activity) and 2-QRS complexes (ventricular activity); in 6:5 block, 5-QRS complexes follow 6-P waves, i.e. the last P wave does not produce any QRS complex.

Aetiology (of 2° heart block)

1. Acute rheumatic fever producing carditis.
2. Ischaemic heart disease.
3. Myocarditis following diphtheria.
4. Digitalis toxicity.
5. May be associated with PSVT or atrial flutter as a 'protective mechanism'.

- 2° heart block may be asymptomatic, or may experience syncope or light-headedness.

III. 3° Heart Block or Complete Heart Block (CHB) (Fig. 4.49)

Here, all the supraventricular impulses are blocked, i.e. no SA impulse is allowed to pass through the AV node barrier (i.e. permanent interruption of AV conduction). Ventricles, therefore, are activated by ectopic pacemaker (idioventricular rhythm) and contract at a regular rate of 30–40/min (idioventricular pacemaker is present in the walls of ventricle close to the AV node). So, there is no relationship between atrial and ventricular pacemaker, and the atrial and ventricular rhythms are asynchronous (there is complete dissociation between P waves and QRS complexes). The atrial rate is that of average regular sinus rhythm. Thus, the P waves and QRS complexes are seen to occur at a different but constant rate (i.e. the P-P and R-R intervals are constant). Usually the rate of the QRS complex is near about half that of the P wave. There is absence of fixed P-R relationship.

If complete heart block develops suddenly and ventricular standstill persists for few seconds, the patient may develop Stokes-Adams syndrome (read the 'Emergency Medicine' section).

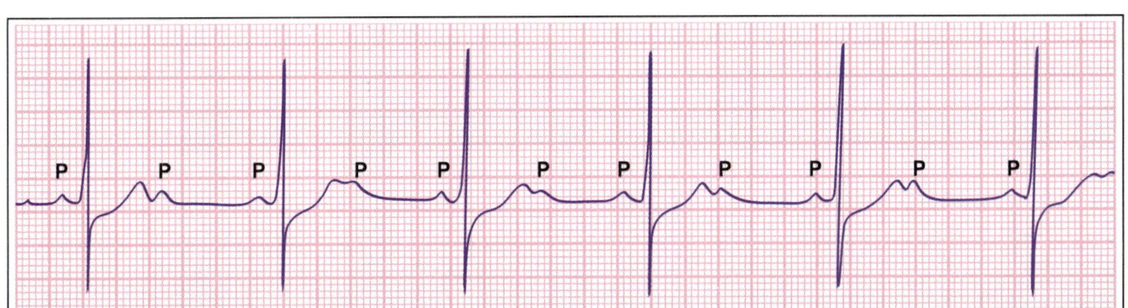

Fig. 4.48: 2° fixed heart block (2:1 type). Every alternate P wave is not followed by QRS complex; clinically mimics bradycardia

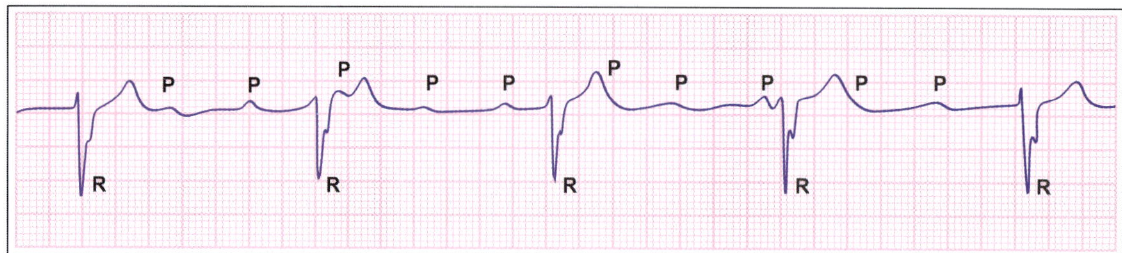

Fig. 4.49: Complete heart block with ventricular rate 43/minute. Atrial rate is 115/minute

Aetiology

1. Coronary artery disease, especially acute inferior wall myocardial infarction.
2. 'Congenital' complete heart block, myotonic dystrophy.
3. Digitalis, quinidine or procainamide overdose.
4. Myocarditis, pericarditis.
5. Calcific aortic stenosis (AS).
6. Association with ASD (ostium primum type) or VSD.
7. Cardiac surgery (near the conducting system).
8. Lenegre's disease (idiopathic sclerodegenerative disease of the conducting system).
9. Lev's disease (fibrocalcific affection of the conducting system).
10. Cardiac tumour, SBE (aortic root abscess), granulomatous infection (tuberculosis, gumma) or parasitic infestations (Chagas disease in central and south America).
11. Idiopathic (especially in India).

- Acute rheumatic fever may be associated with first and second degree heart block but not with complete heart block (CHB).
- Clinically, CHB is associated with bradycardia (36–40/min) with regular pulse rate, varying intensity of S_1 and irregular cannon waves in neck vein.

- **24-hours ambulatory** or **dynamic ECG** (or **'Holter' ECG**, after its inventor): This technique records transient episodes of arrhythmia or ischaemia, e.g. an occasional pause in heart beat or a brief paroxysm of tachycardia in the cardiac cycle, complained by the patient. During the recording, the patient remains ambulatory. Al least 1 lac complexes are recorded in 24-hours and analysed by automatic methods.

F. HEART BLOCK

Classification of Heart Block

1. SA block (Fig. 4.50): The sinus impulse is blocked (exit block) within the SA junction, i.e. neither atrial nor ventricular activation takes place. So, both the P wave and the QRS complexes are absent, and heart will miss a beat as a whole.
2. AV block (read section E).
3. Bundle branch block (read section D).
4. Arborisation or Purkinje block: When the bundle branch block is associated with low amplitude complexes, it is known as arborisation block. This term is uncommonly used at the present moment.

G. MISCELLANEOUS

Wolff–Parkinson–White (W-P-W) Syndrome (Fig. 4.51)

Here, the atrial impulse goes to the ventricles concomitantly via normal as well as anomalous pathway (bundle of Kent). The early activation of the ventricular myocardium is known as **pre-excitation**.

Features

1. Short P-R interval (<0.12 sec).
2. Wide QRS complex (>0.12 sec).
3. Slurred initial upstroke of the QRS complex, known as **'delta wave'**.
4. Secondary ST segment depression and T wave inversion.

- Patients with W-P-W syndrome are prone to attacks of supraventricular tachyarrhythmias.
- WPW syndrome is a congenital abnormality; it may be associated with Ebstein's anomaly, mitral valve prolapse syndrome or hypertrophic obstructive cardiomyopathy (HOCM).

Sick Sinus Syndrome (Structural Nodal Disease) (Fig. 4.52)

It is also known as bradycardia-tachycardia syndrome. Patient with SA node dysfunction may present with dizziness, confusion, fatigue, pre-syncope and syncope, palpitations, chest pain, irritability, etc. It is diagnosed by:

a. Clinical appraisal (symptoms are due to cerebral hypoperfusion and low cardiac output).
b. ECG monitoring (sinus bradycardia, sinus arrest, sinus pause, SA block with the appearance of escape rhythm, AV block or SVT, atrial fibrillation or flutter).

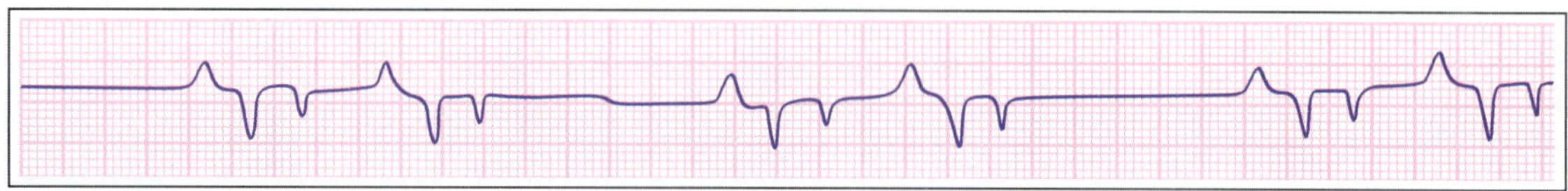

Fig. 4.50: SA block (every third SA impulse is blocked). Incidentally, there is associated first degree AV block (increased P-R interval)

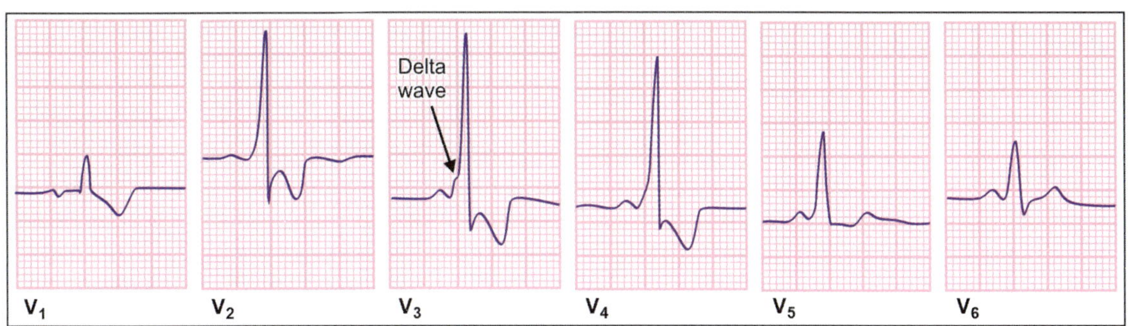

Fig. 4.51: W-P-W syndrome with delta wave

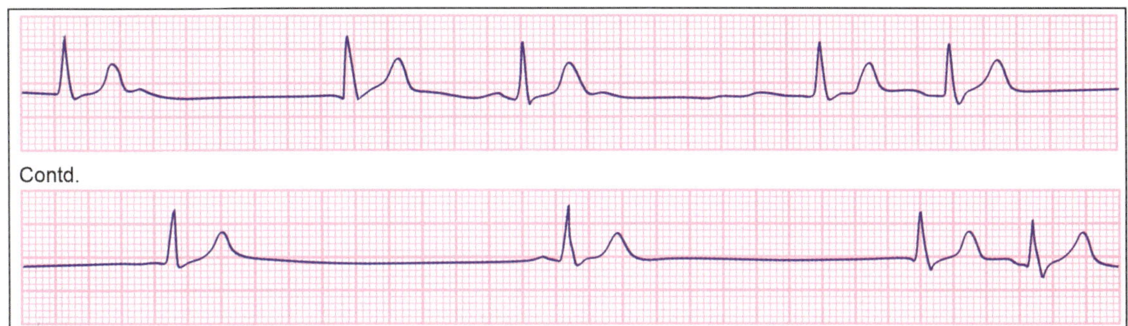

Fig. 4.52: Sick sinus syndrome

Failure of impulse formation in the SA node is known as sinus arrest.

c. Provocative tests: Sinus node recovery time (SNRT: a response to overdrive atrial pacing; normal value of corrected SNRT is <500 miliseconds) and sino-atrial conduction times (normal value is 45–125 milliseconds). These times are prolonged (SNRT >525 milliseconds) in structural SA node disease.

Aetiology

The underlying pathology may involve fibrosis, degenerative changes and/or ischaemia of the SA node.

1. Ischaemic heart disease.
2. Infiltrative or degenerative heart disease.
3. Coronary atherosclerosis with or without systemic hypertension.
4. Cardiomyopathy.
5. Congenital heart disease.
6. Digitalis, quinidine, procainamide-induced.
7. Idiopathic.

ECG manifestations of sinus node dysfunction are often intermittent and thus it is difficult to prove. Ambulatory ECG (Holter) monitoring remains the mainstay in evaluating sinus node function. Treatment of structural nodal disease is done by artificial demand pacemaker into the right ventricle or permanent pacemaker, as well as using various antiarrhythmic drugs (atropine, isoprenaline).

Hypothermia (Fig. 4.53)

Features

1. Sinus bradycardia.

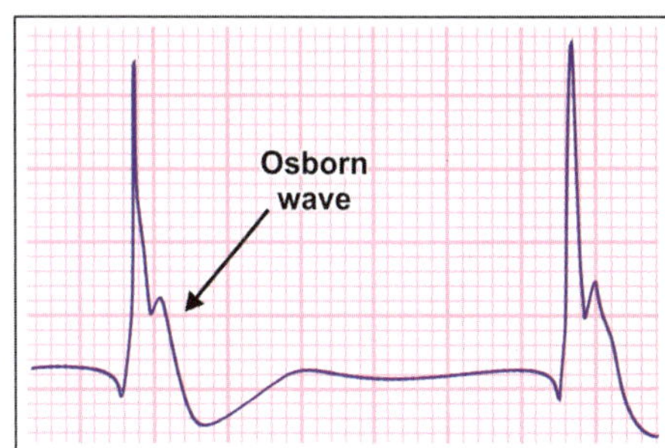

Fig. 4.53: Hypothermia with J wave

2. J wave or **'Osborn wave'**: Narrow hump-like wave superimposed on the terminal part of the distal limb of the QRS complex.
3. Q-T interval is prolonged.
4. Muscle tremor (i.e. shivering artefact).
5. Very low temperature, i.e. 30°C or less may produce ventricular fibrillation.

- Osborn wave is also seen in hypercalcaemia, raised intracranial tension or vasospastic angina.

Electrical Alternans (Fig. 4.54)

Here, the height of the R wave (i.e. QRS complex) alternates every other beat.

Aetiology

1. Pericardial effusion, usually with cardiac tamponade (commonest): Heart may rotate or swing freely within the fluid and the electrical axis of the heart may vary with each beat.
2. Paroxysmal atrial tachycardia (rare).
3. Atherosclerotic heart disease (rare).

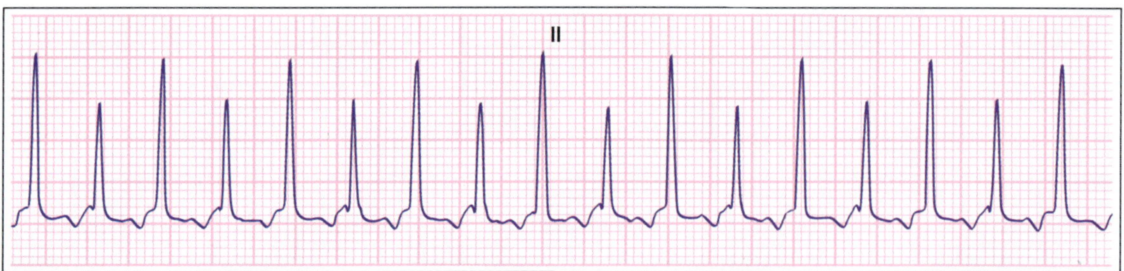

Fig. 4.54: Electrical alternans in a large pericardial effusion

EFFECT OF DRUGS

Digitalis

a. Digitalis Effect (Fig. 4.55)

Digitalis effect in ECG does not indicate the need to reduce the dose of the drug. When the patient reaches adequate digitalisation, these changes may be seen in the ECG.

1. ST segment becomes depressed, rounded and with concave (scooped) configuration. It gives the impresion of T wave inversion: the mirror-image of a 'inverted correction mark' or 'hockey stick pattern'.
2. Shortened Q-T interval.

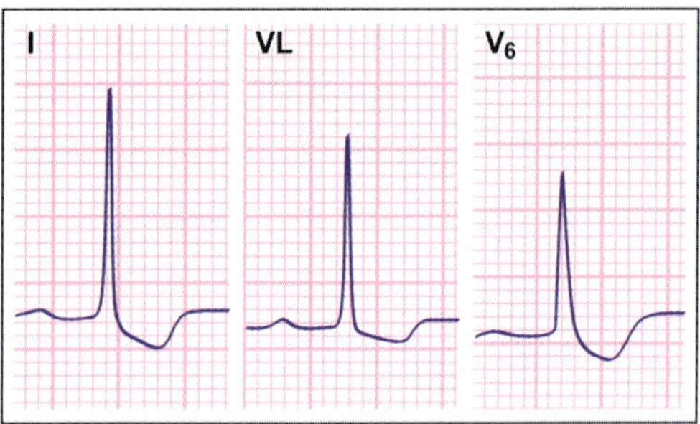

Fig. 4.55: Digitalis effect

b. Digitalis Toxicity (Fig. 4.56)

Overdigitalisation or toxic effect of the drug may be as follows:

1. Sinus bradycardia.
2. First degree, second degree or third degree AV block; SA block and bundle branch block.
3. Isolated VPB which are unifocal or multifocal, or especially ventricular bigeminy.
4. Supraventricular tachyarrhythmias: Paroxysmal atrial tachycardia (PAT) with or without block, atrial flutter, atrial fibrillation.
5. Ventricular arrhythmias: VT, ventricular flutter or fibrillation.

- Digitalis may produce any type of arrhythmia except Mobitz type II AV block and parasystole.

Clinical Wisdom

Digitalis toxicity is increased in the presence of hypokalaemia, renal or hepatic failure, and with advanced heart diseases.

Quinidine

a. Quinidine Effect (Fig. 4.57)

1. ST segment depression with T wave flattening; wide and notched T wave.
2. Prolonged Q-T interval.

b. Quinidine Toxicity

1. SA block; first, second and third degree AV block; bundle branch block.
2. Ventricular arrhythmias: VPB, VT, idioventricular rhythm, ventricular fibrillation and cardiac standstill.
3. AV junctional rhythm.
4. Widened QRS complex.
5. *Marked prolongation of the Q-T interval.*

EFFECT OF ELECTROLYTES

Potassium

a. Hyperkalaemia (Fig. 4.58)

Progressive rise in serum potassium level is associated with the following ECG changes:

1. *Tall, slender and peaked T wave (tented T wave or steeple T wave).*
2. Amplitude of the R wave is diminished. QRS complex widens and merges with the T wave in such a way

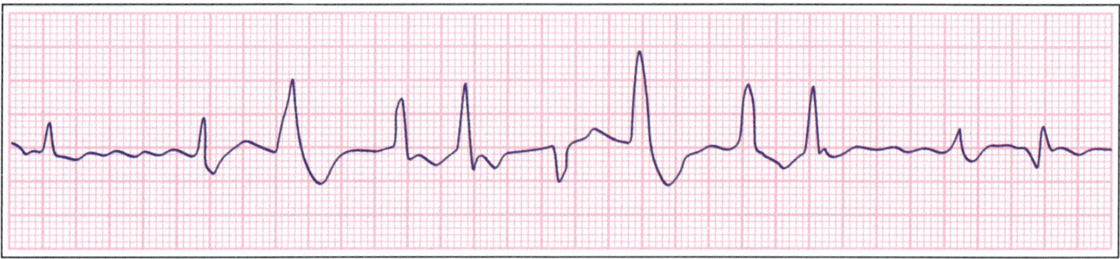
Fig. 4.56: Digitalis toxicity

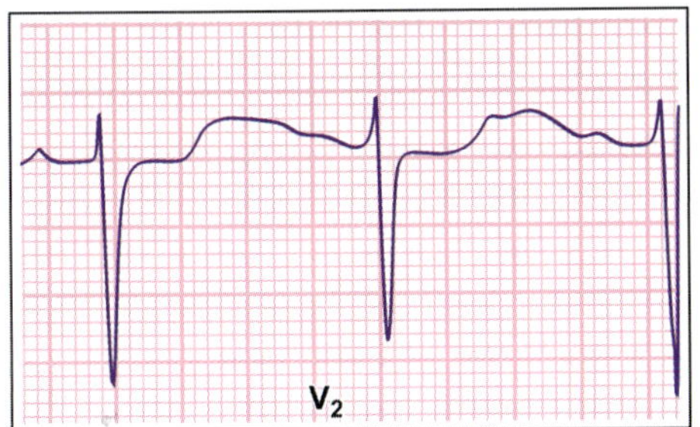

Fig. 4.57: Quinidine effect with prolonged Q-T interval

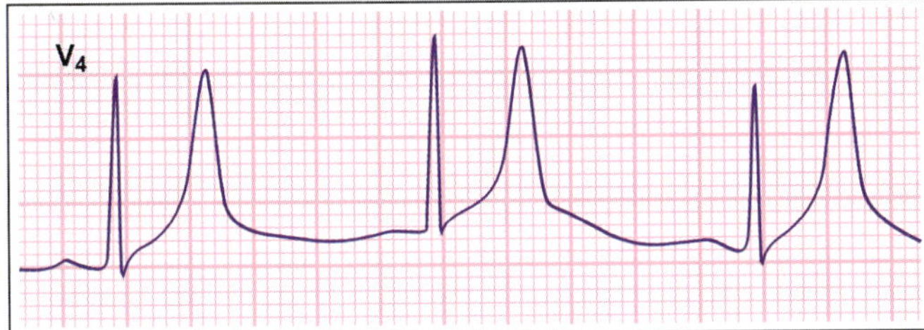

Fig. 4.58: Hyperkalaemia

that it is difficult to detect the ST segment, and producing a bizarre, widened and diphasic deflection of T wave. Shortened Q-T interval.

3. Amplitude of the P wave is diminished and ultimately disappears completely; gradually a 'sine-like wave' is seen.
4. Ventricular arrhythmia (fibrillation or asystole) may be associated with. Sinus bradycardia may be seen.

b. Hypokalaemia (Fig. 4.59)

Progressive diminution in serum potassium level is associated with the following ECG changes:

1. ST depression with flattened or inverted T wave.
2. *Prominent U wave* (camel hump effect).
3. Prolonged P-R interval.
4. Prolonged Q-T interval.
5. Rarely, SA block.

- Normal serum potassium level is 3.5–5 mEq/L. Tented T wave is found in potassium level ≥6.8 mEq/L.

Dextrocardia (Fig. 4.60)

Features

1. P wave is inverted in lead I. QRS complex and T wave are also inverted in lead I. Upright P wave in aVR.
2. Tallest QRS complexes are seen in the right precordial leads, i.e. in V_1 and V_2, and progressively diminished to the left. That is to say, there is gradual diminution of height of R waves from V_1 to V_6.

- In **technical dextrocardia** (i.e. faulty interchange of right and left arm electrode by a technician) lead I, II, III, aVR, aVL and aVF will have similar changes like true dextrocardia; but there will be no alteration of normal ECG pattern in precordial leads (i.e. in V_{1-6}).

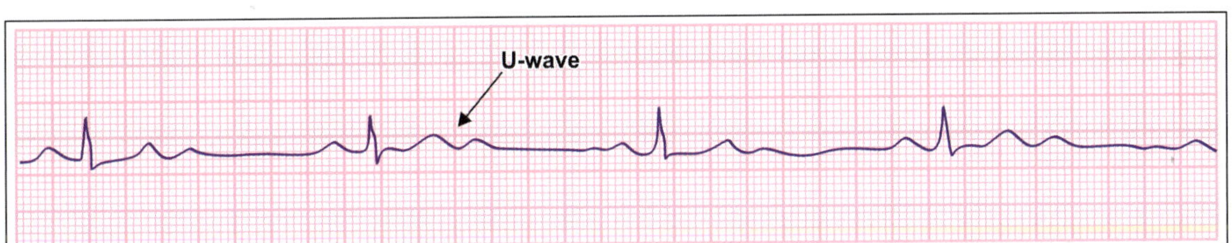

Fig. 4.59: Hypokalaemia with U wave

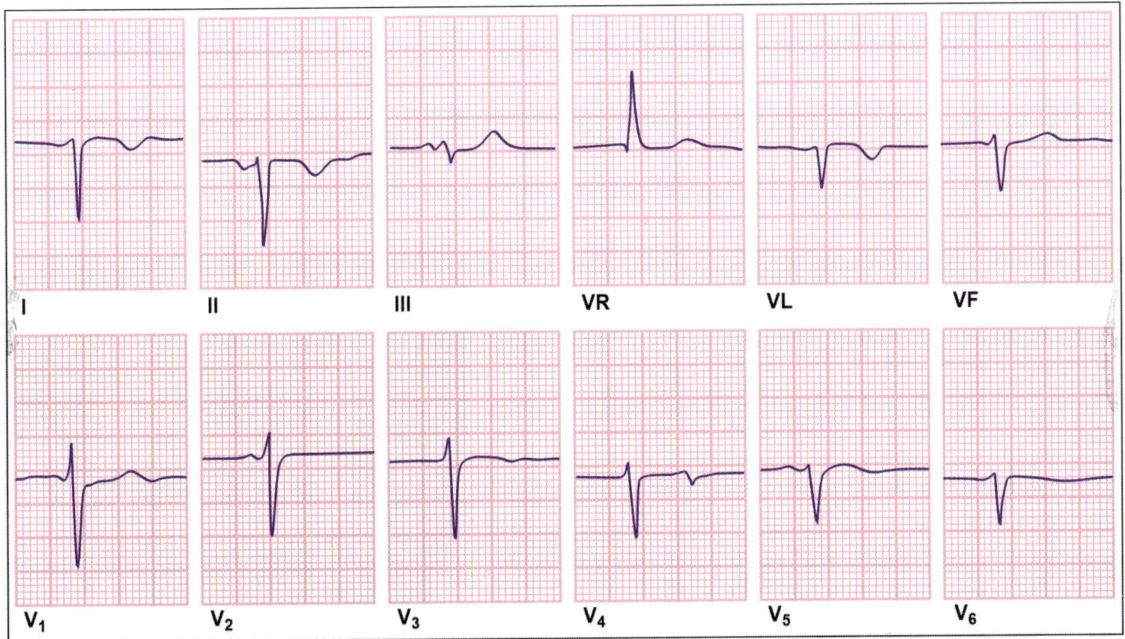

Fig. 4.60: Dextrocardia

Pericarditis

a. Acute Pericarditis (Fig. 4.61)

1. Normal voltage.
2. *Elevated ST segment with concavity upwards* (in contrast to ST elevation with convexity upwards seen in AMI): Saddle-back appearance.
3. T wave remains upright (as there is no myocardial ischaemia). After few days, T wave may be inverted.

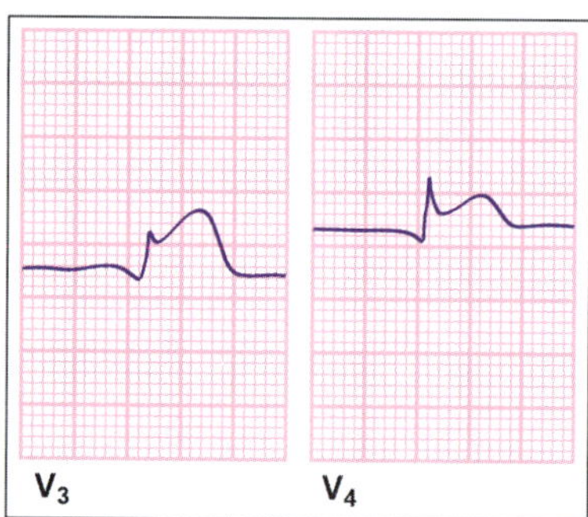

Fig. 4.61: Pericarditis (acute)

b. Chronic Constrictive Pericarditis

1. Low voltage.
2. Low to inverted T wave.

c. Pericardial Effusion (see Fig. 4.54)

1. Low voltage.
2. Low to inverted T wave (sometimes with ST elevation).
3. Electrical alternans may be seen.

Myocarditis

Myocarditis commonly results from secondary to infections (e.g. Coxsackievirus) and produces:

1. Varying degree of heart block, e.g. first degree AV block, bundle branch block, etc.
2. QRS abnormality very often mimics acute myocardial infarction.
3. Various arrhythmias.

Myxoedema (see Fig. 4.6)

1. Sinus bradycardia.
2. Low voltage QRS complexes.
3. Prolongation of the P-R interval.
4. Flattened T waves.

Athlete's Heart

1. Sinus bradycardia.
2. Varying degree of AV block (e.g. first degree AV block).
3. Incomplete RBBB is not uncommon.
4. Non-specific ST elevation along with T wave flattening/inversion in precordial leads.

Cerebral Diseases on the ECG

Abnormal ECG is especially found in cerebral and subarachnoid haemorrhage (i.e. CVA), and the changes are:

1. ST depression, and flat to inverted T waves; precordial T waves may be wide and prominent (bizarre ST-T changes).
2. Prolongation of the Q-T interval.
3. Prominent U waves.
4. Sinus bradycardia.

Pacemaker Complex (Fig. 4.62)

The prime indication of electrical pacing of the heart is Stokes-Adams syndrome (from CHB). The ECG of such a person shows 'pace artefact' or 'pacing spike' (a vertical, sharp, thin line before each complex) in the tracing. If pace artefact is to be removed, a special magnet should be used while recording the ECG.

Permanent pacemaker is indicated in sinus node dysfunction, acquired AV block, post-AMI (with grade II or III heart block), tachyarrhythmias, neurocardiogenic syncope, and congenital heart diseases with heart block.

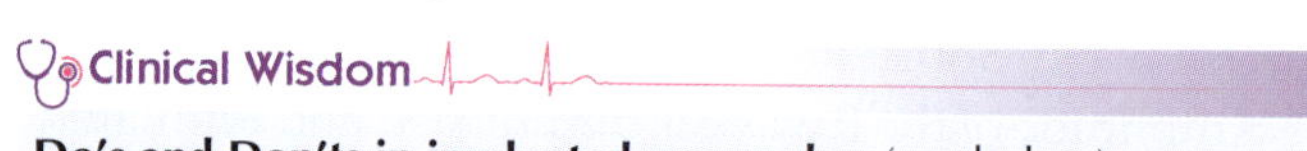

Do's and Don'ts in implanted pacemaker (see below).

Permanent pacemakers are implanted under the layer of skin and fat through surgery, just beneath the left collar bone (Fig. 4.63). Any sort of magnetic device

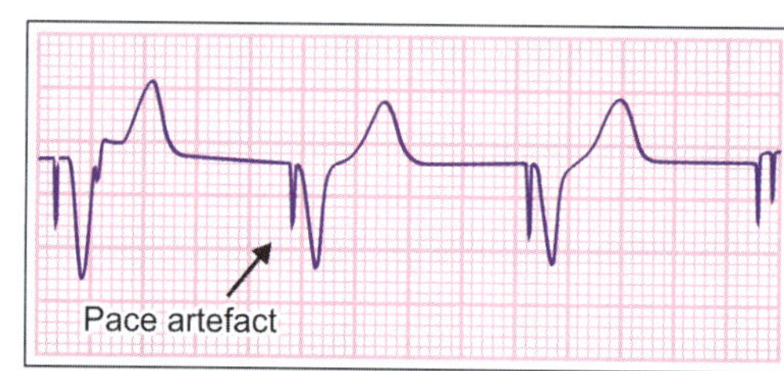

Fig. 4.62: Right ventricular endocardial pacing. **Pace artefact** is seen before each QRS complex

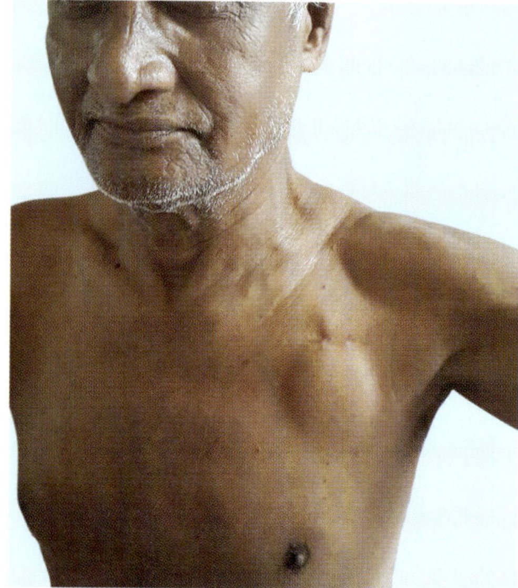

Fig. 4.63: A **pacemaker** is **implanted** surgically about 2 inches below the left clavicle

can interfere with the pacemaker programming. So try to:

1. Avoid MRI machine (pacemaker compatible machine can be used).
2. Avoid metal detector during security check (carry the ID card for pacemaker or wear a medic alert bracelet). Do not linger for too long in shop doorways with anti-theft system, although walking through them is fine.
3. Avoid contact sports (e.g. rugby, boxing).
4. Avoid diathermy (heat therapy), lithotripsy, therapeutic radiation.
5. Use the cellphone in the opposite ear (i.e. left ear for right heart pacemaker, and right ear for left heart pacemaker). Keep the phone in jeans pocket or in a bag.
6. Using properly operating household appliances like microwave ovens or electrical blankets cannot damage the pacemaker.
7. Regular check-up to ensure that the pacemaker is working properly.

Golden Words about ECG

ECG is a simple, painless test that measures the electrical activity of the heart. There is generally no risk associated with this test and as it does not emit electricity, there is no danger of shock. ECG is not 100% accurate because few of the heart diseases are not detectable by ECG. There is no need for regular testing in healthy individuals unless there is inherited risk or it is required in working place or for life insurance requirements.

Analyse – Interpret – Formulate

For example, an ECG showing tall peaked T waves (hyperkalaemia), Q-T prolongation (hypocalcaemia) and left ventricular hypertrophy (from systemic hypertension) may point towards chronic renal failure. So, a simple ECG may be tremendously helpful in assessing a patient clinically.

Always Remember These Golden Lines

ECG is a simple laboratory test and like all laboratory findings, an abnormal tracing reveals significance if correlated clinically. An abnormal ECG tracing does not necessarily mean an abnormal heart and a normal tracing does not rule out pathology. A patient with a normal tracing may be dead after 10 minutes from a coronary attack and another patient with grossly abnormal tracing may survive in this world for many years without having any cardiac symptoms.

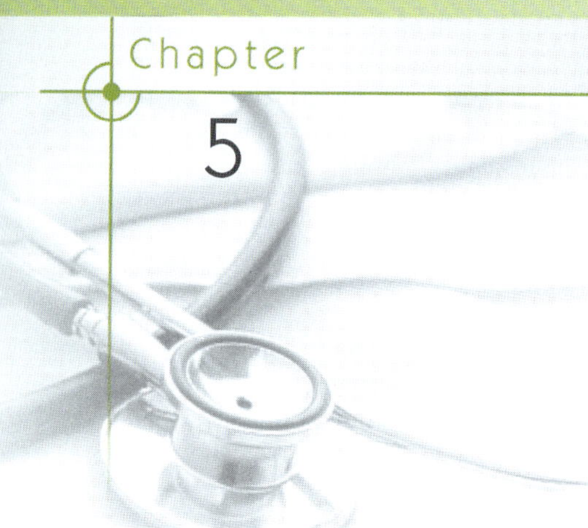

Chapter 5

Emergency Medicine

"Life is short, and art long; the crisis fleeting; experience perilous, and decision difficult."

—**Hippocrates (460 BC-370 BC)**,
an ancient Greek physician, universally recognised as *'Father of medicine'*

EVALUATION AND MANAGEMENT OF COMA

In coma, the patient is deeply unconscious and there is no response evoked by external or internal stimuli. The Greek word *'koma'* means deep sleep.

The common causes of coma are:

1. CVA (e.g. cerebral haemorrhage, massive cerebral infarction with oedema, subarachnoid haemorrhage, hypertensive encephalopathy), encephalitis, meningitis, cerebral abscess, subdural or extradural haematoma, intracranial SOL, tentorial herniation, typhoid state, cerebral malaria, head injury, post-epileptic.
2. Diabetic ketoacidosis, hypoglycaemia, renal failure, hepato-cellular failure, respiratory failure, severe anoxia, myxoedema coma, pituitary apoplexy, adrenal crisis, hyponatraemia, eclampsia.
3. Stokes-Adams syndrome, arrhythmias, tight aortic stenosis, cardiogenic shock (e.g. AMI), hypotension, malignant hypertension.
4. Poisoning (e.g. barbiturate, organophosphorus, morphine), drug or alcohol overdose, hypothermia, heat stroke, extreme cold, snake bite.
5. Severe sepsis.
6. Psychogenic.

- Structural lesion in the brain (affecting reticular activating system in diencephalon, and brainstem), toxic or metabolic derangements, and cardiac problems are the chief causes of coma.
- **Common causes of coma are:** CVA, diabetic ketoacidosis, hypoglycaemia, hyponatraemia, hepatic coma, renal failure, severe anoxia, CO_2 narcosis (e.g. respiratory failure), poisoning/drug overdose, encephalitis or septicaemia.
- Altered consciousness is produced by three basic mechanisms, i.e. diffuse brain dysfunction (e.g. metabolic causes), direct effect within brainstem (e.g. pontine glioma), and pressure effect on the brainstem (e.g. mass lesion within brain) affecting reticular formation, brainstem and cerebral cortex.

Outline of Evaluation

Initial assessment should focus on history (from relatives/associates/eyewitness) and general physical examination.

A. History: Onset, progress, premonitory symptoms, H/o epilepsy, features of increased intracranial tension (IIT), trauma (head injury), alcohol overdose, poisoning, suicidal tendency, high fever, dyspnoea, chest pain, jaundice, haematemesis/melaena, discharge from ear, urinary output, hypertension, diabetes mellitus; circumstances in which the patient was found to be unconscious should be especially asked for.

B. Physical examination: Perform a thorough physical examination. General appearance (flushed face with parotid swelling in chronic alcoholism), odour of breath, ears (for discharge), eyes with special reference to pupil, jaundice, pattern of respiration (frothy sputum coming through nose in organophosphorus poisoning, or Cheyne-Stokes type breathing in metabolic coma), neck rigidity, tongue bite mark, involuntary movements, sweating, soiling of clothes, temperature, pulse (bradycardia in Stokes-Adams syndrome/ IIT), BP, motor response (one side of the face may puff off with expiration in CVA with neurodeficit), hepatosplenomegaly (splenomegaly in cerebral malaria/typhoid state), and fundus examination (diabetic retinopathy, papilloedema in IIT) should be performed. Any injury mark should be carefully examined.

- In coma, plantar response in bilaterally extensor. Often the localisation of side of neurodeficit in CVA is not possible while the patient is in coma.
- **Pupil examination:** Bilaterally equal and normally reactive pupils indicate intact upper brainstem and oculomotor nerve.
  a. Pin-point but reactive pupil: Pontine haemorrhage, organophosphorus poisoning, narcotic (morphine)

overdose. Morphine poisoning also shows features of respiratory depression.

b. Bilaterally dilated and fixed pupil: Severe anoxic encephalopathy, glutethimide or atropine intoxication, dhatura poisoning.

c. Unilateral dilated and fixed pupil (anisocoria): Oculomotor palsy caused by uncal herniation.

d. Midposition (4–5 mm) but fixed pupil: Midbrain lesion.

e. Hutchinson's pupil: Head injury.

f. Horner's syndrome (unilateral): Seen in hypothalamic damage.

- So, a torch must be in hand while the doctor is in emergency. Measure the 'score' (clinical grading of coma) by **Glasgow Coma Scale** (eye opening, best motor response and verbal response). Corneal reflex is absent in coma.

C. Investigations:

a. *Urine:* Especially for sugar, acetone and albumin.

b. *Blood:* Sugar, urea, creatinine, bilirubin, smear for malaria parasite, Na^+, K^+; blood gas analysis. Blood should be sent for metabolic and endocrine studies (e.g. cortisol, TSH), and kept for drug screening (e.g. salicylates, barbiturates).

c. *CSF:* Meningitis, subarachnoid haemorrhage.

d. *Examination of vomitus or gastric contents (i.e. toxicology screening):* Naked eye examination of appearance of undigested tablets, and the odour often clinch the diagnosis of drug overdose or poisoning.

e. *ECG:* Complete heart block, AMI, tachyarrhythmias.

f. *X-ray:* Usually not possible in a comatose patient. X-ray in lying down position may be taken for skull/chest (i.e. in injury).

g. *CT scan:* May detect structural lesion in brain (if facility is available). Early CT scan is often inconclusive in CVA (e.g. cerebral infarction). EEG, radionuclide brain scan or angiography is dependent on the availability of facilities.

Classify Coma on Rapidity of Evolution

a. Abrupt (i.e. within seconds or minutes)

1. Cerebral haemorrhage.
2. Massive cerebral infarction with oedema.
3. Subarachnoid haemorrhage.
4. Cardiac arrest.
5. Epileptic convulsions.
6. Head injury.
7. Psychogenic.

b. Acute (i.e. within a few hours)

1. Cerebral haemorrhage or infarction.
2. Acute poisoning or drug overdose.
3. Hypoglycaemia.

c. Subacute (i.e. within few hours and a few days)

1. Metabolic encephalopathy (hyponatraemia, hepatic or uraemic encephalopathy, anoxia or hypercapnoea, heat stroke, diabetic ketoacidosis, dyselectrolytaemias).
2. Encephalitis, meningitis, brain tumour.
3. Toxic encephalopathies resulting from severe infection, e.g. cerebral malaria.

Outline of Managment

To maintain life, follow a → b → c → d chronologically (*see* below)

1. Place the patient on a soft mattress in supine position; bed with railed cot, if available; change of posture in every two hours. Prone in lateral position may prevent aspiration of gastric contents.
2. Maintain **airway** by neck extension/chin lift; place oropharyngeal airway tube or endotracheal tube; suck the oropharynx to clear off secretions. Always try to prevent the falling back of the tongue.
3. Ensure adequate **breathing**; if necessary, give mouth to mouth ventilation. In a desperate situation give 100% O_2, ventilate with face mask or Ambu bag.
4. Maintain adequate **circulation**; if carotid/femoral pulses are palpable, continue ventilation with O_2. If pulses are not palpable and heart sounds are not audible, deliver a sharp blow to the centre of the chest. If heart does not start immediately, start cardiac massage at a rate of 1/second and ventilate mouth to mouth once/5 massages.
5. After resuscitation by basic life support put a Ryle's tube, insert IV catheter (intracath), apply a Foley's or condom catheter.
6. If necessary (make correction by **drugs**):
   a. Maintain circulation: By 5% dextrose, normal saline or plasma (i.e. hydrate adequately).
   b. Acidosis: Inj. sodium bicarbonate (7.5%) 1 mEq/kg, IV; may be repeated after 10–15 minutes.
   c. To increase renal perfusion and to treat hypotension: By dopamine infusion at the rate of >5 μg/kg/min; 200 mg of inj. dopamine is dissolved in 540 mL of normal saline to run at the rate of 10–12 drops/min.
   d. Suspected hypoglycaemia: 100 mL of 25% glucose, IV.
   e. Suspected morpine poisoning: Inj. naloxone 0.4–0.8 mg, IV.
   f. Convulsions: Inj diazepam 5–10 mg, slow IV; may start inj. phenytoin 13–18 mg/kg in normal saline, not faster than 50 mg/min.
   g. Hypothermia: Cover with blankets, continue O_2, correct acidosis by inj. sodium bicarbonate (7.5%) 1 mEq/kg, IV, to be given over 10 minutes.
   Hyperthermia: Start ice irrigation, ice bag on head, inj. chlorpromazine, 25 mg, IM stat.
   h. Organophosphorus poisoning: Inj. atropine, 1–2 mg, IV to be repeated till the full dilatation of pupil. Start inj. pralidoxime 1–2 g in infusion of 100 mL of normal saline over 30 minutes. Forced alkaline diuresis is started in barbiturate poisoning.
   i. Copper sulphate poisoning: Start D-penicillamine 250 mg, 1 cap 4–6 hourly through Ryle's tube. In

dhatura poisoning, start inj. neostigmine 1 mg, IM stat and repeat 4–6 hourly.

j. Stokes-Adams syndrome: Maintain airway, start inj. atropine 0.6 mg, IV; repeated, if necessary. Now, start isoprenaline drip by 2 mg dissolved in 540 mL of 5% dextrose, IV to maintain the heart rate at 70–80/ min. Permanent pacemaker should be implanted.

k. Drug poisoning: Start gastric lavage, if not applied yet.

l. Administer 100 mg thiamine, IV followed by 5% dextrose, IV, especially in an alcoholic as they are prone to develop Wernicke's encephalopathy.

7. Diabetic ketoacidosis, hepato-cellular failure, renal failure, myxoedema coma, hypertensive encephalopathy, snakebite need special line of management (see afterwards).

8. Inj. hydrocortisone hemisuccinate: 100 mg, IV stat and every 8 hourly. Often helpful in cerebral oedema, Stokes-Adams syndrome and myxoedema coma.

9. **General care of the comatosed patient:**

a. Maintain intake-output chart.

b. Prevention of cutaneous pressure sore (bed sore): Bedsheets should be creaseless, and bed must be made regularly. Frequent change of posture in bed, maintain local hygiene (by alcohol/spirit cleansing); bed should be dry and clean; use air cushions to protect pressure points; apply local antibiotic (with or without povidone iodine and metronidazole ointment) from the beginning of a small bed sore, and consult surgeon.

c. Care of bladder, bowel and mouth: Condom catheter is preferable in male patients as indwelling catheters are common source of UTI. Constipation should be managed by dioctyl sodium sulphosuccinate tablets (100 mg/tablet), 2 tab at bed time or by enema. Mouth care should be done by swabs soaked in boroglycerine/lotio mercurochrome (1%) or by sucker (prevents parotitis); fungal infection should be tackled by oral clotrimazole lotion.

d. Maintain Ryle's tube, IV catheter, condom/ indwelling catheter (with an intake-output chart). Check pulse, respiration, BP, temperature **(vital signs)** regularly including pulse oximetry and continuous ECG monitoring. Recheck serum electrolytes.

e. Start systemic antibiotic in the first chance, if evidenced by UTI, basal pneumonia, etc.

f. Maintain 'nutrition' and hydration by Ryle's tube feeding (3000 calories/day) or IV alimentation.

g. Eye care: Gentamicin or chloramphenicol eye ointment is applied (prevents exposure keratitis); taping of eyelids, irrigation as and when necessary.

h. Start physiotherapy as soon as the patient recovers from coma (e.g. in CVA cases).

i. Inj. ranitidine: 50 mg. IV 3–4 times daily or sucralfate 1 g, 6 hourly, orally to prevent stress ulcer.

j. Maintain normal body temperature.

k. Record improvement by scoring of Glasgow Coma Scale.

l. Move the legs and arms passively thrice daily (or apply compression stockings to legs) to prevent leg vein thrombosis and frozen shoulder respectively.

m. The patient may be shifted to HDU (High Dependency Unit) or ITU (Intensive Therapy Unit).

10. Gastric aspirate and urine should be preserved for possible toxicological screening.

Some Other Facts about Coma

- ***Psychogenic or hysterical coma:***
  1. Very resistant to firm supraorbital or sternal pressure. (Harrey's first sign: When a patient feigns coma or in status epilepticus, the traditional stimulus is to press the thumb into supraorbital notch, or to rub a knuckle over patient's sternum, or to pinch a finger nail-bed, and then stand clear about the situation.) Often shows forced eye closure in response to painful stimuli.
  2. Plantar response: Bilaterally flexor.
  3. May be associated with hyperventilation.
  4. Absence of H/o spontaneous micturition, defecation or tongue bite.
  5. Pupils: Bilaterally normal and reacting equally.
  6. The patient is usually a young female under stress or familial dysharmony.
  7. Increased tone in skeletal muscles in the presence of coma.
  8. Normal caloric test, EEG or CT scan.
- ***Doll's-eye movement (oculocephalic reflex):*** The head of the comatosed patient is quickly rotated from side to side (or rotated vertically) with the eyes kept open, and the positive response observed is conjugate deviation of the eyes to opposite direction to that of the head. For example, in a comatose patient if the head is quickly rotated to the left, the eyes will deviate to the right if the patient has 'intact brainstem' (with release from higher cerebral control). Absence of this reflex indicates severe structural lesion in brainstem or deep metabolic coma. This reflex is not present in normal persons.
- ***'Brainstem functions' are assessed by:***
  1. Level of consciousness.
  2. Pattern of respiration (e.g. Cheyne-Stokes respiration, apneustic breathing or ataxic type of breathing).
  3. Pupillary size and reactivity.
  4. Ocular movements (conjugate deviation, doll's-eye movement).
  5. Oculovestibular reflex (caloric test).

- ***Respiratory patterns in coma (or CNS disorders):***
  1. Post-hyperventilation apnoea (periods of apnoea after 5–10 deep breaths): Indicates bifrontal disease.
  2. Cheyne-Stokes respiration: Indicates supratentorial lesions (massive cerebral lesions).
  3. Central neurogenic hyperpnoea (rather, it is like Kussmaul breathing, i.e. deep, regular breathing with increased rate and depth): Indicates midbrain-upper pontine lesion.
  4. Apneustic breathing (a pause of 2–3 seconds after full inspiration), or
     Biot's breathing (e.g. 3 to 4 respirations without waxing or waning, followed by a pause): Indicates lower pontine-level lesion.
  5. Ataxic breathing (rhythm is chaotic, varying in rate and depth): Indicates lesion in medulla.
  6. Hypoventilation (regular, rhythmic shallow breathing): May have lesion in brainstem.

MANAGEMENT OF HEPATIC PRE-COMA/COMA

Outline of management:

Basic principles of management are:

a. To reduce neurotoxic substances.
b. To remove precipitating factors.
c. To facilitate regeneration of liver.

1. Follow the 'general care of the comatosed patient' (see before).
2. In hepatic pre-coma, patient may be restless. Tie him with gauze and cotton, in a railed cot. Oxazepam (15–30 mg) may be given orally through Ryle's tube.
3. Blood is tested for:
   a. Serum bilirubin and other LFTs
   b. Na^+, K^+, HCO_3^-, Ca^{++}, Mg^{++}, PO_4^{--}
   c. Serum ammonia
   d. Urea and creatinine, sugar (random)
   e. Prothrombin time (coagulation profile)
   f. Blood gas analysis
4. Identify and remove possible precipitating factors, e.g. electrolyte imbalance, infection or drugs consumed with cerebral depressant properties.
5. Protein restricted diet. Replace animal-based protein with vegetable-based protein as it is less ammoniagenic, better tolerated and more laxative.
6. Gut sterilisation with rifaximin (550 mg, BD) or metronidazole (200 mg, QDS) orally is done. Previously neomycin 4 g/day, orally was used.
7. Syrup lactulose 15–30 mL, three times daily to continue, orally or so as to cause two to three semisolid stools daily. Lactitol 30 g daily is compatible in efficacy to lactulose.
8. Inj. mannitol (20%): 100 mL, 8 hourly, IV (few clinicians prefer to run mannitol 300 mL, IV rapidly in 30 minutes). It reduces cerebral oedema in hepatic pre-coma. Mannitol should be withheld in hepatic coma.
9. Maintenance of calorie, fluid and electrolytes:
   a. About 1500–2000 calories/day are required of which 1200 calories/day to be given in the form of 10–25% glucose.
      IV fluid direction (3 bottles/24 hours):
      10% dextrose, followed by 10% dextrose with normal saline, followed by Darrow's solution.
   b. As hypokalaemia is a common complication, 60 mEq/day of K^+ should be given by slow IV route in three divided doses. Half of the dose may be given orally (syrup potassium chloride).
   c. Hypoglycaemia, hypomagnesaemia, hypocalcaemia and hypophosphataemia should be properly dealt with.
10. High bowel wash or enema 8–12 hourly daily for 2–3 days.
11. Inj. vitamin K: 10 mg IM/IV twice daily for consecutive 3 days.
12. Inj ranitidine (50 mg/2 mL): 50 mg, IV, 3–4 times daily till recovery.
13. Miscellaneous: (empirical)
    a. Flumazenil, L-dopa (1–4 g/day, orally in divided doses) may be tried. (empirical)
    b. IV branched-chain amino acid, charcoal haemoperfusion may be beneficial. (empirical)
    c. Bromocriptine: 2.5–15 mg/daily, orally.
    d. Judicious use of diuretics in treating oedema and ascites.
    e. Manage haematemesis/melaena accordingly; Judicious use of sedatives.
    f. Inj. ampicillin: 500 mg, IM/IV, 6 hourly or inj. cefotaxime 1 g, IV, 12 hourly for 5–7 days in systemic infection.
    g. Inj. vitamin B complex: 2 mL, IM/IV once daily.
    h. Fresh blood, fresh frozen plasma or platelet transfusion in case of haemorrhage, if any.
    i. L-ornithine L-aspartate (LOLA) given orally or parenterally promotes hepatic removal of NH_3 along with detoxication (of NH_3).
    j. Zinc supplementation may be helpful.
    k. Others: Polyethylene glycol (PEG), nitrogen scavengers, albumin infusion, probiotics and fecal microbiota transplantation (FMT or 'poop pills') may be tried.
14. A patient in fulminant hepatic failure should be shifted to ICU.

- In hepatic coma, clinical jaundice may be mild.
- Flapping tremor is present in hepatic pre-coma, absent in coma.
- In the management of hepatic encephalopathy (pre-coma/coma), always be careful regarding electrolyte imbalance. It is very often the silent killer (especially hypokalaemia). Paralytic ileus with diminished peristaltic sound is a bedside clue to hypokalaemia.

COMA IN A DIABETIC

The probable causes of coma in a diabetic are:

1. Hypoglycaemic coma (commonest cause).
2. Diabetic ketoacidosis (DKA).
3. Hyperosmolar hyperglycaemic non-ketotic coma (HHNK or HONK).
4. Lactic acidosis (rare).
5. Other causes of coma like:
   a. CVA
   b. Renal failure
   c. Hepatic coma
   d. Drug-induced coma
   e. Septicaemia.

At first, try to differentiate between hypoglycaemic coma and DKA (Table 5.1).

Outline of Management

A. Hypoglycaemic Coma

Symptomatic hypoglycaemia occurs (in diabetes) when the blood level of glucose is less than 55 mg/dL.

1. Inj. dextrose (25%): 50 mL, IV bolus to be followed by 5% dextrose infusion, IV, rapidly until the patient is able to eat a meal. Blood sugar should be preferably kept above 150 mg/dL.
2. As soon as the patient is able to take food orally, start oral feeding with glucose, sucrose or sugar-containing liquids. Frequent monitoring of blood sugar is necessary.
3. In refractory cases, inj. glucagon 1 mg, SC or IM may be given and repeated after 10 minutes if required.
4. If the patient is on insulin or oral hypoglycaemic agents (OHA), re-adjust the dosage schedule and re-educate the patient.

- A normal person may experience hypoglycaemic symptoms if glucose level is <45 mg/dL. All diabetic patients are advised to carry sweets, jaggery, sugar, glucose powder or glucose biscuits.

B. Diabetic Ketoacidosis

Management of DKA should preferably be conducted in ITU (Intensive Therapy Unit). Confirm the diagnosis by level of plasma glucose, metabolic acidosis and positive serum ketones. Success of treatment depends on close monitoring by the physician.

1. In an established case, the patient usually suffers from a fluid deficit of 7–8 litres (sodium loss is 500 mmol). It is better to correct the fluid loss in this way:

Normal saline volume	Time
1 litre	in 30 minutes
1 litre	in next 1 hour
1 litre	in next 2 hours
1 litre	in next 4 hours
4 litres	in next 16 hours

2. Inj. soluble (regular) insulin: Administer short-acting insulin (0.1 units/kg as bolus) or IM (0.3 units/kg), and then 0.1 unit/kg/hour by continuous IV infusion, as long as normal saline drip continues. By this dosage of insulin, blood sugar should fall by 55–110 mg/dL per hour. When the blood sugar level falls to 250 mg/dL, reduce the rate of insulin infusion to 3 units/hour. If the blood glucose concentration does

Table 5.1: Differentiation between DKA and hypoglycaemic coma

Features	DKA	Hypoglycaemic coma
1. History	No insulin; infection	Large dose of insulin, no food; heavy exercise
2. Onset	Gradual	Sudden
3. Symptoms and signs	Pain abdomen, vomiting	Hunger, drenching sweat, tremor, palpitations
a. Tongue and skin	Dry	Moist
b. Pulse	Weak	Bounding
c. BP	Low	Normal or high
d. Respiration	Air hunger	Shallow breathing
e. Tremor	None	Present
f. Dehydration	Present	Absent
g. Reflexes	Diminished	Brisk
4. Urine examination	Sugar +	Sugar –
	Acetone +	Acetone –
5. Blood examination	Sugar ↑	Sugar ↓
	HCO_3^- ↓	HCO_3^- : normal

A patient of lactic acidosis may give H/o regular intake of metformin (biguanides), if associated with severe hepatic or renal disease. HHNK is common in elderly type 2 DM patients.

- DKA patients may have Kussmaul's breathing with smell of acetone in breath.

not fall within 2 hours, the dose of insulin should be doubled.

Another regimen: 20 units IM stat followed by 6 units IM hourly.

3. When the blood sugar level reaches 250 mg/dL, the fluid is changed to 5% glucose (as a prophylactic measure to control late cerebral oedema, to prevent dangerous hypoglycaemia and to supply 'free water'). 12 units of soluble insulin is charged in each bottle to neutralise glucose (5%) present in the solution of the bottle. The rate of the fluid is adjusted according to the degree of dehydration and other parameters.

   When the patient is able to eat and drink normally, start daily subcutaneous insulin regimen four times daily.
4. Inj. potassium chloride: This therapy is usually required after 4 hours of initial therapy (when acidosis tends to be corrected and the K^+ shifts intracellularly by the action of insulin). If plasma K^+ is <5.5 mEq/L, give inj. potassium chloride 10 mEq/hr; administer 40–80 mEq/hr when plasma K^+ is <3.5 mEq/L, or if bicarbonate is given to the patient. If oral feeding is possible, give syrup potassium chloride 2 g, 4 hourly for next 48 hours.
5. If pH goes below 7.0, immediately start 300–500 mL of 1.4% isotonic sodium bicarbonate in place of same volume of normal saline, to run over 30 minutes (to control acidosis). Slow correction of bicarbonate is often beneficial. Repeat, if necessary to bring the pH up to 7.0.
6. Infection is controlled by inj. cefotaxime or inj. ceftriaxone—1 g, IV, 12 hourly.
7. 'General care of the comatosed patient' (see before) is followed meticulously. Blood sugar, serum K^+ and HCO_3^-, pH sugar and acetone in urine, and blood gases should be checked every 2 hourly till the patient regains consciousness.
8. As soon as oral feeding is possible, give fruit juices and frequent small fluid meals. Administer intermediate or long-acting insulin in place of soluble or short-acting insulin.

- Few clinicians prefer 'low-dose insulin' therapy from the beginning by 6-8 units/hour given IV; as the question of insulin resistance (ketosis, acidosis, dehydration, infection and stress may give rise to insulin resistance) can not be ruled out in few patients, many physicians advocate 25–50 units of soluble insulin/hour until the acidosis is reversed. Persistence of acidosis despite several hours treatment with insulin makes the clinician suspicious about insulin resistance.
- As there is phosphate depletion in DKA, potassium may be administered as phosphate salt in the place of potassium chloride, at least initially.
- Plasma expander is used, IV in hypotension. As gastroparesis diabeticorum is common in diabetes, gastric aspiration through a nasogastric tube should be done to minimise the risk of aspiration pneumonia. Central venous pressure (CVP) is monitored in an ideal setting. Catheterisation, if no urine is passed after 3 hours. ECG monitoring in severe cases.
- The body temperature remains normal in DKA. If raised, think of infection. Try to find out the underlying cause (e.g. perianal abscess). A chest X-ray, ECG (to exclude CAD or AMI), urine and blood culture should be performed.
- While managing DKA, a **'flow sheet'** containing timing and amount of parenteral fluid and insulin administered, as well as recording of vital signs, urinary output and blood biochemistries should be maintained.
- Inj. magnesium sulphate (50%) in doses of 2.5–5.0 mL (i.e. 10–20 mEq magnesium), IV can be administered in patients with ventricular arrhythmia.

Clinical Wisdom

DKA is a major medical emergency and remains a serious cause of morbidity and mortality. Other than fluid and electrolytes losses, **complications** encountered are ARDS, cerebral oedema, DIC, thromboembolism (leg veins and pulmonary) and acute circulatory failure.

C. Hyperosmolar Hyperglycaemic Non-ketotic Coma (HHNK or HONK)

In HONK, dehydration is profound and plasma osmolality is high.

1. If plasma osmolality is >350 mOsm/kg, start 1/2 strength, i.e. 0.45% saline until the osmolality becomes normal, when (0.9%) normal saline should be given. The rate of fluid infusion will be judged by monitoring CVP and plasma Na^+ concentration (if osmolality of plasma falls rapidly, there is a chance of developing cerebral oedema).
2. As these patients are usually insulin sensitive, half the dose of insulin advised in DKA should be employed here, at least initially (3 units/hour).
3. Recognition and correction of the precipitating factors (e.g. infection, heat stroke, peritoneal dialysis, high carbohydrate diet, steroids, etc).
4. *Others:* As done in DKA (inj potassium chloride, antibiotic, general care, etc.), sodium bicarbonate requirement is less as it is a non-ketotic coma.

- Usually the fluid deficit is 10 litres or even more in HHNC. The **hyperglycaemic hyperosmolar state** (HHS; a new terminology for HONK) is diagnosed when plasma glucose is >600 mg/dL, osmolality >320 mOsm/kg and there is absence of ketoacidosis (endogenous insulin level is sufficient to inhibit hepatic ketogenesis); the pH of blood is usually >7.3 with HCO_3^- >18 mEq/L. The mortality ranges as high as 20–30% mainly because of the advanced age. As there is absence of 'ketosis', features like pain abdomen, nausea, vomiting and Kussmaul's respiration are absent.

D. Lactic Acidosis

Here, the HCO_3^- deficit is enormous. The pH should be kept over 7.2. Treatment is aimed at:

1. IV sodium bicarbonate: May require 2500 mmol/24 hours.
2. Soluble insulin: As given in DKA.
3. Often haemodialysis is required (if pH does not rise above 7.0 on meticulous treatment).
4. Others (fluid, antibiotic, etc.): As done in DKA.

- Urine may not contain acetone, breath does not smell that of acetone in lactic acidosis. Plasma lactate is high (>5.0 mmol/L) and is diagnostic. The mortality is >50%.

E. Other Causes of Coma

Read respective chapters.

SUDDEN RESPIRATORY DISTRESS

The common causes come in mind are:

1. Acute left ventricular failure (LVF) or acute left atrial failure (i.e. acute pulmonary oedema).
2. Acute exacerbation of bronchial asthma (i.e. acute severe asthma) or COPD (Fig. 5.1).
3. Spontaneous (tension) pneumothorax.
4. Acute laryngeal obstruction (e.g. foreign body).
5. Acute pulmonary thromboembolism (PTE).
6. Cardiac tamponade.
7. Anaphylaxis.
8. Hysterical hyperventilation.

Q. Basic causes of cardio-respiratory dyspnoea:

A. Cardiac

- Myocardial
- Coronary vascular
- Arrhythmias
- Valvular
- Pericardial
- Congenital

B. Respiratory

- Obstructive
- Restrictive
- Alveolar
- Interstitial
- Vascular

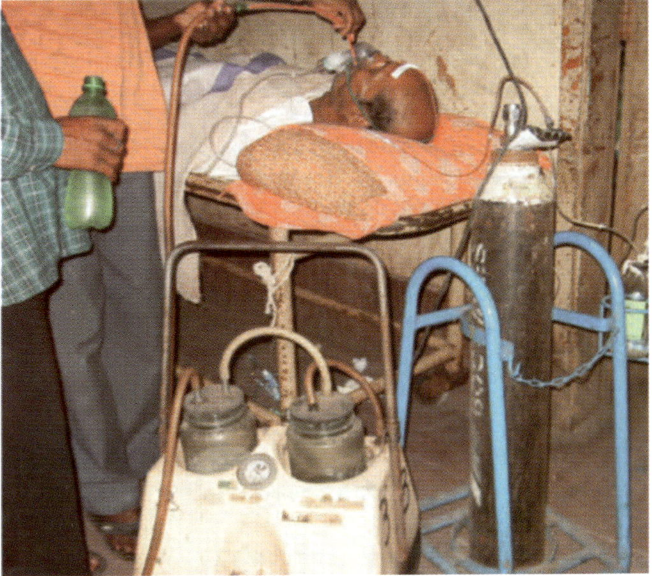

Fig. 5.1: A moribund patient of **COPD with acute exacerbation** is managed in a suburban hospital emergency with the help of nebulisation mask, oxygen cylinder and suction machine

Outline of Evaluation

a. History: Onset (except bronchial asthma and hysterical hyperventilation, all are acute in onset), progress, H/o chest pain (pneumothorax) or ingestion of foreign body, H/o inj. penicillin administration (anaphylaxis), personality disorder (hysteria), and past history (similar episode may occur in LVF or bronchial asthma) should be taken into account.

b. Physical examination: At first, examine the patient for orthopnoea and central cyanosis.

a. Cough ++: Pneumothorax, LVF, foreign body.
b. Pulse: Pulsus alternans in LVF, pulsus paradoxus in acute severe asthma.
   JVP: Raised in cardiac tamponade, LVF; prominent x-trough in tamponade.
c. BP: May be hypertensive in LVF.
d. Respiration: Tachypnoea and even orthopnoea may be evident; hyperactive accessory muscles of respiration. Intercostal suction may be evident in laryngeal obstruction.
e. Urticaria (involving lips, tongue) with itching, and stridor: Anaphylaxis.
f. Stridor: Anaphylaxis and laryngeal obstruction. Wheeze: In other situations.
g. RVH: Acute severe asthma, COPD.
   LVH: LVF.
h. Trachea: Deviated to opposite side in pneumothorax.
i. Percussion: Tympanitic resonance on affected side is obtained in pneumothorax. Obliteration of liver and cardiac dullness may be revealed in acute severe asthma and COPD. Cardiac dullness is increased in cardiac tamponade.
j. Auscultation:
   i. LVF: Rhonchi +, crepitations +++, gallop rhythm; vesicular breath sound with prolonged expiration.
   ii. Acute severe asthma or COPD: Rhonchi+++, crepitations +, heart sounds muffled; may have silent chest.
   iii. Anaphylaxis, acute pulmonary thromboembolism: Vesicular breath sound with prolonged expiration, occasional rhonchi and pleural rub (in PTE).
   iv. Spontaneous pneumothorax: Diminished vesicular or absent breath sound on affected side, no adventitious sound.
   v. Cardiac tamponade: Muffled heart sounds.
k. Hysterical hyperventilation: Pause in-between inspiration and expiration. No cyanosis; exaggerated symptoms in front of relatives. Carpopedal spasm may be seen due to tetany.

C. Investigations: At least, chest X-ray (PA view) and X-ray of neck (foreign body) should be done. Blood gas analysis may be informative.

- Read the differences between cardiac asthma and bronchial asthma from 'Bedside Clinics in Medicine, Part I'.

Outline of Management

A. Acute LVF, Acute LAF or Acute Pulmonary Oedema (Cardiac Asthma)

1. Propped-up position in bed with moist O_2 delivered at a rate of 4–6 litres/min (100%) through face mask or nasal prongs with high flow rates, i.e. up to 10 litres/min. The position in bed should be comfortable to the patient.
2. Inj. morphine sulphate: Slow IV injection in a total dose of 5–10 mg, at a rate of 2 mg/minute or inj. pethidine 100 mg, IM given. Large doses of morphine may produce respiratory depression and it should be aoided if systolic BP is <90 mm of Hg.
3. Inj. furosemide: 40 mg, IV stat (or bumetanide 1 mg, orally, IM or IV injection) and may be repeated after 30 minutes.
4. Inj. aminophylline: It was once commonly used; chance of developing arrhythmia is there; 250–500 mg of the drug should be given IV slowly, in not less than 20 minutes. It relieves bronchospasm and improves cardiac contractility.
5. Digitalis: Needs judicious use (as diuretics produce hypokalaemia and may precipitate digitalis toxicity in turn). Rapid digitalisation is done through IV route, if not contraindicated.
6. One tab. of nitroglycerine (0.5 mg/tab) is given sublingually, may be repeated after 1/2 hour. Inj. nitroglycerine (5–100 μg/min as infusion) may be given IV to reduce the preload.
7. Afterload reduction by IV sodium nitroprusside (20–30 μg/min) may be done if systolic BP is >100 mm of Hg.
8. Dobutamine (2.5–15 μg/kg/min) may be of some help (IV) in cardiogenic pulmonary oedema with shock and hypotension.
9. Phlebotomy or venesection (250 mL) may by required in intractable cases. Rotating tourniquets may be applied in the extremities—it reduce the load in the heart by diminishing venous return. Keep the sphygmomanometer cuff inflated at 80 mm of Hg (i.e. at diastolic pressure) for 15 minutes; inefficient and rarely used.
10. The patient may be transferred to ICU for continuous monitoring of pulse, BP, respiration and cardio-respiratory status.

- This is the treatment schedule of cardiac asthma too.

Few special points in the treatment:

a. The patient is most comfortable in 'trunk up, legs down' position, i.e. patient will be sitting with the legs dangling along the side of the bed. This reduces venous return and central venous pressure. IV fluids should be restricted.

b. Morphine relieves anxiety, reduces venous filling pressure to the heart, shifts blood from lesser to the major circulation (pharmacological phlebotomy) and diminishes adrenergic stimuli to arteriolar as well as venous bed. Morphine-induced emesis can be prevented by metoclopramide.

c. Aminophylline has bronchodilator, vasodilator, diuretic, cardiac inotropic and respiratory muscle inotropic effects.

One amp. of inj. aminophylline (10 mL) contains 250 mg of the drug. Usually it is diluted upto 50 mL with normal saline.

d. If digitalis has not been administered previously 0.5 mg of the drug may be administered by slow IV injection. Later, it may be followed by one tab. of digoxin (0.25 mg/tab) daily.

e. Sodium nitroprusside 50 mg is given in 500 mL of 5% dextrose by slow IV infusion.

f. Correction of precipitating factors, e.g. infection or arrhythmia, and underlying cardiac problem.

g. ACE inhibitors or angiotensin receptor blockers diminish both afterload and preload; especially recommended in hypertensive patients.

h. Control of blood pressure: Hypotensives in high BP and vasopressors in low BP are given.

i. Amrinone and milrinone may be added in severe left ventricular dysfunction.

j. Recombinant brain natriuretic peptide (BNP) to relieve pulmonary oedema, haemodialysis or ultrafiltration for renal failure may be instituted.

- In clinical practice, most common causes of left-sided heart failure are ischaemic heart disease (IHD), hypertensive heart disease, valvular heart disease and chronic kidney disease.
- **High-altitude pulmonary oedema** (a life-threatening form of non-cardiogenic pulmonary oedema) can be prevented by slow ascent, acetazolamide, dexamethasone, calcium-channel blockers, or long-acting inhaled β_2-adrenergic agonists. The situation is treated by immediate descent from altitude, bed rest, O_2 therapy, inhaled nitric oxide and nifedipine.

B. Acute Severe Asthma (Status Asthmaticus)

1. Propped-up position in bed with high concentration O_2 inhalation through an intranasal rubber catheter at the rate of 4–6 litres/min. An IV drip should be started with normal saline.
2. The patient is reassessed. Measure O_2 saturation with a pulse oximeter.
3. Nebulised salbutamol 5 mg or terbutaline 10 mg with O_2 as the driving gas may be started and repeated 2–4 hourly.
4. Inj. hydrocortisone hemisuccinate—IV infusion. Loading dose: 4 mg/kg of body weight for 4 hours.

   Maintenance dose: 3 mg/kg/6 hour for next 24 hours.

   Or, inj. hydrocortisone, 200 mg IV is given 4-hourly for 24 hours from the beginning. Then oral prednisolone 60 mg/day may be given after 24 hours.

5. Inj. aminophylline may also be used—loading dose is 5.8 mg/kg of body weight in 100 mL normal saline over 20 minutes, followed by maintenance dose as mentioned below.
   Patients with CCF or hepatic disorder—0.45 mg/kg/hour. Patients over 50 years of age—0.68 mg/kg/hour. Young patients—0.9 mg/kg/hour.
   If the patient has used the drug sporadically, loading dose will be half in that situation; IV drip is to be continued till the acute crisis is over. However, use of IV **aminophylline is not recommended by pulmonologists** at present though in some cases it may be beneficial.
6. Antimuscarinic bronchodilators, e.g. ipratropium bromide (20–40 μg, 3–4 times daily) or oxitropium bromide (200 mg twice daily) by aerosol inhalation may be started with β_2-adrenoceptor stimulants. Nebulized solution (0.5 mg) may also be used (with nebulised salbutamol or terbutaline).
7. Inj. ampicillin: 500 mg, IM, 6 hourly or inj cefotaxime 1 g, IV, 12 hourly for 5–7 days to prevent pulmonary infection, if any.
8. Maintenance of fluid and electrolyte balance (repeated use of salbutamol may develop hypokalaemia).
9. If no improvement is seen, one of the following IV infusions may be started:
   - Salbutamol 3–20 μg/min,
   - Terbutaline 1.5–5.0 μg/min, or
   - Magnesium sulphate 1.2–2 g over 20 minutes
10. Assisted (mechanical) ventilation in ICU is required if:
    a. i. PaO_2 <60 mm of Hg and falling,
       ii. $PaCO_2$ >45 mm of Hg and rising,
       iii. pH <7.3
    b. Patient goes into coma/respiratory arrest/exhaustion/extreme drowsiness/totally confused.
11. After the acute attack is over, following drugs will continue:
    a. Tab salbutamol (2 mg), terbutaline (2.5 mg) or theophylline (100 mg): 1 tab, thrice daily orally. Doxophylline, 400 mg, BD, orally may be used.
    b. Tab prednisolone (10 mg): Started with 6 tablets in the morning, orally and gradually tapered within 2 weeks. Nowadays, corticosteroids (e.g. beclomethasone, budesonide or fluticasone) are used as inhaler.
    c. Sodium chromoglycate inhalation: 20 mg (i.e. 2 puffs), four times daily or nedocromil sodium inhalation (4 mg, 2–4 times daily)
    d. Ketotifen: 1–2 mg twice daily, orally.
    e. Leukotriene antagonist, montelukast (10 mg, orally, once daily in the evening) or zafirlukast (20 mg, orally, BD) may be used in mild to moderate persistent asthma.
12. Mucolytics (acetyl-cysteine or bromhexine) may be used during the acute attack.
13. Plenty of fluid with semisolid/liquid diet is given orally when the acute attack is over.

- Inhalation of salbutamol/terbutaline/corticosteroid/ipratropium bromide may be used in between the attacks. Never sedate the patient during acute attack. Avoid beta-blockers. The patient should be admitted in the hospital for at least 5 days.

Clinical Wisdom

Monitor acute severe asthma by:
- Repeated PEFR at 15–30 minutes interval.
- SaO_2 should be kept >92% (check by pulse oximetry).
- Blood gas analysis from time to time.
- Exclude pneumothorax by X-ray chest.

C. Spontaneous (Tension) Pneumothorax

Read 'Bedside Clinics in Medicine, Part I'.

D. Acute Laryngeal Obstruction (Foreign Body)

Immediately send the patient to cardio-thoracic surgeon for bronchoscopic removal of the foreign body.

E. Acute Pulmonary Thromboembolism (Acute PTE or acute cor pulmonale)

PTE occurs as a result of blood clots, or fat-foreign body-air-tumour emboli. Diagnosis needs a high index of suspicion. Unexplained chest pain and respiratory distress in a suspicious patient ('predisposing factors for PTE'—see below) should always raise the possibility of PTE. Clinically there are tachypnoea, tachycardia and usually a clear chest on auscultation. Chest X-ray is usually normal. ECG shows non-specific ST-T changes or S_1, Q_3, T_3 pattern; plasma D-dimer levels are high. It is an acute emergency and should be tackled immediately by:

1. Absolute bed rest. High flow moist O_2 (60–100%) inhalation at the rate of 4–6 litres/min.
2. Severe chest pain may be relieved by inj. pethidine 100 mg IM or inj. morphine 15 mg IM (avoid in severe hypotension).
3. Normal saline drip is started.
4. Anticoagulation by inj. heparin sulphate: 10000 units, IV bolus stat, followed by 5000 units IV, 6 hourly, charged in 200 mL of normal saline (via a side connector) for at least 5 days (may be continued up to 10 days). Low molecular weight heparin (LMWH) given in SC route has the same effect as unfractionated heparin (e.g. enoxaparin is used in a dose of 1 mg/kg twice daily subcutaneously; fondaparinux is also used). LMWH is well tolerated, easier to administer, eliminates the need for frequent monitoring of aPTT, and is the treatment of choice in acute PTE. The target INR should be 2.5.
5. Start oral anticoagulation with tablet warfarin sodium (5 mg/tab) from the 2nd day as 1 tab twice daily for at least 3–4 weeks till the patient becomes ambulant, and then tapered gradually (to keep the INR at 2.5–3.0). It may be continued for 6 months. Patients with underlying prothrombotic risk will continue it for life-long.

6. Inj. dopamine infusion in hypotension or shock: 200 mg of dopamine (1 ampoule) is dissolved in 540 mL of normal saline. The bottle runs at the rate of 10–12 drops/min (<10 μg/kg/min) and the systemic BP is maintained near about 90–100 mm of Hg.
7. Thrombolytic (fibrinolytic) therapy: It improves pulmonary perfusion quicker than anticoagulation. In massive embolism with systemic hypotension, sreptokinase or urokinase is injected into the pulmonary artery through a catheter (2.5 lakh units) followed one hourly by 1 lakh unit, IV for 2–3 days; or t-PA (i.e. tissue plasminogen activator), 100 mg given in a drip over 2 hours as an infusion (most preferred agent). The treatment by t-PA is very costly.
8. Digitalis: Digoxin 0.5 mg is given IV, rapidly to increase the right ventricular output.
9. ACE inhibitors are tried but not much beneficial.
10. Surgical: Pulmonary embolectomy is now rarely performed.

Clinical Wisdom

The dose of heparin is adjusted on the basis of clotting time/aPTT (maintained at 1½–2 times of controlled value) and that of warfarin is adjusted by the result of prothrombin time (PT). LMWH needs no monitoring of coagulation profile.

- **Predisposing factors for PTE:**
  1. Prolonged immobilisation in bed (predisposes deep venous thrombosis or DVT).
  2. Post-surgical, pregnancy, post-partum state, old age.
  3. Fracture of long bones of leg.
  4. Carcinoma (especially of pancreas).
  5. Prolonged use of oral contraceptive pills, hypercoagulable states.
  6. Obesity.
  7. Chronic deep venous insufficiency in legs.
  8. LVF and RVF.
  9. Acute myocardial infarction.
  10. Hyperviscosity syndrome (e.g. myeloproliferative disorders), sickle cell anaemia
- Ventilation-perfusion (V/Q) lung scans have traditionally been the main test for suspected PTE and a normal V/Q scan virtually excludes PTE (a V/Q scan mismatch diagnoses PTE); nowadays contrast-enhanced spiral (helical) CT scan of lung is performed. Whenever the clinical data and non-invasive tests are equivocal or contradictory, pulmonary angiography is performed to diagnose PTE; recently CT pulmonary angiography has largely replaced conventional pulmonary angiography. Assay of plasma D-dimer is also helpful (if undetectable, excludes PTE).

  In a patient of DVT, colour Doppler ultrasound of the pelvic or iliofemoral veins remains the investigation of choice.
- Prevention of recurrent PTE: Warfarin sodium is given for 6 months though dabigatran, apixaban and rivaroxaban are newer agents which are also used; and lastly by inferior vena caval filter or clipping.

Clinical Wisdom

Prevention of DVT:
- Avoidance of prolonged immobilisation.
- Adopt frequent change of posture with both active and passive movements of lower limbs. Employ calf and respiratory exercises.
- Wear DVT elastic stockings.
- Try to avoid dehydration or combat dehydration promptly; avoid oral contraceptive pills.
- Prophylaxis by LMWH.

F. Cardiac Tamponade

Immediate pericardiocentesis is done under echocardiographic monitoring (read 'pericardiocentesis' from 'Instruments and bedside procedures' section).

G. Anaphylaxis

Vide 'Syringe (5 mL/50 mL)' in 'Instruments and bedside procedures' section.

H. Hysterical Hyperventilation

1. Reassurance to the patient as well as to the relatives.
2. Rebreathing bag: A paper bag is kept over the mouth of the patient. She/he rebreaths for 5 minutes what has expired out, and this would allow CO_2 retention and correction of acid-base imbalance. This is helpful if the patient develops tetany (hyperventilation → respiratory alkalosis → alkalosis reduces ionic calcium) and syncopal attack after hyperventilation.
3. Often inj. diazepam 5–10 mg, IM is helpful.
4. Psychological counselling.

CONGESTIVE CARDIAC FAILURE (CCF)

Heart failure is a complex syndrome that develops when the heart cannot function as a pump and is not able to maintain an adequate cardiac output for the needs of the body or can do so only at the expense of an elevated filling pressure. The diagnosis of CCF (basically right ventricular failure) should be suspected from clinical presentation. CCF can be acute or chronic.

A. Non-pharmacologic Measures

a. Restriction of physical activity helps to reduce myocardial work load and oxygen consumption. Complete bed rest in propped-up position, if dyspnoeic. O_2 inhalation at the rate of 4–6 litres/minute relieves dyspnoea, reduces the work of breathing, and limits pulmonary vasoconstriction in patients with hypoxaemia. Check pulse and BP regularly. Try to find out the cause of CCF.

b. Salt restricted diet (normal diet contains 10–15 g of NaCl or 4–6 g of Na^+. Salt restricted diet means avoiding table salt or extra salt = 2–4 g of Na^+/day, and salt free diet means avoidance of table plus cooking salt = 1 g of Na^+/day. Restrict the fluid intake <1.5 litre/day, if found to be hyponatraemic (<130 mEq/litre) or presents with volume overload.

B. Pharmacologic Therapy

a. Diuretics: High potency loop diuretic may be used; furosemide (40 mg/tab) 1 tablet daily or bumetanide (1 mg/tab) 1 tablet daily to be taken in the morning (diuretic therapy reduces preload to the heart). Medium potency thiazide diuretics may be used (hydrochlorothiazide 25–100 mg/day, orally, or indapamide 5–10 mg/day, orally, or metolazone 5–20 mg/day, orally), or low potency potassium sparing diuretics may be added to loop diuretics (e.g. spironolactone 50–200 mg/day). Recently, it was noted that spironolactone lowers morbidity and mortality (up to 30% reduction in mortality), improve survival, and decrease hospitalisation in patients with heart failure and severe secondary hyperaldosteronism [spironolactone should not be used with ACE inhibitors, NSAIDs or in renal insufficiency, i.e. serum creatinine >2.5 mg/dL]. The potassium loss by loop diuretics is adjusted by adding spironolactone to it. Eplerenone (in place of spironolactone) 25–50 mg/day may be used.

b. Tab digoxin (0.25 mg/tab) 2–4 tablets on the first day, then 1 tab daily to continue. In old age or in the presence of renal insufficiency, 1 tab may be given daily for '5 days in a week'. One should be careful about the appearance of digitalis toxicity as the toxic: therapeutic ratio of the drug is narrow. These days, digoxin has a limited role in heart failure due to the availability of better alternatives like β-blockers, ACE inhibitors and diuretics. Digitalis is useful in CCF with atrial fibrillation.

c. ACE inhibitors like enalapril (2.5/5/10/20 mg per tablet): 2.5–5 mg tab daily, orally to be taken in the morning or in divided doses. ACE inhibitors improve symptoms and survivals in patients of CCF (reduces preload as well as afterload). The treatment with this drug decreases ventricular filling pressure and thus increases the cardiac output, without little or no change in heart rate or BP. Captopril 6.25 mg, orally, TDS or ramipril, orally, 1.25–2.5 mg daily may also be given. Angiotensin II receptor blockers (e.g. losartan or valsartan) may be useful in patients unable to tolerate ACE inhibitors because of intractable cough or angio-oedema.

   Contraindications of ACE inhibitors are high serum creatinine (>2.5 mg/dL), pregnancy, bilateral renal artery stenosis and previous H/o angio-oedema.

d. β-blockers: These drugs have been shown to relieve symptoms, reduces the risk of arrhythmia and sudden death (mortality). The deleterious effects of endogenous catecholamines on the failing heart (e.g. myocyte toxicity) can be antagonised by beta-blockers, e.g. carvedilol (initiated at a dose of 3.125–6.250 mg, orally BD and is titrated to 25–50 mg, orally, BD), bisoprolol (initiated by 1.25 mg/day, orally and gradually increased to 10 mg/day), metoprolol (initiated by 12.5–25 mg/day, orally and gradually increased to 100–200 mg/day). Nebivolol (1.25–10 mg) is beneficial in stable heart failure in aged patients. A minimum of 2–3 months of therapy is required to observe significant haemodynamic improvement. One must be cautious in using these drugs in heart failure with very low ejection fraction. It is better to avoid β-blockers in patients having bradycardia, severe bronchospasm and heart block.

e. Reduce the dose of digitalis with the appearance of toxicity (may be given 1/2 tab daily and to continue as '5 days in a week' with 2 days rest/week). Periodic check up of urea, creatinine, Na^+, K^+ is necessary.

f. In hospital, all patients may require prophylactic anticoagulation. Treatment of arrhythmia is better controlled with amiodarone. Treatment of the underlying cause should be done. General lifestyle advice should be followed (stop smoking, reduce obesity, restriction of physical activity, etc.).

- Arterial vasodilators (hydralazine, prazosin), venodilators (glyceryl trinitrate) and inotropic agents (dobutamine) are not beneficial in CCF. Vasodilator ivabradine (5 mg daily, orally) slows the heart rate and beneficial in chronic heart failure with LV dysfunction.
- **Specific treatment of heart failures:**
  Forward failure: Vasodilators and inotropes
  Backward failure: Diuretics and venodilators
  Systolic dysfunction: Diuretics and vasodilators
  Diastolic dysfunction: Vasodilators
- **Newer therapeutic options** for CCF are BNP (i.e. brain natriuretic peptide), endothelin antagonist (e.g. bosentan), arginine vasopressin antagonist, neutral endopeptidase inhibitor (e.g. ecadotril), TNF-inhibitors (e.g. etanercept), cardiac assist devices (i.e. ICD or implantable cardioverter defibrillator), revascularisation and cardiac transplantation (with severe intractable heart failure).
- Read different types of **shock** [hypovolaemic, cardiogenic, anaphylactic, obstructive (pulmonary thromboembolism) and septic] and **'systemic inflammatory response syndrome'** (SIRS) from any standard textbook.

REFRACTORY HEART FAILURE

Heart failure is considered refractory when the response to therapy with diuretics, vasodilators and digoxin becomes inadequate, and the patient does not improve in due time. Probable possibilities are:

a. Overlooked underlying otherwise correctable diseases: Silent MS or AS, SBE, systemic hypertension, thyrotoxicosis or constrictive pericarditis.

b. Precipitating cause of heart failure persists: Recurrent pulmonary thromboembolism, hypoxia, anaemia, arrhythmia, silent ischaemia, pulmonary infection, myocarditis, pregnancy.

c. Complications induced by overzealous therapy: Digitalis toxicity, hypokalaemia, hyponatraemia or other electrolyte imbalance.

d. Others: Suboptimal treatment, non-compliance, excess intake of salt.

- The most common complication in CCF results from vigorous therapy with diuretics.

Management

1. Carefully look for and correct the overlooked underlying cause or precipitating cause.
2. Search for complications of overzealous therapy, e.g. hypovolaemia, dyselectrolytaemia or digitalis toxicity.
3. Easing up of salt restriction and diuretic administration temporarily.
4. Hyponatraemia is corrected by temporary cessation of diuretic therapy and restriction of oral water intake.
5. IV sodium nitroprusside plus dopamine/dobutamine (raises cardiac output and lowers filling pressure) are started. As the patient feels better, combination of hydralazine/enalapril and amrinone (a phosphodiesterase inhibitor with positive inotropic and vasodilator actions) is used orally.
6. Biventricular pacing or cardiac transplantation (i.e. final line of treatment) may be considered if all of the above measures fail.

EVALUATION AND MANAGEMENT OF ACUTE CHEST PAIN

The common causes should be considered are:

1. IHD, i.e. angina pectoris and acute myocardial infarction (AMI).
2. Acute dry pleurisy due to any cause/acute dry pericarditis.
3. Pneumothorax.
4. Trauma to the chest wall.
5. Diffuse oesophageal spasm (DES)/oesophagitis.
6. Costochondritis.
7. Malignant deposits on the ribs, rib fracture, intercostal myalgia, herpes zoster on the chest wall, multiple myeloma.
8. Dissection of ascending aorta.
9. Hiatal hernia, gallbladder disease, acute pancreatitis (i.e. referred pain to chest from abdomen)
10. Pulmonary thromboembolism (PTE).
11. Cardiac neurosis (psychogenic).

Outline of Evaluation

a. History: Onset, progress, pain with movement, actual site and character of pain, aggravating and relieving factors, duration, relation with food, associated symptoms (e.g. profuse perspiration and vomiting are present in AMI), dyspnoea present or not (AMI, pneumothorax, PTE, dissection of aorta are associated with dyspnoea), shock (AMI, tension pneumothorax, PTE, etc.), radiation of pain, or any personality disorder should be taken into account.

- **Retrosternal chest pain:** AMI, dissection of aorta, PTE, DES, pericarditis and psychogenic.
- Character:
  a. Tenderness: 2, 4, 6 and 7 (musculoskeletal disorders).
  b. Pleuritic in nature: 2, 3 and 10.
  c. Chest pain with abdominal pain: AMI, basal pleurisy and 9
  d. Retrosternal chest pain with dysphagia: DES
  e. Diffuse chest pain with tenderness all over the chest: Trauma, cardiac neurosis

b. Physical examination: Ashen-grey pallor, pulse, BP, JVP cyanosis, oedema, decubitus, features of shock, vesicles on the chest wall, tenderness, heart sounds, gallop, pericardial rub, breath sound, rhonchi, crepitations, pleural rub should be meticulously searched/examined.

c. Investigations:

a. If one investigation to be done, it is the electrocardiogram (ECG).
b. Chest X-ray (PA view).
c. Others: Cardiac injury enzymes (e.g. CK and CK-MB, AST, LDH, troponin T and troponin I), USG of abdomen, plasma D-dimer assay (e.g. PTE), barium swallow or upper GI endoscopy.

Outline of Management

A. Angina Pectoris (Chronic Stable Angina)

It is the cardiac ischaemia due to fixed atheromatous stenosis.

1. Acute attack:

a. Isosorbide dinitrate (5 mg/tab) or glyceryl trinitrate (GTN; 0.5 mg/tab): 1 tab to be placed sublingually (GTN may be used as spray). Usually pain is relieved within 2–5 minutes. If not relieved, any of the drug may be repeated after 10 minutes. If the chest pain continues after use of 2/3 tablets, think of AMI.
b. Acetyl salicylic acid or aspirin (75–150 mg/tab): 1 tab stat and to be continued indefinitely as 1 tab daily after meal. Clopidogrel (75 mg)—1 tab daily may be started (instead of aspirin) or added with aspirin.
c. Alprazolam (0.25/0.5 mg per tablet): 1 tab stat and sos to allay anxiety. Diazepam (5 mg)—1 tablet may be given instead.

2. Prevention of further attacks:

a. Restful life. Avoid weight gain, smoking, exertion and psychic stress. Salt restricted, fat free, light diet.
b. Continue isosorbide dinitrate (5 mg/tab): 1 tab 4 times daily (may produce headache). Isosorbide-5 mononitrate (20 mg/tab) may be used instead (1 tab twice daily at 8 AM and 3 PM—known as eccentric dosage schedule).

- Propranolol: 40 mg, twice daily, orally, or atenolol: 100 mg, once daily orally, or bisoprolol: 5–10 mg, daily, orally may be continued. Calcium-channel blockers (CCB) like nifedipine: 10 mg, 6–8 hourly daily (or sustained-release form), orally or amlodipine (2.5–10 mg daily, orally) or verapramil (120–240 mg, 8 hourly, orally, daily) or diltiazem (60–120 mg, 8 hourly, orally, daily) may be prescribed. β-blockers reduce myocardial O_2 demand by reducing heart rate and myocardial contractility. CCBs reduce myocardial O_2 demand by relaxing coronary arteries and vasodilatation. Potassium channel activators, e.g. nicorandil (10–30 mg, BD, orally) may also be helpful.

c. Prinzmetal's angina: Add nifedipine 5–20 mg, 8 hourly daily, orally.
d. Regular BP and ECG (resting) check up. Stress ECG (treadmill test) and echocardiography may be performed. The patient is advised to carry isosorbide dinitrate (5 mg/tab) or glyceryl trinitrate (0.5 mg/tab) with him, and to be kept under tongue if there is chest pain. In uncontrolled angina pectoris, coronary angiography should be performed.
e. Associated systemic hypertension, diabetes mellitus, hyperlipidaemia (i.e. comorbidities) should be treated by diet control and drugs. Correct exacerbating factors contributing to angina, e.g. obesity, CCF, anaemia or hyperthyroidism.
f. In intractable angina pectoris: Patient may be advised to do coronary angiography with a view to undergo coronary artery bypass grafting (CABG) or percutaneous transluminal coronary angioplasty (PTCA).

- Angina pectoris was first described by Heberden in the year 1772 (Heberden's angina).
- Internal mammary artery or reversed segments of saphenous vein of patients are used for CABG.
- **Angina without coronary artery occlusion** may be seen in severe myocardial hypertrophy, severe AS or AI, severe anaemia, hyperthyroidism or paroxysmal atrial tachycardia with rapid ventricular rate.

Clinical Wisdom

Mnemonic (ABCDE) for treatment and secondary prevention:
A: Aspirin and anti-anginal therapy
B: Beta-blocker and BP (control)
C: Cessation of cigarette smoking and control of cholesterol
D: Diet (modification) and diabetes (control)
E: Education (for lifestyle modification) and exercise training

B. Acute Myocardial Infarction (AMI)

It is the necrosis of the myocardium due to acute occlusion of a coronary artery resulting from plaque rupture and thrombosis. **AMI is a medical emergency** requiring immediate intervention.

Common **symptoms** of AMI are excruciating retrosternal chest pain, breathlessness, vomiting and collapse (due to cardiogenic shock reflected by ashen-grey pallor, intense perspiration and cold-clammy extremities). The common **signs** are fast and feeble pulse, initially high BP which may be followed by hypotension (in cardiogenic shock), central cyanosis, raised JVP, and muffled heart sounds which may be associated with gallop and basal crepitations in lung.

The **risk factors** for coronary artery diseases are male sex, family H/o IHD, type A personality, systemic hypertension, hyperlipidaemia, diabetes mellitus, tobacco smoking, obesity, physical inactivity, stress or depression, homocysteinaemia and consumption of oral contraceptive pills.

1. First aid:

a. Bed rest. Give reassurance. Moist O_2 inhalation at the rate of 4–6 litres/minute.
b. Tab isosorbide dinitrate (5 mg/tab) or tab glyceryl trinitrate (0.5 mg/tab)–1 tab to be kept under tongue immediately and to be repeated every 5 minutes till relief of chest pain. Discontinue, if hypotension develops.
c. Take brief history. Enquire risk factors. Try to examine the patient, especially the vital signs.
d. Insert IV cannula, if possible.
e. Inj. morphine sulphate (to combat excruciating chest pain)—10 mg, IV stat may be repeated (5 mg, IV) if necessary.
f. Acetyl salicylic acid (aspirin, 150–300 mg/tab): 1 tab stat to be chewed or clopidogrel 300 mg given orally as gel (i.e. loading dose) to relieve chest pain and improve blood flow. Loading dose of prasugrel 60 mg or ticagrelor 180 mg may be given instead.
g. Inj. cyclizine tartrate: 50 mg, IV stat, or inj. metoclopramide 10 mg, IV stat (as an antiemetic).
h. Start slow IV drip of 5% dextrose solution as an emergency IV channel.
i. Carry out 12-lead ECG. Take blood for cardiac enzymes (CK, CK-MB, AST, LDH, troponin T and troponin I), blood count, ESR, electrolytes (Na^+, K^+, Mg^{++}), glucose and lipid profile. Repeat the enzymes study at 12 hours and 24 hours. Remember, **CK-MB is elevated** in AMI, myocarditis or after electrical cardioversion.
j. Patient is shifted to ICU at the earliest opportunity.

2. Specific therapy: If the patient comes within 12 hours (preferably within 6 hours) of the onset of symptoms,

a. Thrombolysis by inj. streptokinase: 1.5 million units dissolved in 100 mL of normal saline and infused by IV route over 1 hour. It is a widely used drug. Side effects are allergic reaction, bleeding and hypotension.

   Anistreplase (30 units, single IV injection given over 5 minutes), alteplase or human tissue plasminogen activator or t-PA (IV infusion schedule as 15 mg bolus followed by 50 mg in the first 30 minutes and then 35 mg in the next 1 hour), urokinase (1.5 million unit bolus plus 1.5 million unit as infusion over 1½, hours) may be substitute of streptokinase. Newer thrombolytic drugs reteplase (r-PA) and tenecteplase (TNK-t-PA) facilitate rapid administration of fibrinolytic therapy.
b. IV atenolol (10 mg) or metoprolol (10 mg) relieves pain, reduces the chance of arrhythmias and also diminishes the size of infarction, if the patient is attended within 12 hours of the onset of symptoms. β-blockers are helpful to combat ongoing chest pain,

tachycardia and hypertension. In hypotension, bradycardia, CCF and heart block, β-blockers can not be used.

- Antithrombin drugs: Inj. heparin, SC, 5000 units twice daily may prevent deep vein thrombosis and left ventricular thrombus formation. After successful thrombolysis, inj. heparin 5000 units, SC, twice daily may be continued for 7 days (in addition to daily oral aspirin). Enoxaparin, a LMWH may be used 1 mg/kg twice daily, subcutaneously instead. Oral anticoagulation with warfarin sodium may follow inj. heparin or LMWH. Unfractionated heparin needs frequent monitoring, which is not required in LMWH. Bivalirudin (a thrombin inhibitor) and fondaparinux (inhibits thrombin generation) are useful alternatives.
- ACE inhibitors reduce mortality. Captopril 6.25 mg, three times daily (may be increased) should be started early (in patients who are haemodynamically stable) and may be continued (to counteract ventricular remodelling) after discharge from the hospital. Enalapril (5 mg, orally daily), ramipril (2.5–10 mg, orally daily) or lisinopril (5 mg, orally daily) may be used instead.
- Though controversial, glucose-insulin-potassium (GIK) 'cocktail' therapy may slow down myocardial injury.

3. Treatment of complications:

a. LVF: See before.
b. CCF: See before.
c. Sinus bradycardia: Elevation of the legs and/or foot end of the bed; inj. atropine 0.6 mg, IV stat.
d. Sinus tachycardia: Inj. propranolol 2.5 mg, IV and may be repeated.
e. Hypertension: Inj diazepam 10 mg, IV may be given.
f. Atrial fibrillation or flutter: Digoxin 0.25 mg, IV stat; synchronised DC shock in rapid ventricular rate with hypotension or circulatory collapse.
g. Paroxysmal atrial tachycardia: Inj. verapramil 10 mg, IV.
h. Ventricular fibrillation: DC shock, cardiopulmonary resuscitation (CPR).
i. Cardiac asystole: CPR; if falls, temporary pacemaker.
j. Heart block: Inj. atropine 0.6 mg, IV stat, repeated if necessary; temporary pacemaker.
k. Ventricular premature beats: Inj. lignocaine 1 mg/kg, IV, followed by an IV infusion of 1–4 mg/min. Serum magnesium level may be measured and repeated if necessary, to reduce the risk of ventricular arrhythmia.
l. Cardiogenic shock: Oxygen (8–10 litres/min), normal saline drip, dopamine infusion (2–20 µg/kg/min), inj. hydrocortisone hemisuccinate (200 mg, IV stat and repeated 100 mg, 4 hourly, IV), intra-aortic balloon counterpulsation may be tried. Arrhythmias should be carefully dealt with.
m. Chest pain: Inj. morphine sulphate, 5 mg, IV stat given and may be repeated after 10–15 minutes. In recurrent chest pain IV nitroglycerine at the rate of 0.6–1.2 mg/hr and IV heparin (1000 unit/hr) are to be infused.

- Ongoing chest pain, arrhythmias, CCF and shock are **common complications in AMI**.
- If percutaneous coronary interventions (PCI) are planned (i.e. percutaneous transluminal coronary angioplasty, i.e. PTCA, or stent placement in the coronary artery), start glycoprotein IIb/IIIa inhibitors (i.e. abciximab, tirofiban, eptifibatide).
- Heart failure as a complication of AMI is assessed by Killip classification.

4. Symptomatic treatment:

a. Constipation: Tablet dioctyl sodium sulphosuccinate 200 mg at bed time/Isabgol husk 2–4 tsf in tepid water at bed time.
b. Restlessness: Diazepam (5 mg/tab), 1 tablet twice daily may be given.

5. General treament:

a. Record vital signs regularly.
b. Low calorie diet, multiple small feeds from the 2nd day onwards (liquid diet on the 1st day). Diet should contain fibres. Stop smoking.

6. Discharge:

a. Usually after 7–10 days (depends on complications) with an advice to restrict physical activities for 4–6 weeks.
b. Advise to liaise with family physician.
c. Diet and lifestyle modifications:
   i. Diet: Consume low calorie, low fat, low cholesterol and high fibre diet.
   ii. Avoid smoking and alcohol (two small pegs/day are permitted).
   iii. Control diabetes and hypertension.
   iv. Regular exercise with control of weight (desirable BMI is 18.5–24.9 kg/m^2).
d. Continue:
   i. Antiplatelet drugs: Tab aspirin (75–150 mg/tab) or clopidogrel (75 mg–150 mg/tab)—1 tab daily after meal to continue indefinitely until further advice. Aspirin reduces post-infarct mortality and reinfarction.
   Instead prasugrel 10 mg daily, orally or ticagrelor 90 mg daily, orally may be given.
   ii. Tab atenolol (25/50/100 mg/tab): 25–50 mg daily to continue until further advice. Metoprolol 25–50 mg orally, twice daily may be given instead.
   iii. Tab isosorbide-5 mononitrate (20 mg/tab): 1 tab twice daily (8 AM and 3 PM; eccentric dosage schedule to prevent nitrate tolerance) to continue until further advice. Tab isosorbide dinitrate (5 mg/tab)—1 tab to be placed sublingually, sos at the onset of chest pain.
   iv. Tab captopril (25 mg/tab): 1/2–1 tab three times daily to continue until further advice. Ramipril (2.5–10 mg) orally daily or lisinopril (5–10 mg) orally daily are other alternatives. Angiotensin receptor blockers are given in those who can not tolerate ACE inhibitors.
   v. Statins: Atorvastatin (5–20 mg) or simvastatin (5–20 mg) orally, daily given at bedtime to control hyperlipidaemia.

7. Review:

a. Usually at 1 month.
b. Carry out exercise test.
c. Review secondary prevention (avoid smoking, control hypertension and diabetes, taking regular exercise, control weight gain, lower lipid level by diet control and statins) and screening of the family.

- Relative contraindications of thrombolytic (e.g. streptokinase) therapy:
  1. Recent major surgery (within 2 month).
  2. Active internal bleeding (e.g. probable active peptic ulcer bleeding) excluding menstruation.
  3. Past H/O intracerebral or subarachnoid haemorrhage.
  4. A recent head injury, even if minor/recent trauma.
  5. Pregnancy.
  6. Severe uncontrolled hypertension.
  7. Diabetic retinopathy (proliferative).
  8. Acute pericarditis or dissection of aorta.
  9. Acute pancreatitis.
  10. Recent streptococcal infection.

- **Aim of initial therapy in AMI** is to relieve pain, reduce the size of infarcted tissue, prevent/treat arrhythmias and mechanical complications.
- Clopidogrel (75 mg)—1 tablet, orally daily may be an alternative to aspirin (may be added to aspirin). Clopidogrel may be used where **aspirin is strictly contraindicated like** acute gastritis, H/O chronic duodenal ulcer, H/o recurrent upper GI bleeding, acute gout (low dose aspirin is contraindicated), dengue fever or incipient renal failure.

- **Right ventricular infarction** is suspected by: ↑JVP, ↓cardiac output and hypotension, Kussmaul's sign, right ventricular S_3 or S_4, absence of pulmonary congestion, presence of TI murmur and oedema in the background of inferior wall infarction. The patient presents with retrosternal chest discomfort, nausea, vomiting and diaphoresis (in LV infarction, there is dyspnoea which is uncommon in RV infarction). The therapy aims at maintenance of patency of infarct-related artery, intravascular volume expansion and inotropic support.
- At present thrombolytic therapy is not recommended for NSTEMI (non-ST-elevation myocardial infarction) and unstable angina.

C. Musculoskeletal Disorders

1. Hot fomentation followed by local analgesic gel application (e.g. diclofenac gel).
2. Analgesics or NSAID, e.g. ibuprofen 400 mg, 8 hourly, orally after meals or etoricoxib 90 mg, orally once daily after meals, plus tab antacid—1 tab, 8 hourly, orally to be taken after meals. Analgesic spray is also very helpful.
3. Alprazolam: 0.25 mg tablet, orally at bed time.

D. Acute Dry Pleurisy

1. Rest in bed.
2. Relief of chest pain by,
   a. Hot fomentation.
   b. Splinting of the chest wall with leucoplast strapping (old practice).
   c. Analgesics, e.g. indomethacin 25 mg, 8 hourly, orally after meal along with tablet antacid.
   d. Sedatives.
3. Treatment of the underlying aetiology.

E. Acute Dry Pericarditis

1. Rest in bed.
2. Hot fomentation, analgesic and sedatives are not of much value.
3. If pericardial effusion develops: Echocardiography-guided pericardiocentesis is to be done.
4. Treatment of the underlying aetiology (viral, tuberculous, uraemic, etc.).

- Cardiac tamponade is a medical emergency; so, treat acute dry pericarditis at the earliest.

F. Herpes Zoster

1. Calamine lotion or povidone iodine solution—as local application; acyclovir cream may be applied 4 hourly for 7 days.
2. Acyclovir (800 mg/tab): 1 tab 5 times daily for 7 days. Valacyclovir 1 g, 8 hourly may be used.
3. NSAID, e.g. indomethacin 25 mg, 8 hourly, orally after meals along with tablet antacid.
4. Post-herpetic neuralgia is managed by amitriptyline/carbamazepine/gabapentin. Transcutaneous electrical nerve stimulation (TENS) with aggressive analgesia is helpful.

G. Diffuse Oesophageal Spasm

1. Nifedipine (5 mg): 1 tab stat, orally, twice daily to continue.
2. Glyceryl trinitrate (0.5 mg/tab): 1 tab to be used sublingually stat and sos.
3. Tranquilisers, e.g. alprazolam 0.25–0.5 mg, orally daily at bed time to continue.
4. Oesophageal dilatation with mercury-filled rubber dilators.
5. Surgery: Longitudinal myotomy of oesophageal circular muscles in intractable cases.

H. Cardiac Neurosis

1. Reassurance to the patient as well as to the relatives.
2. Inj. diazepam: 10 mg, IM stat.
3. Tab alprazolam: 0.25 mg, orally at bed time to continue.
4. Psychological counselling.

Clinical Wisdom

Unstable angina:

It is the ischaemia as a result of dynamic obstruction of a coronary artery caused by plaque rupture with superimposed thrombosis as well as spasm. It is managed by:

1. Absolute bed rest. Continuous ECG monitoring. Rule out AMI by ECG and cardiac enzymes.
2. Aspirin 75–300 mg/day. Clopidogrel (75–150 mg, orally, daily) or ticlopidine (250 mg, BD, orally) may be used.

3. Atenolol 50–100 mg daily or metoprolol 50–100 mg twice daily, orally. If beta-blockers are contraindicated, it is better to start diltiazem (60 mg thrice daily, orally) or verapamil (40 mg thrice daily, orally) with gradual increment of dose later on.
4. If pain persists, anticoagulation is done by IV heparin (1000 unit/hour, adjusted by PTT) or LMWH, and
5. IV nitroglycerine (for refractory pain): Started at 10 μg/min and maintained at systolic BP >100 mm of Hg.
6. Identify exacerbating factors, e.g. ↑BP, arrhythmia, acute infection or chronic heart failure, and treat them accordingly. Statins may be added for plaque stabilisation.
7. Patients refractory to medical treatment are advised to do coronary angiography with a view to undergo CABG or PTCA.

Definitions

a. ***Unstable angina:*** It includes i. recent onset of severe angina (<2 months), ii. angina at rest or with minimal activity, iii. recent increases in frequency as well as intensity of chronic anginal pain, and iv. recurrent angina within several days of AMI without re-elevation of cardiac enzymes.
b. ***Angina decubitus:*** Anginal pain while lying flat.
c. ***Nocturnal angina:*** Unusual form of anginal pain which occurs at night and may be associated with dyspnoea, palpitations or nightmares; commonly seen in aortic regurgitation.
d. ***Postprandial angina:*** Anginal pain after a meal indicates severe CAD and is due to 'intramyocardial steal' phenomenon. Postprandial vasodilatation (due to carbohydrate content of meal) of superior mesenteric artery stealing blood from stenotic coronary artery is also responsible.
e. ***Prinzmetal's or variant angina:*** Pain occurs as a result of coronary arterial spasm and is accompanied by transient ST segment elevation in ECG without any increase in cardiac enzymes.

- **Acute coronary syndromes (ACS)** include unstable angina, ST-elevation myocardial infarction (STEMI) and non-ST-elevation myocardial infarction (NSTEMI). In unstable angina, CK-MB and troponin are not elevated whereas in other two, there are elevation of cardiac enzymes.

DRUG THERAPY IN HYPERTENSIVE EMERGENCIES

Hypertensive crises are life threatening events which demand immediate medical attention. It is an acute perilous state associated with marked increase in peripheral vascular resistance and decrease in tissue perfusion. This syndrome consists of:

1. Malignant hypertension.
2. Hypertensive encephalopathy.
3. Hypertensive acute LVF/acute pulmonary oedema.
4. Dissection of aorta/leaking aneurysm of aorta.
5. Eclampsia.
6. Epistaxis associated with hypertension.
7. CVA (cerebral haemorrhage commonly; also cerebral infarction and subarachnoid haemorrhage).
8. Hypertension-related decreasing renal function (hypertensive nephropathy).
9. Acute coronary syndrome (ACS).
10. Severe hypertension associated with pheochromocytoma.
11. Severe hypertension-related peripheral vascular diseases.

No. 1, 2, 3, 5 and 7 are commonly encountered problems.

Hypertensive 'emergency': Severe elevation in BP (>180/120 mm of Hg) accompanied by impending or progressive acute target organ damage, which must be reduced **within minutes**, ususally with **parenteral medication**. Above mentioned 11 causes are examples of the situation.

Hypertensive 'urgency': Severe elevation in BP without any life-threatening target organ damage, which must be reduced **within hours**, usually with **oral drug therapy**. The examples are postoperative hypertension, uncontrolled hypertension in patients requiring surgery, accelerated hypertension or hypertension associated with severe burn/post-organ transplantation.

Hypertensive 'crisis': In hypertension, initially there is LVH, later it gives rise to LV dilation, which ultimately leads to LVF.

Outline of Management

1. Complete bed rest; propped-up, if necessary. Hospitalisation is a must.
2. Diet: Salt free diet (avoidance of table salt plus cooking salt), i.e. 1 g of Na^+/day is allowed; liquid diet till the crisis is over. Restrict cholesterol, saturated fat; stop smoking, alcohol may be permitted only in moderation; perform isotonic or aerobic exercise regularly (cycling, swimming, jogging) after recovery and are followed life-long (lifestyle modifications).
3. Take detailed history to come to a pin-point aetiological diagnosis. Check BP at 10 minutes interval. Perform ophthalmoscopy.
4. a. Insert IV cannula and send blood for sugar, urea, creatinine, VMA (vanillylmandelic acid for pheochromocytoma).
   b. Inj. diazepam: 10 mg, IM stat given.
5. Primary target is to lower the sustained high level of BP by antihypertensives to prevent further target organ damage (majority are administered through IV route) **(Table 5.2)**:
   a. Sodium nitroprusside: The bottle and tubing have to be protected from light by wrapping in an opaque covering as ultraviolet rays can breakdown it into toxic thiocyanates. Dose—initially 0.3 (μg/kg)/min., IV; usual 2–4 (μg/kg)/min; maximum 10 (μg/kg)/min for 10 min. Overdose may give rise to cyanide poisoning.
   b. Diazoxide: This is given in the dose of 50–100 mg over 5 minutes in slow IV bolus and may be

repeated. It should not be used with H/o coronary insufficiency and CVA (precipitous fall of BP may occur).

c. Hydralazine: 5–10 mg, IV bolus dose is given at every 15 minutes (maximally 50 mg).
d. Nicardipine: Initially 5 mg/hr, titrate by 2.5 mg/hr at 5–15 min intervals; maximum 15 mg/hr. Putting the punctured nifedipine capsule sublingnally for rapid reduction of BP is not practised now as sudden death may supervene due to precipitous fall of BP.
e. Furosemide: 1 amp (2 mL = 20 mg), IV stat in shot push and may be repeated after 1/2 hour, if necessary. Electrolyte imbalance (especially hypokalaemia) may pose a problem.
f. Reserpine (not a very popular drug at present): It can be given in the dose of 2–5 mg, every 3 hourly by IM route. The onset of action is delayed (not prompt like the drugs mentioned above).
g. Enalaprilat (intravenous form of enalapril): The dose is 0.625–1.25 mg, IV, over 5 minutes, and is given stat and every 6–8 hours; maximum 5 mg/dose.
h. Labetalol: 2 mg/min up to 300 mg, or 20 mg over 2 min, then 40–80 mg at 10 min-intervals up to 300 mg total dose.
i. Esmolol: Initially 80–500 µg/kg over 1 min, then 50–300 (µg/kg)/min to be maintained.
j. Nitroglycerine: Initially 5 µg/min, then titrate by 5 µg/min at 3–5 min intervals; if no response occurs at 20 µg/min, one may incrementally increase the dose by 10–20 µg/min.
k. Phentolamine: 5–15 mg bolus dose.

6. Discharge the patient with some advice (mentioned in point No. 2) and antihypertensive medications (ACE inhibitors, calcium-channel blocker, etc.).

Reasons for poor therapeutic response in hypertension:

a. Poor patient compliance, suboptimal dose, inappropriate combinations or non-adherence.
b. Gain in weight, smoking, insulin resistance, sleep apnoea, ethanol intake (>30 mL/day).
c. Volume expansion done by:
   1. Excessive intake of salt.
   2. Secondary to non-diuretic antihypertensive drugs.
   3. Inadequate diuretic therapy.
d. Secondary hypertension (e.g. pheochromocytoma).
e. Using one class of drugs (in that situation, try different classes).
f. Drug antagonism by:
   1. Oral contraceptive pills.
   2. Corticosteroids.
   3. Sympathomimetics.
   4. Carbenexolone.
   5. Nasal decongestants, licorice (as may be found in chewing tobacco), erythropoietin, antidepressants
g. Pseudo-resistance. 'White-coat' hypertension, use of regular cuff on very obese arm.

Q. How to suspect secondary hypertension?

1. Resistant hypertension (i.e. poor response to therapy).
2. Systolic BP >180 mm of Hg and diastolic BP >110 mm of Hg.
3. Onset before 20 years of age.
4. Significant target organ damage within a short period.
5. Lack of control in previously stable patient.

Table 5.2: Different drugs in hypertensive emergencies

Hypertensive emergency	Drug (s) of choice	Drugs to be avoided
1. Hypertensive encephalopathy	Nitroprusside, diazoxide, labetalol	Methyl dopa, reserpine
2. Hypertension with LVF	Nitroprusside, enalaprilat, loop diuretics	Hydralazine, nifedipine
3. Hypertension plus renal failure	Nitroprusside, diazoxide, hydralazine, furosemide	Trimethaphan
4. Malignant hypertension	Nitroprusside, hydralazine, furosemide, enalaprilat	—
5. Hypertension with pregnancy	Methyldopa, labetalol, nicardipine, hydralazine, atenolol	Nitroprusside, diazoxide, enalaprilat
6. Hypertension with subarachnoid haemorrhage	Nitroprusside, nicardipine	Methyl dopa, reserpine
7. Pheochromocytoma	Phentolamine, nitroprusside	All other drugs
8. Dissection of aorta	Nitroprusside, esmolol, labetalol	Diazoxide, hydralazine
9. Hypertension associated with AMI or severe angina	Labetalol, nitroglycerine, nicardipine, esmolol	Nifedipine

- In case of cerebral haemorrhage and infarction (i.e. CVA), immediate reduction of high BP may hamper cerebral autoregulation and exacerbate cerebral damage. So, CVA is an exception among hypertensive emergencies where urgent BP reduction may be injurious to the patient.
- In hypertensive emergency, BP should be reduced gradually so much so to attain the target level of mm of 160/110 Hg within 2–6 hours. Initially BP should be reduced up to 25% within minutes to one hour. Too much rapid and excessive reduction in BP may precipitate cerebral, coronary or renal ischaemia.
- **Target BP** to be achieved: <140/90 mm of Hg in a patient who is <60 years, or patients with diabetes or chronic kidney disease (CKD). Patients >60 years should have BP <150/90 mm of Hg.

6. Absence of family history of hypertension.
7. History or physical examination (e.g. renal artery stenosis) indicates a secondary cause.

MANAGEMENT OF AN UNCONSCIOUS PATIENT WITH BRADYCARDIA

The common causes of bradycardia encountered in day-to-day practice are:

1. Athletes or during sleep.
2. Myxoedema.
3. Obstructive jaundice
4. Increased intracranial tension.
5. Complete heart block (CHB).
6. Drugs like propranolol, digitalis or verapramil.
7. Sick sinus syndrome.
8. Vasovagal attacks.
9. Hypothermia.

Except the CHB, all are established cause of sinus bradycardia. In CHB, there is generation of idioventricular rhythm at the rate of 36–40/minute (obviously it is not sinus bradycardia). Now, while considering **bradycardia in an unconscious patient**, few of the above causes come in mind, e.g.

1. Complete heart block (Stokes-Adams syndrome).
2. Increased intracranial tension.
3. Sick sinus syndrome.
4. Myxoedema coma.
5. Hepatic coma from obstructive jaundice (rare).
6. Hypothermia (rare).

D/D among these causes are easy and overt.

A. Stokes-Adams Syndrome

1. Stoppage of the precipitating agent, e.g. digitalis, propranolol, etc. if any; a sharp blow over the precordium is often enough to start the cardiac impulse. During the attack, cardiopulmonary resuscitation (CPR) should be done. External cardiac massage as well as mouth to mouth respiration may be initiated. If ventricular fibrillation is detected by ECG, cardioversion defibrillation with DC defibrillator is done. Moist O_2 inhalation at the rate of 4–6 litres/minute is started.
2. Before inserting temporary pacemaker, following drugs can be given:
   a. Inj. isoprenaline sulphate: Direct IV injection of 0.1–0.4 mg of the drug, or 2 mg dissolved in 540 mL of 5% dextrose solution to be infused at the rate of 1–10 μg/min (by drip rate approximately 15 drops/minute) so as to keep the heart rate between 70–80/minute. Afterwards, tablet isoprenaline (20 mg) may be prescribed 1 tab thrice daily to be taken orally, or tablet orciprenaline (10 mg) 1 tab thrice daily to be taken orally.
   b. Inj. sodium bicarbonate: 50 mL of 7.5% $NaHCO_3$ IV is given immediately and may be repeated (to combat acidosis).
   c. Inj. hydrocortisone hemisuccinate: 100 mg IV may be given stat to relieve oedema around the AV node, if any (not advocated by all). The drug may be repeated, if necessary.
   d. Inj adrenaline: 0.2–0.5 mL of 1: 1000 solution of the drug may be given IM, IV or even in intracardiac route (be sure by ECG that the asystole is not due to ventricular fibrillation). Few clinicians try inj. atropine 0.6 mg, IV stat.
   e. It is better to transfer the patient in ICU for further management.
   f. Immediate implantation of permanent pacemaker, if facilities are available.

- **It is the management of complete heart block too.**
- **Sequence of events in Stokes-Adams syndrome:** Vertigo and headache at 3 seconds, fainting at 6 seconds, unconsciousness at 9 seconds, convulsions at 12 seconds, death—if cardiac asystole persists for >2 minutes.
- Sudden loss of consciousness may occur without any warning and often results in a fall. During the attack, pallor is observed and flushing appears after recovery; in prolonged bradycardia, pallor may change over to cyanosis. Stokes-Adams syndrome is manifested by sudden loss of consciousness (or syncope or black-out due to ventricular asystole) unrelated to posture and **may arise from** complete heart block (most common), ventricular tachycardia or fibrillation, Mobitz type II block, profound bradycardia or sinoatrial disease.
- Most of the attacks are very brief and may disappear before the physician arrives. The future plan should be to prevent such attacks.

Clinical Wisdom

W Stokes (1804–1877), Professor of Medicine in Dublin, and R Adams (1791–1875), Professor of Surgery in Dublin.

B. Increased Intracranial Tension

See afterwards.

C. Sick Sinus Syndrome

1. Inj. isoprenaline: Direct IV injection of 0.1–0.4 mg of the drug; or inj. atropine—0.6 mg, IV stat given. In structural disease of the SA node, both the drugs are unlikely to be successful.
2. Permanent pacemaker (demand type) is the answer of the 'bradycardia–tachycardia syndrome'. As associated disease of the AV conduction system is not infrequent, pacing from the ventricles is commonly indicated; pacing of the atrium may prevent episodes of atrial fibrillation.

D. Myxoedema Coma

1. Triiodothyronine: 20 μg IV bolus is followed by 10–25 μg every 8 hourly until there is sustained clinical improvement. If thyroxine (T_4) is available, it is given as IV bolus in a dose of 400–500 μg and may be continued in a dose of 100 μg/day by IV or orally.
2. Hydrocortisone hemisuccinate: 100 mg IV stat and continued every 8 hourly (especially if suspicion of

hypopituitarism). It is followed by tapering doses of oral steroids when consciousness is regained.
3. IV saline and glucose infusion to combat hypotension and hypoglycaemia, respectively.
4. Combat hypothermia with 'slow rewarming' of the patient by wrapping with a blanket in a warm room.
5. High-flow oxygen or assisted ventilation (if necessary).
6. Treatment of arrhythmia and heart failure accordingly. Preferably management should be done in an ICU.
7. Inj. ampicillin 500 mg, IV, 6 hourly, or inj. ceftriaxone 1 g, IV, 12 hourly or any broad-spectrum antibiotic since many a time infection is a common precipitating factor.
8. Blood should be sent for T_3, T_4, TSH, cortisol, Na^+, PaO_2, $PaCO_2$, pH and R/E (TC/DC).
9. Try to correct hypotension, hypothermia, hypoglycaemia, electrolyte imbalance and respiratory failure.

- As injection of T_3 and T_4 are not always available, attending physician is often compelled to give:
  a. Tab triiodothyronine (50 μg/tab): 2 tab stat, then 1 tablet 4 times daily through Ryle's tube until clinical improvement occurs (pulse, BP, temperature are the guidelines), or
  b. Tab levothyroxine (100 μg/tab): 2 tab stat and then 1 tab daily through Ryle's tube to continue until clinical improvement occurs.
- It is a life-threatening emergency with a mortality rate of 20–40%. As T_3 is biologically more active than T_4, most physicians recommend IV T_3 over T_4.

E. Hepatic Coma from Obstructive Jaundice

See before

F. Hypothermia (Temp <95°F)

- Mild 95°F–89.6°F, moderate 89.6°F–82.4°F and severe hypothermia <82.4°F.
- Possible causes of hypothermia are:
  a. Accidental exposure to cold weather (especially in alcoholics, elderly, babies, diabetics, street beggars and in mountain climbers).
  b. Malnutrition, sepsis, peripheral circulatory failure due to any cause.
  c. Myxoedema coma, hypothalamic lesions, hepatic coma, Addisonian crisis, hypoglycaemia, CVA.
  d. Drug-induced, e.g. phenothiazines, ethanol, opiates, lithium, benzodiazepines.
  e. Immersion hypothermia, frost bite.
  f. Artificial hypothermia induced in open heart surgery.

Management

1. Move the person out of the cold environment. Remove wet clothings. Cover the patient with blankets in a warm environment (room). A plastic sack or 'space blanket' may be used (if available), if no shelter is available. 'Gradual warming' is done with an aim to increase core temperature by 1°C/hour. Avoid alcohol; give warm fluids orally. Keep the patient horizontal or slightly head down position.
2. O_2 inhalation (warm): 4–8 litres/min.
3. 5% dextrose drip (IV) or warm isotonic saline is started immediately (in an attempt to maintain the blood volume).
4. Internal rewarming technique: Extracorporeal rewarming by haemodialysis and cardiopulmonary by-pass. Inhaled humidified air or peritoneal lavage (with warm liquid) may be done.
5. Inj. sodium bicarbonate: 50 mL of 7.5% of the solution may be given IV, if pH is <7.2.
6. Erythromycin 250 mg, 4 times daily, is started orally to prevent pneumonia. Treat the underlying condition promptly, e.g. sepsis; correct metabolic abnormalities, if there is any.
7. Blood should be drawn for serum Na^+, K^+, HCO^-_3, PaO_2, $PaCO_2$. ECG (arrhythmia) and a chest X-ray (pneumonia) should be done. Always monitor the vital functions with special reference to arrhythmias. Treat in the line of myxoedema coma, if found to be hypothyroid.
8. Arrhythmias are to be treated in ICU. Bretylium tosylate is the drug of choice in ventricular fibrillation. Ventricular tachycardia/fibrillation, or asystole is the usual cause of death. So long the patient is unresponsive to CPR and rewarmed to 89.6°F (32°C), the patient should not be declared dead.

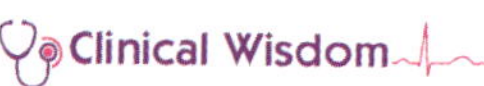

Do not apply direct heat like heating pad, heating lamp or hot water to warm the person.

MANAGEMENT OF A PATIENT OF HYPERPYREXIA (>106.7°F)

The probable causes of hyperpyrexia are:
1. Malaria.
2. Septicaemia.
3. Encephalitis.
4. Pontine haemorrhage.
5. Lobar pneumonia.
6. Heat stroke.
7. Malignant hyperthermia (halothane-induced).
8. Thyroid storm.
9. Neuroleptic malignant syndrome (haloperidol-induced).
10. Rabies.

Malaria will be described in 3 parts, i.e. benign tertian malaria (*P. vivax*), malignant tertian malaria (*P. falciparum*) and cerebral malaria (*P. falciparum*).

A. Benign Tertian Malaria (Uncomplicated Malaria)

Usually caused by *Plasmodium vivax* and rarely by *Plasmodium ovale* or malariae type.
1. Tab chloroquine phosphate (one tablet contains 250 mg of drug, and 150 mg of base): One of the two schedules [between a) and b) below] may be followed:

a. 1st day: 4 tab stat (600 mg base), followed by 2 tablets (300 mg base) after 6 hours, 2nd day onwards: 1 tab (150 mg base) twice daily for 2 more days.
b. 10 mg base/kg stat and followed by 10 mg base/kg at 24 hours and 5 mg base/kg at 48 hours (i.e. 4 tab on the 1st day, 4 tab on the 2nd day and 2 tab on the 3rd day). or

Amodiaquine: 10–12 mg of base/kg daily, orally for 3 days.

- Minimally 3 days treatment should be done.

2. Tab primaquine phosphate: Usually each tablet contains 7.5 mg of base. The recommended dose is 1 tab twice daily for 14 days (radical cure). Transfusion-induced malaria need not receive treatment for radical cure. Tab primaquine is better started after completion of the course of chloroquine (or may be during treatment with chloroquine).
3. Treatment is possible at home. Diet should be adequate with plenty of fluids (glucose-drink is preferred). Use blankets during cold stage and tepid sponging in high rise of temperature. Tab paracetamol (500 mg/tab)1 tab used sos, if the temperature shoots >102°F.

   Dose of chloroquine phosphate in children:
   <5 kg = 1/4th of adult dose
   5–20 kg = 1/2 of the adult dose
   20–40 kg = 3/4th of the adult dose
   > 40 kg = Adult dose

- Before giving primaquine, the patient should be screened for G_6PD deficiency. **In mild G_6PD deficiency**, dose of primaquine will be 45 mg once weekly for 6–8 weeks. Primaquine is absolutely contraindicated in pregnancy and severe G_6PD deficiency.

B. Malignant Tertian Malaria (Uncomplicated *Plasmodium falciparum* Infection)

1. Tab chloroquine phosphate: As used in BT malaria (see no. 1 of previous prescription). If no response occurs within 3 days, probably it is a case of chloroquine-resistant falciparum malaria (chloroquine resistance is being reported from most of the states of India) and start—Tab quinine sulphate (300 mg/tab) in the dose of 2 tab 3 times daily for 7 days. This regimen should be added by:
   a. Combined tablet of sulfadoxine-pyrimethamine (500 mg + 25 mg in a single tablet) to be taken, 3 tablets at a time as single dose therapy, or
   b. Cap tetracycline 250 mg 4 times daily, orally for 7 days or cap doxycycline 200 mg daily orally for 7 days (used in sulphonamide sensitivity), or
   c. Cap clindamycin: 10 mg/kg, BD for 7 days.
2. Alternative to quinine are:
   a. Artesunate (4 mg/kg, daily, orally for 3 days) plus 3 tablets of sulfadoxine-pyrimethamine (500 mg + 25 mg in a single tablet) as a single dose, or
   b. Artesunate (4 mg/kg, daily, for 3 days) plus amodiaquine (10 mg of base/kg, daily for 3 days).
3. Diet and general treatment are same as done in BT malaria. Few clinicians prefer hospital treatment as the patient may be deteriorated at any moment.

- Dose of quinine sulphate in children is 10 mg/kg given three times daily.
- In pregnancy, chloroquine is the safest antimalarial drug; quinine may be used with caution. Tetracycline and doxycycline are contraindicated in pregnancy and children <8 years of age.
- Primaquine phosphate should be given 45 mg 'as a single dose' for gametocidal therapy of *P. falciparum,* after the remission of fever. *P. falciparum* has no persistent exo-erythrocytic cycle; recrudescence occurs due to incomplete elimination of parasite from RBC.
- The terminology of 'malignant' malaria is going to be obsolete nowadays.
- It is important to remember that most of the *P. falciparum*-infected patients are resistant to chloroquine and that is why one may start oral quinine from the very beginning. On the other hand, quinine-resistance is growing slowly and thus most of the internists start treatment with artemisinin.

Clinical Wisdom

The WHO now recommends artemisinin combination regimens as first-line therapy for falciparum malaria in all tropical countries and advocates the use of fixed-dose combinations.

C. Cerebral Malaria (*P. falciparum*-induced encephalopathy) or Severe Falciparum Malaria

It is **a medical emergency** and needs urgent treatment. Cerebral malaria is **defined as** diffuse symmetric encephalopathy in a patient with falciparum malaria which is manifested by diminished consciousness, confusion and convulsions, often progressing to unarousable coma and death, and the encephalopathy is not attributable to any other cause, e.g. metabolic, dyselectrolytaemic or any other inflammation.

The patient may have high fever (may be hyperpyrexic), altered mental status (drowsiness, irritability, unconsciousness), convulsions, pallor and jaundice. On examination, the patient may be obtunded with passive resistance to head flexion (though signs of meningeal irritation are absent), may have splenomegaly, and variable tendon reflex with extensor or flexor plantar response.

1. Due to high prevalence of resistant falciparum infection, artemisinin compounds are now regarded as drug of choice in cerebral malaria.
   a. Artesunate (2.4 mg/kg stat, IV or IM, followed by 2.4 mg/kg at 12 and 24 hours, and then daily for 7 days. If artesunate is unavailable, one of the following (among b, c, d or e) may be used, or
   b. Artemether (3.2 mg/kg stat, IM, and 1.6 mg/kg daily for 2–5 days), or
   c. Arteether (150 mg, IM, once daily for 3 days), or

d. Quinine hydrochloride: 600 mg (2 mL) of the drug is dissolved in 300 mL of 5% or 10% dextrose solution for slow IV infusion (loading dose) to run over a period of 2 hours.

The drug is repeated in the same dose (600 mg) every 8 hours till the patient is conscious.

The loading dose is avoided if the patient has received quinine, quinidine or mefloquine in previous 24 hours. Quinine hydrochloride may be given by IM injection though there is a chance of muscle necrosis. After regaining consciousness (truely, oral medication is started as soon as possible), oral medication is started with tab quinine sulphate (300 mg/tab)–600 mg (2 tab) to be continued 3 times daily for minimally 7 days. Few clinicians advocate IV loading dose of quinine by 20 mg/kg in 500 mL of 5% or 10% dextrose solution to run for 4 hours, and then followed by 600 mg, IV, 8 hourly as described above. It is better to have the cardiac monitoring while the patient is on IV quinine therapy as the drug is myocardial depressant (at least ECG should be done for wide QRS and Q-T prolongation → prolongation of Q-T interval is an indication to discontinue quinine). According to some clinicians, quinine is the treatment of choice in cerebral malaria except in areas with quinine-resistant malaria, or

e. Quinidine (10 mg of base/kg) infused over 1–2 hours, followed by 1.2 mg of base/kg/hour with ECG monitoring.

2. Fluid and electrolyte balance: 5% dextrose drip should run alternating with dextrose-normal saline solution. The volume of fluid should be calculated according to urine output and state of dehydration. Correct metabolic acidosis, if present.
3. Control of cerebral oedema: Inj. mannitol (20%) 100 mL, 8 hourly, IV rapidly over 30 minutes may be tried (not advocated by all). **Dexamethasone (corticosteroid) should not be given.**
4. Control of hypoglycaemia: This is corrected by 5% or 10% dextrose solution (hypoglycaemia results from glucose consumption by malaria parasite and the host, and hyperinsulinaemia as a result of quinine therapy; there is also failure of neoglucogenesis).
5. Control of convulsions: Diazepam is the drug of choice (0.2 mg/kg) and may be repeated every 4 hours. Drip of phenytoin sodium (13–18 mg/kg) at the rate of 50 mg/min, mixed with normal saline solution may be started.
6. Acute pulmonary oedema (acute lung injury): managed by propped-up position, O_2 inhalation, inj. furosemide IV, and stoppage of IV fluid. In moribund patients, intubation and addition of continuous positive airways pressure (CPAP)/ positive end-expiratory pressure (PEEP) are advocated (in life-threatening hypoxia).
7. Plasmapheresis (or PLEX) or exchange transfusion is done in elderly with severe malaria, pregnant woman and >10% parasitaemia.
8. Follow the 'general care of the comatosed patient'.
9. Feeding is continued through Ryle's tube or IV route.
10. Pulse, BP, respiration, temperature, pupil check-up are done hourly. Blood should be sent for sugar, urea, creatinine, Na^+ and K^+, malaria parasite, lactate and arterial blood gas analysis.
11. Follow 'to combat hyperpyrexia' mentioned in heat stroke (see below).
12. Supportive care is given for severe anaemia (blood transfusion), renal failure (haemodialysis is effective in a desperate situation), hypotension, thrombocytopenia, superadded bacterial infection, DIC and hyponatraemia.

- **Artemisinin-based combination therapies (ACT) for malaria:**
  a. Fixed-dose combination tablets available at present: Artemether-lumefantrine, artesunate-amodiaquine, dihydroartemisinin-piperaquine.
  b. Fixed-dose, co-packed, separate tablets: Artesunate-mefloquine, artesunate-sulfadoxine-pyrimethamine.
  c. No combination package available at present: Artesunate + clindamycin, or artesunate + doxycycline. ACT are given in uncomplicated falciparum infection, falciparum infection in pregnancy (in 2nd/3rd trimester) and in infants.
- Toxicity of mefloquine is neuropsychiatric reactions and convulsions, while halofantrine may give rise to cardiac arrhythmias. Corticosteroids are of no value, rather they increase the chance of infection and GI bleeding. Vomiting induced by chloroquine or quinine should be treated by inj. ondansetron (1 mL = 2 mg), 4 mg, IV as and when necessary. Metoclopramide should better be avoided as extrapyramidal syndrome may develop. Treatment of pernicious malaria/ severe falciparum malaria/complicated malignant malaria are similar to treatment of cerebral malaria.
- **Multi-drug resistant (MDR) falciparum malaria is treated by:**
  a. Artemether-lumefantrine (1.5 mg/9 mg)/kg, BD, orally with food for 3 days, or
  b. Artesunate (4 mg/kg), daily, orally for 3 days, plus mefloquine (25 mg of base/kg) as 8 mg/kg, daily, orally for 3 days, or
  c. Dihydroartemisinin-piperaquine (2.5/20 mg/kg), daily, orally for 3 days.

Clinical Wisdom

Parasitaemia is cleared rapidly by **artemisinin derivatives**, e.g. by artesunate, artemether or arterether. Artemisinin (Qinghaosu) is the active component of a herbal medicine, which is being used in China for over 2000 years.

D. Heat Stroke

Heat stroke is manifested by hyperpyrexia along with systemic inflammatory response.

1. Remove clothings. Take the patient to ITU, or in a cool and well-ventilated room (air-conditioned room).
2. Perform vigorous massaging of the body (chiefly the neck and torso) and allow the patient to bath repeatedly in tepid water. For rapid cooling immerse

the patient in ice water, or arrange fanning (to increase convection heat loss), or start gastric lavage with iced saline. The goal is to reduce the core temperature to 102.2°F within 30–60 minutes.
3. Application of ice over the lateral aspect of the trunk.
4. 5% dextrose-saline IV drip (i.e. cold crystalloid IV replacement) should be started immediately and to continue by the guidance of dehydration and central venous pressure.
5. Follow the 'general care of the comatosed patient'.
6. Repeated checking of the rectal temperature (by thermocouple), pulse, BP, respiration and other vital signs. Send the blood sample for estimation of urea, creatinine, sugar, Na^+, K^+, BT and CT, INR, aPTT, platelet count (coagulation profile), Ca^{++}, CK, AST and ALT. Record ECG.
7. **To combat hyperpyrexia (i.e. >106.7°F or >41.5°C):**
   a. Ice water enema. Antipyretics are ineffective as the hypothalamic set point remains normal.
   b. Ice-cap application over forehead.
   c. O_2 at a flow rate of 6–8 litres/min.
   d. Lytic cocktail: Pethidine 100 mg, promethazine 50 mg and chlorpromazine 50 mg in IM route.
   e. Inj. analgin 0.5 g, IM stat and may be repeated, if necessary.
   f. Convulsions (or shivering): Inj. diazepam 10 mg, IV stat and may be repeated, if necessary.
   g. Acidosis: Inj. $NaHCO_3$, 50 mL of 7.5% of the drug may be given IV.

FEVER, UNCONSCIOUSNESS AND NECK STIFFNESS

The probable possibilities strike in mind are:
1. Meningitis of any aetiology (pyogenic, tuberculous, viral or fungal) (Table 5.3).
2. Cerebral malaria.
3. Meningoencephalitis.
4. Typhoid meningism.
5. Subarachnoid haemorrhage (with some cause of pyrexia).

- Other less common causes are Weil's disease, cerebellar tonsillar herniation at foramen magnum and rarely in intracerebral haemorrhage.

A. Pyogenic Meningitis (Meningococcal) (Table 5.4)

1. Immediate hospitalisation, preferably in isolation ward. Recording of vital signs with ophthalmoscopic examination is done. If papilloedema is absent, lumbar puncture is performed and the CSF sample is sent for cell count and type, biochemical, bacteriological and serological examinations.
2. Follow the 'general care of the comatosed patient'.
3. Start normal saline drip; inj benzyl penicillin is started as follows:

   4 megaunits (million unit) of the drug is infused IV every 4 hourly (after proper skin test)

   or

   Inj. cefotaxime 1–2 g, IV, 4–6 hourly according to severity (maximally 12 g of the drug can be given daily) or inj. ceftriaxone 2 g, IV, 12 hourly may be started. The drug should be continued minimally for 10 days.

- Inj. cefotaxime/inj. ceftriaxone **plus** vancomycin (2 g/day, 12 hourly, IV) may be started as empirical therapy in community-acquired suspected bacterial meningitis.

4. Daily monitoring of pulse, BP, respiration, temperature, sensorium, neck rigidity and plantar response should be done. Blood should be sent for TC, DC, electrolytes, urea, creatinine and sugar estimation. CT or MRI scan of brain may be performed, if facilities are there.
5. Management of complications:
   a. High fever: Tepid sponging with 1 tablet of paracetamol (500 mg) through Ryle's tube. Inj. paracetamol (150 mg/mL) is now available.
   b. Convulsions: Inj. diazepam 10 mg, slow IV or inj. phenytoin sodium 5 mg/kg/hour in IV route.
   c. Headache: Paracetamol (500 mg/tab) 1 tab to be given, as and when necessary.
   d. Cerebral oedema: Usually 100 mL of inj. mannitol (20%) is given IV, 8 hourly.
   e. Hypotension and shock (adrenal crisis): Inj. hydrocortisone hemisuccinate 100 mg, IV, 8 hourly till hypotension persists.
   f. Respiratory failure: Needs assisted ventilation.
   g. If hydrocephalus develops as a sequelae, consult neurosurgeon for ventriculo-atrial shunt.

Clinical Wisdom

Palpate for splenomegaly (malaria/typhoid). Plantar response may be extensor in meningoencepalitis and cerebral malaria (even in semicoma stage).

Table 5.3: Clinical clues in different types of meningitis

Possible agent	Clinical clue
Meningococcus	Petechial rashes
Pneumococcus	Skull fracture, otitis media, splenectomy
HIV	Immunocompromised patients
Leptospira (Weil's disease)	Works in drains, polluted water, or recreational swimming
Enterovirus infection	Pleuritic chest pain or rash
Malaria	Travel to tropical countries

Table 5.4: Chemotherapy of bacterial meningitis

Organism	Drugs	Dose	Alternative drugs	Duration
Meningococcus	Benzyl penicillin	See the above prescription	Chloramphenicol, ceftriaxone, cefotaxime	10 days
Pneumococcus	Cefotaxime	See the above prescription	Ceftriaxone, chloramphenicol	10–14 days
H. influenzae	Chloramphenicol	1 g, IV, 6–8 hrly	Cefotaxime	7–10 days
L. monocytogenes	Ampicillin + Gentamicin	1–2 g, IV, 4 hrly + 80 mg, IV, 8 hrly	Rifampicin, co-trimoxazole	3–4 weeks
S. aureus	Oxacillin	12–18 g, IV in divided doses	Nafcillin, vancomycin	10 days
Pseudomonas	Ceftazidime	1–2 g, IV, 6–8 hrly	Cefoperazone, gentamicin	21 days
Unknown cause	Benzyl penicillin or cefotaxime or ceftriaxone	See the prescription above	Chloramphenicol + gentamicin	10 days

Clinical Wisdom

Nowadays, third-generation cephalosporins are drug of choice in all infections resulting in bacterial meningitis.

Dose in children:

a. Crystalline (or benzyl) penicillin: 300000 units/kg/day in IV route.
b. Cefotaxime: 200 mg/kg/day in IV route.

- Treatment of pyogenic meningitis should be started very promptly. Final drug of choice will be dictated by the culture-sensitivity report of CSF.
- Drugs acting against *Pseudomonas aeruginosa* are: Penicillin, ciprofloxacin, aminoglycosides (gentamicin, amikacin, tobramycin), carbenicillin, third generation (cefoperazone and ceftazidime)/fourth generation (cefepime) and fifth generation cephalosporins (ceftobiprole), tricarcillin, piperacillin-tazobactam, aztreonam, azlocillin, mezlocillin, colistin (in MDR pseudomonas infection), imipenem and meropenem.
- As per available evidence, adjunctive dexamethasone therapy (10 mg, IV, 6 hourly for 4 days) may have some benefit in meningitis caused by *H. influenzae* and *S. pneumoniae* in reducing sensorineural deafness and death (avoid in septic shock).

B. Tuberculous Meningitis

1. Follow No. 1, 2 and 4 of previous prescription (pyogenic meningitis).
2. In an unconscious patient, all the drugs should be given through Ryle's tube.
   a. Cap rifampicin: 450 mg/day if <50 kg and aged; 600 mg/day if >50 kg.
   b. Tab INH:
      5 mg/kg/day (adult).
      10 mg/kg/day (children).
   c. Tab pyrazinamide: 20–35 mg/kg/day (maximally 2.5 g).
   d. Inj. streptomycin: 1 g/day, IM if >45 kg; and 0.75 g/day, IM if <45 kg.
   e. Tab prednisolone (5 mg/tab): Initiated by 8 tablets daily for 6 weeks and then tapered off by 5 mg/week, and ultimately stopped at 3 month. Corticosteroids seem to improve mortality.

- a + b + c + d for 2 months (initial phase), and a + b for 7–10 months more (continuation phase) according to discretion of the physician. Treatment is usually continued for 1 year. The drugs a, b, c and d enter CSF readily in the presence of meningeal inflammation.

   f. Tab pyridoxine (40 mg/tab): 1/4 of a tablet to be continued along with INH.
3. Management of complications:
   a. Convulsions (as done in pyogenic meningitis).
   b. High fever and headache (as done in pyogenic meningitis).
   c. Cerebral oedema (as done in pyogenic meningitis).
   d. Vomiting: Inj. metoclopramide 10 mg, IM, as and when necessary.
   e. Cranial nerve palsy: Reduce the 'raised intracranial tension'.
   f. If hydrocephalus develops as a sequelae, consult neurosurgeon (not uncommon) for ventriculo-atrial shunt.

C. Viral Meningitis

1. *Specific treatment:*
   a. HSV_1 and HSV_2: Acyclovir 10 mg/kg, 8 hourly in IV infusion with normal saline (infused over 1 hour) is started immediately and continued for 2–3 weeks; may be followed by oral acyclovir (800 mg, 5 times daily). Instead famcyclovir (500 mg, tds) or valacyclovir (1000 mg, tds) may be given for 2–3 weeks.
   b. Influenza: Tamiflu, rapivap, amantadine and rimantadine may be used.
   c. HIV: Zidovudine 200 mg, 6 times daily in IV infusion with normal saline/orally through Ryle's tube. Actually, the patient should receive highly active anti-retroviral therapy.
2. *General and symptomatic treatment:* As done in pyogenic and tuberculous meningitis. Anticonvulsants treatment for convulsions and dexamethasone for raised intracranial tension are often necessary.

- SIADH may develop in the course of the disease of meningitis (any type). So physician should be careful for the development of hyponatraemia (water restriction and hypertonic saline are the mainstay of treatment of SIADH).

D. Cerebral Malaria

Though passive resistance to head flexion is present (not true neck rigidity), signs of meningeal irritation are absent here.

See before for management.

E. Meningoencephalitis

Along with the signs of meningitis one may get altered level of consciousness, high fever, altered mental state, H/o seizures (focal or generalised), focal or diffuse neurological signs (cranial nerve palsy, aphasia, hemiplegia, Babinski's sign) and involuntary movements (myoclonic jerks).

For management, follow the regimens given in the management of viral meningitis (see above). IV ribavirin (15–25 mg/kg/day) in divided doses given 8 hourly, has been reported to be of benefit in isolated cases of meningoencephalitis.

F. Typhoid Meningism

1. *Specific treatment:*
   a. Inj. chloramphenicol: 50 mg/kg/day in IV route (in shot push within the plastic tube of the dextrose-normal saline drip) in 4 divided doses for 3–7 days. Then cap chloramphenicol (250 mg/cap) 2 cap, 6 hourly is continued for another 7–11 days, or
   b. Inj. ciprofloxacin: 200 mg (200 mg/100 mL) IV, 12 hourly for 3–7 days and then followed by oral ciprofloxacin tablet (750 mg/tab) as 1 tab twice daily for another 7–11 days, or
   c. Inj. ceftriaxone 2 g, IV, 12 hourly may be used for 10–14 days (probably, the drug of choice),

   +

   Inj. hydrocortisone hemisuccinate 100 mg, 8 hourly along with the IV infusion (charged in the bottle) till the patient regains consciousness.
2. Follow the 'general care' of the comatosed patient.

- IV ciprofloxacin 200 mg BD for at least 10 days is a good alternative in MDR typhoid fever.

G. Subarachnoid Haemorrhage

See afterwards.

RAISED INTRACRANIAL TENSION

Treatment of increased intracranial tension (IIT) should be started immediately in patients with cerebral haemorrhage or massive infarction (i.e. CVA), producing midline shift:

1. Propped-up position at 30° (improves jugular venous outflow without impairing cerebral perfusion).
2. Mannitol [reduces cerebral oedema/raised ICT (intracranial tension) by osmotic diuresis, known as 'osmotherapy']: 100 mL (1–2 g/kg) mannitol (20%) IV thrice daily. It is better to start 300 mL, IV rapidly as a bolus dose and then 100 mL, IV, TDS to be continued for 2–3 days. Prolonged use may develop into water loss and hypernatraemia. Many a time, rebound cerebral oedema may pose a problem following cessation of the drip.
3. Inj. furosemide: 40 mg, IV stat, as and when necessary.
4. Oral glycerol: 1–2 g/kg/day in 3 divided doses. Usually it corresponds to 6 tsf three times daily (given with fruit juice). IV glycerol may be given in a dose of 1.5 g/kg as a bolus followed by 50 g in 500 mL of normal saline every 4 hourly (may produce haemoglobinuria). Glycerol is not a very good drug for reduction of ICT.
5. Inj. dexamethasone: 4–6 mg, IM or IV, 4–6 hourly. It may aggravate hypertension and diabetes, if there is any. **Corticosteroid is contraindicated in cytotoxic oedema, head injury and CVA** but reduces vasogenic reactive oedema surrounding a tumour, an abscess, chronic subdural haematoma or brain metastases.
6. Retention enema of magnesium sulphate (not used nowadays). IV $MgSO_4$ reduces the ICT in pre-eclampsia.
7. Hyperventilation → lowering $PaCO_2$ around 25–30 mm of Hg decreases cerebral blood flow by cerebral vasoconstriction → reduction of intracranial blood volume → reduces intracranial tension.
8. Treat hypoxia, hypothermia. High-dose barbiturate therapy is adviced for 'refractory' ICT; barbiturate therapy and hypothermia reduce cerebral metabolism.

- This is the management of **cerebral oedema** too; drugs are used singly or in combination. Cerebral oedema is of three types:
  a. Vasogenic, e.g. tumour, abscess, CVA, purulent meningitis.
  b. Cytotoxic, e.g. hypoxia, Na^+ depletion in SIADH, dialysis disequilibrium syndrome.
  c. Interstitial, e.g. increase water content of brain in hydrocephalus.
- Acetazolamide and/or repeated lumbar puncture may help to lower ICT in idiopathic intracranial hypertension (benign intracranial hypertension or 'pseudotumour cerebri').
- **Surgical management** is done by treating underlying cause, ventriculo-atrial or ventriculo-peritoneal shunt in hydrocephalus, removal of space-occupying lesion or surgical decompression by decompressive craniotomy or limited lobectomies in selected cases.

CEREBROVASCULAR ACCIDENTS (CVA)

A. Cerebral Thrombosis

1. Urgent hospitalisation. Complete bed rest. Draw blood for Hb, TC, DC, sugar, urea, creatinine, Na^+, K^+ and lipid profile (total cholesterol, LDL, HDL, VLDL and triglyceride). Place the patient in a railed cot. Introduce Ryle's tube and Foley's catheter. About 2000 calories should be provided daily. Start with liquid diet (in conscious patient) and gradually change over to normal diet, as the patient recovers.

2. Follow the 'general care of the comatosed patient'.
3. Treat 'raised intracranial tension' (*see* before).
4. Antiplatelet drugs are advised: Aspirin (75–300 mg/day, orally), dipyridamole (50 mg, 8 hourly, orally daily) or ticlopidine (250 mg, 12 hourly, orally daily) for long-term prophylaxis. Tab pentoxifylline (400 mg, 8 hourly), the haemorheology modifier may be used for few weeks. Clopidogrel (75 mg)—1 tablet, orally daily is an alternative to aspirin, or may be combined with aspirin.
5. Reduce hypertension by amlodipine (5 mg/tab): 1–2 tab, once daily, orally. Diuretics or ACE inhibitors may be used. BP should be kept at or just below 185/110 mm of Hg.
6. Control of other comorbid conditions like diabetes mellitus, hyperlipidaemia, CAD, smoking, obesity. Oral contraceptives should be discontinued.
7. Arrangement should be made to perform an early CT scan of the brain.

B. Cerebral Embolism

1. Follow No. 1, 2 and 3 of previous prescription (cerebral thrombosis).
2. Specific treatment:
   a. Inj heparin sulphate: 5000 units, IV infusion, 6–12 hourly for 5 days along with,
   b. Tab warfarin sodium (5 mg/tab): Usually started from the second day as 2 tab daily for 2 days and then 1 tab daily to be continued for 6 months. Inj. heparin sulphate should be withdrawn after 5 days and let warfarin to be continued alone.
3. Treatment of the underlying cardiac disorder (e.g. tablet digoxin in atrial fibrillation).

- Early CT scan should rule out cerebral haemorrhage before giving inj. heparin or thrombolytic therapy. Heparin and warfarin are especially indicated in an 'evolving stroke' when the patient have atrial fibrillation, paroxysmal arrhythmia or cardiac valve lesions. Anticoagulants have no role in completed stroke.
- *In cerebral infarction (cerebral thrombosis or embolism), maintain the BP at or just below 185/110 mm of Hg.* **Reduction of BP should be gradual and should be tried when the acute stage is over.**
- In acute ischaemic strokes, thrombolysis by IV alteplase (r-TPA or recombinant tissue plasminogen activator) is done in few sophisticated centres within first 3 hours of onset. Total dose is 0.9 mg/kg (maximum 90 mg). Thrombolysis reduces the infarct size.

C. Cerebral Haemorrhage

1. Follow No. 1, 2 and 3 from the prescription of cerebral thrombosis. Treatment should be maintained on a stroke unit or neuroscience intensive care unit.
2. Inj sodium nitroprusside (for reduction of blood pressure): 50 mg dissolved in 500 mL of 5% dextrose (100 μg/mL) and infused in the dose of 20 μg/min. Usually the IV infusion dose is 0.25–8.0 μg/kg/min. Protect the bottle from light (to prevent the production of toxic thiocyanates). Many neurologists do not agree to administer sodium nitroprusside. *Maintain the blood pressure just below 160/100 mm of Hg* or mean arterial pressure 130 mm of Hg to preserve the cerebral autoregulatory mechanism.
3. If CT scan shows >3 cm haematoma or the patient progressively deteriorates, consult neurosurgeon for surgical drainage of the haematoma (evacuation of deep cerebral haematoma is rarely beneficial rather surgical consultation is indicated for cerebellar haematoma).

- Cerebral haemorrhage is commonly due to systemic hypertension (commonest), ruptured aneurysm, vascular malformations, blood dyscrasias and vasculitis (SLE and other collagen vascular diseases).
- Early CT scan is advisable in all of the above cases. Physiotherapy should be started in (A), (B) and (C) as soon as the patient recovers from the neural shock stage. Subsequently speech therapy, dysphagia care, lifestyle modification (e.g. smoking cessation) and occupational therapy are looked for.
- *Aspirin and clopidogrel are absolutely contraindicated in cerebral haemorrhage and very big cerebral infarction.* Take care of bladder, bowel, pulmonary infection and bed sores.
- In cerebral ischaemia try to avoid hypoxia, dehydration, corticosteroid and 5% dextrose infusion.

D. Subarachnoid Haemorrhage

1. Follow No. 1, 2 and 3 from the prescription of cerebral thrombosis. Immediate bed rest and supportive measures are mainstay of treatment.
2. Nimodipine tablets (30 mg/tab) should be crushed and introduced through Ryle's tube. Recommended dose is 2 tab 4 hourly to be started within 3–4 days of subarachnoid haemorrhage and usually continued for 3 weeks, or
   Epsilon amino-caproic acid (EACA): The drug was previously used. The usual dose is 24–48 g/day by IV infusion in 5% dextrose-saline infused over 24 hours with the help of a micro-drip apparatus. EACA is a fibrinolytic inhibitor.
3. Hypertension is controlled by diuretics, ACE inhibitors (if mean arterial pressure is >130 mm of Hg).
4. MR angiography should be performed in patients potentially fit for surgery (<65 years) and neurosurgeon may be called for surgical treatment (clipping of the neck of aneurysm, coiling or embolisation).
5. Avoid hypotension, hypovolaemia, hyperglycaemia, hyponatraemia and hyperpyrexia to prevent delayed cerebral ischaemia.

- Nimodipine (calcium-channel blocker) prevents vasospasm and EACA prevents rebleeding.
- According to few clinicians, anticonvulsants (phenytoin sodium) are used for prophylaxis, and inj. dexamethasone for reduction of cerebral oedema as well as for stabilization of blood-brain barrier.

E. Hypertensive Encephalopathy

1. Follow No. 1, 2 and 3 from the prescription of cerebral thrombosis.
2. The initial aim is to lower the diastolic pressure to about 100–105 mm of Hg. Aggressive hypotensive therapy may reduce the BP below autoregulatory range, which may lead to ischaemic events.
3. Sodium nitroprusside or diazoxide is the drug of choice (see the doses from the section on 'Drug therapy in hypertensive emergencies'). Hydralazine, nicardipine or labetalol may be used.
4. Inj. diazepam 10 mg, IV slowly is used for convulsions and may be repeated, if necessary.

Clinical Wisdom

In CVA, rapid reduction of BP hampers autoregulation and thereby enhances neurodeficit.

CONVULSIONS AND OTHERS

A. Febrile Convulsions

1. Place the patient in prone or lateral position. Prevent aspiration and guard against tongue bite by a rubber oropharyngeal tube. Start tepid sponging to bring down the raised temperature.
2. Syrup paracetamol (125 mg/mL): 1/2 to 2 mL orally, according to body weight.
3. Diazepam: Inj. diazepam (0.2–0.5 mg/kg/dose in shot push IV; maximum of 5 mg/dose) or solution of diazepam may be given per rectally in a dose of 0.2–0.4 mg/kg, or phenobarbitone (60 mg/tab)—1/2 to 1 tab stat.
4. Antibiotics may be prescribed, if indicated.

- The age limit of febrile convulsions is 6 months to 5 years. Few pediatricians continue phenobarbitone (30 mg at bedtime) till 5 years of age in a patient of febrile convulsions. An EEG should be done afterwards. Remember, epilepsy may develop in less than 3% of all children with febrile convulsions.

B. Status Epilepticus

When convulsions (seizures) and unconsciousness recur wihout any intervening normal period in-between, it is known as status epilepticus. Actually, it is the occurrence of prolonged serial seizures (two or more) without the patient regaining consciousness between the attacks over a period of 15–30 minutes (recent definition). Practically, it is a serious condition where the duration of seizure, which is more than 5 minutes, and demands prompt use of anticonvulsants. **It is a life-threatening medical emergency** (cardio-respiratory embarrassment, metabolic derangement, hyperpyrexia) and an ITU is essential for optimal management.

1. Railed cot, mouth gag to prevent tongue bite. Avoid head-pillow. Place in any lateral position with foot end raised (to prevent aspiration pneumonia) and head turned sideways. Protect the patient from injury. Try to listen the history of past illness from patient's relatives.
2. Maintain the airway by repeated suction of mouth, nose and throat. Insert one rubber oropharyngeal tube through mouth. Administer O_2, if necessary.
3. Do not try to draw blood samples during convulsions. Blood samples can be taken (sugar, urea, creatinine, glucose, calcium, electrolytes, LFT and for toxicology) afterwards when the patient becomes totally sedated. Take care of pulse, BP, monitor ECG, acidosis, and intubation and ventilation (in an ITU setting).
4. Anticonvulsants:
   a. Start IV lorazepam (0.1 mg/kg, i.e. 3–6 mg) at the rate of 2 mg/min; may be repeated after 5 minutes, or
   IV diazepam (0.2 mg/kg, i.e. 10 mg) at the rate of 5 mg/min: The short duration of action of lorazepam or diazepam needs concomitant administration of maintenance anticonvulsants, i.e. immediately after the first lorazepam/diazepam dose, start IV phenytoin drip (always in normal saline; phenytoin precipitates in 5% dextrose solution; fosphenytoin has no such problem which is a pro-drug of phenytoin where the risk of hypotension is less in comparison to phenytoin, and 1.5 mg fosphenytoin = 1 mg phenytoin), 15 mg/kg to run at the rate of 50 mg/min. Pediatric dose of the drug is 5 mg/kg to run at the rate of 25 mg/min. Monitoring of BP and ECG (to detect hypotension and heart block) should be done (EEG, if possible) during infusion of phenytoin. Fosphenytoin 15 mg/kg, IV given in normal saline to run at 50–100 mg/min.
   b. Consider sodium valproate, IV, 25 mg/kg if seizures continue in spite of inj. phenytoin, or who was taking valproate for the treatment of epilepsy.
   c. Inj. chlormethiazole 0.5–1.2 g/hour, IV by infusion may be tried in diazepam-failure patients.
   d. Thiopentone sodium 100–250 mg, IV slowly may be started and followed by 90–120 mg/hour infusion or phenobarbitone is started 10 mg/kg, IV at a rate of 60 mg/min. These drugs need assisted ventilation.
   e. Lastly, IV anaesthesia with propofol (2 mg/kg loading dose followed by 30–250 µg/kg/min infusion) or midazolam (0.2 mg/kg loading dose followed by 0.75–100 µg/kg maintenance dose as infusion) may be considered.
5. Moist O_2 inhalation to be continued at the rate of 4–6 litres/min.
6. Maintenance drip by normal saline (to act as a route of emergency).
7. 50 mL of 50% inj. glucose, IV often aborts an attack as hypoglycaemia may be an aggravating factor.
8. Discharge the patient from the hospital with tab phenytoin (100 mg/tab): 1 tab three times daily, orally, regularly till further instruction; follow-up at regular interval.

9. Treatment of acidosis (50 mL of 7.5% sodium bicarbonate) and hyperpyrexia (see before) are done accordingly as these may complicate the course of status epilepticus.

- EEG (mandatory), and CT or MRI scan should be done as soon as the acute stage is over.
- A continuous infusion of diazepam (2–4 mg/hr) is often beneficial over phenytoin drip in some patients.
- Lorazepam and diazepam may produce respiratory depression and hypotension.

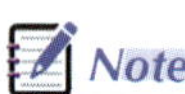

Read different drugs for epilepsy form the section on 'Drugs'.

ACUTE ATTACK OF MIGRAINE

Migraine is a hemicranial, throbbing, periodic, intensely debilitating headache, commonly in women, which may be associated with nausea and vomiting, and is precipitated by some triggering factors (see below). The management goes in the line of:

1. Rest. Reassurance.
2. Avoid stress and triggering factors. Chocolate, cheese, alcohol should be prohibited. Avoid oral contraceptive pills. Oral fluid intake is encouraged. Regulated lifestyle is helpful.
3. Tab ergotamine tartarate (1 mg/tab): 1 tab to be taken orally and may be repeated at 1/2 hour interval, not exceding 3 mg/day (should be taken *in the aura stage* to abort the attack), or

   Tab sumatriptan (25/50/100 mg per tablet): 50–100 mg, orally to be taken *soon after the onset of headache,* and may be repeated, not exceeding 300 mg/day, or inj. sumatriptan (6 mg/0.5 mL) 6 mg, SC, not more than 2 injections in 24 hours may be given (highest efficacy with rapid response). Sumatriptan is a 5-$HT_{1B/1D}$ receptor agonist. Zolmitriptan, almotriptan, eletriptan, frovatriptan, rizatriptan or naratriptan may be used instead by SC route for prompt relief of headache. 'Triptans' may be effective where analgesics do not work.
4. *Prevention for future attacks* (any one or combination):
   a. Flunarizine (5/10 mg per tablet): 10 mg daily, orally in single or divided doses to continue till further advice.
   b. Tab propranolol (40 mg/tab): 1–2 tab, orally three times daily to continue till further advice. Start initially as 1/2 tab twice daily and then increase the dose gradually. Slow release propranolol (80–160 mg) often works better.
   c. Tab amitriptyline (25/50/75 mg per tablet): 25–100 mg, orally at bed time to continue till further advice.
   d. Tab sodium valproate: 500–1500 mg, orally in 2 divided doses.
   e. Pizotifen: 0.5–1.5 mg daily at bed time.
   f. Methysergide: 1–2 mg, thrice daily in resistant cases.
   g. SSRI (selective serotonin reuptake inhibitor) or SNRI (serotinin-noradrenaline reuptake inhibitor), verapramil or topiramate (100–200 mg, daily, orally) may be used.
   h. Gabapentin: 900–3600 mg/day, orally may be used.

- Ergotamine is strictly contraindicated in pregnancy, peripheral vascular disease (e.g. Raynaud's phenomenon) and IHD. Sumatriptan is contraindicated in IHD, severe uncontrolled hypertension and with previous H/o myocardial infarction.
- *Acute attack may also be treated by* aspirin (325–625 mg), ibuprofen (400–800 mg), naproxen (375–750 mg) or paracetamol (500 mg), orally. Prochlorperazine (12.5 mg) IM, metoclopramide (10–20 mg) IV, or domperidone 2 mg IV may be used as antiemetic. Avoid use of opiates.
- **'Triggering factors'** ('anything under the sun including the sun' may be the precipitating factor though it differs from person to person) for migraine are: stress, loud noise and irritating lights, premenstrual tension, lack of sleep/meals and variations in daily routine, strong perfumes, caffeine, tobacco, alcohol, chocolate, cheeze, food additives, e.g. monosodium glutamate, oral contraceptive pills and a time of relaxation (weekend migraine).

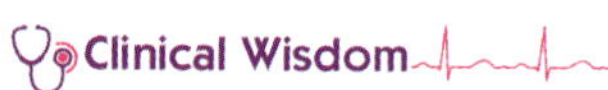

Valproate and **topiramate** are most effective drugs for prophylaxis. Nasal formulations of ergotamine, zolmitriptan, sumatriptan and butorphanol (an opioid) are available for acute migrane. Botulinum toxin (31 small SC injections over scalp, above the ears, temples, and into the neck, and to be repeated every 3 months) is a new entrant for treatment of chronic migraine.

A BOY OF 14 YEARS WITH TWO DAYS H/O PUFFY FACE AND OLIGURIA WHO SUDDENLY BECOMES DYSPNOEIC

Most probably the boy is suffering from acute left ventricular failure (LVF) developing from **acute glomerulonephritis or AGN** (other acute complications of AGN are hypertensive encephalopathy and acute renal failure). At first, urgent treatment of LVF is done, which is followed by treatment of acute poststreptococcal glomerulonephritis.

Management

1. Treatment of acute LVF—See before (page 143).
2. Treatment of AGN:
   a. Complete bed rest until the signs of glomerular inflammation (i.e. proteinuria, RBC in urine) and circulatory congestion (i.e. oedema, hypertension) subside.
   b. Mild protein restriction in azotaemic patients. Salt-free foods are given. The fluid intake is restricted to previous days output plus 500 mL of fluid. Check blood urea, creatinine and electrolytes regularly.
   c. Maintenance of intake-output chart; regular checking of BP and other vital signs.

d. Tab furosemide (40 mg/tablet): 1 tab daily; the dose may be increased according to necessity (to relieve oedema and hypertension).

e. Tab nifedipine (5 mg/tab): 1 tab 8–12 hourly according to the height of BP. Other calcium-channel blockers (e.g. amlodipine), hydralazine or diazoxide may be of help.

f. Inj. crystalline penicillin: 5 lakh, IM twice daily for 7–10 days (after proper skin test) to eradicate residual streptococcal infection. Erythromycin (250 mg, QDS, orally) may also be given instead.

g. Dialysis, if ARF or fluid overload develops.

h. Tonsillectomy may be done after recovery.

- The prognosis of AGN in children is usually good. A small number of adults (who suffered from AGN) may develop hypertension and renal impairment later in life.

MANAGEMENT OF ACUTE PYELONEPHRITIS (UTI)

The treatment of urinary tract infection (UTI) is as follows:

1. Co-trimoxazole (trimethoprim + sulphamethoxazole = 80 mg + 400 mg/tab)—2 tab twice daily orally for 14 days, or cap ampicillin or amoxicillin (500 mg/cap)—1 cap 8 hourly, orally for 10 days, or cap cefuroxime (250 mg/cap)—1 cap 12 hourly for 10 days, or tab norfloxacin (400 mg/tab) or tab ciprofloxacin (500 mg tab)—1 tab 12 hourly for 10 days, or nitrofurantoin 100 mg 12 hourly for 10 days. In severe infection (high fever, loin pain and tenderness), aminoglycosides, e.g. inj. gentamicin IM/IV 3–5 mg/kg/day is given in 3 divided doses for 7–10 days, or inj. amikacin IM/IV 15 mg/kg/day is administered in 2 divided doses for 7–10 days. In severe cases, switching to a further 7 days' oral antibiotic therapy (after receiving aminoglycosides) is done with improvement of symptoms.
2. Rest in bed. Normal diet. Plenty of fluid (at least two litres/day) to be taken by mouth to initiate water diuresis.
3. Ideally, urine sample should be sent for culture-sensitivity test and colony count, before initiating treatment. As soon as the result of sensitivity test is available, treatment is started (or changed, if already started) according to maximum sensitivity. Severe cases may require intravenous therapy. After recovery, often monthly culture of urine is advised.
4. Females, especially postmenopausal women comonly suffer from UTI. Factors predisposing to infection, e.g. obstruction (stasis), neurogenic urinary bladder, calculus, catheterisation, diabetes mellitus or immunosuppression, etc. should be properly identified and treated, if possible. Regular complete bladder emptying, maintenance of adequate perineal hygiene and application of 0.5% cetrimide cream peri-urethrally before intercourse often reduce the incidence of UTI in females.
5. If blood urea and creatinine values rise, modification of dose of antibiotics is necessary.
6. In dysuria:
   a. Tab flavoxate (200 mg tab)—1 tab 8 hourly for 10 days, or
   b. Tab phenazopyridine (200 mg/tab)—1 tab 8 hourly for 10 day (produces red urine).
7. To prevent recurrent infection, suppressive antibiotic therapy by single nightly oral dose of trimethoprim 100 mg, ampicillin/amoxicillin 250 mg, cephalexin 250 mg or nitrofurantoin 100 mg may be continued for few weeks (up to 6–12 months in recurrence). Cranberry juice is said to reduce recurrence of UTI.

- Renal parameters should be normal (i.e. normal urea and creatinine) in patients who are advised aminoglycosides. Patients presenting for the first time should be advised to do USG examination of abdomen to exclude any obstructive lesion.

INTRACTABLE HICCOUGH

Hiccough in an abrupt, involuntary, synchronous contraction of the diaphragm and the inspiratory intercostal muscles, followed by immediate closure of the glottis. The glottic closure is responsible for the production of characteristic inspiratory sound and associated discomfort. The synonyms of hiccough are hiccup or singultus. Hiccough is sometimes considered as myoclonus of the diaphragm.

Management

Recurrent hiccough is very distressing and difficult to manage.

1. *Reassurance:* The patient as well as the relatives should be reassured.
2. *Simple household remedies:* Divert patient's attention (e.g. by conversation, sudden slapping), intake of ice-cold water, breath holding, Valsalva manoeuvre, lifting uvula with cold spoon, breathing in and out in a paper or plastic bag for 5 minutes, induction of vomiting by stimulation of the pharynx, spraying of ethyl chloride under the costal margins, swallowing rapidly one teaspoon of 'dry' granulated sugar, drinking water without taking any breath, coughing, sneezing (nasopharyngeal stimulation often aborts hiccough of postoperative origin).
3. *Local measures:* Intake of local anaesthetic viscus, e.g. lignocaine (15 mL, tds, orally), nasogastric suction followed by ice-cold stomach wash or alkaline stomach wash through a Ryle's tube.
4. *Antacids/H_2-receptor blocker/proton-pump inhibitor (PPI):* Any liquid antacid (preferably containing local anaesthetic oxetacaine) is given 2–4 tsf, 6–8 hourly daily, orally, or ranitidine 150 mg BDAC or omeprazole 20 mg ODAC, orally. It is often advised to take the tablets with little water, and thus irritation of the pharynx may terminate a bout of hiccough.

5. *Drugs:* Chlorpromazine (probably best tried first, as an intravenous bolus; 25 mg, orally, tds or 25 mg IV bolus stat), metoclopramide (10 mg, IM, tds), baclofen (10 mg, orally, tds), haloperidol (5 mg, IM stat or 0.25 mg orally, tds), clonazepam (2 mg, orally, tds) amitriptyline, amantadine, quinidine (200 mg, orally, qds), ondansetron (4 mg, IV, tds), anticonvulsants like phenytoin sodium, carbamazepine, valproic acid are worth trying in resistant cases. Gabapentin is useful in patients with CNS lesions. **Baclofen (beta agonist) is a very effective drug** in the treatment of intractable hiccough.
6. *Surgery:* In stubborn cases, phrenic nerve block by bupivacaine, or nerve section is done surgically.
7. Treatment of the underlying cause.

Common causes of hiccough in clinical practice are:
1. Overdistention of stomach.
2. Acute gastritis.
3. Uraemia.
4. Diaphragmatic pleurisy.
5. CVA.
6. Idiopathic.

MANAGEMENT OF HAEMATEMESIS AND/OR MELAENA

Haematemesis is vomiting out of blood, and melaena is presence of altered blood in stool. Both indicates upper GI haemorrhage and should be tackled immediately.

Q. How to clinically assess blood loss in upper GI bleed?

Clinical assessment is highly important in the management of these patients and is like:
- No symptoms: 500 mL blood loss (except in anaemic and aged patients).
- Syncope, tachycardia and postural hypotension: 1000 mL blood loss.
- Hypotension and profound shock (i.e. pulse >100/min, systolic BP <100 mm of Hg and urine output <30 mL/min): 2000 mL or more of blood loss.

Outline of Management

1. Complete bed rest. Record pulse, BP, respiration, temperature and any sign of shock.
2. Introduce Ryle's tube. O_2 is given through nasal catheter, if the patient is in shock. Try to assess the amount of blood loss from history and orthostatic haemodynamic changes (see below).
3. Make an IV channel. Monitor central venous pressure (CVP). Blood is sent for grouping and cross-matching, and for biochemical tests, i.e. urea, creatinine, sugar, serum electrolytes, coagulation screen and for LFT.
4. Nothing per mouth should be given if the bleeding continues. Liquid and then semisolid diet of low residue may be given when the bleeding has stopped. Tea, coffee, alcohol and smoking are strictly prohibited.
5. Start Ryle's tube suction intermittently and note the character of the aspirate. Gastric lavage is usually done with isotonic saline (ice-cold).
6. I/V fluid therapy goes like this:
   Dextrose solution (10%)—1 bottle
   ↓ ↑
   Ringer's lactate—1 bottle
   Total 4–5 bottles will run in 24 hours depending upon the amount of blood loss. Rate of fluid infusion will be guided by the patient's vital signs. Type of fluid regimen may be changed according to need (e.g. electrolyte imbalance) of the patient. Plasma expanders like low molecular weight dextran is infused to maintain the BP till blood is available for transfusion.
7. Inj. ranitidine (50 mg/2 mL): 50 mg, IV, 3–4 times daily should be given till recovery. As soon as the vital signs improve and active bleeding stops, start tablet ranitidine (150 mg/tab) 1 tab twice daily before meal to continue till further advice. PPI (i.e. omeprazole, pantoprazole or rabeprazole) may be used instead.
8. Inj. promethazine: 25–50 mg, IM stat for restless patients; may be repeated, if necessary.
9. Nowadays upper GI endoscopy can be done at the bedside. It yields high 'diagnostic accuracy', therapeutic capability, and low morbidity. When the patient becomes haemodynamically stable after receiving volume resuscitation, upper GI endoscopy should be performed early in the clinical course. Though it does not reduce the mortality, therapeutic endoscopy definitely reduces transfusion requirements, need for surgery and length of hospital stay.
10. Look for evidence of comorbidities like heart failure, IHD, renal or malignant disease, and be vigilant on them.
11. *a. For bleeding peptic ulcer:*
    i. Blood should be transfused as soon as it is available (**blood transfusion is required, if the** nasogastric aspiration shows active bleeding, the patient is in persistent shock, Hb% is <10 g/dL, systolic BP is <100 mm of Hg and the pulse rate is consistently >100/minute). Maintain the fluid drip after the transfusion is over.
    ii. Liquid antacid containing aluminium hydroxide and magnesium trisilicate is given 4–6 tsf every two hourly daily through the Ryle's tube.
    iii. Upper GI endoscopy (if not done initially) is done as soon as the patient becomes stable.
    iv. If the above measures fail, consider angiography and surgical intervention (ligation of the bleeding vessels).
    v. Endoscopic therapy: Adrenaline injection (1:10000) given quadrantically around bleeding point, or thermal coagulation (by heater probe or bipolar electrocoagulation), or by mechanical

devices (endoscopically placed clips holding the bleeding vessels). Laser therapy may also be done. Therapeutic angiography by intra-arterial vasopressin or embolotherapy with microcoils needs technical efficiency.

b. *For rupture of oesophageal varices:*
   i. Blood should be transfused as soon as it is available (**indications for transfusion are same** as in bleeding peptic ulcer). Maintain the fluid drip after the transfusion is over (if blood is transfused in late hours, patient may precipitate hepatic pre-coma).
   ii. Vasopressin (pitressin): 20 units to be dissolved in 200 mL of 5% dextrose. This will run as a separate drip over 20 minutes and will be repeated again (may repeat hourly). It will continue for another 12–24 hours after the bleeding stops (note facial pallor, abdominal colic and bowel evacuation as indicators of active drug molecule; IHD is a contraindication for its use). The therapeutic dose of vasopressin is 0.1–0.5 units/min. Vasopressin constricts the splanchnic arterioles, and thereby reduces portal pressure and portal blood flow. Inj. terlipressin 2 mg, 6 hourly by IV route, followed by (till bleeding stops) 1 mg, 6 hourly for 24 hours may be used instead of vasopressin. Nowadays, somatostatin infusion (250 µg IV stat followed by 250 µg/hr/IV) is given in few sophisticated centres. Inj. octreotide (somatostatin analogue) 50–100 µg bolus, then 25–50 µg/hour may be infused for 3–5 days. Somatostatin and octreotide increase splanchnic arterial resistance. These are known as vasoconstrictor therapy.
   iii. If bleeding still continues or recurs, introduce a Sengstaken-Blakemore tube (balloon tamponade). The Minnesota modification is preferred because it contains aspiration facility from stomach and oesophagus.
   iv. If bleeding continues after tamponade, emergency endoscopic sclerotherapy or variceal ligation/banding is tried, if feasible.
   v. If bleeding is still not controlled, surgical assistance, e.g. TIPSS (transjugular intrahepatic portosystemic stent shunting) is tried, if in a specialised centre.
   vi. Surgery is done in a desperate situation, e.g. oesophageal transection or shunt surgery (portocaval shunt or distal spleno-renal shunt).
   vii. Antibiotics in bacterial infections (not uncommon): Ciprofloxacin 200 mg, IV, BD for 5 days.
   viii. Inj. Vit K: 10 mg, IM/IV daily for consecutive 3 days. Platelet transfusion may be done. Significant coagulopathy can be corrected by fresh frozen plasma (FFP: 15 mL/kg).
   ix. All cirrhotics are to be graded on Child's criteria as early as possible. Lactulose and rifaximin (see the section on 'Management of hepatic precoma/coma') may be started.

12. Follow-up:
   a. *Bleeding peptic ulcer:* Follow the 'Eradication of *H. pylori* (see **Table 3.1**)' described in 'Gas under the diaphragm' in 'Radiology' section.
   b. *Rupture of oesophageal varices:*
      i. Endoscopic confirmation and grading of varices (if not done initially).
      ii. Endoscopic sclerotherapy, banding/ligation or TIPSS.
      iii. Tab propranolol (40 mg/tab): 1 tab, 8–12 hourly or isosorbide dinitrate (5 mg/tab): 1 tab twice daily, orally may be continued (both are portal hypotensive agents).
      iv. Porto-systemic shunt surgery may be done afterwards. In recurrent variceal haemorrhage, think of liver transplantation.

- Variceal bleeding is a life-threatening medical emergency.
- For other causes of haematemesis/melaena, primarily treat in the line of bleeding peptic ulcer. Do specific management, when upper GI endoscopy clinches the diagnosis.
- **Orthostatic haemodynamic changes:** Drop in systolic BP of >10 mm of Hg, rise in pulse rate of >15 beats/min are seen with loss of 20% of the circulatory volume.

DYSENTERY AND MISCELLANEOUS

It is characterised by diarrhoea where stool is mixed with blood and mucus as a result of acute inflammation of large gut (colicky pain abdomen and tenesmus are associated with dysentery).

A. Acute Amoebic Dysentery

1. Bed rest. Liquid diet. To consume boiled drinking water.
2. Tab metronidazole (400 mg/tab): 2 tab 3 times daily for 7 days; or metronidazole (500 mg/100 mL) IV infusion may be given, as 100 mL 3 times daily till the acute stage subsides; or tab tinidazole (300 mg/600 mg per tablet): 600 mg 2 times daily for 7 days or 2 g single daily dose for at least 3 days; or tab ornidazole: 500 mg 2 times daily for 7 days. These drugs are *followed by*,
3. Tab diloxanide furoate (500 mg/tab): 1 tab 3 times daily for 10 days (to eradicate intestinal cyst), after the treatment with metronidazole or tinidazole is over. Alternative 'luminal agents' are iodoquinol (650 mg tds for 20 days) or paromomycin (500 mg tds for 10 days).
4. Cap tetracycline (250 mg/cap): 1 cap 4 times daily for 5 days along with any one of the drugs described in No. 2 may be prescribed to eradicate luminal amoebae or to treat secondary bacterial infection.
5. Oral rehydration therapy (see afterwards), if dehydration develops.

6. Tab dicyclomine hydrochloride (10 mg/tab): 1 tab stat and sos to be used in colicky abdominal pain. Drotaverine hydrochloride (40 mg/tab) may be used instead.
7. Stool examination should be done after 1 month to confirm eradication of *Entamoeba histolytica*.

- The patient should be warned about the side effects (nausea, vomiting, metallic taste, disulfiram-like reactions, abdominal discomfort) of nitroimidazole compounds (i.e. metronidazole or tinidazole).

B. Acute Bacillary Dysentery (Shigellosis)

1. Complete bed rest in isolation. Liquid diet till acute stage subsides.
2. Record vital signs at 1/2 hourly interval. Ensure normal urine output.
3. Assess hydration. Oral rehydration therapy (see afterwards), if dehydration develops.
4. Stool should be sent for culture-sensitivity test but it is not always possible to get the report of stool before initiating specific antimicrobial therapy.
5. Trimethoprim-sulphamethoxazole (80 mg + 400 mg/tab): 2 tab twice daily for 5 days, or
   Tab ciprofloxacin (500 mg/tab): 1 tab 12 hourly for 5 days, or
   Tab norfloxacin (400 mg/tab): 1 tab 12 hourly for 5 days, or
   Tab nalidixic acid (500 mg/tab): 2 tab 6 hourly for 5 days in adults (especially used in children; in the dose of 55 mg/kg/day in divided doses).
6. Tab dicyclomine hydrochloride (10 mg/tab): 1 tab stat and sos to be used in colicky abdominal pain. Drotaverine hydrochloride (40 mg/tab) may be used instead.
7. Loperamide (2 mg/tab or cap): 1 such stat and 1 tab/cap is used sos with each motion (use cautiously in children and aged as it may precipitate paralytic ileus).
8. In high fever, paracetamol (500 mg/tab): 1 tab stat and sos is used.

- Avoid milk and milk products in dysentery.

AMOEBIC LIVER ABSCESS

It is a collection of pus (liquefactive necrosis) in the liver in response to *Entamoeba histolytica*.

1. Complete bed rest. High calorie nutritious diet. Advise the patient to consume boiled drinking water. Cysts present in water are disinfected by iodination.
2. IV metronidazole: 100 mL (containing 500 mg of the drug) to be infused thrice daily till definite clinical improvement occurs; followed by tab metronidazole (400 mg/tab): 800 mg thrice daily for 7 days, or
   Inj. dehydroemetine (previously used when metronidazole was not available): 60 mg, deep IM daily for consecutive 6 days, gap for 3 days, and again injected IM for consecutive 3 days. Strict bed rest and ECG monitoring is a must during treatment. Emetine is more cardiotoxic than dehydroemetine. Three days gap is given to avoid drug cumulation within the body. These agents are toxic and thus rarely used at present. Their toxic effects are arrhythmia, chest pain, muscle weakness, myalgia, nausea/vomiting, diarrhoea, hypotension and pain at site of infection.
3. If parenteral therapy is not employed, one may start oral treatment with tab metronidazole (400 mg/tab): 2 tab 8 hourly for 10 days, or
   Tab tinidazole (300 mg/600 mg per tablet): 600 mg 8–12 hourly for 10 days or 2 g single daily dose for 3–5 days. Tab ornidazole 2 g single daily dose for 3–5 days may be used instead.
4. Cap tetracycline (250 mg/cap): 1 cap 4 times daily for 5 days as luminal antiamoebic drug or to control secondary bacterial infection.
5. Tab chloroquine (250 mg/tab): 2 tab twice daily for 2 days, and 1 tab twice daily for next 19 days.

- No. 4 and No. 5 are used along with No. 2 or 3.

6. To eliminate intestinal luminal cyst, tab diloxanide furoate (500 mg/tab) 1 tab, orally, 8 hourly to be given for 10 days after the treatment with metronidazole is over.
7. Indications of aspiration (under USG or CT guidance):
   a. Clinical lack of response to 3–5 days' metronidazole treatment.
   b. Very large abscess (>5 cm in diameter).
   c. Abscess in the left lobe likely to rupture into the peritoneum or pericardium.
   d. To rule out pyogenic abscess (especially in patients with multiple lesions).
   e. Threat of imminent rupture of abscess.
8. Maintain nutrition by IV normal saline or dextrose-saline infusion.
9. If the abscess ruptures (confirm clinically and by bedside ultrasound machine), immediately resuscitate the patient by parenteral fluid therapy, which is followed by open surgical drainage.

- Few physicians prefer inj. ciprofloxacin infusion (200 mg/100 mL), 200 mg, 12 hourly infused over 60 minutes to combat secondary pyogenic infection within the abscess. Tablet domperidone (10 mg/tab) 1 tab, 8 hourly, orally in empty stomach for 2–3 days may be advocated in nausea/vomiting.

ACUTE VIRAL HEPATITIS

1. There is *no specific treatment for acute viral hepatitis*. Restrict physical activity. Rest in bed till the patient is symptom-free (physical well-being with return of appetite), the liver is no longer tender, and the serum bilirubin becomes less than 1.5 mg/dL, gradual ambulation.

2. A diet containing 2000–3000 kcal daily is given. Low-fat and high-carbohydrate diet is preferred. The food must be palatable. Plenty of fluid should be taken.
3. Blood should be sent for estimation of serum bilirubin (conjugated and unconjugated fraction), AST, ALT, alkaline phosphatase, serum albumin and prothrombin time. Blood biochemistry, e.g. urea, creatinine and glucose should be estimated. Tests of IgM anti-HAV, Australia antigen (HBsAg), anti-HCV, IgM anti-HEV should be advised.
4. During the acute stage, close physical contacts should be avoided. Avoid sharing comb, rajor, etc. with the patient (especially in type B and C hepatitis). Alcohol, sedatives, oral contraceptive pills are to be totally avoided. Reassurance, as recovery is the rule in majority.
5. Regular surveillance on clinical parameters and close observation regarding development of hepato-cellular failure (abnormality in higher function, pedal oedema, ascites, asterixis, etc).
6. Symptomatic treatment (keep the patient on minimum drugs):
   a. Nausea and vomiting: Domperidone 10 mg, three times daily before meal.
   b. Severe vomiting and fluid loss: Inj. metoclopramide 10 mg, IM stat; 10% dextrose drip should be started and maintained (4 bottles/day) for 2–3 days. In severe vomiting, ondansetron may be given orally (2 and 4 mg/tab) or preferably parenterally (2 mL inj. containing 2 mg/mL).
   c. Pain in the right hypochondrium (due to stretching of hepatic capsule): Tab paracetamol (500 mg/tab), 1 tab sos.
   d. Pruritus (in prolonged cholestatic variety): Read the chart on 'Cholestasis'. Chiefly UDCA, antihistaminics or cholestyramine is advocated.
   e. Weakness: Reassurance; routine vitamins supplement are not necessary. Parenteral injection of vitamin K, 10 mg by IM or IV route may be given daily for consecutive 3 days if prothrombin time is high.
   f. Hepatic pre-coma/coma (from fulminant hepatitis): Read the 'Management of hepatic pre-coma/coma' from early part of 'Emergency medicine'.

- Admission to hospital is rarely necessary (except in clinically severe disease and fulminant hepatitis).
- Corticosteroids have no benefit. There are no controlled data on the efficacy of lamivudine in acute type B hepatitis.
- In acute hepatitis B, patients are advised to monitor their HBV markers. Many hepatologists advice interferon in acute hepatitis C to prevent chronic disease.

ENTERIC FEVER

1. Bed rest with isolation till fever subsides. Care of the mouth, eyes and skin; high calorie, semisolid, low roughage diet with plenty of fluid by mouth should be taken. Tepid sponging is advised in high rise of temperature. Tab paracetamol (500 mg/tab) 1 tab used sos, if the temperature shoots > 102°F.
2. Tab ciprofloxacin (500 mg/tab): 1 tab twice daily or 400 mg IV, BD for 5–7 days.

Other Drugs (any one may be used)

- Cap chloramphenicol (250 mg/cap): 3 cap 4 times daily till fever persists, then 2 cap 4 times daily is continued up to 14–21 days (nowadays, chloramphenicol-resistant *S. typhi* is not uncommon; moreover, there is chance of development of aplastic anaemia. So many physicians avoid this drug). Pediatric dose is 30–50 mg/kg of body weight/day.
- Cap amoxicillin (500 mg/cap): 2–3 cap 4 times daily for 14 days. Pediatric dose is 100 mg/kg of body weight/day.
- Co-trimoxazole (160 mg trimethoprim + 800 mg sulphamethoxazole/tab): 2 tab twice daily for 14 days.
- Ofloxacin (200 mg tab): 2 tab twice daily for 7 days.
- Inj. ceftriaxone: 1–2 g daily, IV for 10–14 days. Pediatric dose is 75 mg/kg of body weight, once daily for 7–10 days.
- Azithromycin (500 mg/tab): 2 tab OD for 5 days.

3. If typhoid state develops, start inj. hydrocortisone hemisuccinate: Read 'Typhoid meningism' from early part of 'Emergency medicine'.
4. For chronic carrier:
   Tab ciprofloxacin (500 mg/tab)—1 tab twice daily continued for 4 weeks or advise cholecystectomy.

- In **multidrug-resistant (MDR) *S. typhi* infection,** the bacteria is resistant to chloramphenicol, co-trimoxazole, ampicillin or amoxicillin, streptomycin, sulphonamides and tetracycline. The drugs used in MDR disease are:
  A. MDR *S. typhi* infection:
     a. Ciprofloxacin 500 mg BD, orally × 5–7 days
     b. Ceftriaxone 2–3 g/d in d/d IV × 10–14 days
     c. Azithromycin 1 g/d, orally × 5 days
     d. Cefixime 400 mg BD, orally × 10–14 days
  B. NARST (Nalidixic acid-resistant *S. typhi*) strain, i.e. quinolone-resistant:
     a. Ceftriaxone 2–3 g/d, IV × 10-14 days
     b. Azithromycin 1 g/d, orally × 5 days
     c. Cefotaxime 4 g/d × 10–14 days

MDR infection as well as quinolone resistance are found in India.

ACUTE PANCREATITIS

It is an acute abdominal medical emergency. Though it is a self-limiting disease (85–90% cases subside spontaneously within 3–7 days of treatment), support through a) analgesia, b) avoidance of oral alimentation, and c) IV fluid therapy to maintain intravascular volume are targeted for a fruitful outcome. The patients should be managed in high dependency unit (HDU) or ITU.

1. Urgent hospitalisation with absolute bed rest.
2. No oral intake until the patient is free of pain abdomen and nausea/vomiting.

3. Intermittent nasogastric suction (prevents abdominal distension and vomitus, and reduces the risk of aspiration pneumonia) through Ryle's tube at 15 minute interval (Fig. 5.2).
4. Catheterisation of urinary bladder by Foley's catheter.
5. Moist O_2 inhalation by nasal catheter at the rate of 4–6 litres/min.
6. IV drip to continue with normal saline, Ringer's lactate or plasma expanders as hypovolaemic shock is very common and early fluid loss may be enormous. Monitor by CVP and measuring urine output.
7. Inj. pethidine: 100 mg, IM, 8 or 12 hourly or inj. tramadol 100 mg, IM, 12 hourly for analgesia (do not use morphine as it causes contraction of sphincter of Oddi; inj. pentazocine should also be avoided) (Fig. 5.3).

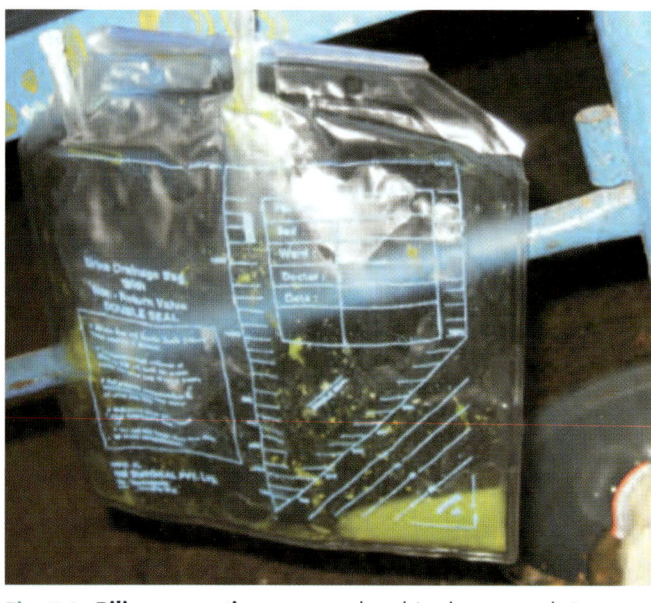

Fig. 5.2: **Bilious secretion**, accumulated in the stomach in acute pancreatitis, is coming out through Ryle's tube and collected in a bag

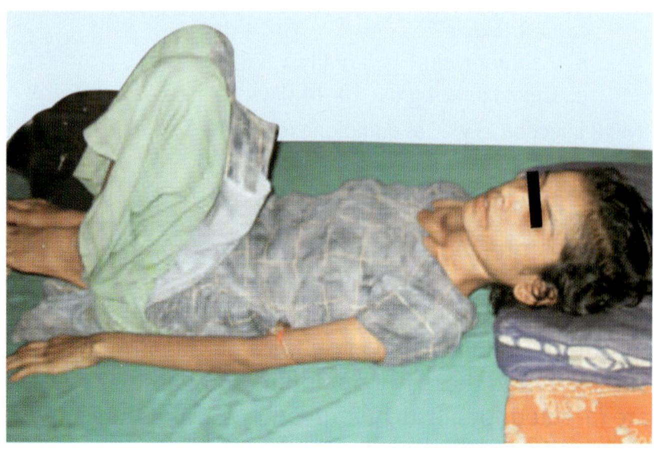

Fig. 5.3: A patient suffering from fibrocalculous pancreatic disease (FCPD) is trying to manage abdominal pain by drawing folded legs over the abdomen—decubitus of **chronic pancreatitis**; she had type 1 diabetes mellitus

8. Blood sample is drawn and sent for haematocrit, TC, DC, amylase, lipase, sugar, calcium, bilirubin, albumin, lipid profile, arterial blood gases, and grouping and cross-matching. Record the vital signs at regular interval.
9. Inj. ranitidine (50 mg/2 mL)—50 mg, IV/IM, 8 hourly to continue till recovery. Acid suppression should be done in critically ill patients with risk of stress ulcer bleeding from stomach.
10. Blood transfusion may be required in haemorrhagic pancreatitis.
11. Antibiotics (prophylactic): Inj. cefotaxime, 1 g, IV, 6 hourly or inj. aztreonam 1–2 g, IV/IM, 6–12 hourly or imipenem 0.5 mg, IV, 6 hourly for 7 days to reduce the risk of infective complications. Use of antibiotic in acute pancreatitis still remains controversial.
12. Inj. trasylol (aprotinin): 5 lacs units as IV bolus may be tried.
13. Inj. glucagon: 1 mg, SC may be given.
14. Inj. calcium gluconate: 10 mL (10%) by IV route in shot push and may be repeated.
15. Inj. octreotide: 50–200 µg, SC, 8 hourly may be of some help (reduces exocrine secretion).
16. NSAID, glucocorticoids and calcitonin are found to be ineffective in the treatment of acute pancreatitis.
17. Diet: Liquid diet is started on the 3rd to 6th day and a regular low-fat diet by the 5th to 7th day.
18. Fulminant and necrotising pancreatitis: Peritoneal lavage/laparotomy with adequate drainage and removal of necrotic tissue are done. Urgent ERCP is indicated in acute severe biliary pancreatitis with organ failure and/or cholangitis; elective ERCP with sphincterotomy is considered in patients with persistent biliary obstruction.

- An urgent USG or CECT scan (preferable) of the abdomen is required to confirm the diagnosis, to exclude other diagnosis (e.g. perforation of viscus) or to see whether phlegmon/abscess has formed or not.
- No. 12, 13, 14, 15 may be given empirically.
- Inj. insulin is given for hyperglycaemia, IV calcium for hypocalcaemia and ventilatory support for ARDS. Low molecular weight heparin (LMWH) is given for prophylaxis of deep vein thrombosis (DVT).
- **Elevated serum amylase** is characteristic of acute pancreatitis, perforation of peptic ulcer, small intestinal obstruction, mesenteric ischaemia, tubo-ovarian mass, renal insufficiency, burn, diabetic ketoacidosis, ectopic pregnancy, mumps and macroamylasaemia.

Clinical Wisdom

An HDU or ITU set up is necessary for porper treatment. In the management of acute pancreatitis APACHE II (Acute Physiology and Chronic Health Evaluation) or dynamic CECT scoring system should be carried out to assess the severity of the attack. BISAP (Bedside Index of Severity in Acute Pancreatitis), which incorporates five clinical and laboratory parameters (e.g. mental status), also useful in assessing severity. There are many more criteria to asess prognosis like modified Marshall scoring system, Glasgow criteria and Ranson criteria. Nowadays, enteral nutrition (by a nasojejunal tube, which crosses stomach and pancreas, and thereby prevents gastric paresis and pancreatic stimulation) is preferred over total parenteral nutrition (associated with a high risk of infection). Lexipafant, a platelet-activating factor inhibitor is advocated by few clinicians though not very effective.

Serum amylase value >150 Somogyi unit/dL, should raise the question of acute pancreatitis. Levels >300 units make the diagnosis more likely, and values >3 times normal virtually clinch the diagnosis. Serum amylase is usually elevated within 24 hours and the level gradually falls back towards normal over the next 3–5 days. Serum lipase levels remain elevated for a longer period of time than amylase.

CHOLERA WITH SEVERE DEHYDRATION

Cholera is a severe acute GI infection, caused by *Vibrio cholerae* (serotype 01) and is characterised by acute onset of diarrhoea (exotoxin-mediated), vomiting, fluid and electrolyte loss, dehydration and acidosis.

Renal failure may complicate the situation. The patient remains mentally clear till to the end. Death is usually as a result of acute circulatory failure.

Management

1. Complete bed rest *in isolation*. The excreta of the patient should be properly disposed off. Notify the municipality/corporation.
2. Record **vital signs**, i.e. pulse, respiration, temperature (rectal), BP, and intake-output chart carefully.
3. Nothing should be given by mouth except the oral rehydration salt.
4. A quick clinical assessment of state and degree of dehydration is made by assessing general appearance, pulse, BP, skin turgor (elasticity), eyes, tears, mucous membrane, thirst, urine output and anterior fontanelle (in infants).
5. IV fluids should be immediately started with **Ringer's lactate solution (fluid of choice in cholera)** at the rate of 50–100 mL/min. A large bore needle (e.g. No. 18) is inserted for this purpose. Ringer's lactate will continue till Dacca solution is available.
6. Dacca solution:

NaCl	5 g
$NaHCO_3$	4 g
KCl	1 g
Distilled water	1 litre

   To start with, 4–5 litres of solution is prepared. This is the recommended fluid for treatment of cholera. The fluid required is calculated every 8 hourly from urinary output, vomitus, stool and estimated insensible loss, which may be up to 5 litre/24 hours in hot and humid climate. The Dacca solution replaces running Ringer's lactate solution till the peripheral pulse are palpable. Then the drip rate is reduced at the rate of 30 mL/min. When the pulse, BP become near normal (i.e. severe dehydration has been corrected), oral rehydration therapy replaces IV fluid treatment.
7. Oral rehydration therapy by oral rehydration salt (ORS): As suggested by WHO, the 'universal formula' is:

NaCl	3.5 g/L
$NaHCO_3$	2.5 g/L
KCl	1.5 g/L
Glucose	20 g/L

   The content of the packet is dissolved in one litre of sterile drinking water. It should be taken frequently as directed by the physician (depends on degree of dehydration). It should be used for next 48 hours or till diarrhoea persists. ORS takes advantage of the hexose-Na^+ co-transport mechanism to move Na^+ across the gut mucosa with actively transported molecule of glucose.
8. Cap tetracycline (250 mg/cap): 1 cap 6 hourly for 3–5 days. Other antimicrobials like ampicillin, fluoroquinolones, nalidixic acid, doxycycline, trimethoprim-sulphamethoxazole, erythromycin or azithromycin may be used.
9. If vomiting is incessant: Inj. metoclopramide (5 mg/mL), 10 mg, IM or inj. promethazine hydrochloride 25–50 mg, IM as and when required. Inj. ondansetron 2 mL (4 mg), IV may be given instead.
10. Acidosis is corrected by 50–100 mL of inj. sodium bicarbonate (7.5%) given IV in shot push, according to the necessity.
11. If acute renal failure develops, send the patient for peritoneal or haemodialysis.

- In severe dehydration, total fluid deficit is usually 100–110 mL/kg.
- If Ringer's lactate is not available: 2 litres of isotonic saline is alternated with 1 litre of isotonic sodium lactate/bicarbonate, and potassium is added to it. Accurate fluid loss may be recorded by the use of 'cholera cot' (hole is made in the cot under patient's buttocks, and a graded bucket is placed there).
- Convulsions (febrile convulsions) in children is treated by inj. diazepam (0.2 mg/kg/IV dose).
- Inj. chlorpromazine: 50 mg, 6 hourly may be helpful in reducing intestinal secretion and fluid loss.

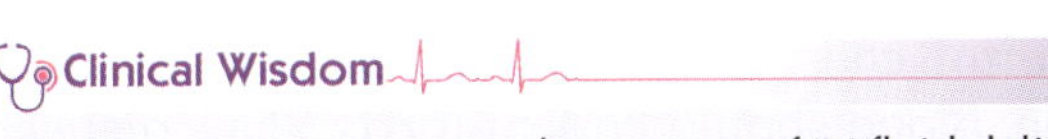

It is important to measure the amount of IV fluid delivered, and to calculate the fluid lost as loose stool and vomitus.

HAEMOPTYSIS

Usually haemoptysis (i.e. coughing out of blood) is scant and stops spontaneously without specific therapy (Fig. 5.4). If haemoptysis is prolonged, massive (>600 mL/24 hours) or alarming, the following treatment should be instituted immediately (Fig. 5.5).

1. Reassurance. Complete bed rest in semi-reclined position with leaning on the affected side (if chest

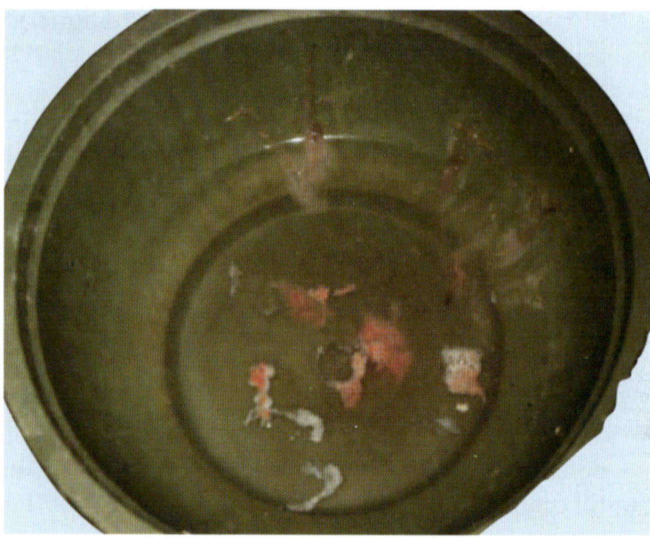

Fig. 5.4: Expectoration mixed with blood **(haemoptysis)** is seen in sputum-bowl in a patient suffering from pulmonary tuberculosis

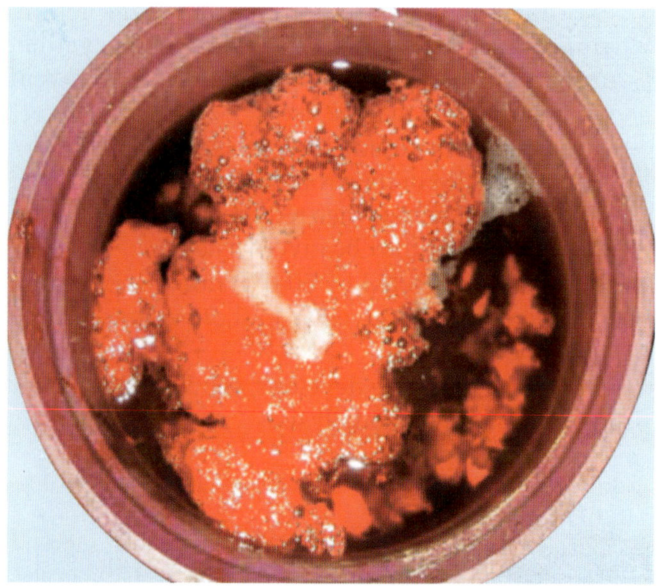

Fig. 5.5: **Massive haemoptysis** in a patient of bronchogenic carcinoma; air bubbles (froth) are seen mixed with blood

pain or chest X-ray indicates the side of lesion); this posture is maintained to prevent asphyxiation due to aspiration of blood into the normal lung. Only liquid diet is allowed.

2. Advise for chest X-ray (PA and lateral view), if feasible. Blood should be sent for TC, DC, platelet count, ESR, sugar, BT, CT, prothrombin time or INR, arterial blood gases, grouping and cross-matching; CT scan of thorax, if feasible.
3. Inj. diazepam (as anxiolytic): 5–10 mg, IM stat given.
4. IV drip of normal saline is started as a 'route of emergency' and let the fluid run at the rate of 15–20 drops/min.
5. Ensure adequate oxygenation. Record **vital signs** (pulse, BP, respiration, temperature) repeatedly. Maintain adequate BP. Measure urine output. Thorough and meticulous general survey, and examination of chest and CVS (with special reference to mitral stenosis) to come to an aetiological diagnosis, should always be tried.
6. If shock supervenes, treat by:
   a. IV normal saline infusion.
   b. Head-low position with intermittent O_2 therapy at the rate of 4–6 litres/minute.
   c. Blood transfusion, as early as possible (as per clinical guidelines of quantity of blood lost, BP, pulse rate, haematocrit and urine output).
   d. Frequent bronchial aspiration to prevent collapse of the lung.
7. Cough suppression: Small and repeated dose of linctus codeine (15 mL, tds) may be given in harassing or troublesome cough as coughing may prevent normal clotting after haemorrhage.
8. Inj. ethamsylate (125 mg/mL): 2 mL, IM/IV stat in severe haemoptysis, as a coagulant. Tab tranexamic acid (500 mg/tab) may be added, 1 tab 3 times daily as fibrinolytic inhibitor.
9. Syrup amoxicillin (125 mg/5 mL): 2 tsf 8 hourly to prevent secondary infection.
10. Treatment of the cause, i.e. antituberculosis drugs for pulmonary tuberculosis, higher antibiotics with proper doses in pneumonia, specific drugs for complicated mitral stenosis should be started. Fresh frozen plasma (FFP) for prolonged PT or elevated INR, and platelet transfusion for thrombocytopenia may be initiated.
11. If respiratory distress starts, think of asphyxiation due to aspiration. Intubation and suctioning are done by sending the patient to 'Respiratory Care Unit' (RCU). Endotracheal intubation is also indicated in ongoing bleeding, poor gas exchange and haemodynamically unstable patients.
12. Further measures to stop bleeding: Ice-cold lavage with local injection of epinephrine through a rigid bronchoscope after suctioning of blood may be employed. Topical coagulation with laser photocoagulation (Nd:YAG) may be tried. Next, a Fogarty balloon catheter is passed through bronchoscope, which may stop bleeding with tamponade technique. Removal of the clot, if the patient suffers from severe airway obstruction, may be done under bronchoscopic supervision. Lastly, surgical help (e.g. ligation of the bronchial artery or resection of the affected lobe or lung) may be sought. Few pulmonologists prefer bronchial artery catheterisation and embolisation in uncontrolled haemoptysis (after bronchial artery angiogram).

Clinical Wisdom

Haemoptysis according to age and time:

- Young—tuberculosis, bronchiectasis, mitral stenosis, bronchial adenoma, arteriovenous malformations.
- Around 40 years—bronchogenic carcinoma.
- Recurrent—chronic bronchitis, bronchial adenoma, bronchiectasis.

SEVERE ANAEMIA

Anaemia is the qualitative or quantitative diminution of RBC and/or haemoglobin concentration in relation to standard age and sex, and is clinically manifested by pallor. When the haemoglobin concentration goes below 40%, i.e. Hb < 6 g/dL, it is designated as severe anaemia.

The patient usually complains of severe weakness, fatigue, light-headedness, giddiness, pre-syncope or fainting, lassitude, anorexia, palpitations, breathlessness, anginal pain, tingling sensation in the extremities (paraesthesia), insomnia and irritability, or dysphagia (Plummer-Vinson syndrome).

Causes

1. *Acute haemorrhage:* Haematemesis and/or melaena, haemoptysis, menorrhagia, epistaxis, haematuria, bleeding haemorrhoids or road-traffic accident.
2. *Acute haemolysis:* Sickle cell crisis, thalassaemia.
3. *Deficiency of iron, folic acid, vitamin B_{12}:* Iron deficiency anaemia, megaloblastic anaemia.
4. *Failure or depression of bone marrow:* Aplastic anaemia, chronic infection, long-continued rheumatoid arthritis, chronic renal failure, lymphoma, disseminated carcinomatosis.

Management

In the presence of cardiac or cerebral symptoms, emergency treatment by blood transfusion is necessary.

1. *Packed cell transfusion:* One unit of packed red cell transfusion (330 mL) usually raises the haemoglobin concentration by about 1 g/dL in an average adult. Transfuse cautiously at the rate of 10–15 drops/minute. If the patient is in cardiac failure, always give IV furosemide 20–40 mg before transfusion. In a suspected patent of IHD, keep the rate of transfusion at 10 drops/minute (i.e. slow transfusion). More than one unit of blood should not be transfused in 24 hours. In non-availability of packed cell, transfuse whole blood and discard the plasma. It is better to transfuse packed cell when Hb concentration is <7g/dL.
2. *Treatment of the underlying cause:* This should be started simultaneously. Treat anaemia by replacement of iron, vitamin B_{12}, folic acid; combat CRF by drugs and haemodialysis, leukaemia by specific chemotherapy, aplastic anaemia by oxymetholone or bone marrow transplant.

- Other indications of blood transfusion are: (1) Hypertransfusion therapy to block production of defective cells, e.g. thalassaemia (2) Exchange transfusion, e.g. haemolytic disease of the newborn.
- In India, one pouch usually contains 350 mL of blood (300 mL blood and 50 mL anticoagulant).

Hazards of Transfusion

About 5% patients receiving blood transfusion will have some reaction. The complications arising out of transfusion are often classified into acute (<72 hrs) and delayed (>72 hrs), but this results in a degree of overlap; thus an alternative classification is made to consider them dividing into two broad groups, immune and non-immune reactions. Antibody-mediated reactions are directed against RBC, WBC, platelet, and immunoglobulins (e.g. IgA). The non-immune reactions are circulatory overload, thrombophlebitis, air embolism, massive transfusion, iron overload and transmission of infectious agents.

The **major hazards of transfusion** are:

1. Febrile or pyrogen reactions with rigors (non-haemolytic).
2. Allergic reactions (urticarial and anaphylactoid).
3. Haemolytic reactions (immediate and delayed).
4. Circulatory (volume) overload.
5. Thrombophlebitis.
6. Air embolism.
7. Transmission of infection.
8. Complications of massive transfusion.
9. Transfusion haemosiderosis.
10. Dilutional coagulation defects.
11. Immunological sensitisation by compatible blood (e.g. Rh-isoimmunisation).
12. Transfusion-related acute lung injury (ALI).
13. Transfusion-associated graft-versus-host disease (GvHD).
14. Hypothermia, plasticizers (components of bag get eluted, into bag's content and enter recipient's body).

Individual Complications are Analysed below:

a. Febrile reactions (pyrogens, antibodies against donor's plasma protein or leucocytes antigens are thought to be responsible): Fever, chills, urticaria, pruritus, etc.

Rx: 1. Slow the drip rate.
2. Cover with blanket; hot drinks.
3. Tab paracetamol (500 mg): 1 tablet orally.
4. Inj. promethazine or inj. diphenhydramine or inj. chlorpheniramine: 1 amp, IM, stat.
5. In recurrent febrile episodes: Transfuse WBC-free and plasma-free red blood cells.
6. If rigor occurs: Inj. diazepam, 1 amp (10 mg), IM may be given. Keep the patient under close vigilance. Rarely, glucocorticoids or adrenaline may be required.

b. Anaphylactic reaction: Read 'Syringe (5 mL/50 mL)' in 'Instruments and bedside procedures' section. It is due to IgA present in donor's blood when the recipient is IgA-deficient or having IgA antibodies. Transfusion is stopped immediately with administration of adrenaline 0.5 mg, i.e. 0.5 mL (1:1000), IM or SC as soon as possible. In future, recipient should receive blood components from IgA-deficient donors.

c. Haemolytic reaction (it is an immediate haemolytic transfusion reaction as a result of transfusing ABO incompatible blood group/haemolysed blood/improper storage of donor's blood): Features of **mismatched blood transfusion** are:

1. Fever.
2. Chill.
3. Aching loin pain.
4. Chest pain.
5. Nausea, vomiting.
6. Tachycardia.
7. Hypotension.
8. Throbbing of the head.
9. Breathlessness.
10. Pallor.

This is the 'stage of shock'. In the post-shock stage, haemoglobinuria develops; jaundice may develop after 12 hours. Ultimately, acute renal failure (ARF as a result of acute tubular necrosis) sets in.

R_x:

1. Immediately stop the transfusion.
2. Collect the clotted and EDTA-treated samples of patient's blood along with the remainder of suspected unit and send them to the blood bank to repeat the cross-matching. Check all documents to identify the source of error.
3. There is massive intravascular haemolysis. Blood should be examined for serum bilirubin and test of DIC (disseminated intravascular coagulation); plasma and freshly voided urine should be tested for free haemoglobin.
4. Management is targeted for preservation of intravascular volume and protection of normal renal function:
   a. Urine output should be 100 mL/hour or greater: By diuretics (inj. furosemide 40 mg IV), IV fluid (normal saline) or mannitol (300 mL of 20%) infusion.
   b. 7.5% inj. $NaHCO_3$ (1 amp = 10 mL) may be added to IV fluid to alkalinize the urine, which will help in excretion of free haemoglobin.
   c. Treat DIC and ARF, accordingly.
5. Inj. hydrocortisone hemisuccinate 100–200 mg, IV stat may be of some help.

Clinical Wisdom

A 'delayed' transfusion reaction occur in alloimmunised patients by previous transfusions. As the haemolysis is extravascular, haemoglobinuria and renal failure do not occur. Patient may develop anaemia and jaundice after 1–2 weeks. Treatment is done by fresh blood transfusion.

d. Circulatory overload: Features:

1. Breathlessness.
2 Tightness of chest.
3. Cough (dry).
4. Basal crepitations.
5. Raised jugular venous pressure.
6. Facial puffiness (late feature).

R_x:

1. Slow the rate of transfusion (stop transfusion, if required).
2. Propped-up position with moist O_2 inhalation.
3. Inj. morphine: Slow IV injection in a total dose of 5–10 mg, at a rate of 2 mg/min.
4. Inj. furosemide: 20–40 mg, IV stat and may be repeated after 30 minutes.
5. Digitalis: 0.5 mg in 10 mL normal saline, IV, given over 10 minutes.
6. The patient may be transferred to ICU for continuous monitoring of pulse, BP, respiration and cardio-respiratory status. In desperate situation, intubation and positive-pressure ventilation may be required.

e. Thrombophlebitis: Manifested by local pain, tenderness and brawny induration, and is being treated by:

1. Tab paracetamol (500 mg, thrice daily) or aspirin (325 mg, thrice daily) or aceclofenac (100 mg, once daily after meal).
2. Elevation of the limb; application of crepe bandage.
3. In severe infection, antibiotics may be required.
4. Tab serratiopeptidase (10 mg, thrice daily) or trypsin-chymotrypsin preparation (thrice daily).
5. Ointment containing heparin and benzyl nicotinate (e.g. thrombophob) to apply locally.

f. Air embolism: The incidence is less with collapsible plastic bags.

Features: Breathlessness, tachycardia, hypotension, cyanosis and syncope.

R_x:

1. The patient is placed on left lateral position.
2. Head-end down with foot-end up position.
3. Help of cardio-thoracic surgeon is sought for.

If these positions are adopted, air may be disloged/displaced from the outflow tract of right ventricle.

g. Transmission of infection:

1. Hepatitis B virus
2. Hepatitis C virus
3. HIV-1
4. HTLV-1
5. Malaria
6. West Nile virus
7. Syphilis
8. Cytomegalovirus
9. Parvovirus B19
10. Yersinia

h. Complications of massive transfusion: Administration of blood products in 24 hours of greater than the normal volume of blood of the patient (e.g. >5 litres) may be associated with **(massive transfusion)**, which is manifested by:

1. Hypothermia: Rapid infusion of chilled blood may produce cardiac dysrhythmias. So, prevent the situation by warming the blood before transfusion (or use 'blood warmer').
2. Citrate intoxication: Patient may develop hypocalcaemia (paraesthesia, tetany, hypotension and low cardiac output) and is usually seen in patients with hepatic dysfunction. Calcium gluconate, IV, 10 mL of a 10% solution may prevent the situation.
3. Hyperkalaemia and acidaemia may occur: Usually not significant.
4. Bleeding complications: This may happen as a result of dilution of platelet and coagulation factors. Transfusion of fresh blood, FFP or platelet concentrates may tackle the situation.
5. Microembolism: May lead to acute lung injury.

i. Iron overload: As each unit of RBC contains 200–250 mg of iron, iron overload features (i.e. endocrine, hepatic and cardiac dysfunction) occur after 100 units of RBC transfusion. So, judicious transfusion is preferable.

j. Transfusion-related acute lung injury (ALI): Anti-leucocyte antibodies present in donor's blood are responsible; usually develops within 4 hours of transfusion and is often indistinguishable from ARDS (acute respiratory distress syndrome).

Features: Breathlessness, hypotension, fever, chills and hypoxaemia.

R_x: By ventilatory support. Usually diuretics are of no help.

k. Transfusion-associated graft-versus-host disease (GvHD): It is invariably fatal but entirely a preventable situation. Rash, fever, diarrhoea or bone marrow failure occurs 1–2 weeks after transfusion. This condition usually occurs in immunocompromised individuals. Treatment is supportive. Prevention is done by irradiation of all cellular blood products before transfusion.

Blood Components and Blood Products

Nowadays, whole blood is rarely used for transfusions and all transfusions are done in the form of blood components. Blood components are prepared from single donations and is usually carried out by simple seperation methods. They are:

a. *Blood components:* Red cell concentrate, platelet concentrate, granulocyte concentrate, fresh frozen plasma (FFP) and cryoprecipitate, etc.
b. *Blood products:* Albumin, coagulation factor concentrates and immunoglobulins are prepared from plasma.

Blood components and blood products are:

- Whole blood.
- Packed RBCs: One unit increases Hb by 1 g/dL, and is used in acute blood loss, bone marrow failure, thalassaemia with severe anaemia. Washed RBCs are transfused in patients with severe reaction to plasma.
- WBC-depleted RBC: Are used for patients with recurrent febrile episodes (non-haemolytic) after transfusion.
- Granulocyte concentrates: Used in severe neutropenia with evidence of bacterial infections.
- Platelet concentrates: One concentrate increases platelet count by 10000/mm^3, and is used in thrombocytopenia, inherited or acquired platelet function defect, leukaemias, DIC, etc.
- Fresh frozen plasma (FFP): Contains clotting factors without platelets. Usual dose is 10–15 mL/kg of body weight, and is commonly used in clotting factor deficiency, DIC, liver disease, snakebite, thrombotic thrombocytopenic purpura.
- Cryoprecipitate: It is a concentrated FFP. It is the concentrate of factor VIII, fibrinogen, von Willebrand (vW) factor, and is useful in DIC and other hypofibrinogenaemic conditions.
- Rh immune globulin: Used to prevent maternal Rh antibody formation.
- Irradiated blood products: To prevent graft-versus-host disease (GvHD).
- Human albumin: Available as 4.5% or 20% solution, and is indicated in severe, acute hypoalbuminaemias, e.g. nephrotic syndrome or hepatic disorders.
- Blood substitute (fluorocarbon synthetic chemicals)—'true' blood substitute is yet to be available.

MANAGEMENT OF CARDIAC ARREST (CPR)

Cardiac arrest is the sudden and complete loss of cardiac function where the pulse is not palpable, BP cannot be recorded, respiration stops and the patient becomes unconscious. Unless promt treatment is started within 4–5 minutes, the patient dies. Worldwide, it is the leading cause of death (by sudden cardiac arrest). Ventricular fibrillation, pulseless ventricular tachycardia, cardiac asystole or electromechanical dissociation are responsible for cardiac arrest. **Cardiopulmonary resuscitation (CPR)**, i.e. basic life support should be immediately instituted to rescue patients with acute circulatory or respiratory failure or both, followed by implementation of advanced life support measures.

Sudden cardiac death (SCD) is an unexpected death due to cardiac causes, which occurs in a short time period (i.e. within one hour of onset of symptom) in a person with known or unknown cardiac disease. There is sudden and irreversible cessation of all biological functions. SCD is one of the largest cause of natural death in the world. SCD is different from 'heart attack' (i.e. acute myocardial infarction). Common causes of SCD are AMI, following coronary artery bypass surgery, hypertrophic cardiomyopathy, cyanotic congenital heart diseases, valvular heart diseases, prolongation of Q-T interval in ECG, diabetes mellitus, etc.

- Causes of cardiac arrest:

1. *Ventricular fibrillation (VF) or pulseless ventricular tachycardia:* Acute myocardial infarction (AMI), drugs (e.g. quinidine or

digitalis toxicity), electrical shock, dyselectrolytaemia (↓K^+ or ↑K^+, ↓Ca^{++}, ↓Mg^{++}).
2. *Ventricular asystole:* Massive AMI, failure of conduction.
3. *Electromechanical dissociation:* Rupture of the heart, massive pulmonary thromboembolism.

Basic life support (BLS) starts immediately:

1. *Check the patient's responsiveness:* Shake and shout.
2. *Airway:* The patient should be placed on a firm, flat surface in face up, i.e. in an extended supine position with elevated legs. Extend the neck (head tilt) and raise the chin (chin lift or jaw thrust). Remove visible vomitus debris or dentures after opening the mouth. If any foreign body is suspected, the patient is rolled over to one side and 4–5 forceful blows are delivered rapidly between two shoulder blades by the heel of the palm; again the patient is placed in supine position. Oropharyngeal aspiration may be needed.
3. *Breathing:* Check breathing (look, listen, feel). Mouth-to-mouth breathing (direct, or indirectly via a ventilation tube) should be started immediately at the rate of 12/minute. Extending patient's neck, pinching patient's nose by index finger and thumb, and placing a gauge piece on patient's mouth, start mouth to mouth respiration. First, take a deep inspiration and then exhale totally on the patient's mouth. Always look at the patient's chest for signs of expansion (i.e. for signs of adequate ventilation). If facilities are available, ventilate with Ambu bag, face mask. Start 100% O_2. In foreign body obstruction within larynx or trachea, **Heimlich's manoeuvre** should be attempted to relieve the obstruction (standing behind the patient, encircle the waist with your arms. A clenched fist is placed against the epigastrium, above umbilicus but below the xiphisternum. After grasping the fist with the other hand, quick upward thrusts are applied into the patient's abdomen several times necessary to clear the airway).
4. *Circulation:* Feel for carotid pulsations and if carotid or brachial pulse is still not palpable, deliver a blow over the chest and start closed **cardiac massage** immediately. With the heel of both hands (one placed above the other), the lower part of the body of sternum is compressed vertically (depresing sternum by 5–6 cm) at the rate of 100–120/minute after placing the patient on a hard surface. For one rescuer, ventilate twice after 15 chest compressions; and for two rescuers ventilate once after 5 chest compressions. Chest compression does not massage the heart, rather thorax acts as a pump and thereby heart maintains the forward circulation. Cardiac massage should be gentle, rhythmic and smooth.
5. *Automated external defibrillator (AED):* Since VF is the major cause of **cardiac arrest**, application of early defibrillation by paramedical staffs or doctors is of paramount importance.
6. Try to record an ECG of the patient to come to an aetiological diagnosis. The BLS should be stopped for 5 seconds at the end of first minute (and thereafter every 2–3 minutes) to assess whether spontaneous breathing or circulation has resumed or not. The BLS should be continued till ALS is made available (for ALS, the patient should be shifted to a hospital or till an 'cardiac ambulance' arrives) for revival. Now start **advanced life support (ALS)** as follows:

A. Cardiac Asystole

Precordial thump or blow, if vital signs do not return

↓

Inj. adrenaline: 5–10 mL of 1: 1000 aqueous solution by IV route

↓

Inj. atropine 3 mg IV, once only

↓

Inj. calcium chloride (10%): 5–10 mL of the solution is given, IV slowly

↓

If electrical activity is yet to be evident, support life by transvenous or transthoracic pacemaker

B. Ventricular Fibrillation

Precordial thump or blow

↓

Defibrillate by DC shock with 200 Joules initially

↓

Repeat DC shock with 360 Joules

↓

Inj. adrenaline: 5–10 mL of 1: 1000 aqueous solution by IV route

↓

Mouth-to-mouth breathing with simultaneous closed cardiac massage

↓

If this fails, start lignocaine 75 mg bolus in IV shot push; then continue 50 mg, IV every 5 minutes up to a maximum dose of 225 mg

↓

Inj. bretylium 5 mg/kg bolus in IV shot push

↓

Defibrillation by DC shock with 360 Joules

- Intubate the patient and resuscitate by assisted ventilation; always try to correct acidosis.
- VF is the most common and easily treatable cause of cardiac arrest. Cardiac asystole is prognostically worse.

C. Electromechanical Dissociation

Inj adrenaline: 5–10 mL of 1: 1000 aqueous solution by IV route

↓

Try to correct acidosis, hypoxia, hypovolaemia, hypothermia, electrolyte imbalance, cardiac tamponade or pulmonary embolism (if present)

↓

Mouth-to-mouth breathing with simultaneous closed cardiac massage

7. Acidosis: Inj. sodium bicarbonate (7.5%) 50 mL, IV stat and 30–50 mL to be repeated every 10 minutes till circulation is restored.
8. Hypotension: Start dopamine infusion (2–20 µg/kg/min) by mixing 200 mg of inj. dopamine in 540 mL of normal saline and to run at the rate of 10–12 drops/min. Try to adjust the systolic BP near about 100 mm of Hg.
9. Cerebral oedema: Inj. hydrocortisone hemisuccinate 500 mg, IV stat.
10. Termination of CPR: If pulse is absent, BP is non-recordable, spontaneous respiration is lacking and the patient remains unconscious for 30 minutes with fixed and dilated pupils—terminate CPR.

A flat ECG diagnoses cerebral death.

- Basic life support (BLS) can be done by anybody, whether medical, paramedical or a lay person.
- Advanced life support (ALS) targets to restore normal cardiac rhythm and to give support to circulation by defibrillation, IV drugs, positive pressure ventilation, etc.

Clinical Wisdom

Do not ignore the warning signals—the 'window period' for cardiac arrest is 5 minutes, for heart attack (AMI) 3 hours, for stroke (CVA) 3 hours and for stoppage of bleeding (anywhere in the body) it is 1 hour. **A, B, C, D, E** in resuscitation stand respectively for airway, breathing, circulation, drugs and examination (repeated).

PAROXYSMAL ATRIAL TACHYCARDIA (PAT)

In PAT, the pulse rate is usually 160–220/min and the rhythm is regular. It is thought to be due to a run of rapidly repeated atrial premature beats. PAT is being managed by:

1. Non-pharmacological (mechanical) measures to increase the vagal tone:
   a. Valsalva manoeuvre in supine position (most effective way).
   b. Carotid sinus massage (after excluding occlusive carotid disease).
   c. Self-induced gagging.
   d. Pressure over the eyeballs, coughing, breath holding, stretching the arms and body, lowering the head between two knees.

- These physical measures delay the AV conduction, blocks the re-entry phenomenon and may terminate the attack.

2. Drugs (if mechanical measures fail):
   a. Adenosine: It is a very short-acting naturally occurring purine nucleoside and a first-choice drug for PAT. The dose is 6 mg, given as a rapid IV bolus, followed by a 10–30 mL saline flush; if necessary, may repeat with 12 mg, IV bolus. Contraindications for its use are 2° or 3° AV block, atrial fibrillation, sick sinus syndrome and ventricular tachycardia. It may produce bronchospasm in asthmatics and other side effects are flushing, chest pain, heaviness in the limbs, transient hypotension or atrial standstill. Usually the attack of PAT is terminated within a few seconds.
   b. Verapramil: If adenosine is not effective, inj. verapramil 5–10 mg, IV is given over 5 minutes which may terminate the attack; if no effect is there, the drug may be repeated after 30 minutes.
   c. Other drugs: Metoprolol (5 mg, IV bolus up to 15 mg), esmolol (500 µg/kg IV bolus, then 50 µg/kg/min), digitalis (0.75–1 mg, IV loading), amiodarone (200 mg) or disopyramide (200 mg) orally may be effective.
3. DC shock: If drugs fail or the patient shows signs of cardiogenic shock (haemodynamically unstable), heart failure or angina—synchronized DC shock (150 Joules) may prove effective.
4. Follow-up: Avoid tea, coffee, smoking, alcohol, exclude underlying valvular heart disease or thyrotoxicosis. Advice tab verapramil (80 mg), 1 tab thrice daily to continue. The patient is then referred to cardiologist for electrophysiological evaluation and long-term management.

- Ideally, the carotid massage, antiarrhythmic treatment and DC shock should be done in an ICU under ECG monitoring.

ACUTE RHEUMATIC FEVER

1. Complete bed rest till fever, arthritis, carditis, WBC count, ESR and tachycardia subside. Prolonged bed rest is necessary for 2–6 weeks in rheumatic carditis.
2. High calorie, salt restricted diet.
3. Chorea is being treated by clonazepam, chlorpromazine, carbamazepine or haloperidol.
4. Symptomatic treatment:
   a. Arthritis, arthralgia, fever: Aspirin (0.3 g/tab; acetyl salicylic acid) is started in a dose of 80–100 mg/kg/day in children and 4–8 g/day in adults in 4–5 divided doses, and is continued for 2 weeks. If symptoms subside, a lower dose of 60–70 mg/kg/day (in children) is continued for further 2–4 weeks. Gastric intolerance may be combated by giving antacid 15–30 min after each dose of aspirin, or proton-pump inhibitor once daily before breakfast. Aspirin is usually given in enteric-coated form. Typically, aspirin should be continued until ESR becomes normal, and then tapered off gradually. Other NSAIDs like naproxen in a dose of 10–20 mg/kg/day gives symptomatic relief.
   b. Patient without carditis: Aspirin is preferred.
   c. Patient with carditis but without heart failure: Aspirin ± glucocorticoid (role of corticosteroids is doubtful in carditis but majority of cardiologists opine that they help in rapid resolution of heart failure). Prednisolone (5 or 10 mg/tab), 1–2 mg/kg/day (maximum of 80 mg) is given orally for a period of 2 weeks and then tapered off over next 2 weeks.

d. Patient with carditis and heart failure: Majority opine that corticosteroid is mandatory over and above aspirin. Treatment of CCF is done accordingly (see before).
e. Antibiotics: Single injection of 1.2 million units of benzathine penicillin, IM is given to eradicate Group A *Streptococcus*, if present (after proper skin test). Oral penicillin V (phenoxymethyl penicillin) 500 mg twice daily (250 mg twice daily for children ≤ 27 kg), orally for 10 days or erythromycin 40 mg/kg/day, orally may be used for 10 days (in patients allergic to penicillin).

5. Secondary prevention of acute rhumatic fever: The **mainstay of controlling rheumatic heart disease is secondary prevention.** The dose of inj. benzathine penicillin is 1.2 million units, IM given at 4 weekly interval (in endemic areas and high-risk cases, the interval is 2–3 weekly). Dose of penicillin in children (≤27 kg) is 0.6 million units. Instead oral penicillin V may be used 250 mg twice daily or oral erythromycin 250 mg twice daily (in penicillin allergy). Controversies exist regarding duration of therapy and the guideline is:
   a. Rheumatic fever without proven carditis: 5 years after the last attack or until the age of 21 years, whichever is longer.
   b. Rheumatic fever with carditis but having minimal residual valve damage: 10 years after the last attack or 21 years of age, whichever is longer.
   c. Rheumatic fever with carditis along with residual heart disease: 10 years after the last episode or until the age of 40, whichever is longer. Few clinicians prefer to give penicillin life long in this situation.
   d. If valvular surgery is done: Penicillin prophylaxis is continued life long.
6. Follow up: Echocardiographic evaluation in assessing subsequent valve lesions, especially in patients with carditis.

- Prophylaxis against infective endocarditis is required in valve damage.
- 'Post-steroid rebound' may be prevented by an 'overlap' course of aspirin when the corticosteroid is being tapered over a 2 week period. Aspirin in then continued for 2–3 weeks more.
- Primary prevention (which means treatment of Group A streptococcal sore throat) is given by a course of penicillin (see above) started within 9 days of onset of sore throat.

TETANUS

The diagnosis of tetanus (infection due to toxin-secreting *Clostridium tetani*) is made on clinical grounds; the neurotoxin is known as tetanospasmin. The disease is characterised by muscular rigidity, spasm of muscles, trismus (lock jaw due to spasm of masticatory muscles), risus sardonicus (facial grimace), neck rigidity, opisthotonus (backward bending of the body like an arc), autonomic disturbances (sweating, tachycardia, labile BP and cardiac arrhythmias) but the consciousness and mental clarity remain intact till to the end.

The patient may die from hypoxia, aspiration, respiratory depression, cardiac arrest or exhaustion. Bad prognostic factors are extremes of ages and short incubation period. It is a preventable disease but if a patient develops tetanus, it should be managed promptly.

Management

1. Isolation; preferably transfered to 'Infectious diseases' ward or hospital.
2. Complete bed rest in a railed cot in a noise-free (quiet), darkroom. There should not be any undue light, sound or cutaneous stimulation for the patient (avoid unnecessary stimuli).
3. If oral feeding is possible, give liquid feed orally. If not possible, insert Ryle's tube. In its failure, maintain nutrition by IV fluid therapy.
4. Skilled nursing is necessary. Check vital signs repeatedly. Maintain intake-output chart. Cleanse the wound (if any) with soap-water/povidone-iodine/normal saline-20% hydrogen peroxide solution; debridement, if necessary.
5. Maintain airway.
6. Inj. Human Tetanus Immunoglobulin (HTIG): IM injection of 3000–6000 units of antitoxin; single dose. It should be given after proper skin test though hypersensitivity reaction is rare. HTIG is administered before manipulating the wound and a portion of HTIG should be injected around the wound. Immune equine tetanus immunoglobulin 10000–20000 units by single IM injection is an alternative to HTIG. HTIG is preparation of choice.
7. Inj. crystalline penicillin: 2 million units, IV, every 4–6 hourly after proper skin test, for 10 days. Metronidazole (500 mg/100 mL)—500 mg, IV, 6 hourly for 7–10 days; erythromycin or clindamycin may be given in penicillin allergy. IV metronidazole is probably the drug of choice.
8. Inj. diazepam (5 mg/mL): 10 mg is given IV stat and may be repeated, if necessary in muscle spasm/convulsions. Larger doses of diazepam may be required (≥250 mg/day); lorazepam and midazolam are other options. Chlorpromazine, phenobarbital, IV magnesium sulphate, baclofen or tizanidine may also be used in muscle spasm. Neuromuscular blockade may be necessary.
9. Labetalol, esmolol, clonidine or verapramil may be considred in autonomic dysfunction.
10. Tracheostomy and assisted ventilation are necessary in asphyxia due to laryngeal spasm or hypoventilation from oversedation.
11. IV fluid therapy is done by 5% dextrose (1 bottle), dextrose-normal saline (2 bottles) and amino acid (1 bottle) infusion. Total 4 bottles/day are required.
12. Inj. tetanus toxoid: It should be given IM (0.5 mL) at a different site of HTIG, and should be repeated (0.5 mL, IM) after 1 month and 6 months.

ORGANOPHOSPHORUS (OP) COMPOUND POISONING

Organophosphorus poisoning is mainly suicidal and it is a medical emergency. These insecticides are potent inhibitors of cholinesterase. They are absorbed quickly after ingestion, inhalation or through the intact skin. Inactivation of acetylcholinesterase allows accumulation of excessive acetylcholine at different neurosynaptic sites like CNS, autonomic ganglia, parasympathetic and motor nerve endings, and thus there is increased muscarinic and nicotinic activity. The **organophosphorus compounds** are malathion, parathion, guthion, chlorothion and diazinon; common **carbamate insectisides** are carbaryl, propoxur and aldicarb.

Management

1. Gastric lavage with normal saline infusion while admitted in a hospital. Forced emesis is not encouraged. The first sample should be kept for toxicology. Change the soiled clothings and preferably, wash the contaminated skin with soap and water. Wash the contaminated eyes with normal saline.
2. 100 g of activated charcoal is mixed in 1/2 bottle of normal saline and introduced into the stomach through Ryle's tube to prevent continued absorption. This is done after a satisfactory stomach wash.
3. Inj. atropine sulphate (0.6 mg/ampoule): It is the drug of choice; 4–5 amp, IV stat and 1–2 amp to be given by slow IV route at every 5–10 min interval till full atropinisation is achieved, i.e. the mouth is dry, pulse becomes >100/min and pupil becomes fully dilated. Afterwards, 1 amp to be given IV, 8 hourly for next 2–3 days. *Atropine counteracts the muscarinic effects* of organophosphorus poisoning. Glycopyrrolate may be helpful when copious secretions are not controlled by atropine alone (according to some studies).
4. Inj. pralidoxime (PAM): 1 g in aqueous solution to be given IV stat over 5–10 minutes, and to be repeated 3–4 times daily (maximum total dose is 4 g) for 2–5 days. Alternatively, an infusion of PAM may be given at the rate of 8–10 mg/kg/hour. **PAM counteracts the nicotinic effects** as well as the muscarinic effects of organophosphorus poisoning. PAM is a cholinesterase reactivator and should be started as early as possible. According to some clinicians, use of PAM is controversial but it helps in revival of neuromuscular transmission. It does not work in carbamate poisoning.
5. Moist O_2 inhalation at the rate of 4–6 litres/min; if required (in respiratory failure), ask for assisted ventilation. Place the patient in a railed cot.
6. Suction of the mouth, oropharynx and nose repeatedly.
7. Inj. diazepam: 5 mg, IV slowly, if convulsions appear. Inj. phenytoin may be used.
8. Inj. furosemide (20 mg/amp): 20 mg, IV stat and may be repeated in non-cardiogenic pulmonary oedema. Few clinicians advocate inj. hydrocortisone hemisuccinate 100–200 mg, IV stat in this situation.
9. Maintain an IV drip with dextrose (5%)–normal saline solution at the rate of 15 drops/min.

- Up to 100 amp. (60 mg) or even more of atropine may be given in quick succession in moribund patient of poisoning by organophosphorus compound.
- PAM is of little value if started after 24 hours of incidence of poisoning.
- Signs of **atropinisation**: Tachycardia, dry mouth (can not spit), fixed and dilated pupil, rise of surface temperature. Signs of over-atropinisation: Restlessness, disorientation, delirium, hyperpyrexia, subsultus tendinum (involuntary movements of fingers) and irrelevant talks. In over-atropinisation, give inj. haloperidol 1 mL (5 mg), IM stat
- Patients of **organophosphorus poisoning** show following features: Nausea, vomiting, diarrhoea, blurring of vision as a result of miosis (pin-point pupil), sweating, lacrimation, salivation, bronchorrhoea, bradycardia, hypotension, chest tightness, involuntary urination and defecation (*muscarinic effects*). They may also have muscular twitching, fasciculations, tachycardia, hypertension, respiratory paralysis, extreme weakness and flaccid paralysis (*nicotinic effects*). The CNS effects are anxiety, restlessness, tremor, convulsions, slurred speech, confusion, delirium and coma. Other effects are pulmonary oedema and hyperglycaemia.

Clinical Wisdom

'Neurological syndromes' of OP poisoning include a) cholinergic crisis, b) intermediate syndrome, and c) delayed polyneuropathy.

Other Important Poisonings

a. Aluminium phosphide: Used as insecticides and rodenticides. Toxic 'phosphine' is liberated when it comes in contact with moisture in the air. Common lethal toxicities are cardiac (arrhythmias, failure), pulmonary oedema, metabolic acidosis, acute kidney injury and peripheral circulatory failure (shock). No specific antidote is available (hence, high mortality), and treatment is symptomatic and supportive. Diagnosis is done by detecting phosphine in exhaled air:

b. Methyl alcohol: Methyl alcohol is often deliberately and illegally mixed with alcoholic beverages as a cheaper alternative to ethyl alcohol. Methanol is used as a solvent, and is metabolised to formaldehyde and formic acid in the liver by alcohol dehydrogenase. Inebriation, drowsiness, blurred vision (progressing to blindness) and metabolic acidosis are well-known complications. Gastric lavage, correction of acidosis, ethanol (loading dose of 5% solution, IV at 15 mg/kg, followed by 2–3 mL/kg/hour orally; IV infusion is also given), or fomepizole (inhibits alcohol dehydrogenase), or haemodialysis (if serum methanol level >50 mg/dL) are mainstay of treatment.

c. Strong acid/alkali (caustic) ingestion (Fig. 5.6)*:* Both of them burn the GI tract by coagulative necrosis (acid) and liquefaction necrosis (alkali). Damage of stomach >oesophagus is caused by acid, while oesophagus

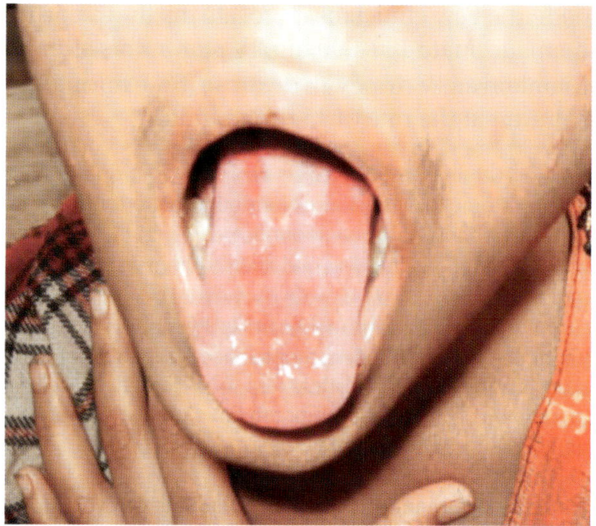

Fig. 5.6: **White slough in tongue** with haemorrhagic spots and erythema (sore tongue) are seen in accidental acid ingestion

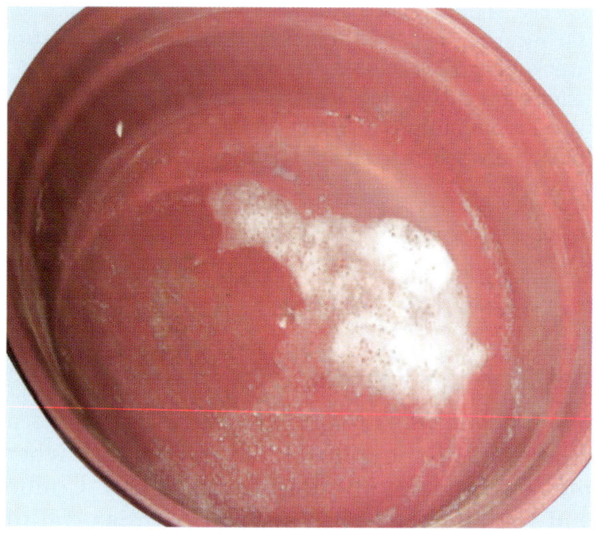

Fig. 5.7: **Profuse saliva** is seen ia sputum-bowl in a patient of suicidal acid ingestion; she had ptyalism or sialorrhoea

>stomach is affected by alkali ingestion. Increased salivation, dysphagia, odynophagia, and cough are common (Fig. 5.7). Mediastinitis (due to oesophageal perforation), peritonitis (due to gastric perforation) are dreaded complications. Oesophageal stricture and gastric outlet obstruction are late complications. Treatment is symptomatic and supportive. Stomach wash, forced emesis, neutralising acid or alkali, or corticosteroids are contraindicated.

d. Salicylates: Aspirin (acetylsalicylic acid) and oil of wintergreen (methyl salicylate) are common offender when taken in large quantity. It stimulates respiratory centre → hyperpnoea → respiratory alkalosis → renal excretion of bicarbonate and potassium → metabolic acidosis → a mixed acid-base imbalance supervenes. Gastric lavage, forced alkaline diuresis, correction of metabolic acidosis (IV, 7.5% sodium bicarbonate), and haemodialysis (in severe renal or respiratory insufficiency, or coma) are the steps of management.

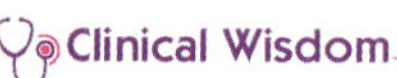

Guideline of quick examination for the poisoned patient:

1. a → b → c → d → e = airway → breathing → circulation → disability → examination.
2. Level of consciousness (by Glasgow Coma Scale).
3. Ventilation: Assess by pulse oximetry.
4. Pulse rate and blood pressure (BP).
5. Pupil: Size and reaction to light.
6. Temperature.
7. Head injury as a complication of poisonings.
8. Try to identify the poison by physical signs (e.g. miosis, hypersecretion, bronchorrhoea, hypersalivation in organophosphorus and carbamate poisoning).

e. Paracetamol (acetaminophen): It is hepatotoxic, and is a common drug used for suicidal attempt in UK, USA and many other countries. Toxic metabolite N-acetyl-p-benzoquinone imine (NAPQI) accumulates resulting from paracetamol-induced depletion of hepatic glutathione. The severity of symptoms are dose-related. A single dose >10 g in healthy persons, or 8 g in chronic liver disease/alcoholics are lethal. Therapy should be begun within 8 hours of ingestion. Acetylcysteine is the specific antidote, oral or IV, depending on the serum acetaminophen level and severity of manifestations. Acetylcysteine (regimen) is given 150 mg/kg dissolved in 200 mL of 5% dextrose over 15 minutes, then 50 mg/kg in 500 mL of 5% dextrose over next 4 hours, and then 100 mg/kg in 1000 mL of 5% dextrose over next 16 hours (total dose is 300 mg/kg over 20 hours).

SNAKEBITE

Venomous snakes are basically of three families:

a. **Viperidae** (with two subgroups): Crotalinae (pit vipers, rattle snakes) and Viperinae (Russell's viper). This group is *vasculotoxic* and presents with haemorrhages from different sites like haematuria (Fig. 5.8) and haemoptysis, vomiting, shock, intense local reaction and acute renal failure.

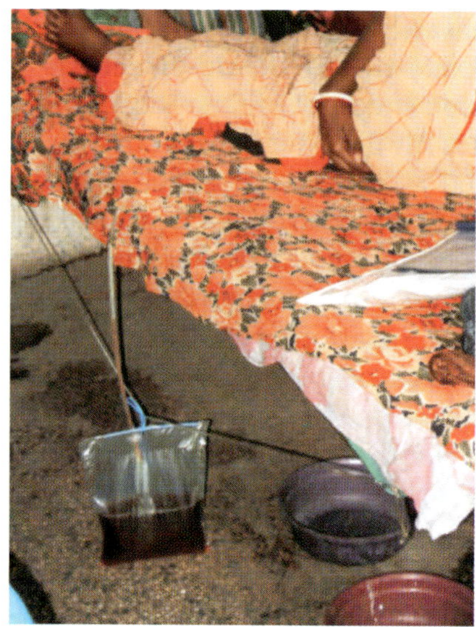

Fig. 5.8: Viperidae snakebite with **haematuria** in an adult

b. **Elapidae** (cobras, kraits, mambas, coral snakes): This group is *neurotoxic* and produces ptosis, facial palsy, bulbar palsy, muscle weakness, paralysis of respiratory muscles, blurred vision and slurred speech.

c. **Hydrophiidae** (sea snakes): This group is *myotoxic*, and produces myalgia, myoglobinuria, acute renal failure; hyperkalaemia due to release of potassium from necrosed muscles may lead to cardiac involvement. In majority of sea snakes, no venom is released (dry bites).

- There are two other venomous snake family called Colubridae which includes mongoose snakes, and Atractaspididae (Natal black snake) which gives rise to coronary vasoconstriction or AV conduction defects.
- Snake venom may contain ≥20 toxins. Generally two puncture wounds with a gap of 0.2 cm to 2.5 cm (fang marks) indicate bite by poisonous snake while non-poisonous snakebite usually leave rows of small scratches, often arranged in an arc.

Management

1. First aid measures (field management): Reassurance; if necessary, mild sedation (alprazolam 1 tablet, i.e. 0:25 mg) is given to allay apprehension. Firm and wide pressure bandaging is applied 5 cm above the bite area which is at least 1–1.5 cm wide, preferably with 'immobilisation' by a splint to keep the affected part in functional position. The tourniquet (even a handkerchief will do) should be so tight (lympho-occlusive dressings) that it would allow the tip of one finger only to pass through, and will obstruct the lymph flow and not the arterial or venous circulation. The tourniquet should be released at 20 minutes interval for 1–2 minutes and reapplied just proximal to the progressing oedematous area.
   Nowadays, application of tourniquet seems to be controversial. It may be used if the transit period is >60 minutes from the time of bite to application of antivenin. In fact, it worsens local tissue necrosis. According to recent trend, tourniquets should not be used as it leads to higher rates of amputation of limb.
2. Try to identify the snake (a photograph of the snake from a distance may help with snake identification and management decisions) and refer the victim to nearby hospital.
3. Inj. polyvalent antivenin serum (AVS): First do the intradermal test by 0.1 mL of the solution (after mixing 1 unit in 10 mL of distilled water). Inj. adrenaline (1: 1000 solution), inj. hydrocortisone and inj. diphenhydramine must be kept ready in hand to combat anaphylaxis. If there is absence of any skin reaction, mix 10 vials (each vial containing 1 unit of antivenin are made into 10 mL solution) in 400 mL normal saline and let it run at the rate of 50–100 drops/min, IV according to severity. Again, 10 vials may be repeated, if necessary. AVS gives maximum benefit, if given within 24 hours. Monovalent serum is more potent.
4. Inj. benzathine penicillin: 1.2 million units IM stat after proper skin test to check secondary infection of the devitalised bitten area.
5. Inj. diclofenac (25 mg/mL): 2 mL, deep IM stat in severe local pain (burning, bursting or throbbing).
6. Inj. Human Tetanus Immunoglobulin (HTIG): If the patient did not receive full course of inj. tetanus toxoid earlier, give 250 units stat by IM route (after proper skin test).
7. Inj. tetanus toxoid: 0.5 mL, IM stat and to be repeated after 1 month (0.5 mL, IM) and 6 month (0.5 mL, IM).
8. Blood transfusion, if the patient is in shock or there is profuse internal haemorrhage.
9. *Shock and hypotension:* Albumin (5%) infusion is better than dextrose or normal saline. Dopamine infusion (2–20 µg/kg/min) or even inj. hydrocortisone hemisuccinate 200 mg, IV slowly or fresh frozen plasma (FFP), may be started. Moist O_2 inhalation is given at the rate of 4–6 litres/min.
10. *Acute renal failure (or acute kidney injury):* Try to correct the electrolyte imbalance and give sufficient fluid parenterally. Inj. mannitol (20%) 300 mL is infused over 3 hours or large dose of furosemide (100–200 mg) IV is given. If not corrected by above measures, the patient may require *peritoneal or haemodialysis*.
11. In Elapidae (cobras) group of snake bite: Inj. neostigmine 0.5 mg (1 mL) is given, IV every half an hour for 4–6 injections until the ptosis or neurodeficit is corrected (here, the toxin blocks neuromuscular junction). Then injection neostigmine is given every one hourly and ultimately to be given at 2–3 hours interval till all signs of paralysis have disappeared. Every injection of IV neostigmine should be preceded by 0.6 mg (1 amp) of inj. atropine given by IV route. Carefully watch for relapse of paralysis.
12. *Respiratory failure:* In respiratory muscle paralysis (by Elapidae group), ventilation by a respirator and proper control of blood gases should be employed.
13. Lately surgical debridement, fasciotomy or skin grafting may be needed.

- As the outcome of snake bite is unpredictable in the initial stage, all cases should be carefully monitored for at least first 12 hours. Dose of antivenin serum (AVS) in children is either equal or a bit more than the adult dose. Antibiotics covering gram-negative organisms and anaerobes are advocated in local infection.
- Spreading blisters suggest a massive dosage of venom. Vomiting, hypotension, bleeding from different sites are signs of systemic envenomation. Shock and AKI are common in Viperidae group. Wound debridement and skin grafting afterwards may be required, especially in cobra and viper bites. If no pulse is felt in a bitten limb, 'compartment syndrome' should be suspected and surgical help should be immediately sought for.

- **Conventional dosage schedule of AVS:**
  a. Only local swelling, no systemic symptoms—2–5 units.
  b. Systemic symptoms/haemorrhagic abnormalities—5–9 units.
  c. Severe systemic manifestations/shock—10–15 units.
- **Do not do:** Cruciate incision and suction over the fang marks, applying ice packs, tight ligatures and local antivenin infiltration, giving the victim alcoholic beverage or applying electric shock.
- In positive antivenin (AVS) skin test, pre-treat with H_1 and H_2 blockers and dilute the antivenin. Treat anaphylaxis with inj. adrenaline and inj. hydrocortisone. In spite of reactions, in a desperate situation, start the 'diluted' antivenin in a 'slow' infusion.

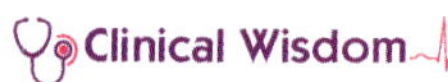

Do it 'RIGHT' in snakebite: **R**eassurance, **I**mmobilization of the extremity, **g**o to the **h**ospital and tell the doctor **t**elltale symptoms and signs.

DOG BITE

Dog bite may lead to rabies or tetanus infection and thus an immediately medical care is required.

Management

1. Bite wounds from dogs can range from minor to life-threatening. Immediately cleanse and scrub the wound vigorously with scap water, then flush with normal saline solution. Chemical treatment with any virucidal agent, e.g. alcohol, tincture iodine or povidone-iodine may now be done. Chemical cleansing with 1–4% benzalkonium chloride or 1% centrimonium bromide may be effective in inactivating the virus. If necessary, debride surgically. Do not put any suture to close the wound (i.e. left open).
2. Confine the dog and observe for at least 10 days, if possible.
3. Inj. Human Rabies Immunoglobulin (HRIG) 10 IU/kg is infiltrated around the bite and another 10 IU/kg is given by IM route in the gluteal region. If hyperimmune animal serum is available, double the dose. Always do intradermal test for any hypersensitivity reaction before giving the HRIG.
4. Inj. Human Diploid Cell Vaccine (HDCV): It is the safest and recommended vaccine, and 1 mL is given IM in the deltoid, on days 0, 3, 7, 14, 28 and 90. The dose on the day 90 is the booster dose. The first dose should be given as early as possible after the bite. According to few specialists, 5th dose on day 28 is no longer recommended (only for immunocompromised persons). Local reactions, e.g. swelling, erythema and induration at the injection site are not uncommon. This vaccine is costly. Pregnancy is not a contraindication for vaccination.
5. Inj. Human Tetanus Immunoglobulin (HTIG): 250 units by IM route stat (after skin test).
6. Inj. tetanus toxoid: 0.5 mL, IM stat and to be repeated after 1 month (0.5 mL, IM) and 6 month (0.5 mL, IM).
7. Inj. crystalline penicillin: 10 lac units, IM twice daily for 7 days after proper skin test. Co-amoxyclav (amoxycillin 500 mg + clauvulinic acid 125 mg) 625 mg, tds for 5 days is an alternative to penicillin. Moxifloxacin 400 mg, once daily, orally may be given in suspected mixed aerobic and anaerobic infection.
8. Observe the patient for development of any neurological abnormality. Allow normal diet.
9. If the dog dies or is killed, the brain should be examined for Negri bodies by immunofluorescence test in a specialised centre. In this situation, report to the concerned physician.

- HRIG is not given in every case. If the dog is suspected to be rabid, immediately start HRIG. If the dog is found to be healthy even after 10 days, probably it does not have rabies.
- Pre-exposure prophylaxis by HDCV in IM route may be given (persons at risk) on days 0,7, and 21 or 28 (3 doses in deltoid).
- If 7 days have elapsed after dog bite, it is not necessary to give HRIG because endogenous antibodies have already being produced.

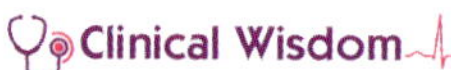

Infected dog bite may result in **rabies**, a disastrous viral disease affecting the central nervous sytem. Rabies may also result from bite of foxes, wolves, bats, cats and racoons. Hydrophobia (i.e. extreme or irrational fear of water) is a common symptom of rabies. It is a fatal disease, if not treated early.

SCORPION BITE (STING)

Scorpion stings pose a big problem in many regions of the world, often reported from rural areas, especially in developing countries like India. Common poisonous scorpions in India are black scorpion (Palamnaeus) and red scorpion (Mesobuthus). Scorpion stings are very painful but rarely life-threatening.

Black scorpion bite causes local symptoms while red scorpion bite develops into 'autonomic storm' (affecting parasympathetic system at the initial part while stimulating sympathetic nervous system later on).

Common symptoms are vomiting, sweating, hypotension, piloerection, abdominal colic, anxiety, cold extremities and diarrhoea. The signs of systemic involvement may be delayed for 24 hours.

Management

1. Wash the sting with soap and water. Apply ice packs to the wound. Apply tourniquet proximal to the site of bite. Reassurance.
2. Inj. pheniramine maleate 15 mg, IM stat or inj. promethazine hydrochloride 50 mg, IM stat is given.
3. Inj. tetanus toxoid: 0.5 mL, IM stat and to be repeated after 1 month (0.5 mL, IM) and 6 month (0.5 mL, IM).
4. Local infiltration (ring block) by inj. lignocaine hydrochloride (2%) without adrenaline usually

ameliorates the severe local pain. The usual dose is 2–5 mL which may be repeated after 1/2 hour. Local emetine or dehydroemetine also relieves pain but may produce tissue necrosis. NSAID (parenteral, IM) may be used to relieve pain.

5. Inj. antivenin (serotherapy): May be given IV in cranial nerve dysfunction and increased involuntary activity in sketetal muscles. Practically, this is not required in most of the patients. Specific antivenin, if available, should be administered at the earliest.
6. Inj. diazepam: 5–10 mg, IM stat if the patient becomes restless and anxious.
7. *Prazosin* (1 mg/tab), 1 tab stat and 0.25–0.5 mg every 4–6 hourly may be administered to control hypertension. It is the sheet-anchor and most promising drug in the prevention of cardio-pulmonary complications (e.g. pulmonary oedema) of scorpion bite. Prazosin is usually indicated in extremes of ages and severe poisoning.
8. Corticosteroid may be given in severe cases. Management of DIC (disseminated intravascular coagulation) should be done, if present. Infusion of glucose-insulin solution may be beneficial in systemic envenomation.
9. Others: IV fluid for dehydration, IV electrolytes for dyselectrolytaemia, dopamine infusion for hypotension, intubation and ventilation for respiratory failure, and furosemide for acute pulmonary oedema. Treatment for shock, DIC and mental obtundation are done accordingly. Always monitor the patient for arrhythmia, conduction abnormalities and arterial O_2 saturation.

Chapter 6

Drugs

"If every drug in the world were abolished, a physician would still be a useful member of the society"

— **Sir William Withey Gull (1816–1890)**

19th century English physician and an outstanding clinical teacher

Drugs	Dosage		Indications	Contraindications	Adverse effects
	Oral	Parenteral			
DRUGS ON AUTONOMIC NERVOUS SYSTEM					
ADRENALINE	—	0.2–0.5 mL, SC/IM (1 in 1000 in 1 mL)	1. Anaphylaxis 2. Cardiac resuscitation 3. Bronchial asthma 4. Arrest of haemorrhage in epistaxis or after tooth extraction	1. IHD 2. Systemic hypertension 3. Tachycardia 4. Cardiac dysrhythmia	1. Pain chest (angina) 2. Pallor, palpitation, anxiety, tremor, headache 3. Sudden elevation of BP 4. Ventricular dysrhythmia in patients with infarction
DOPAMINE	—	2.5–5 µg/kg/ min (diuresis) 5–10 µg/kg/ min (stimulates cardiac contraction)	1. Cardiogenic shock 2. Hypotension 3. Cardiac arrest 4. Refractory heart failure	Hypertrophic cardiomyopathy	1. Nausea, vomiting 2. Chest pain 3. Palpitations 4. Arrhythmias
DOBUTAMINE	—	2.5–10 µg/kg/min	Same as dopamine	Same as dopamine	Same as dopamine
BETA-BLOCKERS a. **(cardioselective:** atenolol, metoprolol, acebutol, bisoprolol, betaxolol, celiprolol, nebivolol, esmolol) b. **(Beta-blockers used in heart failure:** Carvedilol, metoprolol, bisoprolol, bucindolol)	Widely varies according to aetiology and beta-blocker with different mode of action, e.g. **propranolol** 10–320 mg, labetalol 200–800 mg	—	1. Migraine (prophylaxis) 2. Anxiety neurosis 3. Thyrotoxicosis 4. Glaucoma (open angle) 5. Portal hypertension (variceal bleeding) 6. Angina, systemic hypertension, SVT, anoxic spells of Fallot's tetralogy, IHSS, AMI 7. Pheochromocytoma 8. Essential tremor 9. Reduction of infarction (myocardial) size	1. Bronchial asthma 2. CCF 3. Heart block 4. Cardiogenic shock 5. Bradycardia 6. Patients on oral hypoglycaemic agents 7. Peripheral vascular disease	1. Bradycardia, heart block 2. Bronchospasm 3. CCF 4. Hypoglycaemic unresponsiveness in diabetes mellitus 5. Fatigability, depression 6. Constipation 7. Cold extremities 8. Nightmare, skin rash 9. Impotence

*Beta-blockers with intrinsic sympathomimetic activity are pindool and acebutol

Contd...

Drugs	Dosage: Oral	Dosage: Parenteral	Indications	Contraindications	Adverse effects
ATROPINE	0.6 mg tablet	0.6–12 mg (0.6 mg/mL)	1. Organophosphorus poisoning 2. Dysmenorrhoea and intestinal colic 3. Complete heart block 4. Pre-anaesthesia 5. For mydriasis and cycloplegia 6. For ophthalmoscopy 7. As an antidote to neostigmine	1. Glaucoma 2. Enlarged prostate 3. Psychosis 4. Pyloric stenosis 5. Paralytic ileus	1. Palpitation 2. Retention of urine 3. Blurring of vision 4. Psychosis 5. Precipitation of glaucoma 6. Paralytic ileus 7. Dry mouth
NEOSTIGMINE	15–30 mg	0.5–2 mg, SC or IM	1. Myasthenia gravis 2. Snakebite (Elapidae gr.) 3. Supraventricular tachycardia 4. Retention of urine, paralytic ileus 5. Curare poisoning	1. Hypersensitivity 2. Peritonitis	1. Salivation, sweating 2. Pain abdomen or diarrhoea 3. Pain chest 4. Tremor 5. Fasciculation
OXIMES (pralidoxime)	—	1 g, 8 hourly, IV slowly	Organophosphorus poisoning (malathion, parathion)	1. Hypersensitivity 2. Carbamate poisoning	1. Thrombophlebitis 2. Drowsiness 3. Diplopia 4. Palpitations 5. Giddiness
EPHEDRINE	30 mg	30 mg, SC or IM	1. Bronchial asthma 2. As a nasal decongestant 3. As a mydriatic 4. Nocturnal enuresis	Same as adrenaline	Same as adrenaline
EDROPHONIUM	—	10 mg, IM (10 mg/mL)	To diagnose myasthenia gravis	Same as neostigmine	Same as neostigmine
DRUGS USED IN BRONCHIAL ASTHMA/AIRWAYS OBSTRUCTION					
SALBUTAMOL	4 mg, 8 hourly	100 µg per puff by inhalation	1. Bronchial asthma 2. Hyperkalaemic periodic paralysis	1. Cardiac tachyarrhythmia 2. Narrow angle glaucoma	1. Tremor 2. Palpitations 3. Nervousness 4. Hypokalaemia
TERBUTALINE	5 mg, 8 hourly	500 µg per puff by inhalation	Bronchial asthma	Same as salbutamol	Same as salbutamol
ISOPRENALINE	5–20 mg, sublingually	0.5 mL of 1: 200 solution by inhalation. 1–10 mg/min by IV route	1. Bronchial asthma 2. Stokes-Adams syndrome 3. Heart block 4. Severe bradycardia 5. Shock	1. IHD 2. Tachycardia 3. Recent AMI	1. Tremor, flushing 2. Arrhythmia 3. Chest pain 4. Anxiety 5. Headache
AMINOPHYLLINE	—	Loading dose: 6 mg/kg Followed by: 0.5–1 mg/kg/hr (mixed with N. saline or 5% dextrose)	1. Bronchial asthma 2. Cardiac asthma 3. As a diuretic 4. Sometimes in heart failure 5. Sometimes in COPD	1. Convulsions 2. Arrhythmia 3. Vomiting 4. Palpitation	1. Vomiting 2. Collapse 3. Convulsions 4. Headache
EPHEDRINE	See drugs on autonomic nervous system				

Contd...

Drugs	Dosage: Oral	Dosage: Parenteral	Indications	Contraindications	Adverse effects
THEOPHYLLINE	100–600 mg	3-5 mg/kg, IM or IV	Bronchial asthma	Same as aminophylline	Same as aminophylline
DISODIUM CROMOGLYCATE (OR NEDOCROMIL SODIUM)	—	20 mg, 6 hourly by inhalation (or 4 mg, QDS/d)	Prophylaxis for acute episode of br. asthma	1. Acute asthmatic attacks 2. Status asthmaticus 3. Allergic rhinitis	1. Local irritation 2. Wheezing, breathlessness
IPRATROPIUM BROMIDE	—	20 µg/puff by inhalation, 2 puffs, 8 hourly	1. COPD 2. Acute bronchial asthma, especially with coexistent cardiac disorders 3. Acute attack of chronic bronchitis	1. Very old age 2. Where rapid action with highest potency is required	Mild anticholinergic side effect may occur
KETOTIFEN	1–2 mg, 12 hourly/day	—	1. Prophylaxis of bronchial asthma 2. Allergic rhinitis or conjunctivitis	1. Hypersensitivity 2. Glaucoma	1. Drowsiness 2. Increased appetite 3. Weight gain 4. Thrombocytopenia (rare)

*Systemic corticosteroids like prednisolone, betamethasone, dexamethasone or hydrocortisone may be used; beclomethasone dipropionate (100 µg, QDS), budesonide (100 µg, BD) or fluticasone (up to 2000 µg/day) may be administered by inhaler. Anticholinergic drugs used are ipratropium bromide, tiotropium bromide or oxitropium bromide. Leukotriene antagonist like montelukast (10 mg, orally, once daily) or zafirlukast (20 mg, orally, BD) or zileuton (800 mg, OD) controls mild to moderate persistent bronchial asthma.

Drugs	Dosage: Oral	Dosage: Parenteral	Indications	Contraindications	Adverse effects
DRUGS USED IN SYSTEMIC HYPERTENSION					
ALPHA METHYLDOPA	250–750 mg, 8 hourly	—	1. Syst. hypertension 2. Malignant hypertension 3. Hypertension with pregnancy	CVA (the drug produces drowsiness)	1. Sedation 2. Haemolytic anaemia 3. Diarrhoea 4. Gynaecomastia 5. Chronic active hepatitis 6. Lupus-like syndrome
CLONIDINE	0.1–0.6 mg, 2–4 times/day	—	1. Syst. hypertension 2. Prophylaxis of migraine 3. Autonomic neuropathy in diabetes mellitus (nocturnal diarrhoea)	1. Hepatic coma 2. Sick sinus syndrome 3. Pheochromocytoma with hypertension	1. Postural hypotension 2. Drowsiness 3. Impotence 4. Dry mouth 5. Rebound hypertension after abrupt withdrawal
NIFEDIPINE (not used commonly)	5–20 mg, 8 hourly	—	1. Syst. hypertension 2. Hypertensive emergencies (rarely used) 3. IHD (chronic stable angina, Prinzmetal's angina) 4. Raynaud's phenomenon	1. Hypotension 2. Cardiogenic shock 3. Acute myocardial infarction 4. 2nd or 3rd degree heart block	1. Tachycardia 2. Ankle oedema 3. Flushing 4. Hyperplasia of gum 5. Hyperkalaemia 6. Headache 7. Constipation
AMLODIPINE	2.5–10 mg, 12–24 hourly	—	Same as nifedipine	Same as nifedipine	Same as nifedipine

Contd...

Drugs	Dosage: Oral	Dosage: Parenteral	Indications	Contraindications	Adverse effects
*CAPTOPRIL	12.5–75 mg, 12 hourly	—	1. Systemic hypertension 2. CCF 3. Renal crisis of scleroderma 4. Diabetic nephropathy 5. Postmyocardial infarction	1. Pregnancy 2. Renal failre 3. Bilateral renal artery stenosis 4. Aortic stenosis	1. Cough (dry) 2. Hyperkalaemia 3. Pancytopenia 4. Disturbance of taste 5. Fever, pruritus, rash
*Other ACE inhibitors are **ramipril** (1.25, 2.5, 5, 10 mg), perindopril (2, 4, 8 mg), **lisinopril** (5, 10, 20, 40 mg), benazepril (5, 10, 20, 40 mg), fosinopril (10, 20 mg) and quinapril (5, 10, 20, 40 mg).					
ENALAPRIL	2.5–40 mg daily	—	Same as captopril		
BETA-BLOCKERS	—	—	See drugs on autonomic nervous system (atenolol and metoprolol mainly)		
INDAPAMIDE (a diuretic)	2.5 mg/day	—	Essential hypertension	1. Severe renal or hepatic failure 2. Hypokalaemia	1. Hyperuricaemia 2. Na^+, K^+ and H_2O depletion 3. Dizziness
PRAZOSIN (alpha-blocker)	1–10 mg,12 hourly	—	1. Syst. hypertension 2. CCF 3. Pheochromocytoma 4. Benign hypertrophy of prostate	1. CCF due to mechanical obstruction 2. Hypotension	1. Postural hypotension 2. Dry mouth 3. Sudden syncope 4. Palpitations 5. Dizziness
RESERPINE (not used now)	0.05–0.25 mg daily	0.5–2.5 mg, IV or IM	1. Syst. hypertension 2. Hypertensive emergencies	1. Peptic ulcer 2. Depression 3. Suicidal tendency 4. Epilepsy	1. Nasal congestion 2. Depression 3. Diarrhoea 4. Dyspepsia 5. Parkinsonism 6. Postural hypotension 7. Impotence
HYDRALAZINE	10–75 mg, 6 hourly	10–50 mg, IV or IM	1. Syst. hypertension 2. Renal diseases with hypertension 3. Malignant hypertension 4. Hypertension with pregnancy	1. Severe IHD 2. SLE	1. Angina pectoris 2. Lupus-like syndrome (SLE) 3. Headache 4. Dizziness 5. Palpitation
SODIUM NITROPRUSSIDE	—	0.5–8 μg/kg/min, IV	1. Malignant hypertension 2. LVF, not responding to other drugs	Hypersensitivity	1. Sweating 2. Cyanide toxicity 3. Apprehension
DIAZOXIDE	—	1–5 mg/kg upto 150 mg rapidly; repeated after 5 min.	1. Malignant hypertension 2. Hypertensive emergencies	1. Severe IHD 2. SLE 3. CVA	1. Angina pectoris 2. Hirsutism 3. Hyperuricaemia 4. Hyperglycaemia 5. Fluid retention
*LOSARTAN POTASSIUM (specific angiotensin-II receptor blocker—ARB)	25–50 mg, once daily	—	1. Systemic hypertension 2. Hypertension with gout	1. Pregnancy 2. Hypersensitivity 3. Renal failure	1. Dizziness 2. Orthostatic hypotension 3. Palpitations 4. Dry mouth 5. Cough (rare) 6. Skin rash
*Other ARBs in this group are candesartan (4, 8, 16, 32 mg), irbesartan (75, 150, 300 mg), valsartan (40, 80, 160, 320 mg), **telmisartan** (20, 40, 80 mg), eprosartan (400, 600 mg) and **olmesartan** (5, 20, 40 mg).					

Contd...

Drugs	Dosage: Oral	Dosage: Parenteral	Indications	Contraindications	Adverse effects
LABETALOL	200–400 mg/ day	—	1. Hypertensive emergencies 2. Syst. hypertension 3. Hypertension with pregnancy 4. Clonidine withdrawal	1. 2nd and 3rd degree heart block 2. Bronchospasm 3. Cardiogenic shock	1. Headache 2. Postural hypotension 3. Nightmares
DIURETICS					
FUROSEMIDE	20–80 mg, 8 or 12 hourly/ day (40 mg/tab)	Same as oral dosage (20 mg/2 mL)	1. Mild syst. hypertension 2. Oedematous states 3. CCF 4. Acute pulm. oedema (LVF) 5. Cerebral oedema 6. Forced diuresis 7. Hypertensive emergencies	1. Hypotension 2. Hypokalaemia 3. Hepatic precoma	1. Hyponatraemia 2. Hypokalaemia 3. Hyperglycaemia 4. Pancreatitis 5. Tinnitus (high dose) 6. Hyperuricaemia 7. Weakness
BUMETANIDE	0.5–2 mg/day	0.5–1 mg once, IV or IM	Same as above but it is more potent (1 mg bumetanide = 40 mg furosemide)		
HYDROCHLORO-THIAZIDE	12.5–25 mg, 8 or 12 hourly/day	—	Same as above. Acts best in cardiac oedema		
SPIRONOLACTONE (aldosterone antagonist)	100–400 mg/ day	—	1. Cirrhosis of liver 2. Renal oedema 3. Congestive cardiac failure 4. Primary hyper-aldosteronism 5. To counteract K^+ loss due to loop diuretic and thiazides	1. Hyperkalaemia 2. Addison's disease	1. Gynaecomastia 2. Hyperkalaemia 3. Diarrhoea 4. Menstrual irregularities 5. Confusion
*Eplerenone, like spironolactone, is another aldosterone receptor antagonist.					
TRIAMTERENE	100–200 mg/ day	—	Same as spironolactone	Same as spironolactone	1. Leg cramps 2. Nephrolithiasis 3. Hyperkalaemia 4. Diarrhoea 5. Dry mouth
AMILORIDE	5–10 mg/day	—	Same as spironolactone	Same as spironolactone	1. Dry mouth 2. Hyperkalaemia 3. Muscle cramps
ACETAZOLAMIDE	250–500 mg/ day in divided dosage	—	1. As diuretic 2. Glaucoma 3. Resistant epilepsy 4. Periodic paralysis 5 Prevention of high-altitude pulmonary oedema	1. Hepatic disorders 2. Hyperchloraemic acidosis	1. Hypokalaemia 2. Acidosis (metabolic) 3. Bone marrow depression 4. Drowsiness 5. Paraesthesia
MANNITOL (20%)	—	1.5–2 mg/kg, IV very rapidly	1. Cerebral oedema 2. Poisoning (e.g. barbiturate) 3. Acute renal failure (pre-renal shutdown) 4. Hepatic pre-coma 5. To reduce intraocular tension (when others fail) 6. Forced diuresis in haemolytic reaction after blood transfusion	1. Cerebral haemorrhage 2. Electrolyte disturbance	1. Electrolyte disturbance (hyponatraemia, hypokalaemia) 2. Rebound increase in intracranial tension 3. Pulmonary oedema

*__Loop diuretics__ are furosemide, bumetanide, ethacrynic acid (25–100 mg, BD/TDS, orally), mefruside (12.5–50 mg once a day, orally) and torsemide (5–100 mg/ day, once orally). **Thiazide diuretics** are hydrochlorothiazide, chlorthalidone (12.5–50 mg, once daily, orally), metolazone (0.5–20 mg, OD, orally) and indapamide (1.25–5 mg, once daily, orally). **Potassium-sparing diuretics** are spironolactone, triamterine and amiloride. **Carbonic anhydrase inhibitor** is acetazolamide, and **osmotic diuretic** is mannitol.

Contd...

Drugs	Dosage		Indications	Contraindications	Adverse effects
	Oral	Parenteral			
ANTI-ANGINAL DRUGS					
NITRATES: a. Glyceryl trinitrate	0.2–0.6 mg, sublingual 2.5–6.5 mg, oral	2% skin ointment	1. Angina pectoris 2. LVF 3. Pulmonary hypertension 4. Unstable angina 5. Cyanide poisoning	1. Glaucoma 2. Hypertrophic cardiomyopathy 3. Hypotension	1. Headache 2. Flushing 3. Dizziness 4. Syncopal attack
b. Isosorbide dinitrate	2.5–5 mg, sublingual 10–40 mg, oral	—	1. As above 2. Portal hypertension 3. Achalasia cardia	As above	As above
c. Isosorbide mononitrate	10–20 mg, orally at 8 AM and 3 PM—eccentric dosage schedule	—	1. As isosorbide dinitrate 2. Pulmonary hypertension 3. Postmyocardial infarction	As above	1. As above 2. Sweating 3. Palpitation 4. Throbbing headache
d. Pentaerythritol tetranitrate	40–80 mg/day, orally	—	Same as above (principally used in IHD)	As above	As above
OXYFEDRINE	24–48 mg/day	—	1. Angina pectoris 2. Acute myocardial infarction	1. Obstructive cardiomyopathy 2. Aortic incompetence	1. Giddiness 2. Nausea 3. Constipation 4. Headache
NIFEDIPINE	Vide antihypertensive drugs				
AMLODIPINE	Vide antihypertensive drugs				
ATENOLOL	50–100 mg/day, single daily use	—	Vide drugs on autonomic nervous system		
PROPRANOLOL	80–240 mg/day in divided dosage	—	Vide drugs (beta-blockers) on autonomic nervous system		
TRIMETAZIDINE	40–60 mg/day in divided dosage	—	1. Angina pectoris (stable) 2. Unstable angina 3. Postmyocardial infarction	Hypersensitivity	1. Headache 2. Nausea and vomiting 3. GI disturbance
VERAPRAMIL	40–80 mg, 8 hourly	10 mg, IV in PSVT	1. Angina pectoris 2. PSVT, atrial fibrillation or flutter 3. Extrasystoles 4. Hypertensive emergencies 5. Portal hypertension 6. Angina due to obst. cardiomyopathy	1. 2nd and 3rd degree heart block 2. CCF 3. Sick sinus syndrome 4. Hypotension 5. AMI	1. Headache 2. Palpitations 3. Hypotension 4. Constipation
DILTIAZEM	30–240 mg/day in divided doses 60–120 mg, 12 hourly in sustained release form	20 mg, IV bolus in PSVT	As above	1. As above 2. WPW syndrome	1. Dry mouth 2. Headache 3. CCF 4. Bradycardia 5. Flushing

Contd...

Drugs	Dosage: Oral	Dosage: Parenteral	Indications	Contraindications	Adverse effects
NICORANDIL (K^+ channel activator)	10–30 mg in twice daily dose	—	Angina pectoris	1. Hypotension 2. LVF 3. Cardiogenic shock	1. Headache 2. Flushing 3. Tachycardia 4. Vomiting
RANOLAZINE (inhibitor of late inward Na^+ current)	500–1000 mg in twice daily dose	—	Chronic angina pectoris who continues to be symptomatic despite a standard medical treatment	1. Hepatic failure 2. Renal failure 3. Drugs producing QT-prolongation (quinidine and with ketoconazole	QT-prolongation in ECG
IVABRADINE	5–7.5 mg, twice daily	—	Chronic stable angina pectoris without heart failure	1. Bradycardia 2. Sick sinus syndrome 3. Heart failure 4. With CCBs	1. Bradycardia 2. Dizziness 3. Blurred vision 4. Headache 5. Heart block

*__Calcium-channel blockers (CCBs)__ are classified into three groups according to their chemical structure like:

- Benzothiazepines—Diltiazem
- Phenylalkylamines—Verapramil
- Dihydropyridines—Amlodipine, nifedipine, nicardipine, felodipine, nisoldipine, bepridil, lacidipine, lercanidipine and isradipine

ANTIARRHYTHMIC DRUGS

Drugs	Dosage: Oral	Dosage: Parenteral	Indications	Contraindications	Adverse effects
QUINIDINE	200–400 mg, 4–6 hourly	IV, 800 mg diluted in 50 mL of 5% dextrose and given at 1mL/min	1. Atrial fibrillation and flutter 2. PSVT 3. Ventricular premature beats 4. VT, ventricular fibrillation 5. Hiccough (intractable) 6. Malaria	1. Heart block 2. Hypotension 3. Myasthenia gravis	1. Bradycardia 2. Hypotension 3. Vomiting, diarrhoea 4. Cinchonism 5. Convulsions 6. Thrombocytopenia, anaemia
PROCAINAMIDE	250–500 mg, 4–6 hourly	IV: 500 mg loading dose, followed by 2 mg/kg/hour IM: 100–500 mg	Same as quinidine	Same as quinidine	1. Pancytopenia (especially agranulocytosis) 2. Lupus-like syndrome (SLE) 3. Psychosis 4. QT-prolongation
DISOPYRAMIDE	100–300 mg 6–8 hourly	—	Same as quinidine	Same as quinidine	1. Blurred vision 2. Constipation 3. Retention of urine 4. Feeling faint 5. Myoc. depression 6. Dry mouth
LIGNOCAINE (LIDOCAINE)	—	1 mg/kg as bolus dose followed by 0.5 mg/kg bolus at 8–10 min interval to 3 mg/kg, IV in 5% dextrose	1. Ventricular premature beats 2. VT, ventricular fibrillation (especially in the setting of AMI) 3. Nerve block, anaesthesia	1. Heart block 2. Cardiac decompensation	1. Confusion 2. Convulsions 3. Respiratory arrest 4. Drowsiness 5. Hypotension
MEXILETINE	400 mg initially; then 200–250 mg, 6–8 hourly	250 mg, IV slowly	Same as 1 and 2 of lignocaine	1. Heart block 2. Cardiogenic shock	1. Nausea, vomiting, bad taste 2. Drowsiness, confusion, blurred vision 3. Hypotension, bradycardia

Contd...

Drugs	Dosage		Indications	Contraindications	Adverse effects
	Oral	Parenteral			
PHENYTOIN SODIUM	100–200 mg, 6 hourly	100 mg, slow IV, in every 5 minutes	1. SVT and VT 2. Ventricular extrasystoles 3. Digitalis-induced arrhythmias	1. Sinus bradycardia 2. SA block 3. Stokes-Adams syndrome	1. Gum hypertrophy 2. Megaloblastic anaemia 3. Cerebellar ataxia 4. Hirsutism 5. Hypotension 6. Confusion
PROPRANOLOL	10–200 mg, 6 hourly	IV: 0.5–1 mg/min to 0.15–0.2 mg/kg	Vide autonomic nervous system (beta-blockers)		
VERAPRAMIL	40–80 mg, 8 hourly	—	Vide anti-anginal drugs		
AMIODARONE	200–600 mg, 6 hourly	IV given for VT–15 mg/min as infusion for 10 min followed by 1 mg/min for 6 hrs for next few days	1. Vent. arrhythmias refractory to other treatment 2. VT 3. Tachyarrhythmia due to WPW syndrome 4. Atrial fibrillation and flutter 5. Paroxysmal tachyarrhythmia	1. Heart block 2. Cardiogenic shock	1. Hepatitis 2. Pulmonary fibrosis 3. Microdeposits in cornea 4. Bluish skin 5. Bradycardia 6. QT-prolongation 7. Thyroid abnormalities 8. Photosensitivity
DILTIAZEM	120–360 mg/day	IV: 5–15 mg/hr	Vide anti-anginal drugs		
DIGOXIN	0.25–1.5 mg over 24 hrs	0.5–1 mg	1. CCF 2. Atrial fibrillation and flutter 3. PSVT 4. Sometimes in LVF 5. As an inotropic drug	1. AMI 2. Partial heart block 3. Myocarditis 4. Ventricular tachycardia (VT) 5. High output failure	1. All types of cardiac arrhythmia except Mobitz type II block and parasystole 2. Especially ventricular bigeminy 3. Anorexia, nausea, vomiting 4. Yellow vision 5. Gynaecomastia
ADENOSINE	—	IV: 6–12 mg bolus; if no response, after 2 minutes give 12 mg bolus	Supraventricular tachyarrhythmias	1. Hypotension 2. Bronchial asthma 3. 2°/3° AV block 4. Atrial fibrillation	1. Transient atrial standstill 2. Hypotension 3. Flushing 4. Chest pain
ISOPRENALINE	—	2 mg in 500 mL of 5% dextrose solution	1. 2° AV block 2. Ventricular tachycardia with block 3. Beta-blocker overdose 4. Bronchial asthma	1. Tachyarrhythmias 2. Recent AMI 3. Angina	1. Flushing, headache 2. Palpitations 3. Angina 4. Anxiety 5. Tremor
ANALGESICS, ANTIPYRETICS AND ANTI-INFLAMMATORY DRUGS					
ACETYL SALICYLIC ACID (aspirin)	300–500 mg, 8 hourly; up to 4–8 g/day	—	1. Analgesic 2. Antipyretic 3. Anti-inflammatory 4. IHD (75–300 mg/day) 5. TIA (75–300 mg/day) 6. Rheumatic fever	1. GI bleeding 2. Gout (in low dose) 3. Bronchial asthma 4. Bleeding tendency 5. Dengue fever	1. Nausea, vomiting, GI bleeding 2. Salicylism (vertigo, tinnitus) 3. Wheeze and breathlessness 4. Reye's syndrome 5. Bleeding tendency

Contd...

Drugs

Drugs	Dosage		Indications	Contraindications	Adverse effects
	Oral	Parenteral			
PARACETAMOL	500–1 g/day; up to 4 g/day	Pre-filled vial 1000 mg/ 100 mL—1000 mg, 8 hourly	Analgesic (e.g. headache, toothache, osteoarthritis) and antipyretic actions	Hepatic pre-coma	1. Skin rash 2. Nausea and vomiting 3. Large doses (10 g) produce hepatic failure 4. Leucopenia (rare)
NIMESULIDE (not recommended in children)	100 mg, 12 hourly	—	1. 1, 2 and 3 of aspirin 2. Any painful condition in the body	1. Active peptic ulcer 2. Severe hepatic impairment	1. Heartburn and epigastric distress 2. Nausea and vomiting 3. Dizziness 4. Pruritus
INDOMETHACIN (banned in many countries	50–200 mg/day in divided doses	—	1. Acute gout 2. Rheumatoid arthritis 3. Osteoarthritis 4. Ankylosing spondylitis 5. Dysmenorrhoea 6. Bartter's syndrome 7. PDA in neonates	1. Active peptic ulcer 2. Bronchial asthma	1. Pain abdomen 2. Haematemesis, melaena 3. Breathlessness 4. Giddiness, blurred vision 5. Skin rash
PENTAZOCINE	25–100 mg	60–120 mg, IM or IV	Chronic/recurrent pain associated with: 1. Surgery, colic, burn, trauma 2. Pre-anaesthesia 3. Intense headache 4. Often used in the place of morphine in acut LVF or AMI	1. Respiratory depression 2. Head injury 3. Raised intra-cranial tension	1. Respiratory depression 2. Hallucination and nightmares 3. Dizziness, confusion and drowsiness 4. Nausea and vomiting
MORPHINE	10–15 mg	10–15 mg, IM, IV or SC	1. Analgesic, hypnotic and sedative 2. Antitussive 3. Acute LVF 4. Pre-anaesthesia 5. Relief of prolonged and intractable pain	1. Acute hepatic disorder 2. Respiratory depression 3. Paralytic ileus 4. COPD or bronchial asthma	1. Respiratory depression 2. Bronchoconstriction 3. Constipation 4. Drug dependence and tolerance 5. Retention of urine (old age) 6. Nausea, vomiting
PETHIDINE	—	50–100 mg IM or IV	Same as morphine	Same as morphine	Same as morphine
ANTIHISTAMINICS AND ANTI-5HT DRUGS					
A. ANTIHISTAMINICS: 1. Chlorpheniramine maleate 2. Promethazine 3. Diphenhydramine 4. Pheniramine maleate 5. Dimetindene maleate 6. Hydroxyzine 7. Azatadine 8. Clemastine 9. Mizolastine 10. Ketotifen	5–20 mg 10–25 mg 25–75 mg 25–75 mg 1–2 mg, 8 hourly 10–25 mg, 8 hourly 1 mg, 12 hourly 1 mg, 8 or 12 hourly 10 mg 1–2 mg, 12 hourly	5–20 mg, IM 25–50 mg, IM 10 mg, IM — — — — — — — —	1. Allergic disorders: Pruritus, urticaria, rhinorrhoea, hay fever, angio-oedema, drug rash, common cold 2. Motion sickness (diphenhydramine) 3. As hypnotic 4. Pre-anaesthesia	1. Hypersensitivity 2. Skillful works like drivers, machine operators, pilot	1. Sedation, fatigue 2. Dry mouth, blurred vision 3. Excitation (children) 4. Urinary difficulty

Contd...

Drugs	Dosage: Oral	Dosage: Parenteral	Indications	Contraindications	Adverse effects
B. ANTIHISTAMINICS: (non-sedative effect) 1. Astemizole 2. Terfenadine 3. Loratidine 4. Cetrizine 5. Fexofenadine 6. Desloratadine 7. Levocetrizine	 10 mg 60 mg, 12 hourly 10 mg 5–10 mg 120 mg 5 mg 5 mg	 — — — — — — —	Same as above	—	As above (less or no sedation)
C. ANTI-5HT: 1. Cyproheptadine	4–20 mg	— —	1. As above 2. For stimulation of appetite 3. Prophylaxis of migraine 4. Diarrhoea in carcinoid syndrome	As above	As above
2. Methysergide	6–8 mg		As cyproheptadine	As cyproheptadine	As cyproheptadine

*$5HT_3$-antagonists are ondansetron and granisetron, which are used in chemotherapy-induced nausea and vomiting.

SEDATIVES AND ANTIPSYCHOTIC DRUGS

Drugs	Oral	Parenteral	Indications	Contraindications	Adverse effects
PHENOTHIAZINES (e.g. chlorpromazine)	100–800 mg	25 mg/mL, IM	1. Schizophrenia 2. Anxiety, mania 3. Hyperexcitability 4. Aggressive disorder 5. Hiccough 6. Porphyria 7. Nausea 8. Hyperpyrexia 9. Tetanus	1. Coma 2. Along with other CNS depressants 3. Bone marrow depression	1. Drowsiness 2. Obstructive jaundice 3. Leucopenia and thrombocytopenia 4. Tardive dyskinesia 5. Skin pigmentation 6. Hypotension
HALOPERIDOL	0.25–20 mg, 8 hourly	2–10 mg, IM or IV	1. Schizophrenia 2. Manic disorders 3. Organic psychosis 4. Highly agitated patients	Same as above but with less sedative effect	
DIAZEPAM	5–10 mg, 8 hourly	10–20 mg, IV	1. Tranquilliser 2. Pre-anaesthesia 3. Muscle relaxant 4. Sleep disorder, anxiety, delirium tremens 5. Convulsive disorders 6. Tetanus 7. Eclampsia 8. Status epilepticus	1. Respiratory depression 2. Acute narrow-angle glaucoma 3. Myasthenia gravis	1. Drowsiness 2. Respiratory depression 3. Ataxia 4. Blurred vision 5. Slurred speech 6. Confusion 7. Change in libido 8. Addiction
ZOPICLONE	3.75–7.5 mg at bed time	—	1. Transient, situational or chronic insomnia 2. Physical and mental stress	1. Myasthenia gravis 2. Severe sleep apnoea syndrome 3. Pregnancy, lactation	1. Metallic after-taste 2. Impaired judgement 3. Dry mouth 4. Dependence
ZOLPIDEM	10 mg at bed time	—	Short-term treatment of insomnia	Same as zopiclone	Same as zopiclone

Contd...

Drugs	Dosage: Oral	Dosage: Parenteral	Indications	Contraindications	Adverse effects
IMIPRAMINE	50–150 mg	—	1. Depression 2. Nocturnal enuresis 3. Narcolepsy 4. Diabetic neuropathy 5. Migraine 6. Bulimia 7. Irritable bowel syndrome	1. Manic phase of MDP 2. Acute myocardial infarction 3. Benign hypertrophy of prostate	1. Drowsiness 2. Dry mouth and other anti-cholinergic effects 3. Palpitations 4. Weight gain 5. Constipation
AMITRIPTYLINE	75–150 mg	—	Same as imipramine	Same as imipramine	Same as imipramine
FLUOXETINE (SSRI)	20 mg	—	1. Depression (where sedation is not wanted) 2. Obsessive compulsive disorders	1. Mania 2. Severe renal impairment	1. Insomnia 2. Fatigue 3. Sexual dysfunction
SERTRALINE (SSRI)	25–100 mg	—	1. Depression with anxiety 2. Panic disorders 3. Obsessive compulsive disorder	1. Concurrent administration of MAOI 2. Hepatic insufficiency	1. Dry mouth 2. Tremor 3. Dizziness 4. Rash 5. Insomnia
DULOXETINE (SNRI)	20–120 mg	—	1. Fibromyalgia 2. Musculoskeletal pain 3. Depression 4. Stress incontinence (urinary) 5. Neuropathic pain	1. Hypersensitivity 2. With MAO inhibitors 3. With thioridazine	1. Dry mouth 2. Dizziness 3. Agitation 4. Tiredness 5. Increased sweating 6. Sexual problems
*SNRI—Serotonin-noradrenaline reuptake inhibitor.					
LITHIUM	900–1500 mg (therapeutic blood level: 0.5–1.3 mEq/L)	—	1. Acute hypomania, mania 2. Recurrent depression 3. SIADH 4. Cluster headache 5. Prophylaxis of MDP 6. Idiopathic thrombocytopenic purpura	1. Electrolyte disturbance 2. Dehydration 3. Severe renal impairment	1. Confusion and incoordination 2. Blurred vision 3. Nausea and diarrhoea 4. Ataxia, slurred speech 5. Goitre 6. Diabetes insipidus
OLANZAPINE	5–20 mg	—	1. Schizophrenia and related psychosis 2. Acute mania in bipolar disorder	1. Narrow-angle glaucoma 2. Lactation	1. Somnolence 2. Weight gain 3. Akathisia 4. Tardive dyskinesia
ESCITALOPRAM (SSRI)	10–20 mg once daily		1. Depression 2. Panic disorder with or without agoraphobia 3. Obsessive compulsive disorder	1. Pregnancy and lactation 2. <18 yrs of age 3. Serotonin syndrome 4. Within 14 days of use of MAOI	1. Suicidal tendency 2. Worsening of depression 3. Acute psychosis 4. Sexual dysfunction
*SSRI—Selective serotonin reuptake inhibitor.					
THIORIDAZINE	150–600 mg	—	1. Schizophrenia 2. Mania 3. Behavioural disturbances	1. Extrapyramidal reactions 2. Severe hepatic or renal dysfunction	1. Drowsiness, dry mouth 2. Retinal damage 3. Unsteadiness 4. Sexual dysfunction

Contd...

Drugs	Dosage: Oral	Dosage: Parenteral	Indications	Contraindications	Adverse effects
RISPERIDONE	(Initial dose: 2 mg/d); 4–16 mg in d/d	—	1. Schizophrenia 2. Bipolar mania 3. Autism 4. Mood stabilizer	1. Hypersensitivity 2. Tardive dyskinesia 3. Parkinsonism 4. Breast carcinoma	1. Unsteadiness 2. Dizziness 3. Drooling 4. Weight gain 5. Drowsiness 6. Neuroleptic malignant syndrome (NMS) 7. Risk of suicide
ALPRAZOLAM	0.25–0.5 mg, 8 or 12 hourly	—	1. Anxiety disorders 2. Panic and phobic disorders	1. Acute narrow-angle glaucoma 2. Myasthenia gravis	1. Drowsiness 2. Lack of coordination 3. Impairment of memory
BARBITURATES	See antiepileptic drugs				
ANTIEPILEPTIC DRUGS					
PHENOBARBITONE	60–180 mg in divided doses	60–400 mg, IV	1. Epilepsy (tonic-clonic and focal) 2. Ecclampsia 3. Mania 4. As sedative and hypnotic 5. In jaundice to increase conjugation of bilirubin 6. Pre-anaesthesia	1. Sinus bradycardia 2. AV block 3. Acute porphyria	1. Drowsiness 2. Confusion 3. Fixed drug eruption 4. Addiction 5. Megaloblastic anaemia
PRIMIDONE	125 mg QDS to 250 mg QDS/day (it is converted to phenobarbitone in the body)	—	Used alone or with other medications for treating grand mal, psychomotor or focal epileptic seizures	1. Allergy to barbiturates 2. Porphyria (acute) 3. Megaloblastic anaemia	1. Drowsiness 2. Headache 3. Vertigo 4. Ataxia
PHENYTOIN SODIUM	300–400 mg, usually in divided doses	13–18 mg/kg, IV (in N. saline)	1. Epilepsy (tonic-clonic, focal, complex partial) 2. Trigeminal neuralgia 3. Cardiac arrhythmia 4. Diabetic neuropathy 5. Chorea	1. SA block, Stokes-Adams syndrome 2. Acute porphyria	1. Gum hyperplasia 2. Lymphadenopathy 3. Megaloblastic anaemia 4. Hirsutism 5. Osteomalacia 6. CNS depression 7. Ataxia, incoordination, confusion
CARBAMAZEPINE	100–200 mg, 8 hourly	—	1. Epilepsy (tonic-clonic, focal, complex partial) 2. Trigeminal neuralgia 3. Diabetic neuropathy 4. Post-herpetic neuralgia 5. Lightening pain of tabes 6. Movement disorders 7. Diabetes insipidus	1. Bone marrow depression 2. Jaundice	1. Bone marrow depression 2. Stevens-Johnson syndrome 3. Vertigo 4. Ataxia, diplopia, dizziness 5. Hepatotoxicity

Contd...

Drugs	Dosage: Oral	Dosage: Parenteral	Indications	Contraindications	Adverse effects
SODIUM VALPROATE	750–1250 mg/day	—	1. Epilepsy (absence, atypical absence attack, psychomotor and myoclonic epilepsy) 2. To prevent febrile convulsions in children 3. Prophylactic treatment of migraine	1. Hepatic disorder 2. Thrombocytopenia	1. Sedation 2. Fulminant hepatitis 3. Alopecia 4. Bone marrow depression
GABAPENTIN	300 mg on 1st day, 600 mg on 2nd day 900 mg on 3rd day and continued as 900 mg/day	—	1. Adjunctive therapy of partial seizures, not controlled by other drugs 2. Neuropathic pain	Hypersensitivity	1. Somnolence 2. Ataxia 3. Tremor 4. Nystagmus 5. Headache
CLONAZEPAM	1–12 mg/day	—	Epilepsy, e.g. infantile spasm, myoclonic, atonic, absence seizures; panic attacks, as sedative (0.25–0.5 mg)	1. Respiratory depression 2. Hypersensitivity	1. Drowsiness 2. Unsteadiness 3. Forgetfulness 4. Confusion 5. Lethargy
DIAZEPAM	5–40 mg	10 mg, IV bolus	Vide sedatives and antipsychotic drugs		
PREGABALIN	75–600 mg daily (usually 75–150 mg) in divided doses	—	1. Adjunctive therapy in partial seizures 2. Neuropathic pain (e.g. carpal tunnel syndrome, root pain) 3. Fibromyalgia	1. Lactation 2. Skillful works, e.g. pilot	1. Somnolence, euphoria, confusion 2. Decreased libido, fatigue
*Newer antiepileptic drugs tiagabine (4–12 mg tds/d), vigabatrin (1–3 g/d), lamotrigine (100–500 mg/bd), felbamate (2400–3600 mg/day) and topiramate (300–600 mg/day) are used in refractory epilepsy. **Levetiracetam** (500 mg–3 g/d) is an effective antiepileptic drug.					
ANTI-PARKINSONIAN DRUGS					
LEVODOPA	3–6 g/day	—	Parkinsonism	1. Closed-angle glaucoma 2. Melanoma 3. Hypertension 4. Severe psychosis	1. Nausea and vomiting 2. Dyskinesia 3. Postural hypotension 4. 'On-off phenomenon' 5. Hallucinations 6. Palpitation
SELEGILINE (MAO-B ↓)	10 mg/day in divided doses	—	Parkinsonism	1. Epilepsy 2. Tardive dyskinesia	1. Confusion 2. Involuntary movements 3. Palpitations 4. Psychosis 5. Sexual dysfunctions
AMANTADINE	100 mg daily or 12 hourly	—	1. Parkinsonism (except drug-induced) 2. Post-encephalitic sequelae 3. Prophylaxis of influenza A	1. Epilepsy 2. Renal disorder	1. Mental confusion 2. Ankle oedema 3. Oculogyric episode 4. Suicidal tendency 5. Livedo reticularis
BENZHEXOL	2 mg, 8 or 12 hourly	—	Parkinsonism (even in the presence of IHD or hypertension)	1. Glaucoma 2. Enlarged prostate 3. Paralytic ileus	See the adverse reaction of atropine

Contd...

	Dosage				
Drugs	**Oral**	**Parenteral**	**Indications**	**Contraindications**	**Adverse effects**
BROMOCRIPTINE	2.5 mg, 8 hourly (up to 50–100 mg/day)	—	1. Parkinsonism 2. Galactorrhoea 3. Inhibition of lactation 4. Acromegaly 5. Premenstrual syndrome 6. Prolactinoma	1. Uncontrolled hypertension 2. Eclampsia	1. Headache 2. Constipation 3. Abnormal movements 4. Nausea and vomiting 5. Digital vasospasm 6. Alcohol intolerance 7. Postural hypotension
ANTITUBERCULOUS DRUGS					
INH (ISONICOTINIC ACID HYDRAZIDE)	Adult: 300 mg (5 mg/kg) Children: 10 mg/kg	—	Tuberculosis	1. Hypersensitivity 2. Severe jaundice 3. Convulsions	1. Drug fever 2. Peripheral neuropathy 3. Hepatitis 4. Convulsions 5. Psychosis
RIFAMPICIN	Adult (<50 kg): 450 mg Adult (>50 kg): 600 mg Children: 10–20 mg/kg (daily doses)	—	1. Tuberculosis 2. Leprosy 3. Prophylaxis of meningitis against *H. influenzae, Legionellla, N. meningitidis* 4. Meningococcal carrier	1. Severe hepatic disorder 2. Severe vomiting	1. Flu-like syndrome 2. Hepatitis 3. Vasculitis 4. Nausea, vomiting 5. Purpura (rare) 6. Orange-red coloured urine
ETHAMBUTOL	25 mg/kg for 2 months, 15 mg/kg thereafter	—	Tuberculosis	1. Hypersensitivity 2. Optic neuritis	1. Optic neuritis 2. Nausea and vomiting 3. Hypersensitivity reaction
PYRAZINAMIDE	Adult: 20–35 mg/kg (max — 2.5 g) Children: 40 mg/kg (max — 2 g)	—	Tuberculosis	1. Hepatitis 2. Gout 3. Fever 4. Skin rash 5. Arthralgia	1. Hepatitis 2. Hyperuricaemia
STREPTOMYCIN	—	Adult: 0.75–1 g, IM Children: 20 mg/kg, IM	1. Tuberculosis 2. Plague, brucellosis, tularaemia 3. UTI, RTI 4. Chancroid and granuloma inguinale 5. SBE, Meningitis	1. Diseases in the ear, e.g. CSOM 2. Hypersensitivity	1. Giddiness (ototoxicity) 2. Deafness 3. Loss of renal function 4. Exfoliative dermatitis
* INH, rifampicin, ethambutol, pyrazinamide and streptomycin are first-line drugs. Rest are included in the second line.					
CYCLOSERINE	Adult: 1 g/day Children: 10 mg/kg/day	—	Tuberculosis (second-line agent)	1. Epilepsy 2. Psychosis 3. Depression	1. Depression 2. Convulsions 3. Psychosis 4. Megaloblastic anaemia 5. Tremor
PARA-AMINO SALICYLIC ACID (PAS)	10–15 g/day Children: 300 mg/kg	—	Tuberculosis (especially in multi-drug resistant or MDR-TB)	1. Hypersensitivity 2. Goitre	1. Nausea, vomiting, diarrhoea 2. Hypothyroidism, goitre 3. Leucopenia, eosinophilia 4. Acute renal failure

Contd...

Drugs	Dosage Oral	Parenteral	Indications	Contraindications	Adverse effects
CIPROFLOXACIN	250–750 mg, 12 hourly	100–200 mg, IV, 12 hourly	1. UTI, prostatitis, ear infection 2. Enteric fever, septicaemia, gonorrhoea 3. 2nd line of anti-tuberculosis drug 4. Skin and soft tissue infection, pyogenic liver abscess, intra-abdominal infection, osteomyelitis 5. Diarrhoea	1. Convulsions 2. Patient receiving theophylline (relative contra-indication) 3. Hypersensitivity 4. G_6PD deficiency	1. Arthralgia 2. Convulsions 3. Stevens-Johnson syndrome 4. Tremor 5. Insomnia
ETHIONAMIDE/ PROTHIONAMIDE	0.75–1 g/day	—	2nd line agent against tuberculosis	1. Hypersensitivity 2. Gout	1. Nausea 2. Jaundice 3. Metallic taste 4. Neuropathy 5. Gout 6. Pellagra-like syndrome
BEDAQUILINE	400 mg, OD/day for 2 weeks, then 200 mg thrice weekly for 22 weeks (total 24 weeks)	—	As part of combination therapy for pulmonary MDR-TB	1. Q-T prolongation 2. Abnormal LFT 3. Severe renal impairment	1. Nausea, headache, arthralgia 2. Q-T prolongation 3. Haemoptysis
*Rifabutin (150 mg/day) is given in HIV-associated TB or MDR-TB.					
ANTILEPROSY DRUGS					
DAPSONE	2 mg/kg (not exceeding 100 mg/day)	—	1. Leprosy 2. Dermatitis herpetiformis 3. Vasculitis 4. Erythema nodosum (stubborn cases)	Hypersensitivity to sulpha drugs	1. Rash, drug fever 2. Exfoliative dermatitis 3. Agranulocytosis, haemolytic anaemia 4. Psychosis 5. Hepatitis 6. Hypoproteinaemia
RIFAMPICIN	600 mg, once or twice monthly	—	See antituberculous drugs		
CLOFAZIMINE	50 mg/day	—	1. Leprosy 2. Chronic skin ulcer (Buruli ulcer) 3. Erythema nodosum leprosum	Hypersensitivity	1. Brown discolouration of skin 2. Abdominal pain 3. Pruritus 4. Anorexia, nausea, vomiting 5. Phototoxicity
THIACETAZONE	150 mg/day	—	1. Tuberculosis 2. Leprosy	1. Hypersensitivity 2. Immunodeficiency (e.g. AIDS)	1. Skin rash, Stevens-Johnson syndrome 2. Nausea, vomiting 3. Bone marrow depression
PROTHIONAMIDE	See antituberculous drugs				
OFLOXACIN	200–400 mg/day	—	1. Similar to ciprofloxacin (Ref: antituber-culous drugs) 2. Leprosy	1. Hypersensitivity 2. Convulsions	1. Similar to ciprofloxacin 2. Pseudomembranous colitis

Contd...

Drugs	Dosage		Indications	Contraindications	Adverse effects
	Oral	Parenteral			
DRUGS FOR KALA-AZAR					
SODIUM ANTIMONY GLUCONATE	—	20 mg/kg, IV or deep IM daily for 28 days; 1 mL of inj. contains 100 mg of drug	Kala-azar	1. G_6PD deficiency 2. Hepatic and renal impairment	1. Nausea, vomiting diarrhoea 2. Anaphylaxis 3. Hepatitis 4. 'Nitritoid crisis' 5. Renal failure 6. Arthralgia
MEGLUMINE ANTIMONIATE	—	50 mg/kg/day, for 15 days	Same as above		
PENTAMIDINE ISETHIONATE	—	2 mg/kg, thrice weekly for 7 days	1. Kala-azar 2. Blastomycosis	1. Hypersensitivity 2. Hypoglycaemia	1. Hypoglycaemia 2. Hypotension 3. Peripheral neuropathy 4. Fever, rigor
AMPHOTERICIN-B	—	0.5–1 mg/kg, IV slow infusion on alternate days (total 1–3 g)	1. Systemic mycoses 2. Fatal fungal infection and intestinal moniliasis 3. Resistant kala-azar	Hypersensitivity	1. Pain at inj. site 2. Renal impairment 3. Cardiovascular toxicity (arrhythmia) 4. Convulsions, deafness, diplopia
MILITEFOSINE	2.5 mg/kg/day in dividied doses for 28 days	—	Resistant kala-azar	1. Pregnancy 2. Lactation	1. Mild and transient GI disturbances 2. Motion sickness 3. Reversible elevations of creatinine, AST and ALT
ALLOPURINOL	20–30 mg/kg/day (dose in kala-azar)	—	1. Chronic gout, urate nephropathy, recurrent urate stone formation 2. In anti-cancer therapy 3. In resistant kala-azar with sodium antimony gluconate 4. American trypanosomiasis	1. Hypersensitivity 2. Recent acute attack of gout	1. Fever, chill 2. Headache 3. Vasculitis 4. Rash 5. Toxic epidermal necrolysis (TEN) 6. Granulomatous hepatitis
ANTIMALARIAL DRUGS					
QUININE	Q. sulphate 300–600 mg, 8 hourly for 7 days	Q. hydrochloride (300 mg/mL) 10 mg/kg, IV, 8 hourly	1. Chloroquine resistant malaria (Pv or Pf) 2. Cerebral malaria 3. Nocturnal muscle cramp 4. Quinidine-like effect on heart	1. Hypoglycaemia 2. G_6PD deficiency 3. Pregnancy (relative contraindication)	1. Cinchonism, tinnitus, vertigo, deafness 2. Nausea, vomiting 3. Haemoglobinuria and ARF 4. Idiosyncrasy (pruritus) 5. Photosensitivity 6. Hypoglycaemia 7. Arrhythmias
CHLOROQUINE	10 mg base/kg followed by 5 mg base/kg at 6, 24 and 48 hours (in malaria)	5 mg/kg, IV	1. Treatment and prophylaxis of malaria 2. DLE and SLE 3. Hepatic amoebiasis 4. Rheumatoid arthritis 5. Photoallergic reaction	1. Psoriasis 2. Porphyria 3. G_6PD deficiency	1. Nausea, vomiting 2. Blurred vision 3. Retinopathy 4. Ototoxicity 5. Psychosis and convulsions

Contd...

Drugs	Dosage		Indications	Contraindications	Adverse effects
	Oral	Parenteral			
PRIMAQUINE	15 mg daily for 14 days	—	1. Radical cure of Pv or Po 2. Gametocidal for Pf (45 mg as a single dose)	1. SLE 2. G_6PD deficiency 3. Pregnancy	1. Abdominal discomfort 2. Methaemoglobinaemia 3. Anaemia and leucopenia
PROGUANIL	200 mg/day, continued for 6 weeks	—	1. Prophylaxis of Pf malaria 2. Suppression of transmission of malaria	1. G_6PD deficiency 2. SLE	1. Gastric intolerance 2. Mouth ulcer 3. Reversible alopecia 4. Renal impairment 5. Skin reaction
MEFLOQUINE	25 mg/kg totally (as 8 mg/kg, daily for 3 days)	—	1. Chloroquine sensitive/resistant malaria due to Pv or Pf 2. *Prophylaxis against Pv or Pf—250 mg (1 tab) weekly	1. Convulsions 2. Psychosis 3. Hypersensitivity to quinine 4. Pregnancy	1. Neuropsychiatric dysfunction 2. Vomiting, diarrhoea 3. Rash, itching 4. Convulsions
*One week prior and 4 weeks after leaving endemic areas					
AMODIAQUINE	10 mg/kg, daily for 3 days	—	Treatment and prophylaxis of malaria	1. G_6PD deficiency 2. Hypersensitivity	1. Nausea and vomiting 2. Agranulocytosis 3. Skin rash 4. Headache
ARTEMETHER	—	Loading dose of 3.2 mg/kg, IM, then 1.6 mg/kg, IM daily for 2–5 days to a total of 640 mg	1. Multidrug resistant Pv/Pf malaria 2. Malaria with end-organ damage	1. Hypersensitivity 2. Prolonged Q-T on the ECG	1. Bradycardia, 1° AV block 2. Leucopenia 3. Nausea, vomiting, abdominal cramps 4. Neurotoxicity
ARTEETHER	—	150 mg IM once a days for 3 days	Same as artemether	Same as artemether	Same as artemether
ARTESUNATE	Day 1: 100 mg BD Day 2–5: 50 mg BD Total: 600 mg	2.4 mg/kg, IV stat followed by 2.4 mg/kg at 12 and 24 h, and then daily for 7 days if necessary	Same as artemether	Hypersensitivity	1. Bradycardia, 1° AV block 2. Transient elevation of transaminases
HALOFANTRINE	500 mg at 6 hours interval for 3 doses in a day; with fatty meal	—	Same as artemether	1. Cardiac arrhythmias 2. Hypersensitivity 3. Pregnancy	1. Diarrhoea 2. Abdominal pain 3. Q-T prolongation in ECG 4. Arrhythmias
*Artemether-lumefantrine combination (1.5 mg/9 mg)/kg BD for 3 days with food is effective in multidrug-resistant falciparum malaria. **Arteether, artesunate and artemether are **Qinghaosu (artemisinin) derivatives.**					
PYRIMETHAMINE	25 mg per dose (for malaria)	—	1. Treatment and prophylaxis of malaria (along with sulphadoxine 500 mg) 2. Toxoplasmosis 3. Actinomycetomas 4. Prophylaxis of *P. jirovecii* pneumonia	1. Megaloblastic anaemia due to folate deficiency 2. Hypersensitivity 3. Caution in patients with G_6PD deficiency	1. Agranulocytosis 2. Megaloblastic anaemia 3. Sore throat 4. Loss of appetite

Contd...

Drugs	Dosage		Indications	Contraindications	Adverse effects
	Oral	Parenteral			
LIPID LOWERING AGENTS					
LOVASTATIN	10–80 mg/day at bed time	—	1. Primary hypercholesterolaemia 2. Combined hypercholesterolaemia and hypertriglyceridaemia	1. Active liver disease 2. Hypersensitivity	1. Nausea, flatulence 2. Myopathy 3. Headache 4. Sleep disorder 5. Fatigue 6. Memory loss 7. Transaminitis
SIMVASTATIN	10–40 mg/day at bed time	—	Hypercholesterolaemia	Same as lovastatin	Same as lovastatin
ATORVASTATIN	10–80 mg/day at bed time	—	1. Hypercholesterolaemia 2. Mixed hyperlipidaemia	Same as lovastatin	Same as lovastatin
ROSUVASTATIN (super-statin)	10–20 mg/day at bed time	—	1. Hypercholesterolaemia 2 Mixed dyslipidaemia	1. Severe renal disease 2. Same as lovastatin	Same as lovastatin
FENOFIBRATE	200 mg once daily with food	—	1. Hyperlipidaemia (e.g. hypertriglyceridaemia) 2. Dislipidaemia in diabetes	1. Renal or hepatic disease 2. Gallbladder disease 3. Pancreatitis	1. Elevated liver enzymes 2. Muscle toxicity 3. Gallstones 4. Photosensitivity
EZETIMIBE	10 mg/day	—	1. Adjunct to diet in hypercholesterolaemia 2. With a statin or as monotherapy	Hepatic impairment	1. Myalgia 2. ↑ in serum transaminases 3. Nausea 4. Angio-oedema
GEMFIBROZIL	600 mg BD, 30 min before meal	—	1. Hypertriglyceridaemia 2. ↑ VLDL	Sever hepatic or renal dysfunction	1. GI upset 2. Myopathy 3. Gallstone formation 4. Blurred vision 5. Headache
NICOTINIC ACID	500 mg at betime, gradually increasing to 1–2 g at bedtime	—	1. Hypercholesterolaemia (↑ LDL) 2. ↑ VLDL 3. ↓ HDL	Hyperuricaemia	1. Gout 2. Flushing 3. GI upset 4. LFT abnormalities
CHOLESTYRAMINE (bile acid sequestrants)	4–24 g/d in divided doses	—	↑ LDL	1. Hypertriglyceridaemia 2. Autonomic neuropathy 3. Constipation	1. GI upset 2. ↑ VLDL
CLOFIBRATE	2–3 g/d	—	1. Hyperlipidaemia 2. Atherosclerotic arterial disease	1. Pregnancy, lactation 2. Peptic ulcer	1. Nausea, diarrhoea 2. ↑ in SGOT

*Hypersensitivity may develop in any drug; thus, hypersensitivity is the common contraindication of all. Except digitalis, all drugs can produce drug fever. Read anti-bacterial (e.g. antibiotics), anti-viral and anti-fungal agents from standard textbooks.

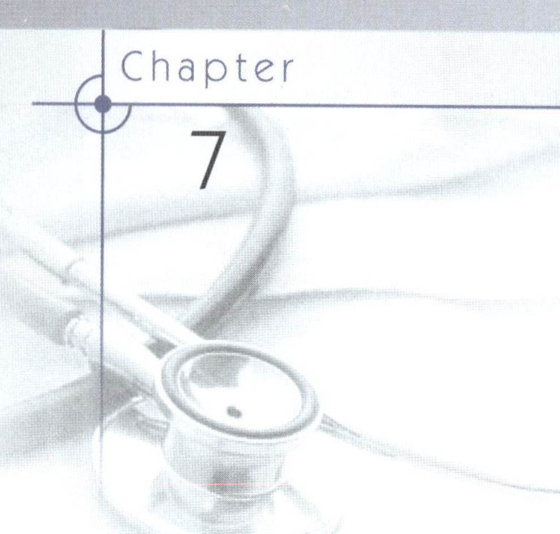

Chapter 7

Charts (Data Analysis)

"War is 90% information."—**Napoleon Bonaparte** (1769–1821)
A French military general who crowned himself the first emperor of France. His Napoleonic Code remains a model for governments worldwide

CHARTS ON HAEMATOLOGY

Introduction

Hematology is the study of blood and blood disorders. Haematology tests (a panel of evaluation that includes blood and bone marrow cells in a special situation) are performed by the Pathology Department and Laboratory Medicine of the Center by the hematologists and hematopathologists. The *hematological tests* help in diagnosis of anaemia, leukaemia, different infections, coagulation disorders, etc.

RBC

a. Total count (TC):
   1. Male: 4.5–6.3 millions/mm^3
   2. Female: 4.2–5.4 millions/mm^3
b. Haemoglobin (Hb):
   1. Male: 13–17 g/dL
   2. Female: 12–15 g/dL
c. Reticulocyte count—0.2–2% of RBC. Increased reliculocyte count indicates bone marrow stimulation with new red cells production, e.g. haemolytic anaemia or acute blood loss.
   Reticulocyte index = Reticulocyte % $\times \frac{\text{Patient's PCV}}{\text{Normal PCV}}$
d. Haematocrit or packed cell volume (PCV):
   a. Male: 42–52%
   b. Female: 37–47%
e. Haemoglobin content of RBC is assessed by:
   Mean corpuscular haemoglobin (MCH): 29.5± 2.5 pg
   Mean corpuscular haemoglobin concentration (MCHC): 35 ± 3 g/dL
   The term 'colour index' is obsolete nowadays rather the 'chromicity' of RBC is assessed by MCH and MCHC.
f. Size of RBC:
   Anisocytosis: Change in size
   Mean diameter: 7.2 microns, and the normal shape is biconcave (as RBC has no nucleus)
   Mean corpuscular volume (MCV): 87± 7 cubic microns
   Macrocyte >100 cubic microns
   Microcyte <70 cubic microns

- Anaemia with normal MCV suggests acute blood loss or anaemia of chronic diseases (e.g. any chronic disease like tuberculosis, chronic inflammation or malignancy).
- Anaemia with low MCV suggests iron deficiency anaemia or thalassaemia.
- Anaemia with high MCV suggests vitamin B_{12}, or folate deficiency.

g. Shape of RBC: The normal RBC is circular with central pallor. Variations in shape is known as *poikilocytosis*. Target cell, spur cell, helmet cells are examples of change in shape of RBC. Distortion of size and shape indicates dyshaemopoiesis.
h. Life span 120 days.
i. FSR (Westergren): Males 0–15 mm/hour and females 0–20 mm/hour.
j. **Anaemia:** It is qualitative or quantitative diminution of RBC and/or haemoglobin concentration in relation to standard age and sex, and is clinically manifested by pallor. Anaemia is divided into mild (9–12 g/dL), moderate (6–9 g/dL), and severe (<6 g/dL) grades clinically.

WBC

a. Total count (TC): 4.3–10.8 × 10^9/L or 4300–10800/mm^3

Leucopenia	<4000/mm^3
Leucocytosis	>11000/mm^3

b. Differential count (DC):

Neutrophils	45–74%
Lymphocytes	16–45%
Monocytes	4–10%
Eosinophils	0–7%
Basophils	0–1%

c. Half-life:

Neutrophils	8 hours
T lymphocytes	100 days
B lymphocytes	10 days

Platelets

a. Total count 1.5–4 lac/mm^3
   Critical count <10000/mm^3 (recent view)
   Thrombocytopenia <1 lac/mm^3
   Thrombocytosis >4 lac/mm^3

b. Half life: 3 days (life span 10 days)

Coagulation Profile

Bleeding time (BT): 2.5–10 minutes (Ivy)
Clotting time (CT): 9–15 minutes (glass tubes)
Prothrombin time (PT): 12–16 seconds
Activated partial thromboplastin time (aPTT): 32–46 seconds.

- Anticoagulants used while collecting blood sample for different examinations are:
  a. Oxalate (mixture of ammonium oxalate and potassium oxalate in a ratio of 3:2).
  b. Citrate (trisodium citrate solution)—Useful for ESR estimation and coagulation study.
  c. EDTA (ethylenediamine tetra-acetic acid)—For cellular morphology and platelet count.
  d. Heparin (used for osmotic fragility test and electrolyte estimation).
  e. ACD (acid citrate dextrose) solution (used in blood banking).

- Haemoglobin is estimated by:
  a. Sahli's or acid-haematin method
  b. Cyanmethaemoglobin method
  c. Alkali-haematin method, or
  d. Oxyhaemoglobin method
- ESR is estimated by:
  a. Wintrobe's, or
  b. Westergren's method
- RBC and platelet are counted by:
  a. Visual method, or
  b. Electronic cell counters
- RBC and WBC counts are done in Neubauer's chamber.
- Extrinsic coagulation pathway is assessed by PT and intrinsic coagulation pathway by aPTT. Heparin therapy is monitored by aPTT and that of warfarin by PT.
- For haematological investigations, venous blood is collected usually from the antecubital vein. Blood smear is then prepared on a clean slide with the help of another slide. To prevent haemolysis of RBC, the air-dried blood smear may be 'fixed' by covering the film with acetone-free methyl alcohol for 1 minute. The slide is now stained with Romanowsky dyes (e.g. Leishman's, Giemsa's stain) and lastly examined under the microscope. Thick smear is required for detection of malaria parasites and microfilaria.

Clinical Wisdom

Complete blood count is a blood test, which evaluates:
RBC count, haematocrit and RBC indices
Reticulocyte count
WBC count (TC, DC, band count)
Platelet count
Peripheral smear (cell size and shape, Hb content, polychromasia)

IRON DEFICIENCY ANAEMIA

Hb	5.4 g/dL
RBC	4.4 million/mm^3
WBC	8700/mm^3
Polymorphs	63%
Lymphocytes	34%
Monocytes	2%
Eosinophils	1%
Basophils	0%
Reticulocytes	1%
Anisocytosis	++
Poikilocytosis	++
Platelets	3.2 lac/mm^3
MCH	22 pg
MCHC	24 g/dL
MCV	68 cubic microns

Interpretation

1. *Anaemia:* Severe (Hb 5.4 g/dL, i.e. approximately 35%); RBC count is reduced to 90% approximately (slight reduction). So the cells are likely to be hypochromic.
2. MCH is low, MCHC is diminished; MCV is less too.
3. Anisocytosis and poikilocytosis indicate dyshaemopoiesis, or marrow stimulation, e.g. haemolytic anaemia, deficiency disorder or infiltration of marrow by malignant cells.
4. WBC series, platelet and reticulocyte count show no abnormality.

Inference

It is a case of microcytic hypochromic anaemia probably iron deficiency anaemia (IDA).

Q. Possible causes with rational approach:

1. Iron deficiency anaemia (all features present).
2. β-thalassaemia (reticulocyte count will be high).
3. Sideroblastic anaemia (dimorphic picture with sideroblasts seen).
4. Lead poisoning (basophilic stippling noted).
5. Anaemia of chronic diseases (ACD) (WBC series show changes in TC and DC).

- Common causes of IDA are nutritional deficiency, chronic blood loss and increased demand due to pregnancy, lactation. Acute blood loss usually produces normocytic normochromic anaemia or macrocytic anaemia.
- Causes No. 1–5 produce microcytic hypochromic anaemia.

Q. What is Mentzer index?

Mentzer index (MCV/RBC), i.e. mean corpuscular volume per red cell is:

a. >13 = Iron dificiency anaemia.
b. <13 = β-thalassaemia trait.

Q. Causes of chronic blood loss:

1. Pediatric age group: Hookworm infestation, polyp.
2. Adult:
   a. Males: Haemorrhoids, peptic ulcer, oesophageal varices.
   b. Females: Menorrhagia, uterine fibroid.
3. Elderly patient:
   a. Males: Carcinoma of GI tract.
   b. Females: Dysfunctional uterine haemorrhage.

Q. Ferrokinetics:

Serum iron: 70–140 μg%

Total iron binding capacity (TIBC): 270–335 μg%; transferrin saturation: 20–50%

Serum ferritin: 30–300 ng/mL.

Total body iron content:

Males: 50 mg/kg of body wt

Females: 35 mg/kg of body wt

Daily intake: 10–20 mg (1–2 mg/day is absorbed)

Iron requirement: 1 mg in men, 2 mg in women and 3 mg during pregnancy.

- It is assumed that 250 mg of iron is required to increase the Hb level by 1 g/dL. One unit of blood (450 mL) supplies 250 mg iron.
- Dietary sources of iron: Red meat, liver, bone marrow, egg yolk, green leafy vegetables (e.g. spinach), dry fruits, nuts, dates, apples and outer layer of cereals. Milk contain very little iron.

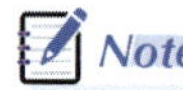
Note

MCH, MCHC and MCV may not be supplied in all haematological data analysis.

Q. Classical picture of iron deficiency anaemia:

Haemoglobin is reduced. It is a microcytic hypochromic anaemia with low MCV, MCH and MCHC. Anisocytosis, poikilocytosis or target cells are seen in severe cases. Usually reticulocyte count is normal but if increased, one should think of blood loss where the patient has enough iron stores in body. Serum iron is low and TIBC is raised; plasma transferrin level is elevated but serum ferritin level is reduced. Bone marrow study reveals moderate erythroid hyperplasia and marrow iron stores (stained by Prussian blue technique) are found to be reduced or absent.

In **'anaemia of chronic diseases (ACD)'**, i.e. caused by infections (tuberculosis, osteomyelitis), collagen vascular diseases, malignancy or rheumatoid arthritis, there will be low serum iron, low TIBC, low transferrin, and normal or elevated serum ferritin level **(Table 7.1)**.

MEGALOBLASTIC ANAEMIA

Hb	5.9 g/dL
RBC	1.5 million/mm^3
WBC	7500/mm^3
Polymorphs	55%; hypersegmentation +
Lymphocytes	40%
Monocytes	3%
Eosinophils	2%
Basophils	0%
Reticulocytes	1%
Anisocytosis	++
Poikilocytosis	++
Platelets	2.5 lac/mm^3
MCH	33 pg
MCHC	39 g/dL
MCV	102 cubic micron

Interpretation

1. Anaemia: Severe (i.e. Hb is 40%); RBC count is reduced to 30% and thus the cells are likely to be hyperchromic.
2. MCH, MCHC and MCV are increased (i.e. the cells are larger than normal and a bit hyperchromic).
3. Anisocytosis and poikilocytosis point towards dyshemopoiesis.
4. WBC series, platelet count and reticulocyte count are within normal limit

Inference

It is a case of macrocytic anaemia probably megaloblastic anaemia (hyperchromic RBC and hypersegmentation of polymorphs with six or more lobes in the nucleus also point towards this diagnosis).

Table 7.1: Iron kinetics in different microcytic hypochromic anaemia

Values	IDA	Sideroblastic anaemia	β-thalassaemia trait	β-thalassaemia major	Anaemia of chronic diseases
Serum iron	↓	↑	Normal	↑	↓
Scrum ferritin	↓	↑	Normal	↑	↑
TIBC	↑	↓	Normal	Normal	↓

Clinical Wisdom

In acute blood loss, Hb and haematocrit remain normal in early stages but haemodilution usually prevails after 24–36 hours resulting in anaemia.

Q. Causes of macrocytic anaemia:

Macrocytic anaemia is of two types, megaloblastic and non-megaloblastic, depending on the bone morrow findings:

1. Megaloblastic anemia (mainly vitamin B_{12}, and folic acid deficiency).
2. Liver diseases (needs liver function tests).
3. Aplastic anaemia (WBC count and platelets will be reduced).
4. Haemolysis or acute blood loss (leucocytosis, thrombocytosis and increased reticulocyte will be present).

So, the present chart probably deals with megaloblastic anaemia.

- Cause Nos 2, 3, and 4 produce macrocytic anaemia which is normoblastic (non-megaloblastic), and the other causes are alcoholism, hypothyroidism, pregnancy, myelodysplastic states and drug-induced (e.g. zidovudine).

Q. Addisonian pernicious anaemia:

It is a special variety of megaloblastic anaemia which results from failure of secretion of intrinsic factor by the stomach, other than from total gastrectomy done in the past.

Q Sources and daily requirements of vitamin B_{12} and folic acid:

a. Vitamin B_{12}: Meat, egg, fish, liver, milk, cheese and dairy products.
   Daily requirement is 1–2 μg.
b. Folic acid: Fruits, green leafy vegetables and animal protein (liver, kidney, yeast).
   Daily requirement is 200 μg.

- Vegetables are deficient in vitamin B_{12}.

Q. Common conditions associated with vitamin B_{12} and folic acid deficiency:

a. Vitamin B_{12} deficiency: True vegetarians (vegans), tropical sprue, blind loop syndrome, fish tapeworm infestation, pernicious anaemia, Crohn's disease, gastrectomy.
b. Folate deficiency: Poor intake of vegetables, old age, pregnancy, chronic haemolytic anaemia, coeliac disease, phenytoin or methotrexate-induced, myeloproliferative disorders.

- **Vegan**—A person who consumes vegetarian diet that excludes meat, eggs, dairy products and all other animal-derived ingredients.

Clinical Wisdom

Neurological manifestations of vitamin B_{12} deficiency are peripheral neuropathy, subacute combined degeneration (SCD) and dementia. It is known that folate appears as methyl tetrahydrofolate in plasma, which is converted into tetrahydrofolate with the help of vitamin B_{12}. So, clinically, folic acid should not be used simultaneously to treat vitamin B_{12} deficiency anaemia because it may precipitate severe neurological damage like SCD (by utilising residual vitamin B_{12} for conversion of folate, and resulting in its absolute deficiency)

- Knuckles in the hands are hyperpigmented in megaloblastic anaemia.

Q. Treatment of vitamin B_{12} and folic acid deficiency:

a. Vitamin B_{12} deficiency: Hydroxycobalamin 1000 μg, deep IM, in 5 doses at 2–3 days apart (i.e. a total of 5 mg), followed by maintenance therapy of 1000 μg every 3 months for rest of the life. Alternatively, oral vitamin B_{12} mg/day can be given as per recent recommendation. Recently, vitamin B_{12} nasal spray is available in the market.
b. Folate deficiency: Oral folic acid 5 mg dally for 4 months to replace body stores, while 5 mg once weekly is sufficient for maintenance therapy.

Q. Enumerate the investigations performed to diagnose macrocytic anaemia:

1. Peripheral blood film (hypersegmented polymorphs are early changes).
2. FSR (increases in malignancy).
3. Thyroid function tests (for hypothyroidism).
4. Serum B_{12} level (normally 200–600 pg/mL).
5. Red cell folate level (normal value is 150–450 ng/mL).
6. Bone marrow study:
   a. Megaloblastic: Vitamin B_{12} or folate deficiency.
   b. Normoblastic: Liver diseases, hypothyroidism.
   c. Abnormal erythropoiesis: Aplastic anaemia, leukaemia.
   d. Increased erythropoiesis: Haemolysis, acule blood loss.
7. Schilling test (helps to identify the cause of vitamin B_{12} deficiency; now considered obsolete).

- ESR is increased in anaemia due to any aetiology except sickle cell anaemia.

ACUTE LEUKAEMIA

Hb	7.5 g/dL
RBC	2.5 million/mm^3
WBC	46000/mm^3
Polymorphs	43%
Lymphocytes	26%
Monocytes	0%
Eosinophils	1%
Basophils	0%
Blast cells	30%
Reticulocytes	1%
Anisocytosis	+
Poikilocytosis	+
Platelets	68000/mm^3

Interpretation

1. Anaemia is moderate and seems to be normochromic. RBC count is proportionately reduced. Anisocytosis and poikilocytosis suggest dyserythropoiesis. Reticulocyte count is normal.
2. WBC count reflects marked leucocytosis. The DC is distributed amongst polymorphs, lymphocytes and blast cells. Huge number of blast cells (30%) in peripheral blood indicate either acute leukaemia (AML/ALL) or blast crisis of chronic leukaemia (CML mainly/rarely CLL).
3. Platelet count is markedly reduced.

Inference

Probably it deals with a chart of acute leukaemia.

- The character of blast cell, bone marrow examination and lineage confirmation by immunophenotyping determine the type of leukaemia (i.e. AML or ALL).

Q. Other probabilities with rational approach:

This chart may well fit in patients with (a) Leukaemoid reaction, and (b) Blast crisis of CML.

Leukaemoid reaction: TC of WBC matches with leukaemoid reaction but presence of anaemia, absence of polymorphonuclear leucocytosis, presence of a large number of blast cells and low platelet count, and absence of metamyelocytes or myelocytes point against the diagnosis.

Blast crisis of CML: 30% blast cells match the diagnosis but absence of myelocytes, metamyelocytes, basophilia do not corroborate with the diagnosis. In blast crisis of CML, a higher total count of WBC is present.

- Leucocyte alkaline phosphatase (LAP) score is high in leukaemoid reaction but low in blast crisis of CML.
- The blast cells of AML contain Auer rods which are not seen in blast crisis of CML or leukaemoid reaction.

Q. Classification of acute leukaemias:

a. Acute myeloid leukaemia (AML): The French-American-British (FAB) classification:
   M0: Minimally differentiated leukaemia
   M1: Without maturation
   M2: With maturation
   M3: Acute promyelocytic
   M4: Myelomonocytic
   M5: Monocytic
   M6: Erythroleukaemia (Di Guglielmo's disease)
   M7: Megakaryocytic
b. Acute lymphoblastic leukaemia (ALL): The French-American-British (FAB) classification:
   L1: Small cells which are usually homogeneous with scanty cytoplasm
   L2: Large cells which are heterogeneous with more cytoplasm
   L3: Large cells which are homogeneous with prominent cytoplasmic vacuolization (also known as 'Burkitt cell leukaemia').

Nowadays, ALL is classified as:

- Common type (Pre-B; 75%): FAB subtype L_1, L_2
- T Cell (20%): FAB subtype L_1, L_2
- B Cell (5%): FAB subtype L_3
- Undifferentiated (rare)

- WHO classification of acute leukaemia is a bit different, and it reviews chromosome translocations and evidence of dysplasia. Read the classification from any standard textbook of medicine.
- **Blast cell** is an immature precursor of myeloid or lymphoid cell. There is an immature nucleus. The cells are larger than normal counterparts and are very rarely seen in normal persons **(Table 7.2)**.

CHRONIC MYELOID LEUKAEMIA

Hb	10 g/dL
RBC	2.7 million/mm^3
WBC	2.3 lac/mm^3
Myelocytes	26%
Metamyelocytes	20%
Promyelocyte	2%
Polymorphs	40%
Lymphocytes	4%
Monocytes	1%
Eosinophils	3%
Basophils	2%
Myeloblasts	2%
Anisocytosis	+
Poikilocytosis	+
Platelets	4.8 lac/mm^3

Table 7.2: Differentiation between myeloblast and lymphoblast

Features	Myeloblast	Lymphoblast
1. Nuclear–cytoplasm ratio	Low	High
2. Number of nucleoli	3 or more	1 or 2
3. Auer rods in cytoplasm	Present (10–20%)	Absent
4. Cytochemical staining:		
a. Myeloperoxidase	+ve	–ve
b. Sudan Black B	+ve	–ve
c. Chloracetate esterase	+ve	–ve
d. Periodic Acid Schiff (PAS)	+ve in <25% cells	+ve in >50% cells

Interpretation

1. There is mild anaemia which seems to be normochromic. Anisocytosis and poikilocytosis indicate some amount of dyserythropoiesis.
2. The total amount of WBC is much increased with large number of myelocytes and metamyelocytes. There is presence of 2% myeloblast too. Basophilia is present.
3. The platelet count is increased.

Inference

The marked leucocytosis with presence of myelocytes and metamyelocytes, associated with basophilia in the peripheral blood smear virtually clinch the diagnosis of chronic myeloid leukaemia (CML). Platelet count may be high initially but ultimately the count falls gradually.

- In CML, the peripheral blood film may contain up to 10% myeloblasts.

Q. What is leukaemoid reaction?

It is the extreme degree of elevation of WBC count (usually 30000–50000/mm^3 with many immature cells; rarely >50000/mm^3) which is composed of mature and/or immature neutrophils and is known as leukaemoid reaction. It reflects the response of normal healthy bone marrow to various stresses. The common causes are:

1. Disseminated tuberculosis (especially in children) or any severe infection (e.g. septicaemia).
2. Malignant infiltration of bone marrow (breast, lung, kidney).
3. Severe haemolysis or after haemorrhage.
4. Burns, eclampsia, mercury poisoning.
5. Application of cytokines (G-CSF or GM-CSF).

There may be presence of myelocyte or few myeloblasts in the peripheral blood. RBC, eosinophil, monocyte, basophil and platelet counts usually remain normal in leukaemoid reaction. The leucocyte alkaline phosphatase (LAP) score is high; there is absence of splenomegaly. Bone marrow is hyperplastic.

Q. Enumerate different haematopoietic growth factors:

a. Factors work early in stem cell differentiation: Interleukin (IL)-1, IL-3, IL-6, IL-7 and IL-11.

b. Factors work later in cellular differentiation cascade: Erythropoietin (EPO), granulocyte colony-stimulating factor (G-CSF), granulocyte macrophage colony-stimulating factor (GM-CSF) and thrombopoietin (TPO). These are used therapeutically in different diseases.

Q. What are myeloproliferative diseases?

These are chronic interrelated conditions associated with clonal proliferation of erythroid precursors, myeloid cells or megakaryocytes in the marrow. There may be progression from one disease to another disease process. The conditions are:

1. Chronic myeloid leukaemia.
2. Polycythemia vera.
3. Essential thrombocythemia.
4. Myeloid metaplasia (myelofibrosis).

- These conditions may give rise to acute leukaemia in course of time.

Q. Classify chronic leukaemias:

a. Chronic myeloid leukaemia (CML): The FAB classification goes like this:
   - Ph^a +ve
   - Ph^a –ve, BCR^b +ve
   - Ph^a –ve, BCR^b -ve
   - Eosinophilic leukaemia

- a = Philadelphia chromosome
- b = Breakpoint clusture region

b. Chronic lymphocytic leukaemia (CLL): The FAB classification goes like this:
   - Common B cell CLL
   - Rare T cell CLL
   - Hairy cell leukaemia
   - Prolymphocytic leukaemia (T cell)

Q. Causes of basophilia:

Basophilia is abolute basophil count >100/mm^3. This is commonly found in:

1. Myeloproliferative disorders (especially CML and polycythemia vera).
2. Allergic disorders.
3. Chronic inflammatory disorders.
4. Malignancy, myxedema, post splenectomy.

Basopenia (i.e. a form of agranulocylosis with a deficiency of basophils) is found in urticaria, anaphylaxis, ↑ level of glucocorticoid, and ovulation.

Q. Leukaemoid reaction induced by various bacterial infections:

1. The smear shows large number of immature neutrophils (non-segmented neutrophils), i.e. there is a 'shift to the left'. It is a benign reactive leucocytosis.
2. Toxic granulations appear within the cytoplasm of the neutrophils.
3. Often small, oval bodies appear within the neutrophils, and is known as Döhle bodies.

PANCYTOPENIA

Hb	7.8 g/dL
RBC	2.6 million/mm^3
WBC	2600/mm^3
Polymorphs	28%
Lymphocytes	70%
Monocytes	2%
Eosinophils	0%

Basophils	0%
Reticulocytes	1%
Platelets	40000/mm^3

Interpretation

1. Moderate anaemia, probably normochromic in type. Reticulocyte count is normal (i.e. haemolysis or marrow infiltration is absent).
2. Marked leucopenia is noted. There is presence of neutropenia, eosinopenia, monocytopenia and lack of basophil associated with relative lymphocytosis.
3. The platelet count is very low.

Inference

Presence of anaemia, leucopenia and thrombocytopenia constitutes the diagnosis of pancytopenia.

- **Pancytopenia:** A decrease in number of all cell lines in blood (i.e. RBC, WBC and platelets). If any two of the series are affected, it is called bicytopenia.

Q. Causes of pancytopenia:

a. **Aplastic anaemia:** Idiopathic, chemical and physical agents (benzene, lonising radiation, alkylating agents, chloramphenicol, pesticides), immunologically-mediated, infections like hepatitis, chronic kala-azar or overwhelming sepsis.
b. Pancytopenia associated with increased or normal bone marrow cellularity: Hypersplenism, myelodysplastic syndromes, severe infection, vitamin B_{12} and folic acid deficiency.
c. Paroxysmal nocturnal haemoglobinuria (PNH).
d. Bone marrow infiltration like carcinomatosis, lymphoma, disseminated tuberculosis, myelofibrosis.
e. Systemic lupus erythematosus (SLE).

- Combination of pancytopenia with fatty and empty bone marrow clinch the diagnosis of aplastic anaemia.

Q. Drugs responsible for aplastic anaemia:

1. Chloramphenicol.
2. Phenylbulazone.
3. Sulphonamides.
4. Phenytoin sodium.
5. Alkylating agents (cyclophosphamide).
6. Chlorpropamide.
7. Carbamazepine.
8. Zidovudine.
9. D-penicillamine.
10. Ticlopidine.

Q. Outline of management of aplastic or hypoplastic anaemia:

The treatment depends on providing 'supportive care' while awaiting for bone marrow recovery and 'specific therapy' to accelerate recovery of marrow. These patients are more susceptible to infections.

1. General measures: Withdrawal of aetiologic agent, strict aseptic precautions, prophylactic use of oral antibiotics; cautious use of razors, gentle brushing of teeth, avoiding injury and falls; avoidance of intramuscular injections and drugs like aspirin. 'Barrier nursing' is strictly employed (shifting the patient to Intensive Therapy Unit or ITU, if necessary).
2. Packed red cells transfusion (to keep haematocrit above 25%), granulocyte transfusion (in <200/mm^3 granulocyte count), and platelet transfusion (in <20000/mm^3 platelet count).
3. Broad-spectrum antibiotic therapy is started in the presence of fever or any sign of infection anywhere in the body.
4. Androgen therapy (e.g. oxymetholone in a dose 3–5 mg/kg/day for 3–6 months) in a target to increase the erythropoietin production may be initiated.
5. Haematopoietic growth factors (GM-CSF, G-CSF or erythropoietin) may be tried.
6. Immunosuppression by:
   a. Antilymphocyte/antithymocyte globulin (ALG/ATG): Horse ATG (40 mg/kg/day for 4 days) or rabbit ALG (3.5 mg/kg/day for 5 days), given in IV route may help in haematological recovery in 50% cases.
   b. Cyclosporine orally in a dose of 12 mg/kg/day with subsequent adjustment (if the patient can not afford ALG or ATG). Tacrolimus may be an alternative of cyclosporine.
   c. Combination of ALG or ATG, with cyclosporine (standard medical treatment).
   d. ALG/ATG + androgens + corticosteroids (especially in females with severe disease).
7. Allogenic bone marrow transplantation (with HLA-matched siblings): the only curative treatment for patients under 40 years of age. Patients over 40 years of age have a high risk of graft-versus-host disease (GvHD) as a complication.
8. Miscellaneous: Corticosteroids (controversial; to treat serum sickness due to ALG infusion or in children with pure red cell aplasia); splenectomy may be tried in cases with pancytopenia.

AGRANULOCYTOSIS

Hb	14.5 g/dL
RBC	5.1 million/mm^3
WBC	1600/mm^3
Polymorphs	12%
Lymphocytes	88%
Monocytes	0%
Eosinophils	0%
Basophils	0%
Platelets	3 lac/mm^3

Interpretation

1. There is no anaemia. Hb content and RBC count are within normal limit.

2. The WBC count shows gross reduction, i.e. leucopenia is present (<4000/mm^3).
3. Differential count reflects reduction of granulocyte series. Marked neutropenia is present. The absolute count of neutrophil in this chart is 192/mm^3 which is much below the expected lower limit (2000/mm^3) of neutrophil count. Though the lymphocyte count shows lymphocytopenia (1408/mm^3), in this chart it reflects relative lymphocytosis.
4. The platelet count is within normal limit.

Inference

There is leucopenia as well as neutropenia. Anaemia and thrombocytopenia are absent. This is a chart of agranulocytosis.

Q. Causes of agranulocytosis:

1. Drugs like chloramphenicol, sulphonamides, chlorpropamide, chlorpromazine, propylthiouracil, cytotoxic drugs or antimetabolites, oxyphenbutazone, phenytoin, carbimazole, and gold salt (previously used in rheumatoid arthritis).
2. Ionising irradiation.
3. As an integral part of pancytopenia.
4. Idiopathic agranulocytosis (rare), and cyclic neutropenia.

- In acute leukaemia (or aleukaemic leukaemia), neutropenia is associated with low haemoglobin and low platelet count.

Q. Salient features in agranulocytosis:

1. History of exposure to one of the drugs or agents.
2. The onset may be acute (sudden) or chronic (gradual). Acute patients present with **sore throat** (agranulocytic angina), fever with chill and rigor, severe prostration associated with malaise and weakness. The throat and mouth reveal multiple necrotic ulceration with little evidence of pus (sterile) formation; there is halitosis. The fulminating cases die of septicaemia and toxaemia.

The chronic patients present with recurrent malaise. fatigability, low grade fever and sore throat.

Q. How will you manage a case of agranulocytosis?

1. Immediate stoppage of the offending drug or agent.
2. Transfer the patient in intensive therapy unit (ITU) and start barrier nursing.
3. Blood culture should be done but usually it comes out to be sterile. Prophylactic antibiotic therapy may be started. If the absolute neutrophil count is less then 200/mm^3, parenteral antibiotic therapy using an aminoglycoside together with mezlocillin, and judicious administration of corticosteroid may be employed. If anaerobic infection is suspected, metronidazole may be given.
4. White blood cell transfusion from a compatible adult relative donor often relieves fever dramatically.
5. Candidiasis in the mouth, if present, may be dealt with gentian violet, nystatin; for systemic candidiasis, parenteral therapy with amphotericin B, fluconazole, itraconazole, voriconazole, flucytosine or caspofungin is employed. Oral hygiene should be properly maintained.

Clinical Wisdom

Actually, patients taking the drugs mentioned above (chloramphenicol, carbimazole, etc.) should be repeatedly warned to report the physician, if any fever or sore throat appears.

Q. What to do in carbimazole-induced agranulocytosis?

The drug carbimazole is used in thyrotoxicosis. Though mild transient leucopenia (10%) may occur with carbimazole, agranulocytosis (0.2%) is rarely seen. Usually these effects are observed within 7–28 days of starting treatment. As agranulocytosis cannot be predicted by routine blood count, *patients should always be warned for the development of sore throat, fever and mouth ulcers*. If the absolute neutrophil count goes below 1500/mm^3, antithyroid medication should be stopped.

Q. Absolute count of different cells of WBC series:

Polymorphs	2000–7500/mm^3
Lymphocytes	1500–4000/mm^3
Monocytes	80–200/mm^3
Eosinophils	40–500/mm^3
Basophils	10–100/mm^3

Q. Causes of lymphocytosis and monocytosis:

a. Lymphocytosis:

1. Infections, e.g. tuberculosis, whooping cough, brucellosis, viral infections (e.g. CMV), infectious mononucleosis.
2. ALL and CLL; NHL
3. Thyrotoxicosis.
4. Adrenal insufficiency.
5. Serum sickness.
6. Relative: All causes of neutropenia.

b. Monocytosis:

1. Chronic infections like tuberculosis, syphilis, kala-azar, brucellosis.
2. Collagen vascular diseases.
3. Acute monocytic and myelomonocytic leukaemia, Hodgkin's lymphoma.
4. Sarcoidosis.
5. Inflammatory bowel disease.
6. Convalescence from acute infections.

Q. Causes of neutrophilia and neutropenia:

a. Neutrophilia:

1. Physiological: Pregnancy, stress, exercise, neonates.
2. Infections (i.e. pyogenic) and non-infective inflammations.
3. Trauma, post-surgery, acute haemorrhage, myocardial infarction, burn, pulmonary thromboembolism.

4. Myeloproliferative disorders, malignancy.
5. Drugs: Corticosteroids, G-CSF.

b. Neutropenia:

1. Infections: Typhoid, measles, malaria, different viral infections like hepatitis, chickenpox, influenza, HIV, etc..
2. Bone marrow failure like aplastic anaemia, myelodysplastic syndrome, myelofibrosis.
3. Drugs: Sulphonamides, antibiotics, bone marrow depressants; irradiation and chemical agents (e.g. benzene).
4. Autoimmune diseases like SLE, rheumatoid arthritis, Wegener's granulomatosis.
5. Starvation and debility.

- **Lymphopenia** is common in severe bone marrow failure, irradiation, Hodgkin's disease and immunosuppressive therapy.

TROPICAL EOSINOPHILIA

Hb	14 g/dL
RBC	5 million/mm^3
WBC	19000/mm^3
Polymorphs	42%
Lymphocytes	25%
Monocytes	1%
Eosinophils	32%
Basophils	0%
Platelets	2.8 lac/mm^3

Interpretation

1. There is no anaemia. Hb content and RBC count are within normal limit.
2. The WBC count shows leucocytosis. The absolute eosinophil count is 6080/mm^3 which is much above the expected maximum value (500/mm^3).
3. The platelet count is within normal limit.

Inference

This is a chart of eosinophilia, probably tropical eosinophilia.

Q. What is tropical eosinophilia?

When the absolute eosinophil count goes above 500/mm^3, it is known as eosinophilia. The diagnosis of tropical eosinophilia is confirmed by:

1. Patient is a prolonged habitat of an endemic area (e.g. Asian subcontinent).
2. Absolute eosinophil count in blood is above 3000/mm^3.
3. Absence of microfilariae in peripheral blood, examined by concentration technique both in day and night.
4. Presence of filarial antibodies in high titre. The filarial complement fixation test is positive in almost every patient.
5. Plasma level of IgE is high (at least 1000 U/mL).
6. Response to diethylcarbamazine citrate (DEC) therapy within 7 to 10 days when the drug is continued in a dose of 100 mg tds for 14 days.

- Tropical eosinophilia is an atypical host response to different filariae including *Wuchereria bancrofti, Brugia malayi, Loa loa, Brugia pahangi, and Dirofilaria immitis.*

Q. Features of tropical eosinophilia:

1. Paroxysmal dry cough with wheezing which is often nocturnal (commonest presentation): Tropical pulmonary eosinophilia.
2. Low grade pyrexia, loss of weight, lassitude, myalgia.
3. Splenomegaly and lymphadenopathy, rarely (Meyers-Kouwenaar syndrome).
4. Male: Female ratio is 4:1; cough with nocturnal bronchospasm and wheeze, where the chest X-ray shows millary mottlings (Weingarten syndrome): Mid- and lower zones are mostly affected with prominent bronchovascular markings.
5. Treatment is done by DEC with 4–6 mg/kg of body weight/day for at least 14 days.

Q. What is 'pulmonary eosinophilia'?

These are a group of disorders of varied aetiology where the pulmonary lesion shows chest X-ray abnormality along with pulmonary eosinophilia, which may or may not be associated with peripheral blood eosinophilia. The entities are:

1. Eosinophilic pneumonia (acute or chronic).
2. Allergic bronchopulmonary aspergillosis (ABPA): Hypersensitivity reaction to fungus *Aspergillus fumigatus.*
3. Parasitic infestations (filaria, roundworm, *Toxocara*).
4. Drug reactions (nitrofurantoin, PAS, sulphonamides, penicillin).
5. Loeffler's syndrome (due to *Ascaris lumbricoides* infestation).
6. Tropical pulmonary eosinophilia.
7. Hypereosinophilic syndrome.
8. Churg-Strauss syndrome.

Q. Common causes of eosinophilia:

1. Allergic disorders like bronchial asthma, hay fever, urticaria, angioneurotic oedema, eczema, pemphigus, allergic vasculitis, serum sickness, food sensitivity.
2. Parasitic infestations like hookworm, schistosomiasis, toxocariasis, ascariasis, strongyloidiasis. filariasis, trichinosis, cysticercosis and tropical eosinophilia.
3. Drugs like aspirin, iodides, penicillin, nitrofurantoin, sulphonamides.
4. Hypereosinophilic syndromes like Loeffler's syndrome, eosinophilic leukaemia.
5. Malignancy like Hodgkin's disease, mycosis fungoides, CML.

6. Collagen vascular diseases like polyarteritis nodosa, Churg-Strauss syndrome (vasculitis).
7. Addison's disease, dermatitis herpeteformis, eczema, psoriasis.

Q. What is hypereosinophilic syndrome?

It is a heterogeneous group of disorder with the common features of prolonged eosinophilia (absolute eosinophil count may go up to 50000–100000/mm^3) of unknown cause and is usually associated with dysfunction of organs like heart (endomyocardial fibrosis, tricuspid valve involvement, CCF), kidney, lungs, gastrointestinal tract, CNS, skin and even bone marrow. The patient commonly complains of pyrexia, weight loss, non-productive cough and respiratory distress. They usually die of congestive cardiac failure (CCF). Treatment by glucocorticoids and hydroxyurea/chlorambucil/vincristine, and management of organ dysfunction by specific drugs may be of value in some cases.

THALASSAEMIA

Hb	7.2 g/dL
RBC	3 million/mm^3
WBC	12900/mm^3
Polymorphs	63%
Lymphocytes	32%
Monocytes	2%
Eosinophils	3%
Basophils	0%
Reticulocytes	12%
Anisocytosis	++
Poikilocytosis	++
Target cells	+
Tear-drop cells	+
Normoblasts	+
Platelets	2.2 lac/mm^3
MCH	21 pg
MCHC	22 g/dL
MCV	66 cubic microns

Interpretation

1. There is moderate anaemia (Hb 7.2 g/dL, i.e. approximately 50%), RBC count is reduced to 60% approximately). So the cells are likely to be hypochromic.
2. Moreover MCH, MCHC and MCV are low, reflecting microcytic hypochromic anaemia.
3. The WBC count shows leucocytosis. The differential count is within normal limit.
4. Reticulocyte count is high (normal value 0.2–2%). Reticulocytosis and presence of normoblasts probably indicate either erythroid hyperplasia or bone marrow infiltration.
5. Anisocytosis and poikilocytosis indicate dyserythropoiesis.
6. Target cells and tear-drop cells are abnormal findings, and indicate either erythroid hyperplasia or infiltration of bone marrow. The platelet count is within normal limit.

Inference

Common causes of microcytic hypochromic anaemia are:

1. Iron deficiency anaemia.
2. Chronic haemolytic anaemia (e.g. thalassaemia).
3. Sideroblastic anaemia.
4. Sometimes seen in lead poisoning.

In sideroblastic anaemia, very often normocytes predominate; reticulocyte count is normal and sideroblasts are seen in peripheral blood. Absence of these facts negate the diagnosis of sideroblastic anaemia.

Again, erythroid hyperplasia (as there is presence of reticulocytosis and normoblasts) and dyshaemopoiesis (as there is presence of anisocytosis and poikilocytosis) point towards chronic haemolytic anaemia or iron deficiency anaemia with recent iron therapy.

The patients of lead poisoning will have specific occupational history like inhalation of fumes as from burning storage batteries, solder or paint spraying, or H/o ingestion of lead-containing material like paint. These patients reveal mild anaemia and basophilic slippling in the peripheral blood.

In iron deficiency anaemia (with iron therapy), usually reticulocyte count is not too high and leucocytosis is seldom present. Rather leucocytosis (often indicates pulmonary infection) may be present in chronic haemolytic anaemia.

So, this chart is probably dealing with chronic haemolytic anaemia. Presence of hypochromia as well as the grade of anaemia indicate the aetiology of anaemia towards thalassaemia major.

Q. What is a reticulocyte?

These are premature or young red cells, which are disc-shaped and contain ribosomal material (RNA). Condensation of the ribosomes to form reticular material (for identification) is best observed by:

a. Supravital stain (cresyl blue, new methylene blue), or
b. Romanowsky stain.

Normal reticulocyte count is 0.2–2% of RBC. An absolute increase in reticulocyte count (reticulocytosis) usually reflects 'increased erythropoiesis' (e.g. therapeutic response to therapy with iron, folic acid or vitamin B_{12}) or haemolytic anaemia. Rarely, when under stress, reliculocyte count may increase (released from marrow) without having increased erythropoiesis. *Low reticulocyte count is seen* in aplastic anaemia and megaloblastic anaemia.

- The normoblasts in a blood film usually indicate excessive or abnormal blood formation, or irritation of bone marrow by infiltration.

- **In clinical practice, reticulocytosis commonly indicates haemolytic anaemia.** *Reticulocyte count is also increased* following therapy in iron/folic acid/vitamin B_{12} deficiency anaemias, and in acute blood loss.
- **Sideroblasts:** The mitochondria, surrounding the nucleus of a normoblast, becomes iron-laden and appears as rings (known as ring sideroblast) with Prussian blue staining. Ring sideroblasts are seen in bone marrow.

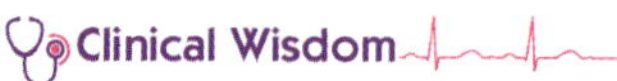

Corrected reticulocyte count in anaemia: Suppose, the reticulocyte count in an adult patient is 2% with 10 g/dL Hb → it does not reflect a true marrow response and thus, the corrected reticulocyte count will be:

$$\frac{\text{Patients Hb} \times \text{estimated reticulocyte count}}{\text{Normal Hb for that age and sex}} = \frac{10 \times 2}{15} = 1.3\%$$

Q. Causes of target cells in peripheral blood film:

1. Thalassaemia.
2. Iron deficiency anaemia.
3. Cholestatic jaundice.
4. Post-splenectomy or hyposplenism.

Q. How do the target cells look like?

These are flat red blood corpuscles with a central mass of haemoglobin (dense zone), surrounded by a ring of pallor (pale zone) and an extreme outer ring of haemoglobin (dense zone).

Q. Clinical triad of chronic haemolytic anaemia:

Triad of chronic haemolytic anaemia is anaemia, jaundice and splenomegaly.

Q. What is meant by punctate basophilia or basophilic stippling?

With Romanowsky staining, scattered deep-blue dots may be seen in the cytoplasm of abnormally damaged red cells. This type of basophilic suppling is commonly seen in chronic lead poisoning, beta-thalassaemia major and in any patient with severe anaemia (e.g. megaloblastic anaemia).

- Read 'Thalassaemia' from 'Bedside Clinics in Medicine, Part I' for further details.

THROMBOCYTOPENIA

Hb	8.9 g/dL
RBC	3.1 million/mm^3
WBC	8200/mm^3
Polymorphs	55%
Lymphocytes	35%
Monocytes	6%
Eosinophils	4%
Basophils	0%
Reticulocytes	1%
Anisocytosis	Nil
Poikilocytosis	Nil
Platelets	68000/mm^3
Bleeding times	13 min
Clotting time	5 min

Interpretation

1. There is moderate anaemia which seems to be normochromic. Anisocytosis and poikilocytosis are absent (i.e. no dyshaemopoiesis).
2. Total and differential count of WBC, and reticulocyte count are within normal limit.
3. There is thrombocytopenia. Bleeding time (BT) is increased in the presence of normal clotting time (CT).

Inference

Presence of anaemia (probably due to bleeding), normal leucocyte count, low platelet count, increased BT and normal CT clinch the diagnosis of thrombocytopenia, probably immune or idiopathic thrombocytopenic purpura (ITP).

Q. Critical platelet count:

It is 20,000/mm^3 (old view); the recent view is 10000/mm^3 and platelet count below this level may endanger the life of the patient by spontaneous haemorrhage in vital organs.

Q. How do a patient of ITP presents?

Women usually between 20–40 years of age (the acute form affects children between 2 and 6 years of age) present with gradually developing petechiae-purpura over skin, bleeding from gum, menorrhagia, epistaxis or haematuria (easy bruisability and spontaneous subcutaneous haemorrhage are most common). Pyrexia and malaise are not uncommon.

On examination, bleeding spots over the skin is noted. There is neither any lymphadenopathy nor any sternal tenderness present. The spleen is not palpable in 90% patients. Hess' capillary test (tourniquet test) may be positive.

[Bone marrow shows normal or increased numbers of immature megakaryocytes, which are otherwise normal].

Q. Possible causes of thrombocytosis:

1. Post-splenectomy.
2. Malignancy, Hodgkin's disease, chronic inflammatory disorders.
3. After severe haemorrhage, tissue damage.
4. Myeloproliferative disorders (CML, polycythemia vera, etc.).

Q. Significance of BT, CT, PT, PTT and IT

1. Bleeding time (BT): Increased in thrombocytopenia and platelet functional defect (thrombasthenia); von Willebrand (vW) disease.
2. Clotting time (CT): Increased in coagulation disorders (e.g. haemophilia) and afibrinogenaemia.

3. Prothrombin time (PT): Increased in factor VII deficiency (extrinsic pathway); factors II, V and X deficiency (common pathway); commonly seen in obstructive jaundice, haemorrhagic disease of the newborn, liver diseases, coumarin therapy, vitamin K deficiency.
4. Activated partial thromboplastin time (aPTT) or kaolin cephalin clotting time (KCCT): Increased in factors XII, XI, IX and VIII deficiency (intrinsic pathway); factors II, V and X deficiency (common pathway). Commonly seen in haemophilia, Christmas disease, heparin therapy, DIC, vW disease, antiphospholipid syndrome (APS).
5. Thrombin time (TT): Increased in afibrinogenaemia or dysfibrinogenaemia.

Q. Causes of thrombocytopenia:

A. Impaired production:

a. Aplastic anaemia (idiopathic).
b. Bone marrow failure: Radiation, cytotoxic drugs, multiple myeloma, leukaemia and lymphoma, metastasis from carcinoma.
c. Myelodysplastic syndromes.
d. Myelofibrosis.
e. Miscellaneous: Vitamin B_{12}/folate deficiency, HIV infection, rare congenital defects.

B. Increased consumption of platelets:

a. Immune: ITP, viruses (Epstein-Barr virus, HIV), drugs (penicillin, thiazides, heparin), SLE, CLL, DIC, TTP.
b. Non-immune: Hypersplenism (causing sequestration), massive transfusion (dilutional).

- Thrombocytopenia is primary (ITP) and secondary (A and B above).

Q. If ITP is suspected, what other diseases you will consider to be excluded?

SLE, leukaemias and antiphospholipid antibody syndrome.

Q. Non-thrombocytopenic purpura:

a. Vessel wall abnormalities, i.e. vasculitis. Henoch-Schönlein purpura, senile purpura, scurvy, uraemia, meningococcaemia, paraproteinaemia and drugs (e.g. sulphonamides); BT is usually normal, rarely increased. Platelet count is normal.
b. Platelet functional defect (thrombasthenia): BT is increased though platelet count remains normal.

Platelet functional defects are of two types:

a. Inherited: Glanzmann's thrombasthenia, Bernard-Soulier syndrome and storage pool disease.
b. Acquired: Myeloproliferative disease, renal and liver disease, paraproteinaemias, drugs (e.g. NSAIDs).

Q. Modalities of treatment adopted in ITP:

The patients usually require no treatment as long as the platelet count is >30000/mm^3 unless they undergo a surgical procedure.

1. Platelet or fresh blood transfusion, usually reserved for intracranial or other extreme haemorrhage. Children usually do not require treatment. Supportive care is employed. In adults, persistent thrombocytopenia is common, and they are being treated by:
2. Prednisolone (1 mg/kg of body weight/day) for 4–6 weeks, and then tapered.
3. IV immunoglobulin (1 g/kg of body weight for 3–5 days): Used temporarily to raise the platelet count (e.g. before surgery).
4. Rho(D) immune globulin therapy in a dose of 25 μg daily, IV for 3 days are helpful.
5. Splenectomy (with pneumococcal, *H. influenzae* and meningococcal vaccination): Majority of patients respond.
6. Vincristine, cyclophosphamide, cyclosporine, azathioprine or mycophenolate mofetil; danazol, dapsone are also tried.
7. Specific monoclonal antibodies, e.g. rituximab [anti CD-20 (B cell) antibody], and recombinant thrombopoietin (TPO) are promising.
8. Eltrombopag (thrombopoietin receptor agonist) and romiplostim (a novel thrombopoiesis protein) have shown encouraging results in refractory cases.

- Read the chapter on 'Haemorrhagic spots' from 'Bedside Clinics in Medicine, Part 1'.

CHARTS ON GLUCOSE TOLERANCE TEST (GTT)

Introduction

Diabetes mellitus is a clinical syndrome characterised by high blood sugar level (hyperglycaemia) and glycosuria due to relative or absolute deficiency of insulin secretion and/or action, or insulin resistance that leads to disturbances in carbohydrate, protein and fat metabolism, as well as disturbance of water and electrolyte homeostasis.

Oral GTT is an estimation of the capacity of a person to dispose off orally administered glucose (i.e. the glycaemic response). Nowadays, **it is not regarded as a very sensitive test to diagnose diabetes mellitus** as several large studies suggest that most of the patients (approximately 75%) with impaired GTT do not develop diabetes mellitus. GTT has a tendency to overdiagnose diabetes mellitus though it may still have a place in research works; moreover, oral GTT is time-consuming with low reproducibility. However, **GTT may be indicated** in 1) diagnosis of gestational diabetes mellitus (GDM), 2) diagnosis of pre-diabetes, i.e. IFG (impaired fasting glucose) and IGT (impaired glucose tolerance), and 3) evaluation of unexplained nephropathy, neuropathy or retinopathy when random glucose concentration is <140 mg/dL.

Q. Procedure of the test:

1. The patient is starved overnight (at least 8 hours) after 3 days of unrestricted carbohydrate diet (at least 150 g/day).
2. The patient should take ½ an hour rest in the laboratory and abstain from smoking but is allowed to drink water; 2 mL of fasting venous blood is drawn, and urine is collected before the test ('zero hour').
3. Now 75 g of glucose dissolved in 300 m1L of water is taken by mouth in 5 minutes in a case where the patient is non-diabetic or not on any therapy. For treated diabetic patients, postprandial blood should be drawn 2 hours after his recommended diabetic meal at scheduled time with usual drugs or insulin.
4. Thereafter blood and urine samples are collected every half-hourly for at least 2 hours. Quantitative estimation of sugar in blood and qualitative estimation of sugar in urine are carried out.
5. A curve is now plotted on a white paper by time in hours against blood level of sugar in mg/dL or mmol/L.

- So, 5 samples of blood and urine each are required for the test.
- While performing GTT, a diabetic patient on drugs or insulin need not take 75 g of glucose, instead he can consume his usual diet in which he is accustomed in his day-to-day life. The patient must receive his drugs as per schedule on the day of the test.

Q. Diagnostic criteria for diabetes mellitus:

- Symptoms of diabetes plus 'random' blood glucose concentration ≥200 mg/dL, or
- 'Fasting' plasma glucose ≥126 mg/dL, or
- '2-h postload' plasma glucose ≥200 mg/dL during an oral GTI, or
- HbA_{1c} ≥6.5%.

The **diagnostic criteria for pre-diabetes and diabetes** are:

In these criteria, the categories of FPG are:

- FPG <100 mg/dL = Normal fasting glucose
- FPG ≥100 mg/dL and <126 mg/dL = Impaired fasting glucose (IFG)
- FPG ≥126 mg/dL = Provisional diagnosis of diabetes (on more than one occasion)

The corresponding categories when the oral GTT is used, are as follows:

- 2 hPG <140 mg/dL = Normal glucose tolerance
- 2 hPG ≥140 mg/dL and <200 mg/dL = Impaired glucose tolerance (IGT)
- 2 hPG ≥200 mg/dL = Provisional diagnosis of diabetes (must be confirmed on a subsequent day)

- FPG = Fasting plasma glucose; 2 hPG = 2-h postload glucose
- The prognostic significance and outcome (i.e. accuracy) are same whether it is FPG >126 mg/dL or 2 hPG ≥200 mg/dL (i.e. in diabetics). This is why, in clinical practice, the FPG test is mostly preferred nowadays because of ease of administration, convenience, acceptibility to patients and its lower cost.

- Venous blood glucose < capillary blood glucose; and whole blood glucose <plasma glucose.
- Blood glucose concentration in mg/dL should be divided by 18 to get the value in mmol/L, e.g. 110 mg/dL = 6.1 mmol/L, 126 mg/dL = 7 mmol/L, 140 mg/dL = 7.8 mmol/L, and 200 mg/dL = 11.1 mmol/L.
- **'Fasting'** is defined as no calorie intake (i.e. overnight) for at least 8 hours. **'Random'** is defined as any time of the day without regard to time since the last meal. HbA_{1C} is currently the gold standard of glucose monitoring.
- In most laboratories, plasma or serum is used for glucose estimation whereas most methods for self-monitoring of blood glucose (SMBG), the whole blood is used (by glucometer).

Clinical Wisdom

As glucometer is available in the market, oral GTT is not a routine practice at present. One should read these charts to learn analysis of facts on diabetes mellitus.

NORMAL GTT (Fig. 7.1)

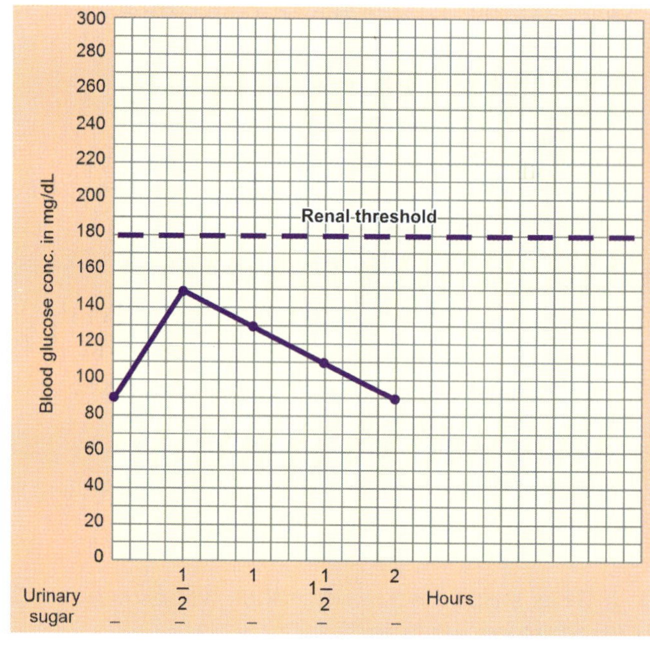

Fig. 7.1: Normal GTT curve

Interpretation

1. The fasting plama glucose level is below 100 mg/dL (i.e. normal).
2. The highest level is reached near 150 mg/dL. All the ½, 1, 1½ and 2-hour levels are below 180 mg/dL (normal renal threshold is 180 mg/dL).
3. The baseline is reached within 2 hours.
4. All the urine samples are sugar-free.

- **'Renal threshold'** is the capacity of the renal tubules to reabsorb glucose from the glomerular filtrate: If the plasma glucose concentration exceeds renal threshold, glycosuria occurs. Normal renal threshold is approximately 180 mg/dL but wide individual variation may exist.

Inference

This is a normal curve following a glucose tolerance test.

IMPAIRED GTT/IFG (Fig. 7.2)

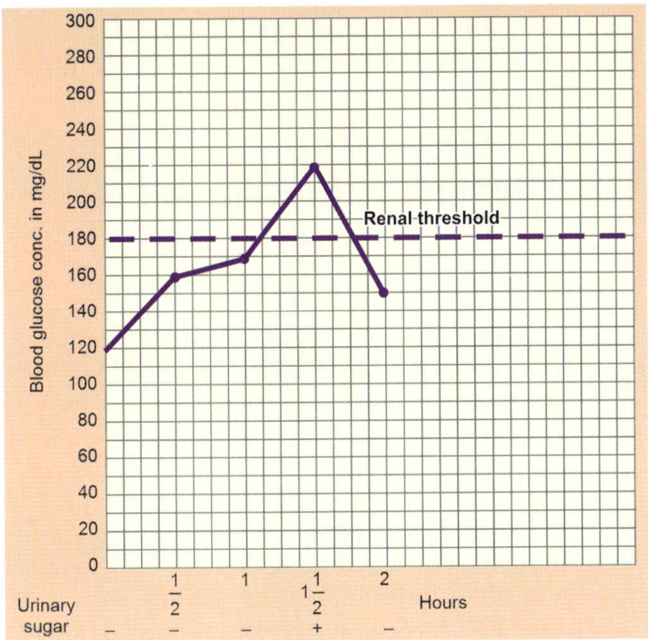

Fig. 7.2: Impaired glucose tolerance with impaired fasting glucose

Interpretation

1. The fasting plasma glucose level is above 100 mg/dL but below 126 mg/dL (i.e. IFG present).
2. The ½ and 1-hour levels are below the renal threshold but the 1½-hour level has crossed 180 mg/dL and is near about 220 mg/dL.
3. Renal threshold is normal, i.e. 180 mg/dL.
4. The 2-hour level is 150 mg/dL (i.e. in between 140–200 mg/dL).
5. The 1½-hour urine sample contains sugar. Other samples are sugar-free.

Inference

As the 2-hour test value is 150 mg/dL (i.e. in-between 140–200 mg/dL) and FPG is 120 mg/dL (i.e. ≥100 mg/dL, but <126 mg/dL), the chart is dealing with both IGT and IFG.

Q. Importance of impaired GTT:

Patients with impaired glucose tolerance (IGT), and/or impaired fasting glucose (IFG), and/or HbA_{1C} of 5.7–6.4% are now referred to as having **'pre-diabetes'** which indicates the relatively high risk for development of diabetes in future for these patients. Though they are not diabetic at the present moment, pre-diabetes indicates the need for further evaluation (future surveillance). Proper history taking is important and the patient may be kept under observation; the test may be repeated on a later date.

RENAL GLYCOSURIA (Fig. 7.3)

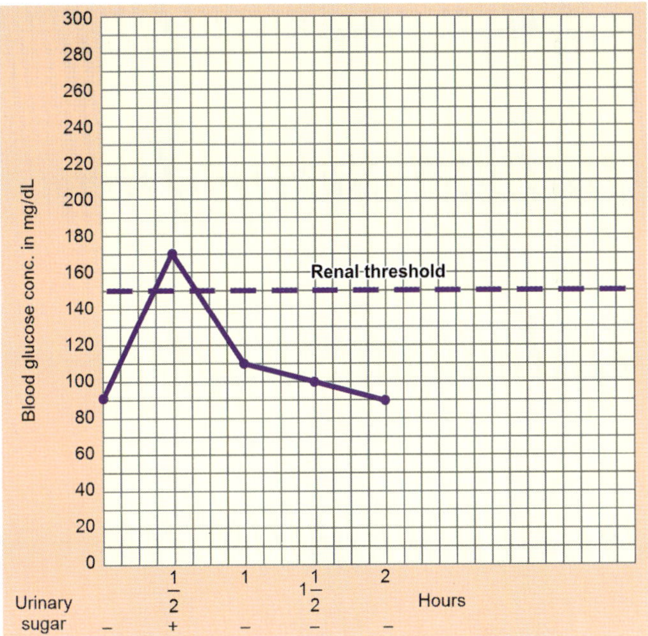

Fig. 7.3: Renal glycosuria

Interpretation

1. The fasting plasma glucose level is 90 mg/dL. The ½, 1, 1½, and 2-hour level is below 180 mg/dL, i.e. the normal level of renal threshold.
2. Renal threshold is 150 mg/dL (i.e. lower than normal).
3. Though the ½-hour level is 170 mg/dL, the urine sample shows presence of sugar, probably due to presence of low renal threshold for glucose.
4. The 2-hour level has touched the baseline.

Inference

It is a curve of renal glycosuria.

Q. What is renal glycosuria?

It is a cause of glycosuria due to lowered renal threshold. There is absence of both hyperglycaemia and the classical symptoms of diabetes mellitus (polyuria, polyphagia and polydipsia). This is a benign condition and is often temporarily *seen in pregnancy*. Renal glycosuria is diagnosed by **Marble's criteria** (glycosuria in the absence of hyperglycaemia, normal storage and utilisation of carbohydrates, normal oral GTT, identification of urinary reducing substance as glucose, and constant glycosuria with little fluctuation related to diet). Probably it is a genetic disorder (autosomal recessive). Rarely, glycosuria may be severe enough to produce polyuria and polydipsia.

ALIMENTARY GLYCOSURIA (Fig. 7.4)

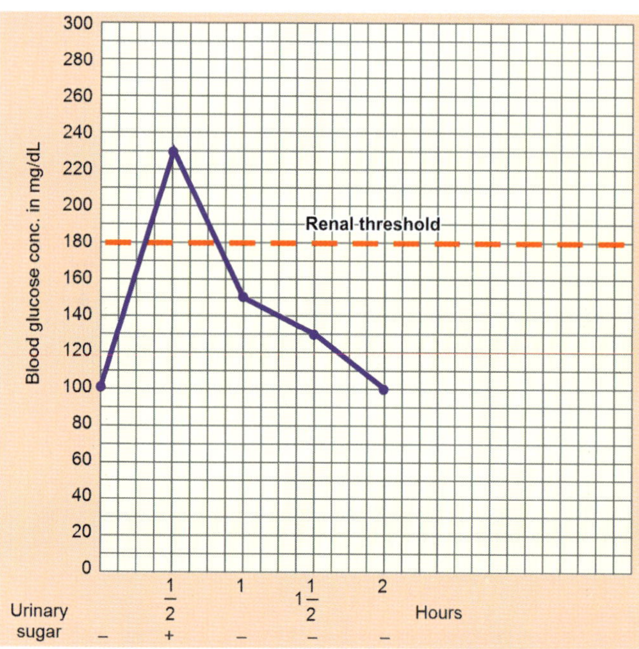

Fig. 7.4: Alimentary glycosuria

Interpretation

1. The fasting plasma glucose level is 99 mg/dL (i.e. normal fasting blood sugar),
2. The 2-hourly level is 100 mg/dl and thereby excludes the diagnosis of diabetes mellitus.
3. The renal threshold is normal (180 mg/dL) and thus the urine sugar is absent in 0, 1, 1½, and 2-hour samples.
4. As the ½-hour blood glucose level is 230 mg/dL (urine sample contains sugar), the possibilities of impaired GTT and alimentary glycosuria come in mind. As the 2-hourly blood level of glucose touches the baseline, question of impaired GTT does not arise. So, probably this is a curve of alimentary glycosuria.

Inference

The GTT deals with alimentary glycosuria or lag storage curve.

Q. What is alimentary glycosuria or lag storage curve?

It is seen that in some persons there is rapid but temporary rise in blood glucose level following a meal and the level usually exceeds the normal renal threshold, and thus the urine sample contains sugar too; the fasting and 2-hour values remain normal. This benign condition is not related to diabetes mellitus. Lag storage is due to defective glycogen synthesis in the liver or some defect lying in the GI tract, and is commonly found in hepatic disorders. Alimentary glycosuria is a better term than 'lag storage'.

Q. Conditions associated with alimentary glycosuria:

1. Normal individual.
2. After gastric surgery (e.g. partial gastrectomy leads to rapid gastric emptying and thereby facilitate increased glucose absorption).
3. Hyperperistalsis due to any cause (e.g. peptic ulcer).
4. Hepatic disorders (e.g. hepato-cellular failure).
5. Hyperthyroidism.

- Remember, **dumping syndrome** may produce sudden hyperglycaemia as is seen in alimentary glycosuria (partial gastrectomy → rapid emptying of sugar containing meals into proximal small intestine → abrupt increase in blood glucose concentration → release of excess insulin stimulated by high blood sugar level → subsequent hypoglycaemia with vasomotor symptoms) but in that situation, the 1/2 to 3-hour samples will show low blood glucose level (hypoglycaemia). However, the GTT may have to be continued for 3 hours instead of 2 hours to diagnose late dumping syndrome.

Q. What is glycosuria of pregnancy?

Glycosuria is a common finding in pregnancy because of drop in renal threshold for glucose as a result of increase in GFR. Sometimes, lactose is found in urine in late pregnancy. As high blood sugar level in pregnancy is associated with increased perinatal morbidity and mortality, all patients with glycosuria of pregnancy should be properly screened to exclude **gestational diabetes mellitus** (GDM).

GDM is defined as glucose intolerance of variable degree with onset or first recognition during pregnancy. This includes pre-existing type 1 or type 2 DM (may be clinically undiagnosed). The majority of women with GDM can expect to go back to normal glucose tolerance immediately after pregnancy. However, GDM is associated with an increased risk of later development of T_2DM. GDM complicates ~7% (1–14%) of pregnancies. A high maternal blood glucose promotes fetal insulin production which stimulates fetal growth. Macrosomia of the fetus may complicates labour and delivery. GDM is treated with insulin as oral hypoglycaemic drugs cross the placenta and may be a potential risk for the fetus.

There are many diagnostic criteria for GDM. The International Association of Diabetes and Pregnancy Study Groups (IADPSG) criteria to diagnose GDM after taking 75 g of oral glucose is (at 24–28 weeks of pregnancy):

- FPG ≥92 mg/dL.
- 1-hour postload plasma glucose ≥180 mg/dL.
- 2-hour postload plasma glucose ≥153 mg/dL.

- A positive diagnosis requires that test results satisfy any one of this criteria.

Q. Reducing agents in urine (positive Benedict's test):

a. Glucose (commonest): Diabetes mellitus, impaired GTT, renal glycosuria, alimentary glycosuria, Fanconi's syndrome.
b. Non-diabetic melituria: Lactose (pregnancy and during lactation), fructose (fructosuria), galactose (galactosuria), pentose (pentosuria after consumption

of grapes, cherries, plums), homogentisic acid (found in alcaptonuria, a rare inborn error of metabolism).

c. Spurious: Patient treated with ascorbic acid, nalidixic acid, cephalosporins or aspirin.

- Sucrose is not a reducing agent. Galactosuria and fructosuria may result from inborn error of metabolism. **Melituria** is the presence of any kind of sugar in urine.

Q. Positive Rothera's test (nitroprusside test) in urine:

1. Ketone bodies.
2. Cystinuria.
3. Homocystinuria.
4. False positive (spurious): Drug treatment with salicylates, levodopa, captopril, penicillamine.

DIABETIC CURVE (Fig. 7.5)

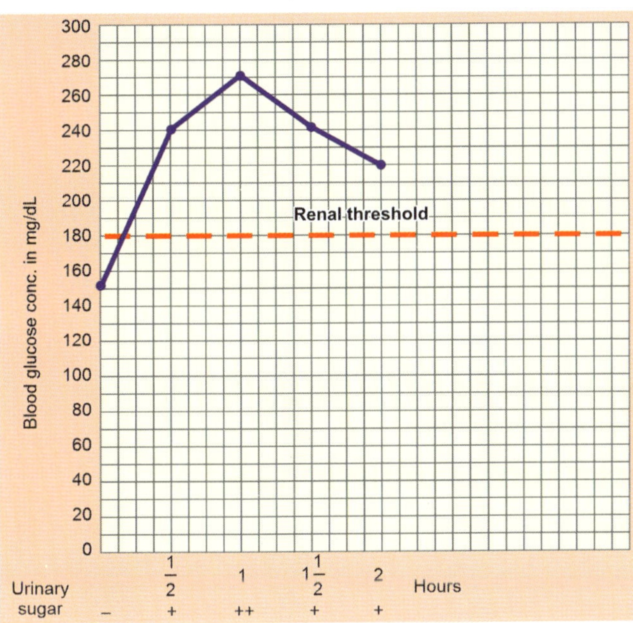

Fig. 7.5: Diabetic curve

Interpretation

1. The fasting plasma glucose level is 150 mg/dL and that of 2-hour postprandial (PP) level recorded is 220 mg/dL (i.e. >200 mg/dL). The 1/2, 1 and 1½, hour levels are well above the renal threshold level (i.e. >180 mg/dL), and virtually above 200 mg/dL.
2. The 1/2, 1, 1/2 and 2-hourly urine samples show presence of sugar (all the corresponding blood glucose level is above the renal threshold).

Inference

This is the curve of a patient who is suffering from diabetes mellitus of moderate severity.

Q. Aetiological classification of diabetes mellitus by American Diabetes Association (ADA):

i. Type 1 diabetes (β-cell destruction, usually leading to absolute insulin deficiency):
   a. Immune-mediated.
   b. Idiopathic.

ii. Type 2 diabetes (insulin resistance ranging from insulin deficiency to secretory defect).

iii. Other specific types:
   a. Genetic defects of β-cell function: Chromosome 12, *HNF-1α (formerly MODY 3); chromosome 7, glucokinase (formerly MODY 2): chromosome 20, HNF-4α (formerly MODY 1); insulin promoter factor-1 (MODY 4); HNF-1β (MODY 5); NeuroD1 (MODY 6); mitochondrial DNA; mutant insulins; hyperproinsulinaemia.
   b. Genetic defects in insulin action: Lipoatrophic diabetes, leprechaunism.
   c. Endocrine disorders: Acromegaly, Cushing's syndrome, pheochromocytoma, hyperthyroidism, glucagonoma, somatostatinoma, aldosteronoma, and others.
   d. Disease of the exocrine pancreas: Pancreatitis, trauma, pancreatectomy, cystic fibrosis, haemochromatosis, fibrocalcific pancreatic disease (FCPD), neoplasia, and others.
   e. Drug- or chemical-induced: Vacor (rat poison), thiazides, glucocorticoids, phenytoin, nicotinic acid, pentamidine, α-interferon, diazoxide, asparaginase, protease inhibitors.
   f. Infections: Congenital rubella, cytomegalovirus, coxsackievirus.
   g. Uncommon immune-mediated disorders: Anti-insulin receptor antibodies, 'stiff-person' syndrome.
   h. Genetic syndromes associated with diabetes: Down's syndrome, myotonic dystrophy, Klinefelter's syndrome, Turner's syndrome, Friedreich's ataxia, Prader-Willi syndrome, Huntington's chorea.

iv. Gestational diabetes mellitus (GDM).

- *HNF, Hepatocyte nuclear transcription factor; MODY, Maturity-onset diabetes of the young.
- In this classification, the older terms like IDDM (insulin dependent diabetes mellitus) and NIDDM are eliminated because many patients with NIDDM (non-insulin dependent diabetes mellitus) eventually would require insulin.
- T_1DM is Type 1 diabetes mellitus and T_2DM means Type 2 diabetes mellitus.

CHARTS ON STOOL/FECES

Introduction

Important information about diseases that affect the gastrointestinal system can be obtained with stool (loosely called as 'poo') examinations. Stool can be examined macroscopically, microscopically, chemically, immunologically and microbiologically. Many a time, a simple sample of stool can give clinical clues of the 25 feet long intestine. *Stool analysis is indicated in* gastrointesinal infections, bowel carcinoma, pancreatic disorders, malabsoption with malnutrition, occult blood test, etc. Stool samples should always be collected in a clean container.

A. Naked-eye Examination or Macroscopic Examination

1. Amount: Copious (e.g. bulky in steatorrhoea) or scanty.
2. Colour: Yellowish brown due to the presence of stercobilinogen/stercobilin (normal), black (melaena, ingestion of bismuth, iron or licorice), red (ingestion of beets/mixed with blood/haematochezia), pale (absence of bile, rapid passage through the intestine in diarrhoea, high fat content due to malabsorption), green (in the presence of diarrhoea, unaltered bile may be there due to rapid passage).
3. Consistency: Well-formed stool (normal), harder than normal (constipation), liquid or watery (diarrhoea), tarry or sticky (melaena), semisolid (normal), slimy or jelly like (due to the presence of excess mucus), soft and frothy (steatorrhoea) or ribbon-like stool in gut obstruction. Does the stool floats in water (e.g. steatorrhoea)?

- The **Bristol stool chart** (1997), used as a clinical assessment tool for bowel health, has 7 types of feces.

4. Odour: Normal fecal odour (due to aromatic substances indole and skatole, etc. and H_2S), odourless (cholera, acute bacillary dysentery), offensive (acute amoebic dysentery, malabsorption syndrome, melaena, jaundice, giardiasis, partial gut obstruction). In nursing infants, stool gives a sour odour due to presence of fatty acids.
5. Parasites: Worms or segments of worms may be present, e.g. roundworm, threadworm, tapeworm.

B. Chemical Examination

1. *Reaction:* Usually it is neutral or slightly acidic (normal), alkaline stool may be found in acute bacillary dysentery, salmonella enteritis, etc. Highly acidic stool may be present in lactase deficiency, after lactulose ingestion in hepatic pre-coma, or in sprue.
2. *Orthotolidine test:* Detects presence of blood (occult or overt) in stool. Before performing this test, patient should have been on a meat-free diet for 3 days and should not have been taking vitamin C and aspirin (NSAID).

C. Microscopic Examination

1. RBC (presence of blood, overt or occult).
2. WBC (acute bacillary dysentery, *Campylobacter*, enteroinvasive or enterohaemorrhagic *E. coli*. *Clostridium difficile*, *Salmonella* infection).
3. Macrophages: Acute bacillary dysentery, acute infectious colitis, pseudomembranous colitis.
4. Eosinophils: Acute amoebic dysentery, eosinophilic enteritis.
5. Parasites, cyst: Intestinal amoebiasis, giardiasis or helminthiasis.
6. Bacteria: Acute bacillary dysentery (shigellosis), acute infectious colitis.
7. Flakes of mucus: Acute amoebic dysentery, acute bacillary dysentery, ulcerative colitis, irritable bowel syndrome, infection by *Campylobacter jejuni*, cholera, malabsorption syndrome.
8. Epithelia: Found in tropical sprue, acute bacillary dysentery.
9. Pus cells: In dysentery of any aetiology.
10. Charcot-Leyden crystals: Acute amoebic dysentery.
11. Undigested food material: Malabsorption syndrome.

- Varieties of different stools: Rice watery stool: Cholera; pea-soup diarrhoea: Enteric fever; china-clay stool: Obstructive jaundice; toothpaste stool: Stricture or Hirschsprung's disease; red currant jelly stool (i.e. mixed with blood and mucus): Intussusception.
- Volume of stool: Small bowel diarrhoea: High volume diarrhoea with uniform watery consistency; colonic diarrhoea: Low volume diarrhoea, the stool usually contains numerous small pieces of feces (*see* **Table 1.5**).
- Under microscope: During microscopic examination, a small portion of feces is taken on the glass slide with the help of a broom-stick and emulsified with a drop of isotonic saline, and lastly coverslip is applied over it (saline preparation).
- Hanging-drop preparation: A bit of diluted fecal matter is taken on a coverslip and the coverslip is then inverted on a slide, and examined under a microscope. By this way, darting motility of Vibrio cholerae can be nicely seen.

Clinical Wisdom

In health, osmolality of stool is 290 mOsmol/kg of water.

ACUTE AMOEBIC DYSENTERY (Table 7.3)

Naked-eye Examination

Amount	Relatively copious
Colour	Dark red; fecal matter seen
Consistency	Liquid yellow stool; fecal matter streaked with blood and mucus. Fecal matter is not adherent to the bottom of the container
Odour	Offensive

Chemical Examination

Reaction	Acidic
Orthotolidine test	++

Microscopic Examination

RBC	+, in clumps
WBC	Very few
Macrophages	Nil
Eosinophils	Present
Parasite/cyst	Trophozoites of *E. histolytica*, often with ingested RBC
Bacteria	Few
Pus cells	Scanty
Epithelia	Absent
Charcot-Leyden crystals	Present

Table 7.3: Differentiation between amoebic and bacillary dysentery

Features	Amoebic dysentery	Bacillary dysentery
1. Number of motions/day	6–8	>10
2. Amount	Copious	Small
3. Colour	Dark red	Bright red
4. Odour	Offensive	Odourless
5. Fecal matter	Present	Minimal
6. Reaction	Acidic	Alkaline
7. Consistency	Non-adherent to the container	Adherent to the container
8. RBC	Clumps	Discrete
9. Pus cells	Scanty	Plenty
10. Macrophage	Very few	Numerous
11. Eosinophils	Present	Absent
12. Charcot-Leyden crystals	Present	Absent
13. Parasites	*E. histolytica*	Absent
14. Bacteria	Nil	Motile bacteria

Interpretation

1. Liquid stool mixed with blood and mucus points towards acute dysentery. Infection by some organism is suggested by the presence of offensive odour. Formation of mild inflammatory exudate (pus cells and WBC are scanty) indicates the presence of very low fibrin content and thus the stool is not adherent to the container.
2. Presence of Charcot-Leyden crystals along with above features suggest acute amoebic dysentery. Positive orthotolidine test confirms presence of blood in the stool.
3. Trophozoites (vegetative form) of *E. histolytica* confirms the diagnosis of acute amoebic dysentery.

Inference

This is a chart of acute amoebic dysentery (amoebiasis).

Q. Describe an amoebic ulcer in intestine:

Usually superficial (does not extend beyond muscularis mucosae), round or oval, from a pin's head to one inch or more, with ragged and undermined margin having overhanging mucous membrane (appearance of flask-shaped ulcer in vertical section), and the base of the ulcer is filled-up by necrotic material and yellowish slough.

Q. Organs involved in amoebiasis:

a. Intestine: Mainly the ileo-caecal region (mimic acute appendicitis), rarely the sigmoido-rectal region.

b. Extraintestinal sites: Liver, lung, brain (acanthamoeba and Naegleria fowleri), spleen, genitourinary tract, skin and cornea (keratitis caused by acanthamoeba).

Q. Laboratory diagnosis of amoebiasis:

a. Stool examination:

1. Naked-eye examination.
2. Microscopic examination (4–6 specimens should be examined). Microscopic examination of fresh stool or colonic exudate revealed by sigmoidoscopy is the simplest way to diagnose colonic affection by amoebiasis. Motile trophozoites containing RBCs confirm the diagnosis

b. Blood examination: May show moderate leucocytosis (in symptomatic patients).

c. Serological tests:

1. Indirect haemagglutination test.
2. Fluorescent antibody test (for amoeba).
3. Complement fixation test.
4. ELISA (Dot ELISA is often preferred).
5. Counterimmunodiffusion.
6. Agar gel diffusion.

- Remember, the 'trophozoite or vegetative' form of *E. histolytica* is the infective form, while the 'cystic' form is present in the carriers.
- Read 'amoeboma' (i.e. large local lesion of amoebic granuloma in bowel) and amoebic liver abscess. Read the treatment of 'acute amoebic dysentery' from the section of 'Emergency medicine'.

Q. Pathological situations with 'ulcers in intestine':

Amoebiasis, typhoid fever, tuberculosis, ulcerative colitis, Crohn's disease, malignancy, Zollinger-Ellison syndrome, bacillary dysentery, drug-induced (e.g. enteric-coated potassium tablet), ischaemic colitis and mesenteric artery occlusion (abdominal angina).

Q. Presence of 'mucus in the stool':

1. Acute amoebic dysentery, acute bacillary dysentery.
2. Ulcerative colitis.
3. Irritable bowel syndrome.
4. Malabsorption syndrome.
5. Small amount may be present in normal person.

ACUTE BACILLARY DYSENTERY (Table 7.3)

Naked-eye Examination

Amount	Scanty
Colour	Bright red
Consistency	Liquid, mainly blood, mucus and pus. Scanty fecal matter which is adherent to the bottom of the container
Odour	Non-offensive (odourless)

Chemical Examination

Reaction	Alkaline
Orthotolidine test	++

Microscopic Examination

RBC	+++; discrete
WBC	+++
Macrophages	Numerous and many of them have RBC within
Eosinophils	Virtually absent
Parasite/cyst	Absent
Bacteria	Plenty of motile bacteria
Pus cells	Plenty
Epithelia	Present
Charcot-Leyden crystals	Absent

Interpretation

1. Liquid stool mixed with blood and mucus points towards acute dysentery. Presence of RBC, WBC, pus cells, macrophages indicate massive inflammatory exudate and thus the fecal matter is adherent to the container as a result of high fibrin content.
2. Scanty fecal maller, presence of blood, mucus and pus, and alkaline reaction (as a result of presence of frank blood) are highly suggestive of acute bacillary dysentery. Positive orthotolidine test confirms presence of blood in the stool.
3. Presence of plenty of motile bacteria are probably due to *Shigella* (producing acute bacillary dysentery) or *E. coli* (may be present normally). Absence of parasite/cyst as well as vegetative form of *E. histolytica* denies acute amoebic dysentery.
4. Other features are also corroborative of acute bacillary dysentery.

Inference

This chart deals with acute bacillary dysentery (shigellosis).

Q. Common causes of dysentery (acute diarrhoea with 'blood and mucus in the stool'):

1. Acute bacillary dysentery (there are four main pathologic strains of *Shigella* like *S. dysenteriae*, *S. flexneri*, *S. boydii* and S. sonnei)
2. Acute amoebic dysentery (*E. histolytica*).
3. Infection of large gut by *Campylobacter jejuni*, *Salmonella enteritidis* or *Yersinia enterocolitica*.
4. Enteroinvasive and enterohaemorrhagic *E. coli*.
5. Dysentery caused by *Schistosoma mansoni*.
6. Ulcerative colitis, Crohn's disease.
7. Pseudomembranous colitis caused by *Clostridium difficile*.
8. Mesenteric vascular disease.
9. Intestinal tuberculosis.
10. Diverticulitis.
11. Carcinoma of the large intestine (lower).
12. Necrotising enterocolitis.

Q. Investigations performed in chronic loss of blood and mucus in stool:

1. Stool examination (naked-eye and microscopic) with culture and sensitivity.
2. Proctoscopy, sigmoidoscopy/colonoscopy, and barium enema examination.
3. Biopsy of the intestine.

Q. Complications of acute shigellosis:

1. Haemorrhage, perforation, toxic dilatation of colon.
2. Bacteraemia.
3. Endotoxic shock.
4. Haemolytic-uraemic syndrome.
5. Pneumonia, meningitis, seizures (rarely seen).
6. Reactive arthritis.

- Diagnosis of bacillary dysentery depends on isolation of the organism from stool cultures.
- Read the treatment of 'Shigellosis' from the section of 'Emergency medicine'.

GIARDIASIS

Naked-eye Examination

Amount	Sufficient for examination
Colour	A bit whitish
Consistency	Greasy
Odour	Offensive

Chemical Examination

Reaction	Acidic
Orthotolidine test	–ve

Microscopic Examination

RBC	Nil
WBC	+
Macrophages	+
Eosinophils	Present
Parasite/cyst	*Giardia lamblia* present
Bacteria	Few
Pus cells	Absent
Epithelia	Absent

Interpretation with Inference

Presence of *Giardia lamblia* in a specimen of stool which is greasy, a bit whitish and offensive clinches the diagnosis of 'giardiasis'.

Q. Describe the clinical features of giardiasis:

Commonly it affects the children in endemic areas (tropics), tourists, persons with poor hygiene, immunosuppressed individuals (e.g. IgA deficiency), male homosexuals and persons with achlorhydria. Mode of spread is through fecal-oral route (ingestion of cysts) and the incubation period is 1–3 weeks. The patient passes cyst with stool, which remain viable in water. The sites of involvement are duodenum and jejunum. The clinical manifestations range from asymptomatic carrier to fulminant diarrhoea and malabsorption. The patient may complain of abdominal pain, anorexia, nausea, vomiting, weakness, pallor and loose offensive stools; there may be abdominal tenderness with distension. There is acquired lactose intolerance. These features may continue for weeks or months, and the patient loses weight, becomes lethargic and complains of flatulent dyspepsia.

Q. How to investigate this patient?

1. **Examination of stool** (at 2–3 days interval on 3 seperate occasions) for cysts.
2. Doudenal or jejunal fluid is aspirated through Ryle's tube or endoscope, and examined for parasites/cyst.
3. Jejunal biopsy (the mucus should be examined fresh): Shows *G. lamblia* over the surface of the epithelium.
4. Tests to detect *G. lamblia* antigen in the stool: May be done.
5. Other investigations to exclude different causes of malabsorption (e.g. tropical sprue, coeliac disease).

Q. Treatment:

1. Single dose of tinidazole 40 mg/kg in the range of 0.5–2 g, may be repeated after 1 week, or
2. Metronidazole 250 mg thrice daily for 5 days, or
3. Quinacrine hydrochloride 0.1 g, thrice daily for 5 days, or
4. Furazolidone 100 mg four times daily for 10 days, or
5. Nitazoxanide 500 mg twice daily for 3 days.

OCCULT BLOOD IN STOOL

Naked-eye Examination

Amount	Sufficient for examination
Colour	Yellowish
Consistency	Semisolid
Odour	Fecal odour

Chemical Examination

Reaction	Acidic
Haemoccult test	+++

Microscopic Examination

RBC, WBC, macrophages	Absent
Ova, parasite, cyst	Absent

Interpretation

All the features indicate normal stool except the presence of positive haemoccult test. As the colour and consistency of the stool is not black, tarry, and the odour is not very offensive, it is not the stool of melaena. So there is presence of occult blood in stool specimen.

Inference

This is a chart of stool containing occult blood.

Q. Common causes of occult blood in stool:

1. Chronic duodenal or gastric ulcer.
2. Erosive gastritis (NSAID, corticosteroids).
3. Variceal bleeding.
4. Carcinoma of the stomach.
5. Hookworm infestation.
6. Colo-rectal malignancy.
7. Mesenteric ischaemia.
8. Angiodysplasia of the colon.

- Intake of NSAID, hookworm infestation and colo-rectal cancer are common causes of occult blood in stool.

Q. Describe stool of melaena (alterted blood in stool):

The characteristics of **melaena stool** is described below:

1. Black tarry stool (due to production of acid haematin); sticky too.
2. Offensive (acid haematin is altered by bacteria), and with a characteristic odour.
3. Semisolid in consistency; often it is difficult to flush out.
4. Red-coloured fluid comes out from the stool after addition of water in it.
5. Usually associated with vertigo, dizziness or syncopal attack during defecation.

- Approximately 60 mL of blood is required to produce a 'single black stool' and blood should remain for at least 8 hours within the gut lumen to produce melaena.

Q. In which forms blood may be present in the stool?

1. Frank blood or haematochezia.
2. Altered blood or melaena.
3. Invisible or occult blood (detected chemically).

Q. Prerequisites for occult blood test in stool (Guaiac test):

As bleeding from GI tract may be intermittent, the test should be performed for several (usually three) consecutive days.

1. To avoid false-positive results, 3 days high-fibre and meat-free diet is advocated.
2. To avoid false-negative result, patient should not have been taking vitamin C.
3. NSAID should not be taken (may produce erosive gastritis). Tooth-brush may be avoided for 3 days. Medicinal iron should be stopped.

- In modern haemoccult test, medicinal iron does not interfere with the test. Fecal blood loss in normal individuals may vary up to 2.5 mL, which does not change the colour of stool (i.e. no melaena). Upto 2.5 mL of 'normal' fecal blood loss may be measured by radioactive chromium.

Q. How do you proceed to diagnose a case with positive occult blood in stool?

1. Detailed history taking (intake of NSAID, anorexia for gastric malignancy, etc.) and meticulous clinical examination (e.g. degree of iron deficiency anaemia suggests the duration of illness, lymphadenopathy pointing to occult carcinoma, abdominal mass indicating GI malignancy, splenomegaly for portal hypertension).
2. Stool examination for hookworm ova/parasite.
3. To diagnose the site of blood loss sigmoidoscopy, colonoscopy or barium enema should be followed by upper GI endoscopy.
4. Barium follow-through examination of the GI tract.
5. If diarrhoea or steatorrhoea is present, investigations for malabsorption is performed.
6. USG or CT scan of whole abdomen.
7. Angiography; radiolabeled erythrocyte scanning.

- Digital examination, proctoscopy and sigmoidoscopy are important manoeuvres/investigations in the aetiological diagnosis of haematochezia.

CHARTS ON URINE

Introduction

Complete urinalysis is done in a laboratory ('to urinate' is loosely termed as 'pee'). It usually involves three steps, i.e. macroscopic, chemical (using a test strip) and microscopical assessment. A simple chemical test of urine which shows mild proteinuria can reflect early kidney involvement with ominous prognosis in collagen disorders like SLE.

Urinalysis is indicated in different kidney diseases, diabetes mellitus, systemic hypertension, UTI, coagulation disorders, collagen vascular diseases, cardiac disorders, pregnancy, etc.

A. Routine Examination (R/E) of Urine Consists of:

I. Naked-eye examination, macroscopic examination or physical examination:

a. Volume or quantity per day
b. Colour and transparency
c. Odour
d. Specific gravity

II. Chemical examination:

a. Reaction or pH
b. Proteins
c. Sugars
d. Ketone bodies
e. Blood and haemoglobin
f. Bile pigments and bile salts

III. Microscopic examination:

a. RBC
b. WBC and pus cells
c. Epithelial cells
d. Casts
e. Crystals
f. Microorganism, spermatozoa

- For microscopical examination, 10–15 mL of urine is centrifused at a speed of 3000 rpm, for at least 3 minutes, and the deposit is examined under microscope.

B. Special Examination of Urine Consists of:

Culture and sensitivity tests (bacteriological examination): >100 000 bacteria/mL of mid-stream urine indicates urinary tract infection. Antibiotic sensitivity is known as 'antibiogram'.

Each component is discussed below in a nutshell:

1. Volume of urine in 24 hours: The normal daily urinary output is 400 ml–3 litres, depending on the fluid intake. Average output in a healthy adult is 1.5 litre per day. Urine volume <400 mL per day is **oliguria** and no urine formation for 12 hours is **anuria**, while **polyuria** is urinary output >3 litres per day.
2. Colour and transparency: Normally fresh urine is clear to straw-yellow coloured. The colour varies from person to person and from day to day. The specific gravity and voided amount of urine often determine the depth of colour. Colour changes may occur in diseases or after ingestion of drugs, like:
   a. Red: Blood, haemoglobin, myoglobin, ingestion of beet roots, phenolpthalein in alkaline medium, drug like penazopyridine, and porphobilinogen (porphyria).
   b. Pink or dark orange: Rifampicin (Fig. 7.6), senna.
   c. Milky white: Chyluria.
   d. Black: Alkaptonuria (darkens on standing due to presence of homogentisic acid), intake of methyl

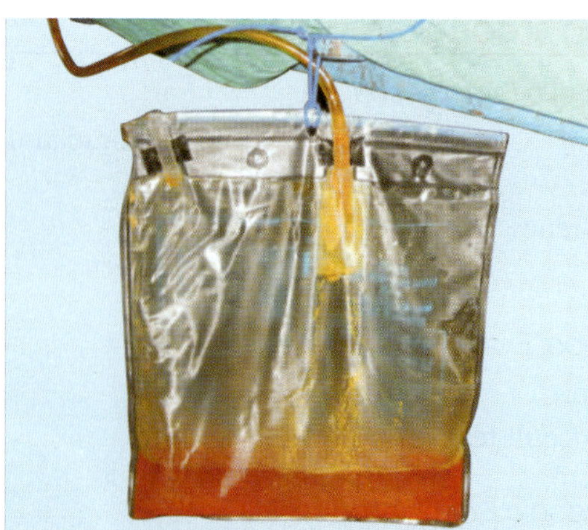

Fig. 7.6: **Orange-yellow coloured urine** collected in urosac in a patient of caries spine who is on rifampicin

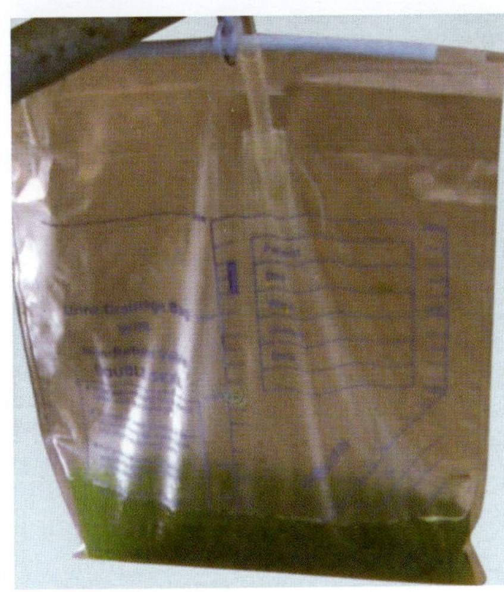

Fig. 7.7: Green urine in *Pseudomonas aeruginosa* infection

dopa, iron therapy (IM), melanoma (melanogen), tyrosinosis.

e. Yellowish-brown: Furazolidone, nitrofurantoin, tetracyclines, riboflavin or sulfasalazine.
f. Deep yellow: Concentrated urine, jaundice.
g. Greenish: Pseudomonas infection in urine (Fig. 7.7), drugs (amitriptyline, methylene blue, propofol).
h. Cloudy: Presence of pus, blood, cellular debris or crystals (phosphates or urates).

- The colour of the normal urine is given by urochrome and uroerythrin. Normally urine darkens on standing because of oxidation of colourless urobilinogen to coloured urobilin.

3. Odour: Normally urine has ammoniacal smell due to bacterial decomposition. *E. coli* infection gives rise to fishy smell, and smell of acetone may come out from the urine of a patient having diabetic ketoacidosis; diabetics have 'fruity' odour in their urine, and even garlic, alcohol and coffee can change the smell of urine.
4. Specific gravity: Minimally 50 mL of urine is required to measure the specific gravity. The specific gravity varies from 1002 to 1035 in a healthy person, depending on the state of hydration. Usually it is within 1015–1025, signifying **normal tubular ability** for concentrating urine. Normal osmolality of urine is 400–750 mOsmol/kg of water.
   - Very high specific gravity: Diabetes mellitus, severe dehydration, massive proteinuria.
   - Very low specific gravity: Diabetes insipidus, psychogenic polydipsia.
   - Fixed specific gravity at 1010—End-stage renal disease (i.e. CRF).
5. Reaction or pH: Normal urine is nearly always acidic in reaction (5–7.2). If the urine reaction repeatedly becomes neutral or alkaline, think of consumption of alkali, alkalosis, loss of tubular function to eliminate acid, patient on high vegetarian diet or UTI by organism other than *E. coli* (especially *Proteus*). Remember, acidic urine turns blue litmus paper to red, while alkaline urine turns red litmus into blue colour.
6. Protein: Presence of protein in urine signifies defect in the **glomerular function**. Normal adult may excrete up to 150 mg of protein in 24 hours, and of this 15 mg is albumin. Proteinuria can be divided into mild (150–500 mg/day), moderate (500 mg–2 g/day) and massive types (>2 g/day). Proteinuria is in the 'nephrotic range' when crosses 3.5 g/day. The pathophysiological types of proteinuria are:
   Glomerular proteinuria: >1.5 g/day, usually albumin and high-molecular weight protein; **tubular** proteinuria: <2 g/day, mainly of low-molecular weight protein rather than albumin, and **overflow** proteinuria: like Bence Jones protein, myoglobin or haemoglobin in urine.
   Proteinuria is divided into selective (steroid-responsive) and non-selective types. Selectivity is estimated by comparing the clearance of IgG with that of transferrin. If the clearance of IgG is >20% of transferrin, it represents 'non-selective' proteinuria. If the value is <10%, it indicates 'highly selective' proteinuria. The range between 10–20% is of little discriminatory value. 'Highly selective' proteinuria is found in minimal lesion nephropathy. The degree of selectivity gives an indication of the amount of glomerular damage.
7. Sugars: Several reducing sugars may be found in urine sample (glucose, lactose, fructose, pentose, galactose) of which glucose is the most improtant. Presence of glucose in urine is known as glycosuria (e.g. alimentary glycosuria, renal glycosura, diabetes mellitus). Sucrose is a non-reducing sugar.
8. Ketone bodies: Ketone bodies are acetone, acetoacetic acid and β-hydroxybutyric acid. Ketone bodies may be found in urine in conditions like starvation, diabetic ketoacidosis, severe vomiting, diet enriched in fat and very low in carbohydrate, acute hepatic necrosis, and in alcoholic ketoacidosis.
9. Blood and haemoglobin, i.e. haematuria. For its causes, read the chapter on 'Acute glomerulonephritis' in 'Bedside Clinics in Medicine, Part I'. Initial haematuria (at the beginning of micturition) is due to penile urethral cause, terminal haematuria (at the end of micturition) is due to bladder neck or prostatic urethral cause, and total haematuria (blood in urine throughout micturition) is due to bladder or urinary tract disease, or systemic causes (malignant hypertension, snakebite, etc.).
10. Bile pigments and bile salts: In jaundice.
11. RBC: Normal urine contains <1 red cell per high power field (HPF) of centrifuged urine and not more than 3 red cells/mm^3 of uncentrifuged urine. Urine collection in menstruating female patients should be done cautiously to avoid contamination. Patients on anticoagulant therapy may have RBC in urine.

12. WBC: Normally uncentrifuged urine in men may contain <3 leucocytes/HPF and females may have <10 leucocytes/HPF. If number of WBC is increased above the aforesaid level, think of urinary tract infection (UTI), renal calculi, renal tuberculosis, and send the urine for culture and sensitivity tests. A positive 'leucocyte esterase test' (commonly signifies UTI) results from the presence of WBC either as whole cells or as lysed cells. A negative test means that UTI is unlikely.
    Even a single eosinophil in urine reflects interstitial nephritis.
13. Epithelial cells: Size and shape of the cells often indicate the site of origin but otherwise they are not of much significance. Normal uncentrifuged urine contains not more than 3 cells/HPF.
14. Casts: Casts are coagulated protein (inside the tubules) and their presence during urinalysis indicate that the proteinuria has its origin in the kidney. Hyaline casts (the basic cast) are found in normal persons or in heavy proteinuria, RBC cast in acute glomerulonephritis, fatty cast in nephrotic syndrome, WBC cast in chronic pyelonephritis, and granular cast may signify acute or chronic inflammation of the kidney (usually CRF).
15. Crystals: Calcium oxalate crystals are often found in normal acidic urine and tripple phosphate (ammonium magnesium phosphate) may be present in alkaline urine. Uric acid and urates, cysteine, leucine and tyrosine crystals may be found in acidic urine. Usually crystals are of no pathological significance.

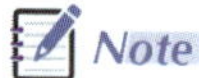
Note

Read proteinuria, haematuria, anuria, oliguria, polyuria from 'Bedside Clinics in Medicine, Part I'.

Chemical Examination of Urine

1. Test for protein (Heat coagulation test): Three-fourth of a test tube is filled-up with the urine. Now holding the bottom, incline the test tube slightly and boil the top 2 cm over a flame. A white cloudy precipitate indicates the presence either of protein or of phosphates. On addition of 10% acetic acid drop by drop, the precipitate due to phosphates disappear; if it persists on adding 10% acetic acid, it is precipitated protein.

2. Test for sugar (Benedict's test): (This is not a specific test for glucose and any reducing substance like lactose, pentose, fructose or galactose present in the urine sample gives positive reaction).

Five (5) mL of Benedict's reagent is taken in a test tube. It is heated to boiling point and then allowed to cool. To it, 8 drops of urine is added. The test tube is now boiled for 2 minutes and then allowed to cool in running tap water. If the urine sample does not contain sugar, the colour of the solution remains unchanged (blue) but a precipitate appears in the presence of reducing substance (sugar), varying from light green turbidity—green precipitate—yellow precipitate—to brick red precipitate (these colour changes of precipitates indicate the approximate concentration of sugar as 0.1 to 0.5 g/dL—0.5 to 1.0 g/dL—1.0 to 2.0 g/dL—to 2.0 g/dL or more, respectively).

3. Test for ketone bodies (Rothera's test): Five (5) mL of urine is taken in a test tube and saturated with ammonium sulphate by adding excess of its crystals. Then 3 drops of freshly prepared solution of sodium nitroprusside is added to it. Now 2 mL of strong ammonia solution is poured very gently by the side of the inclined test tube. A deep purple ring appears at the junction of the two fluids, if the urine sample contains ketone bodies. If ketone bodies are absent, Rothera's test becomes negative.

Clinical Wisdom

Ketone bodies are acetone, acetoacetic acid and β-hydroxybutyric acid. Positive Rothera's test is given by the first two ingredients and not by β-hydroxybutyric acid.

4. Test for bile salts (Hay's surface tension test): Ten (10) mL of urine is taken in a clean test tube and finely powdered sulphur particles are sprinkled over it. If the urine sample contains bile salts, sulphur powder sinks at the bottom of the test tube but the sulphur powder remains on the surface of the urine if the sample does not contain bile salts (bile salts lower surface tension and hence cause sulphur powder to sink).

5. Test for blood:

a. Benzidine test: Urine sample (2–3 mL) is mixed with an equal amount of saturated solution of benzidine in glacial acetic acid. Now, hydrogen peroxide is added to the mixture when a blue colour denotes the presence of blood.
b. Orthotolidine test: Similar to benzidine test; here, instead of benzidine in glacial acetic acid, 0.5 mL of 1% orthotolidine solution in glacial acetic acid is used.

ACUTE GLOMERULONEPHRITIS

Naked-eye Examination

Quantity	350 mL/24 hrs.
Colour	Smoky
Specific gravity	1028

Chemical Examination

pH	6.6
Albumin	++
Blood	++
Sugar	Nil
Ketone bodies	Nil
Bile	Nil

Microscopic Examination

RBC	Plenty in number
WBC/pus cells	2/HPF

Casts:

Hyaline cast	+
RBC cast	++
Epithelial cast	+
Bacteria	Nil
Crystals	Nil

Interpretation

1. Quantity indicates oliguria (<400 mL/24 hrs). Smoky urine points towards microscopic haematuria. High specific gravity reflects normal functioning renal tubules.
2. Moderate proteinuria (glomerular dysfunction), RBC and RBC casts (inflammatory basis of the disease process), presence of blood (injury to glomerulus) suggest acute glomerulonephritis. Presence of pus cells may reflect an inflammatory procedure.

Inference

Presence of:
1. Oliguria,
2. Smoky urine,
3. RBC and RBC cast, and
4. Moderate albuminuria, all together confirm the diagnosis of acute glomerulonephritis (AGN).

Q. How will you assess the 'renal function' in a patient?

A. The **'glomerular function'** is assessed by:

a. Glomerular filtration rate (GFR): The usual GFR in average adult is near about 120 mL/minute. Glomerular function is best assessed by renal clearance, where clearance C = UV ÷ P; now, U and P are respectively the urinary and the plasma concentration of a specific substance, and V is the urine volume formed per minute. Classically the substance used are inulin or ^{51}Cr-EDTA but practically the clearance of creatinine is used in clinical practice.

Calculation of creatinine clearance (CrCl) may he done by (mL/min):*

$$\text{CrCl (male)} = \frac{(140 - \text{age}) \times \text{body weight (in kg)}}{\text{Serum creatinine (mg/dL)} \times 72}$$

CrCl (female) = 0.85 × CrCl (males)

- This is **'Cockcroft-Gault equation'** of CrCl*

b. Serum concentration of urea and creatinine (normal level of urea and creatinine are respectively 20–40 mg/dL and 0.6-1.2 mg/dL).

c. Glomerular damage is often indicated by significant proteinuria.

B. The **'tubular function'** is assessed by:

a. Change in the urinary specific gravity by water deprivation test or administration of vasopressin (reflects urine concentrating defects).

b. Renal acidifying ability is judged by ammonium chloride test.

c. Conservation of electrolytes after administration of fludrocortisone.

d. Phosphaturia, uricosuria, aminoaciduria (all markers of proximal tubular defects), and glycosuria.

Clinical Wisdom

MDRD (Modification of Diet in Renal Disease) equation calculates GFR from 4–6 variables (e.g. age, sex, race, serum creatinine ± urea, albumin). It helps in detection of eGFR. For MDRD calculator, one may see the website www.nephron.com. In the OPD setting, serum creatinine is sometimes used as surrogate (i.e. a substitute) for GFR.

Q. Common causes of ARF or AKI:

1. Hypovolaemia (e.g. acute gastroenteritis).
2. Acute glomerulonephritis (AGN).
3. Septicaemia.
4. Malignant hypertension.
5. Snake bite (Viperidae family).
6. Septic abortion.
7. Eclampsia.
8. Mismatched blood transfusion.
9. Acute interstitial nephritis.
10. Nephrotoxic drugs.

Q. Common complications of acute glomerulonephritis:

1. Acute renal failure (ARF) or acute kidney injury (AKI).
2. Hypertensive encephalopathy.
3. Acute left ventricular failure (LVF).
4. Infections: Urinary tract, respiratory tract, etc.
5. Fluid and electrolyte imbalance.
6. Rapidly progressive glomerulonephritis (RPGN).

Q. Types of ARF:

ARF is of two types: oliguric and non-oliguric

A. Oliguric—has three phases like:
   a. Oliguric phase (1–2 weeks),
   b. Diuretic phase (1 week), and
   c. Recovery phase (2–3 weeks).

B. Non-oliguric—having features like:
   a. No oliguria. Usually the urine output is >1 litre/day.
   b. Low urinary osmolality, e.g. 350 mOsmol/kg of water.
   c. 25–50% patients of ARF suffer from non-oliguric type.
   d. Diuretic phase is usually short (average <1 week).
   e. Dyselectrolytaemia is less common.
   f. Progressive rise in urea and creatinine level.

- **Acute renal failure** (ARF) or acute kidney injury (AKI) is a syndrome mainfested by abrupt deterioration of renal function with rapid decline of GFR (within hours to days) with retention of nitrogenous waste products and disturbance of extracellular fluid balance, electrolyte, and acid-base homeostasis, which is usually reversible within days or weeks.

Q. Metabolic alterations in ARF or AKI:

a. Increased serum concentration of urea, creatinine, potassium, magnesium, phosphate, uric acid, H^+ concentration and fluid volume. Though there is sodium retention, increased fluid volume leads to dilutional hyponatraemia.
b. Low serum level of calcium.

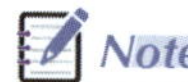

Read AGN in details from 'Bedside Clinics in Medicine, Part 1'.

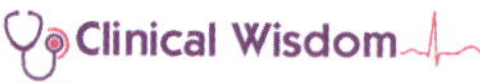

Cystatin C (a biomarker for kidney function) may be used as an alternative to creatinine, which may be useful in early detection of renal dysfunction. Normal serum level is 0.5 1.0 mg/L.

NEPHROTIC SYNDROME

Naked-eye Examination

Quantity	1500 mL/24 hrs.
Colour	Clear
Specific gravity	1016

Chemical Examination

pH	6.4
Albumin	++++
Blood	Nil
Sugar	Nil
Ketone bodies	Nil
Bile	Nil

Microscopic Examination

RBC	Nil
WBC/pus cells	1/HPF
Casts:	
Hyaline cast	+
RBC cast	Absent
Fatty cast	++
Bacteria	Nil
Crystals	Nil

Interpretation

1. Quantity, colour and specific gravity of urine shows no abnormality.
2. Massive proteinuria points the disease process towards nephrotic syndrome.
3. Hyaline cast may be a normal finding but presence of fatty cast (glomerular dysfunction) is highly suggestive of nephrotic syndrome.

Inference

Presence of:

1. Macroscopically normal urine.
2. Massive albuminuria, absence of RBC, and
3. Fatty cast, all together suggest the diagnosis of nephrotic syndrome.

Q. Define nephrotic syndrome:

It is a clinical syndrome characterised by:

a. Massive proteinuria (albuminuria).
b. Hypoalbuminaemia (hypoproteinaemia).
c. Generalised oedema or anasarca, and
d. Hyperlipidaemia (hypercholesterolaemia).

- Proteinuria >3.5 g/1.73 m^2 per day is considered to be in the nephrotic range. Normal body surface for a reference man is 1.73 m^2. According to few clinicians, lipiduria and hypercoagulability are new additions in the clinical complex of nephrotic syndrome (though not essential for diagnosis).
- Proteinuria is the hallmark of nephrotic syndrome.

Q. Classify proteinuria:

Mild: 150–500 mg/day (+)
Moderate: 500 mg–2 g/day (++)
Massive: >2 g/day (+++); if the armount crosses 3.5 g/day, it is designated as 'nephrotic range'.

- Normally, up to 150 mg of protein may be excreted in 24 hours. Proteinuria often makes the urine frothy.

Q. Lipids alteration in nephrotic syndrome:

All types of lipid fraction are altered in nephrotic syndrome. Total cholesterol (both free and ester form), triglyceride, phospholipid and even chylomicron levels are elevated. Free fatty acid levels are usually reduced. LDL, VLDL are increased but HDL level may be normal, elevated or diminished (low HDL level is associated with severe nephrotic syndrome). Lipiduria is common and it is why fatty casts in urine are a characteristic feature.

Q. Why the patient suffers from anasarca?

Fluid comes out from the vascular compartment (due to low oncotic pressure as a result of hypoproteinemia) into the tissue spaces and makes the patient oedematous.

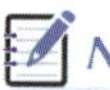

Read 'Nephrotic syndrome' from 'Bedside Clinics in Medicine, Part I'.

CHRONIC GLOMERULONEPHRITIS OR CHRONIC KIDNEY DISEASE (CKD) (Table 7.4)

Naked-eye Examination

Quantity	4 litre/24 hrs
Colour	Clear
Specific gravity	1010

Chemical Examination

pH	6.2
Albumin	+
Blood	Nil
Sugar	Nil

Table 7.4: Stages of chronic kidney disease (CKD)

Stage	Description	GFR (mL/min/1.73 m²)
1	Kidney damage with normal or ↑GFR	≥90
2	Kidney damage with slightly ↓ GFR	60–89
3	Moderate ↓GFR	30–59
4	Severe ↓GFR	15–29
5	Kidney failure	<15 (or dialysis)

- Stage 5 is known as end-stage renal disease (ESRD); in ESRD, renal replacement therapy (either dialysis or renal transplantation) is compulsory to prevent death.

Ketone bodies	Nil
Bile	Nil

Microscopic Examination

RBC	Nil
WBC/pus cells	2/HPF
Casts:	
Hyaline cast	+
RBC cast	Absent
Granular cast	++
Bacteria	Nil
Crystals	Nil

Interpretation

1. Quantity indicates polyuria (>3 litre/24 hrs). Specific gravity is lower than normal (1015–1025) indicating tubular dysfunction.
2. Presence of proteinuria may suggest glomerular dysfunction.
3. pH is normal. Other biochemical findings are within normal limit.
4. Presence of granular cast suggests chronic glomerulonephritis, i.e. renal parenchymal involvement.

Inference:

Presence of:
1. Low specific gravity at 1010.
2. Albuminuria, and
3. Granular cast, all together suggest chronic glomerulonephritis [or chronic kidney disease (CKD)].
4. As the chart shows polyuria, it may be concluded that chronic glomerulonephritis has progressed to chronic renal failure (CRF).

- **'Broad casts'** (casts of unusual width presumed to arise from dilated tubules) are often found in CRF.

Q. Why the specific gravity in CRF is fixed at 1010?

Normally, the concentration of the urine (reflected by specific gravity) changes from time to time. As the patient progresses to CRF, the kidneys lose their ability to concentrate and dilute the urine; thus the specific gravity becomes lower, and approximates to 1010, i.e. equivalent to the specific gravity of the glomerular filtrate. Thus, ultimately the urine becomes isotonic with plasma water **(isosthenuria)**.

Q. Different casts in urine:

1. Hyaline cast: Normal persons, pyrexia, strenuous exercise, heavy proteinuria, concentrated urine, dehydration.
2. RBC cast: Acute glomerulonephritis.
3. Fatty cast: Nephrotic syndrome.
4. Granular cast: Chronic glomerulonephritis, may be non-specific.
5. WBC cast: Pyelonephritis, interstitial nephritis, transplant rejection.
6. Broad cast: Chronic renal failure: (CRF).
7. Crystals in cast: Hypercalcaemia, hyperuricosuria.
8. Waxy cast: Advanced renal failure.
9. Tubular epithelial cast: Renal tubular necrosis, kidney transplant rejection.
10. Pseudocasts: Clumped WBC, bacteria and artefacts.

Q. Common causes of CRF:

1. Chronic glomerulonephritis
2. Malignant hypertension
3. Diabetes mellitus.
4. Chronic pyelonephritis.
5. Nephrotic syndrome.
6. Polycystic kidney disease.
7. Collagen vascular diseases.
8. Obstructive uropathy.
9. Interstitial nephritis.
10. Analgesic nephropathy.
11. Gout, multiple myeloma.
12. Renal tuberculosis.
13. Renal artery stenosis.
14. Amyloidosis.

- **Chronic renal failure (CRF)** refers to long-standing, progressive and irreversible deterioration in renal function developing over a period of years.

Q. CRF with enlarged kidneys:

CRF patients usually have bilateral, small and contracted kidneys. Enlarged kidneys are seen in:
1. Polycystic kidney.

2. Hydronephrosis (bilateral).
3. Diabetes mellitus with CRF.
4. Amyloidosis.
5. Multiple myeloma.
6. HIV infection.

Q. Mention the common complications/abnormalities seen in CRF (uraemia):

1. Haematologic and immunologic:
   a. Refractory anaemia.
   b. Lymphocytopenia; abnormality in WBC formation and function.
   c. Bleeding tendency.
   d. Increased susceptibility to infection.
2. GI tract:
   a. Anorexia, nausea, vomiting.
   b. Uraemic gastritis (nausea, vomiting).
   c. Peptic ulcer and GI tract haemorrhage.
   d. Uraemic fetor.
   e. Ascites.
3. Cardio-pulmonary:
   a. Systemic hypertension.
   b. Acute left ventricular failure.
   c. Accelerated atherosclerosis.
   d. Pericarditis.
   e. Uraemic lung (pulmonary oedema).
4. Neuromuscular:
   a. Peripheral neuropathy.
   b. Convulsions.
   c. Coma.
   d. Flapping tremor.
   e. Encephalopathy.
   f. Myopathy.
   g. 'Restless legs syndrome'.
   h. Dialysis dementia and dialysis disequilibrium syndrome (dialysis-induced).
5. Endocrine and metabolic:
   a. Secondary hyperparathyroidism.
   b. Renal osteodystrophy.
   c. Hyperuricaemia.
   d. Amenorrhoea, loss of libido, infertility.
6. Fluid and electrolytes:
   a. Metabolic acidosis.
   b. Hypocalcaemia.
   c. Volume contraction from polyuria. Na^+ level may be high, normal or low.
   d. K^+ level is usually high.
   e. Oedema.
7. Dermatological:
   a. Pallor.
   b. Hyperpigmentation.
   c. Ecchymosis.
   d. Generalised pruritus.
   e. Uramic frost.
8. Miscellaneous:
   a. Malnutrition (↓ albumin).
   b. Dry skin.
   c. Polyuria.
   d. Hydrothorax.
   e. Cardiac dysrhythmia.
   f. Dyslipidaemia (↑ TG, ↑LDL).
   g. Impotence.
   h. Calciphylaxis (calcific uraemic arteriolopathy).

Q. What are azotaemia and uraemia?

These, more or less similar terms, are defined as:

- Azotaemia: Elevated urea and creatinine level but there is no symptom; GFR is usually 20–50% of normal.
- Uraemia: Worsening of renal functions with appearance of symptoms (urea and creatinine levels are very high); GFR is usually <20% of normal.

Q. Anaemia in CRF:

Anaemia in CRF is due to:

1. Decreased erythropoiesis due to relative deficiency of erythropoietin.
2. Reduced dietary intake due to loss of appetite.
3. Decreased red cell survival.
4. Diminished erythropoiesis due to uraemic toxins.
5. Reduced intestinal iron absorption.
6. Increased blood loss due to abnormal platelet function and increased capillary fragility.
7. Hypoproteinaemia leading to decreased transferrin level.
8. Vitamin B_{12} and folic acid deficiency.

- Anaemia is being treated by recombinant human erythropoietin (EPO) or darbepoetin alfa.

Q. 'Reversible factors' in CRF, if there is any:

1. Systemic hypertension.
2. Obstructive uropathy.
3. Urinary tract infection.
4. Reduced renal perfusion due to hypotension, or renal artery stenosis.
5. Renotoxic medications.

Q. Outline of treatment in renal failure:

Renal replacement therapy is done by haemodialysis/haemofiltration, peritoneal dialysis and renal transplantation.

A. Acute renal failure (ARF):
   a. Conservative treatment.
   b. Continuous arterio-venous or veno-venous haemofiltration.
   c. Haemodialysis.
   d. Peritoneal dialysis.

B. Chronic renal failure (CRF):
   a. Conservative treatment.

b. Haemodialysis.
c. Continuous ambulatory peritoneal dialysis (CAPD).
d. Renal transplantation (cadaveric or living donor transplantation).

Q. D/D between ARF (AKI) and CRF at the bedside:

A provisional diagnosis may be done by:

1. History [short in ARF and prolonged in CRF; ARF is often precipitated by diarrhoea, snakebite, septic abortion, pre-eclampsia or drugs (e.g. aminoglycosides)].
2. Patient is bloated (oliguric phase of ARF); patient of CRF is usually volume depleted from polyuria.
3. Severe anaemia clinches the diagnosis of CRF.
4. Though systemic hypertension may be present in both the types, target organ damage due to hypertension is evident in CRF only, e.g.
   a. Cardiomegaly.
   b. Retinopathy.
5. Presence of bone pain (renal osteodystrophy) and peripheral neuropathy suggest CRF.
6. Ultrasonography shows bilateral contracted kidneys with loss of cortico-medullary differentiation in CRF; kidneys are usually of normal size in ARF.
7. A very rapid rate of rise in serum urea and creatinine suggests ARF. A report of previous urinalysis (normal in ARF) is also helpful for diagnosis.

- 'Acute on chronic renal failure' is precipitated by infection, obstruction (e.g. stone, blood clot), dehydration and nephrotoxic drugs (e.g. aminoglycosides).

Q. Common nephrotoxic drugs:

1. NSAIDs (e.g. diclofenac)
2. Aminoglycosides (e.g. streptomycin, gentamicin, kanamycin).
3. Cisplatin.
4. Amphotericin B.
5. Cyclosporine.
6. Polymyxins (polymyxin B and colistin) and bacitracin.
7. Contrast dye.

Q. Indications of dialysis in ARF (AKI) or CRF:

1. Progressive metabolic encephalopathy.
2. Uncontrolled hyperkalaemia (>7 mEq/L).
3. Intractable overload of fluid, e.g. pulmonary oedema not responding to diuretics.
4. Uraemic pericarditis (most important clinical indicator), or symptomatic uraemia (e.g. fits, confusion).
5. Very high urea (usually above 300 mg/dL) and creatinine (usually above 7 g/dL) levels.
6. Creatinine clearance <15 mL/minute.
7. Refractory metabolic acidosis (pH <7.2), pulmonary oedema not responding to medical treatment, high catabolic state with rapidly progressive renal failure, significant bleeding diathesis, hypertension poorly-responsive to non-dialytic therapy.

Clinical Wisdom

Most useful marker of renal function is **serum creatinine** as it is primarily eliminated by glomerular filtration. Blood urea is modified independent of renal function, e.g. ↑ **urea or BUN** (blood urea nitrogen) is seen in high protein diet, catabolic states, GI bleeding, and ↓ **urea or BUN** is observed in liver disease, malnutrition, etc.

URINARY TRACT INFECTION

Naked-Eye Examination

Quantity	1600 mL/24 hrs.
Colour	Cloudy (Fig. 7.8)
Odour	Fishy
Specific gravity	1016

Chemical Examination

pH	6.1
Albumin	Trace
Blood	Nil
Sugar	Nil
Ketone bodies	Nil
Bile	Nil

Microscopic Examination

RBC	4/HPF
WBC/pus cells	40/HPF
Casts	Nil
Bacteria	Few motile organism
Crystals	+

Interpretation

1. Parameters in macroscopic examination reveals fishy odour which probably reflects the presence of

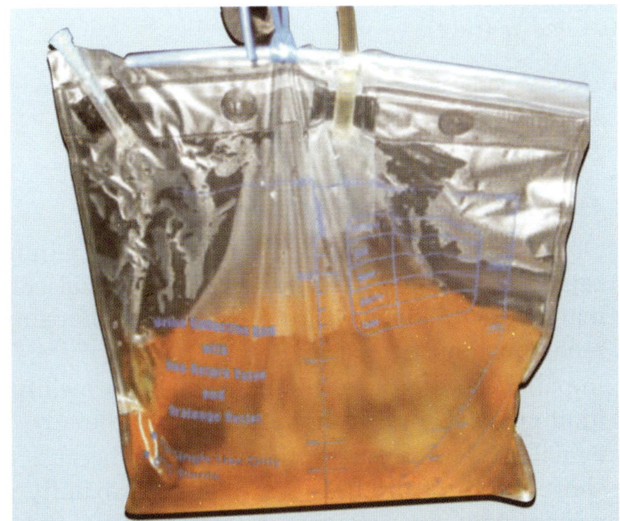

Fig. 7.8: **Cellular debris** present in **urine** is collected in the urosac in a patient of severe urinary tract infection (UTI)

sulphides in urine as a result of urinary tract infection (UTI), and cloudy appearance as a result of plenty of pus cells.
2. Trace proteinuria may be a normal finding or due to UTI. The pH reflects acidic reaction of urine.
3. The presence of plenty of pus cells, few RBC and moreover, few motile bacteria indicate an inflammatory basis of the disease process.
4. Presence of motile bacteria (commonly due to *E. coli*) along with plenty of pus cells suggest urinary tract infection.

Inference

Urinary tract infection (UTI) probably due to *E. coli*.

Q. Reaction of urine:

A. Acidic:
  a. Commonly a normal finding.
  b. Urinary tract infection with *E. coli*.
  c. Acidification of urine done by vitamin C or NH_4Cl.
  d. Acidosis (e.g. diabetic ketoacidosis, uraemia).

B. Alkaline:
  a. Consumption of alkali.
  b. Alkalosis.
  c. Urinary tract infection with *Proteus*.
  d. Loss of tubular function to eliminate acid (e.g. renal tubular acidosis).
  e. Patient is on high vegetarian diet.

Q. Common organisms responsible for UTI:

1. *E. coli*.
2. Streptococci.
3. *Staphylococcus epidermidis*.
4. *Klebsiella*.
5. *Proteus*.
6. *Pseudomonas*.
7. *Chlamydia trachomatis*.
8. *Enterobacter*.
9. *Serratia*.
10. *Candida* (rare).

- Outside hospital: *E. coli* is the commonest organism and is usually derived from fecal reservoir; nosocomial infection: *Klebsiella*, streptococci, *E. coli*.

Q. Predisposing factors in UTI:

1. Obstructive uropathy, renal stone, self-retaining catheter, neurological disorders (e.g. spinal cord injury), cystic kidney, vesico-ureteric reflux, impaired renal function.
2. Impaired body resistance due to diabetes mellitus, immunodeficiency, immunosuppressive therapy.
3. **Females are more susceptible to males** because of short length of urethra (4 cm), close proximity of urethra with anus, pregnancy (chance of retention), absence of bactericidal prostatic secretions, and urethral trauma during sexual intercourse.

Q. Types of UTI:

a. Lower tract infection: Urethritis, cystitis and prostatitis.
b. Upper tract infection: Acute pyelonephritis.

Q. Investigations to be performed in suspected UTI:

1. Routine examination (R/E) of urine.
2. Urine for culture and sensitivity test (C/S) along with colony count.
3. Blood for TC, DC, ESR.
4. Blood for sugar (fasting and postprandial), urea and creatinine.
5. Ultrasonography (USG) to exclude calculi, cyst, obstruction, congenital anomaly, anatomical abnormality. Nowadays, USG is preferred to IVP.
6. IVP, micturating cysto-urethrography and cystoscopy in selected cases.

Q. What should be the 'colony count' in a symptomatic UTI?

Colony count = Number of bacteria present per millilitre of urine sample examined.

Demonstration of >100000 organism/mL grown from a properly collected mid-stream 'clean catch' urine sample strongly suggests infection (100000 organism = 10^5 organism).

Usually, colony count <10000/mL does not signify any infection but there is no absolute rule of thumb regarding the colony count as in a symptomatic patient, a smaller number of bacteria (1000–10000/mL of mid-stream urine) may indicate infection.

Q. Clinical features of UTI:

a. Urethritis: Burning pain during micturition (due to acid reaction of urine), increased frequency of micturition, dysuria.
b. Cystitis: Dysuria, increased frequency, urgency, strangury (due to spasm of the internal sphincter), haematuria, incontinence or retention of urine, suprapubic pain and tenderness. Renal angles may be tender in ascending infection to kidneys.
c. Systemic: Fever with chill and rigor, nausea, vomiting.

- In febrile UTI in male: Think of acute epididymitis, acute prostatitis, or acute pyelonephritis.

Q. What is 'acute urethral syndrome'?

When dysuria, urgency and increased frequency of micturition are not accompanied by significant bacteriuria, it is known as acute urethral syndrome. It is commonly seen in women. Antibiotics are usually not indicated.

Q. How to collect urine for culture and sensitivity (C/S) test?

Mid-stream urine is taken for examination in both the sexes. First, clean the external genitalia with distilled water and then collect the urine aseptically in a sterile container after discarding the first part of urine. Do not touch the container in the genitalia, particuairty in case of female patients. In a special situation, catheterised specimen or urine collected by suprapubic puncture may be taken for examination.

The C/S report takes 5–7 days to reach the physician.

Q. What are the different types of urinary pain?

1. Renal pain: It is dull aching or boring in character, and present in the flanks or renal angle (i.e. in loin) and extends along the rib margin towards the umbilicus. It is usually due to distension or irritation of renal capsule (e.g. AGN or big oxalate stone in the kidney).
2. Ureteric pain: If is acute, severe, colicky in nature and is often associated with nausea, vomiting, chill and rigor, excessive perspiration and rigidity of abdominal muscles. Ureteric pain is due to smooth muscle spasm or distension.
   a. High ureteric pain: Characteristically radiates to groin, testicles (or vulva) and inner aspect of thigh (i.e. along distribution of genitofemoral nerve, $L_{1,2}$).
   b. Mid uretric pain: Usually felt in the lower quadrant of the abdomen on the affected side; may radiate upto groin.
   c. Low ureteric pain: Felt deep into the pelvis.
3. Vesical pain: It is usually due to overdistension of a normal bladder. A dull aching pain is felt in the hypogastrium which is relieved by micturition. A stone impacted in the intramural part may have referred pain to the tip of the penis.

Clinical Wisdom

Pain in the loin may be due to renal stone/malignancy/infection, polycystic kidney, acute cholecystitis, acute pancreatitis or ruptured spleen.

Q. Complications of acute and chronic pyelonephritis:

a. Acute pyelonephritis:
   1. Acute papillary necrosis.
   2. Septicaemia.
   3. Chronic pyelonephritis.
   4. Chronic renal failure.

b. Chronic pyelonephritis:
   1. Hypertension.
   2. CRF.
   3. Pyonephrosis.
   4. Renal calculi.

Q. Causes of increased frequency of micturition:

1. Cystitis, urethritis, small contracted bladder, vesical calculus, benign hypertrophy of prostate (BHP).
2. Balanitis, pinhole meatus, phimosis.
3. Polyuric conditions, pregnancy, psychogenic, pressure in the bladder from adjacent structures.

- Diabetes mellitus, benign hypertrophy of prostate and UTI are common causes in clinical practice. Diabetics suffer from increased frequency of micturition to clean-up the polyuria or as a complication of UTI.

Q. Causes of sterile pyuria (pyuria associated with sterile culture):

1. Incompletely treated UTI.
2. Infections, e.g. *M. tuberculosis*.
3. Calculi in the urinary tract.
4. Interstitial nephritis.
5. Chemical cystitis.
6. Prostatitis.
7. Papillary necrosis.
8. Analgesic nephropathy.
9. Pregnancy.
10. Glucocorticoid therapy.

- Pyuria is commonly due is pyelonephritis, cystitis (infective) and urethritis.

DIABETIC KETOACIDOSIS

Naked-eye Examination

Quantity	3800 ml/24 hrs.
Colour	Clear
Odour	Smell of acetone
Specific gravity	1038

Chemical Examination

pH	4.9
Albumin	+
Blood	Nil
Sugar	+++
Ketone bodies	+++
Bile	Nil

Microscopic Examination

RBC	Nil
WBC/pus cells	2/HPF
Casts	Hyaline cast present
Bacteria	Nil
Crystals	Nil

Interpretation

1. The chart reflects polyuria and high specific gravity as well as smell of acetone in the macroscopical examination of urine.
2. Reaction of urine is acidic. Ketonuria associated with glycosuria is virtually diagnostic of diabetic ketoacidosis. Mild proteinuria indicates development of early diabetic nephropathy.
3. Microscopical examination is within normal limit, except for the presence of hyaline cast (indicate glomerulopathy).

Inference

It is a chart of diabetic ketoacidosis in a patient of early diabetic nephropathy.

Q. Definition of diabetic nephropathy:

It is the presence of persistent proteinuria (>500 mg protein/24 hrs; >300 mg albumin/24 hrs) in a patient suffering from diabetes mellitus in the absence of other renal disease, UTI or heart failure. Diabetic nephropathy (microvascular complication) includes all the lesions occurring in the kidneys of patients suffering from DM (e.g. glomerulosclerosis, interstitial nephritis, arterionephrosclerosis, etc.)

Q. What is microalbuminuria?

A normal person excretes <20 µg of albumin per minute (i.e. <30 mg in 24 hours). By convention, microalbuminuria is defined as urinary albumin excretion ratio (UAER) between 20–200 µg/min (i.e. 30–300 mg/day) in an overnight or 24-hour urinary collection demonstrated in at least 2–3 occasions within a period of 6 months. Microalbuminuria in diabetes mellitus usually develops around the 5th–10th year. *In type 1 DM, It is an early predictor of nephropathy and in type 2 DM, it usually predicts future development of malignant angiopathy and cardiovascular complications.* It is measured by radioimmunoassay. Microalbuminuria responses well with drugs like ACE inhibitors.

Instead of 24-hours urine collection, a random sample is used in clinical practice where urinary albumin concentration is related to urinary creatinine concentration. An **albumin: creatinine ratio** (ACR) of 2.5–20 corresponds to albuminuria of 30–300 mg daily respectively.

The causes of microalbuminuria are:

1. DM with early renal involvement (indicates endothelial dysfunction).
2. Systemic hypertension.
3. Congestive cardiac failure.
4. Urinary tract infection.
5. Moderate to strenuous physical exercise.
6. As an acute phase response, pyrexia or haematuria.

Q. Conditions associated with reducing substances and ketone bodies in urine:

Read 'Alimentary glycosuria' of 'Charts on GTT', and 'Introduction' of 'Charts on urine'.

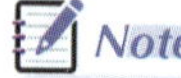

Note

Read 'Management of diabetic ketoacidosis' from the 'Emergency medicine' section.

CHARTS ON CSF

Introduction

Initially, read the 'CSF dynamics and other details' of CSF from 'Lumbar puncture needle' under 'Instruments and bedside procedures' section. To summarise: CSF is a clear fluid circulating in the intracranial and spinal compartments. CSF sample is collected through lumbar puncture. Examination of CSF is relevant in neurological disorders like infections (meningitis, encephalitis), subarachnoid haemorrhage, spinal block, demyelinating disorders (e.g. multiple sclerosis), etc. for diagnosis, and assessment of severity and prognostication. Analysis of CSF consists of opening pressure measurement, biochemical analysis, cytology, biomarkers assay and microbiological evaluation.

A. Naked-eye (macroscopic) examination:

1. Pressure:
   60–150 mm of CSF (lying position), and
   150–250 mm of CSF (sitting position)
   CSF pressure may be:
   a. High: Cerebrovascular accidents (CVA), intracranial tumour, meningitis, meningism, encephalitis, cerebral abscess, benign intracranial hypertension, circulatory block like aqueduct stenosis or hypertensive hydrocephalus, head injury, hypoxic encephalopathy.
   b. Low: Spinal subarachnoid block, severe dehydration, thick CSF (e.g. in pyogenic meningitis), partially blocked needle, after repeated lumbar puncture, bad needle placement.
2. Colour or appearance: Crystal clear or colourless. The common variations in appearance are:
   a. Clear: Normal, tuberculous and viral meningitis, meningism.
   b. Turbid: Turbidity usually indicates high leucocyte count and is seen in pyogenic meningitis, rarely in carcinomatous meningitis and subarachnoid haemorrhage.
   c. Straw-coloured: Tuberculous meningitis.
   d. Haemorrhagic or red: Subarachnoid haemorrhage, trauma, extensive cerebral haemorrhage; rarely due to haemorrhagic encephalitis, bleeding diathesis.
   e. Xanthochromia: See the chart on 'Xanthochromia'.
3. Coagulum formation on standing: Normally, the CSF does not clot on standing and if it happens so, one should think of presence of high protein and fibrinogen in the CSF. Traumatic puncture clots on standing.
   a. Cobweb coagulum (forms after few hours; indicates mild to moderate rise of protein along with fibrinogen in CSF): Tuberculous meningitis (most important cause, and the coagulum is a rich source of tubercle bacilli), acute anterior poliomyelitis and neurosyphilis.
   b. Big coagulum (forms immediately or shortly after withdrawal, indicates very high protein in CSF): Spinal subarachnoid block, GB syndrome.

B. Chemical (biochemical) examination:

1. Total protein: 20–40 mg%. Normally the ratio of albumin and globulin in CSF is 8:1; the total protein

may be 'very high' in conditions like GB syndrome, total spinal block, meningitis (especially tuberculous) and acoustic neurofibroma.

Normally CSF IgG is <15% of the total protein concentration. IgG is increased in multiple sclerosis, neurosarcoidosis, neurosyphilis and in some connective tissue diseases. CSF globulin can be detected by different tests like Pandy's test, Nonne-Apelt reaction, Noguchi's test, Lange's colloidal gold curve reaction and immunoelectrophoresis.

2. Sugar: 40–80 mg% (usually 1/2–2/3rd of the random blood sugar concentration). CSF sugar is increased in diabetes mellitus and following IV glucose infusion, while is sugar is decreased in pyogenic and tuberculous meningitis.
3. Chloride: 720–750 mg% (120–170 mmol/L). Normal plasma chloride value is 98–106 mmol/L. CSF chloride becomes markedly reduced in tuberculous meningitis (probably due to fall in the plasma level as a result of prolonged vomiting) and slightly reduced in pyogenic meningitis. CSF chloride is increased in uraemia.
4. pH: 7.31–7.34

C. Microscopic examination: Normally the cells are mononuclear cells (70% lymphocytes and 30% monocytes) in the range of 0–5 cells/mm^3. There are no polymorphis.

If the increased cell count shows polymorphs and is above 75% of the total, it is known as *polymorphonuclear pleocytosis;* and if more than 90% lymphocytes are found, it is designated as *lymphocytic pleocytosis*.

D. Bacteriological (includes staining and culture): Normally CSI is sterile. Pathogens can be isolated by different staining techniques (Gram stain, Ziehl-Neelsen stain, India ink preparation) or cultures.

E. Serological: VDRL, Kahn test, Wassermann reaction help in the diagnosis of neurosyphilis. Nowadays, different serological tests are available for bacterial, mycobacterial and fungal infections.

F. Special: Lange's colloidal gold curve reaction—a positive reaction (indicating high globulin in CSF) is found in tabes dorsalis (tabetic curve), GPI (paretic curve), and meningitis (meningitic curve). Polymerase chain reaction (PCR) to identify bacteria are available.

- To diagnose and interpret CSF study, a close liaison between physician and microbiologist is essential. Adenosine deaminase (ADA) activity in CSF in tuberculous meningitis is >10 U/L.

ACUTE PYOGENIC MENINGITIS

Naked-eye Examination

Pressure	++
Appearance	Turbid/cloudy
On standing	No coagulum formation

Chemical Examination

Protein	180 mg%
Sugar	12 mg%
Chloride	695 mg%

Microscopic Examination

Total cells	4000/mm^3
Polymorphs	90%
Lymphocytes	10%

Bacteriological Examination

Gram +ve cocci seen in pairs or short chains.

Interpretation

1. The CSF pressure is high indicating abnormality in the CNS. Turbidity is probably due to large number of polymorphs.
2. Total protein is 'moderately' increased, sugar content is much reduced and the chloride concentration is a bit lower than normal.
3. High total count of cells with polymorphonuclear pleocytosis suggests pyogenic infection of the central nervous system (CNS).
4. Presence of gram +ve cocci in pairs or short chains indicates infection produced by *Pneumococcus*.

Inference

The CSF chart deals with acute pyogenic meningitis probably caused by *Pneumococcus* (*S. pneumoniae*).

Q. Organisms involved in acute pyogenic meningitis:

Worldwide, the three major pathogens are *H. influenzae*, *N. meningitidis* and *S. pneumoniae*, which account for approximately 70–80% cases of pyogenic meningitis.

a. Neonates (<1 month): Gram –ve bacilli (*E. coli*), streptococci.
b. Children (1 month to 15 years): *H. influenzae*, *N. meningitidis*, *S. pneumoniae*, *M. tuberculosis*.
c. Adults: *N. meningitidis*, *S. pneumoniae*, *Staphylococcus*, *M. tuberculosis*, gram –ve bacilli.

Q. Causes of alteration in sugar content of CSF:

A. High: Diabetes mellitus and other hyperglycaemic states, rarely in cerebral haemorrhage.
B. Low (hypoglycorrhachia):
   a. Marked reduction: Pyogenic meningitis.
   b. Moderate reduction: Tuberculous, fungal and carcinomatous meningitis, neurosarcoidosis, lymphomatous infiltration, hypoglycaemia.
C. Normal: In health, viral meningitis, encephalitis.

Q. Classical features of acute pyogenic meningitis:

1. Intense headache (generalised or holocranial/nuchal), high fever, meningismus, nausea, vomiting, profuse sweating, rigors, myalgia and photophobia may be present.

2. The meningismus is accompanied by **positive neck rigidity (stiffness), Kernig's sign, and Brudzinski's sign (especially in children)**. Fever, nuchal headache and neck rigidity are the *classical triad of meningitis*.
3. Features of cerebral dysfunction (mental obtundation) like altered sensorium, confusion, delirium or coma are not uncommon.
4. Convulsions, bilateral VIth nerve palsy as a false localising sign due to raised intracranial tension; focal neurodeficit evidenced by dysphasia, visual field defects, hemiparesis, extensor plantar response may be present.
5. Meningococcal meningitis may be suggested by the presence of skin rash (erythematous → macular or morbilliform → petechial → purpuric) mainly present over the extremities (may be present over the conjunctiva). Herpes labialis may be found. Acute adrenal failure (Waterhouse-Friderichsen syndrome) may be noted as a complication.
6. Special features in neonates and young infants:
   a. Neck rigidity (stiffness) and Kernig's sign may be absent.
   b. Listlessness, high-pitched cry, refuse to suck, irritability.
   c. Fever may be absent.
   d. Poor muscle tone, persistent vomiting, a vacant state, circulatory collapse.
   e. Anterior fontanelle may or may not be bulging.

Q. Complications of acute pyogenic meningitis:

a. Systemic: Waterhouse-Friderichsen syndrome, SIADH, septicaemia, acute renal failure, circulatory collapse, disseminated intravascular coagulation (DIC).

b. Neurological: Focal fits, mental retardation, neurodeficit (aphasia, blindness, deafness), brain abscess, auditory impairment, internal hydrocephalus, subdural effusion, cranial nerve palsy.

Q. Clinical associations in different types of pyogenic meningitis:

1. Pneumococcal: Pneumonia, mastoiditis, sinusitis, olitis media, endocarditis; splenectomised patients, multiple myeloma, head injury with basilar fracture of the skull, hypogammaglobulinaemic patients are more prone.
2. Meningococcal: Usually occurs in epidemics; fulminant; children living in overcrowded houses are predisposed.
3. Staphylococcal: Neonates (umbilical infection, pyoderma, septicaemia); older children (otitis media mastoiditis, fracture of the skull, septic lesion in scalp).
4. *H. influenzae:* Convulsions are commonly seen. Auditory impairment is a residual complication.

Q. Possible causes of aseptic and recurrent meningitis:

a. Aseptic meningitis: Meningitis induced by Echovirus, Coxsackievirus, HSV-2, HIV and Arbovirus; Weil's disease, carcinomatosis, drugs or contrast medium, subarachnoid haemorrhage, neurosarcoidosis.

b. Recurrent meningitis: Herpes simplex virus (commonest), chemical meningitis due to leakage into CSF of contents from an epidermoid tumour, craniopharyngioma; due to primary inflammatory conditions like SLE, Behcet's syndrome, drug hypersensitivity, Mollaret's meningitis or Vogt-Koyanagi-Harada disease.

 *Note*

Vide the 'Management of pyogenic meningitis' from 'Emergency medicine' section of this book.

TUBERCULOUS MENINGITIS

Naked-eye Examination

Pressure	++
Appearance	Clear
On standing	Formation of cobweb coagulum (fine clot)

Chemical Examination

Protein	600 mg%
Sugar	30 mg%
Chloride	580 mg%

Microscopic Examination

Total cells	450/mm^3
Polymorphs	8%
Lymphocytes	92%

Bacteriological Examination

Ordinary culture shows no growth (sterile).

Interpretation

1. The CSF pressure is raised indicating abnormality in the CNS. The clear appearance may be due to tuberculous or viral meningitis, or meningism. Cobweb coagulum strongly suggests meningitis due to tuberculous aetiology.
2. Total protein is 'much' raised, sugar content is slightly reduced and the chloride content is very much reduced.
3. High total cell count with lymphocytic pleocytosis seen.
4. Ordinary culture is sterile (probably needs special and appropriate culture media).

Inference

High CSF pressure, clear appearance, very low chloride content, cobweb coagulum with lymphocytic pleocytosis strongly indicate tuberculous meningitis (TBM). Though lymphocytic pleocytosis is often observed in viral meningitis, it is not associated with low sugar content in CSF. Moreover, sterile ordinary culture points towards tuberculous aetiology too.

- Very high level of protein often indicates block to CSF flow due to tuberculous meningitis (TBM).

Q. Is it tuberculous meningitis or 'partially treated' pyogenic meningitis?

Points in favour of TBM are:

1. Duration of illness is usually >5–6 days.
2. H/o intense headache; squint may be evident.
3. CSF: Appearance clear, WBC <1000/mm^3, lymphocytes >30% with protein >100 mg%.
4. Enlarged ventricles in CT or MRI scan of brain.
5. CSF adenosine deaminase activity is usually >10 U/L.

Q. What is pleocytosis?

It is the cellular preponderance in CSF.

a. Polymorphonuclear pleocytosis: Acute pyogenic meningitis.
b. Lymphocytic pleocytosis: Meningitis of tuberculous or viral actiology, syphilitic or fungal meningitis, multiple sclerosis, viral encephalitis, neurosarcoidosis, rarely in partially treated pyogenic meningitis.
c. Mixed pleocytosis: Early phase of viral meningitis (often in the first 36 hours, few neutrophils may be seen), sometimes in tuberculous meningitis.

Q. Common clinical features of TBM:

This condition commonly occurs shortly after a primary infection in childhood or as a part of miliary tuberculosis.

a. Children: Lassitudes, anorexia, constipation, headache, lack of interest in toys or talking.
b. Adults: Low grade pyrexia, malaise, intense headache, vomiting, convulsions, coma.

Q. How will you investigate a case of TBM?

1. Lumbar puncture: CSF is drawn out for macroscopic, chemical and microscopic examination (sometimes repeated CSF examinations are necessary). Detection of AFB (tubercle bacilli) from the centrifused deposit of CSF or from the testing of cobweb smear—examination by Ziehl-Neelsen stain is done. CSF may be cultured in Lowenstein-Jensen (L-J) media or Middlebrook agar media. Guineapig inoculation test takes much time to give result. As culture in L-J media may take more than 6 weeks time, BACTEC system of culture technique may be adopted which gives the result within 7 days.
   Newer modes of diagnostic avenues may be of some help in quicker diagnosis from CSF:
   a. Adenosine deaminase assay (>10 U/L).
   b. Polymerase chain reaction (PCR): To detect mycobacterial DNA.
   c. Detection of tuberculostearic acid.
   d. ELISA (not very sensitive).
   e. CB-NAAT/GeneXpert test (cartridge-based nucleic acid amplification test).
2. Blood for R/E (Hb, TC, DC, ESR), chest X-ray (PA view), Mantoux test (may be negative) are done. Lymphocytosis and high ESR may indicate towards tuberculous aetiology. Chest X-ray shows evidences either of primary complex or miliary tuberculosis. Sputum examination for AFB in concomitant pulmonary tuberculosis should be performed.
   Primarily, a high index of suspicion by the attending physician is necessary for a quick diagnosis.
3. CT scan or MRI scan of brain may reveal hydrocephalus, brisk meningeal enhancement on enhanced CT or a tuberculoma.

Q. Adenosine deaminase activity to diagnose tuberculous meningitis:

Adenosine deaminase (ADA) activity, an enzyme associated with disorders that induce cell-mediated responses, in CSF is useful for the diagnosis of tuberculous meningitis. High ADA activity in CSF may found in:

1. Tuberculous meningitis (commonest cause).
2. CNS lymphoma with meningeal involvement.
3. Neurobrucellosis.
4. Sarcoidosis.
5. Subarachnoid haemorrhage.

- In pleural, pericardial or ascitic fluid ADA activity in tuberculosis: 40–60 U/L is borderline activity, whereas >60 U/L is high activity. In CSF, ADA >10 U/L favours tuberculous aetiology.

Q. What are the predisposing factors for acquiring tuberculosis?

Tuberculosis remains a major global problem and a serious public health issue. The risk factors are:

1. HIV infection (risk increases 100-times more than normal).
2. Recent infection (probably within the past 2 years) with *M. tuberculosis*.
3. Diabetes mellitus (risk increases 3-times than normal).
4. Prolonged corticosteroid treatment or Cushing's syndrome, other immunosuppressive therapy.
5. IV drug abusers (e.g. heroin addict).
6. Silicosis.
7. leukaemias, lymphomas.
8. Gastrectomy or intestinal by-pass surgery.
9. End-stage renal disease.
10. Malignancy of head and neck region.

Q. Classification of neurological tuberculosis?

1. Tuberculous meningitis.
2. Tuberculous arachnoiditis.
3. Tuberculoma (intracranial).

4. Tuberculous abscess (intracranial).
5. Tuberculous encephalopathy.
6. Non-osseous spinal cord tuberculosis.

Q. Complications of TBM:

Untreated or lately treated cases may prove to be fatal. Mortality ratio is moderately high and the survivors may be left with serious disabling sequelae like mental retardation, epilepsy, blindness, deafness and obstructive hydrocephalus.

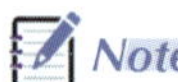
Note

Read the 'Management of tuberculous meningitis' from 'Emergency medicine' section of this book.

ACUTE VIRAL MENINGITIS

Naked-eye Examination

Pressure	++
Appearance	Clear
On standing	No coagulum formation

Chemical Examination

Protein	150 mg%
Sugar	65 mg%
Chloride	730 mg%

Microscopic Examination

Total cells	140/mm^3
Polymorphs	10%
Lymphocyles	90%

Bacteriological Examination

Ordinary culture shows no growth (sterile).

Serological Examination

VDRL and Kahn test of CSF are negative.

Interpretation

1. High pressure in the CSF indicates some abnormality in the CNS. The colour is clear and there is no coagulum formation on standing.
2. Though the total protein content is 'moderately' increased, the sugar and chloride concentration remain unchanged.
3. High total cell count with lymphocytic pleocytosis seen.
4. Negative serology virtually excludes neurosyphilis.
5. Sterile ordinary culture raises the possibilities of tuberculous, viral or fungal meningitis, or aseptic meningitis.

Inference

High CSF pressure, clear appearance, absence of cobweb coagulum, moderately high protein with normal sugar and chloride content as well as lymphocytic pleocytosis strongly suggest acute viral meningitis.

Normal sugar and chloride content excludes tuberculous meningitis, and negative serology rules out the diagnosis of neurosyphilis.

Aseptic meningitis is usually due to a viral infection of the meninges, and may be confused with partially treated bacterial meningitis; however, question of bacterial meningitis does not come here (as there is lymphocytic pleocytosis). Fungal meningitis needs special culture medium. Possibility of acute viral meningoencephalitis may be there and can be ruled out after meticulous clinical examination (with added features of encephalitis).

Q. Viruses producing meningitis:

Acute viral infection of meninges is probably the commonest cause of meningitis. Though less serious than acute pyogenic meningitis, it may prove fatal if associated with encephalitis. Usually it is a benign and self-limiting disease.

Viruses responsible:

1. Enteroviruses—commonest.
2. Mumps virus.
3. Arboviruses (Togavirus and Bunyavirus).
4. Herpes simplex virus (HSV).
5. Lymphocytic choriomeningitis (arenavirus).
6. Influenza viruses.
7. HIV.
8. Rabies virus.
9. Epstein-Barr virus (EBV).
10. Varicella zoster virus.

Aseptic meningitis commonly occurs due to enteroviruses, arboviruses, HIV and HSV-2 (see the chart of 'Acute pyogenic meningitis' described earlier).

- Enteroviruses are Echovirus, Coxsackievirus and Poliovirus.

Q. Investigations performed in acute viral meningitis:

1. Blood for routine examination (R/E) reveals leucopenia along with relative lymphocytosis.
2. Examination of CSF.
3. Detection of antiviral antibodies (IgM) in both serum and CSF. Often the ratio of CSF/serum antibody increases the sensitivity of the diagnosis.
4. CSF PCR has become the primary diagnostic test for CMV, EBV, HSV or enteroviruses.
5. Amplification of viral-specific DNA or RNA from CSF.

Q. Classify neurosyphilis:

Neurosyphilis is very rare nowadays and only considered as a theoretical possibility.

A. Meningovascular

1. Cerebral:
   a. Asymptomatic neurosyphilis.
   b. Acute syphilitic meningitis.
   c. Cerebral pachymeningitis.

d. Cerebral leptomeningitis.
e. Cerebral endarteritis obliterans (may produce hemiplegia).
f. Cerebral gumma (behaves like a SOL).

2. Spinal:
   a. Pachymeningitis hypertrophic cervicalis.
   b. Chronic meningomyelitis.
   c. Erb's spastic paraplegia.
   d. Spinal endarteritis obliterans.
   e. Syphilitic amyotrophy.
   f. Syphilitic radiculitis.

B. Parenchymatous

1. General paresis of insane (GPI): Cerebral.
2. Tabes dorsalis: Spinal.
3. Taboparesis (tabes dorsalis plus GPI).

Q. Clue to diagnosis of fungal meningitis:

Lymphocytic pleocytosis with low sugar level may suggest fungal meningitis (indicates tuberculous aetiology too). The CSF may show the fungus, e.g. it is seen as budding yeast cells and surrounded by a gelatinous capsule in 'India ink preparation' in case of Cryptococcus meningitis. *Cryptococcus neoformans* (commonest cause of fungal meningitis) or *Histoplasma capsulatum* meningitis are common in immunodeficiency (e.g. AIDS).

- Remember, in viral meningitis focal neurological signs are rare though high pyrexia is associated with. In comparison to pyogenic meningitis, headache is a prominent feature here.

MENINGISM

Naked-eye Examination

Pressure	++
Appearance	Clear
On standing	No coagulum formation

Chemical Examination

Protein	35 mg%
Sugar	70 mg%
Chloride	730 mg%

Microscopic Examination

Total cells	4/mm^3
Polymorphs	Nil
Lymphocytes	100%

Bacteriological Examination

Ordinary culture shows no growth (sterile).

Interpretation

All the parameters in macroscopic, chemical, microscopic and bacteriological examination are within normal limit except the raised CSF pressure.

For all probabilities, no specific diagnosis can be given. In the presence of raised CSF pressure, the most likely diagnosis is meningism which requires clinical correlation.

Inference

The chart deals with meningism.

Q. What is meningism?

It is synonymous with meningeal irritation as a result of some local or systemic infection without any direct infection/inflammation of CNS. The symptoms of meningism often mimic meningitis.

Clinical associations:

1. Enteric fever.
2. Pneumonia (commonly atypical variety).
3. Empyema thoracis.
4. Diphtheria.
5. Acute pyogenic tonsillitis.
6. Viral encephalitis; any viral illness.
7. Weil's disease.
8. Leukaemia, lymphoma, malignancy.

One may find positive neck rigidity in meningism which is usually painless. Meningitis produces painful neck rigidity. Kernig's sign is less pronounced in meningism.

Though passive resistance to head flexion is present in cerebral malaria, signs of meningism are always absent.

SUBARACHNOID HAEMORRHAGE

Naked-eye Examination

Pressure	++
Appearance	Blood-stained and uniformly red on standing
On prolonged standing	Supernatent fluid is yellow

Chemical Examination

Protein	500 mg%
Sugar	70 mg%
Chloride	725 mg%

Microscopic Examination

Total cells	Plenty
Polymorphs	Few
Lymphocytes	Few
RBC	10000/mm^3, few are crenated

Bacteriological Examination

Ordinary culture shows no growth (sterile).

Interpretation

1. CSF pressure is high. The fluid is blood-stained and on prolonged standing, supernatent fluid becomes yellow. These findings are highly suggestive of subarachnoid haemorrhage.

2. Total protein is raised probably due to added protein from blood. Sugar and chloride content are within normal limit.
3. Total cell count is raised. Plenty of RBC are seen of which few are crenated. They indicate the diagnosis of subarachnoid haemorrhage.

Inference

The chart deals with subarachnoid haemorrhage (SAH).

- D/D of this chart is traumatic haemorrhage in the CSF. In traumatic haemorrhage, CSF pressure is not altered and the CSF protein content is not so high (see **Table 1.1**).

Q. Causes of haemorrhagic CSF:

The common possibilities are:

1. Subarachnoid haemorrhage.
2. Trauma.
3. Extensive cerebral haemorrhage (dissecting).
4. Haemorrhagic encephalitis.
5. Bleeding diathesis.

For *differntiation between subarachnoid haemorrhage and trauma*, read the 'Lumbar puncture needle' from the 'Instruments and bedside procedures' section. Extensive cerebral haemorrhage may develop into secondary subarachnoid haemorrhage. CSF shows lymphocytic pleocytosis in haemorrhagic encephalitis. Bleeding diathesis is diagnosed clinically and by coagulation profile.

Q. Aetiology of subarachnoid haemorrhage:

A. Primary: Rupture of:

a. Saccular or berry aneurysm: Congential defect; commonest.
b. Arteriovenous malformations or dural arterio-venous fistula.
c. Mycotic aneurysm (may arise from endocarditis).
d. Traumatic/dissecting aneurysm.
e. Atherosclerotic aneurysm.
f. Neoplastic aneurysm.
g. Angioma.
h. Bleeding diathesis or use of anticoagulants.

B. Secondary:

a. Dissecting intracerebral bleed: Especially in a hypertensive subject.
b. Haemorrhage into cerebral infarct.
c. Haemorrhage into cerebral tumour.

- The berry aneurysms are commonly located at:
  1. Posterior communicating-internal carotid artery junction.
  2. Anterior communicating-anterior cerebral artery junction.
  3. Middle cerebral artery bifurcation region.
- Hypertension, smoking and alcohol consumption are important risk factors. SAH causes severe reduction of cerebral blood flow, diminished cerebral autoregulation and acute cerebral oedema.

Q. Congenital malformations associated with berry aneurysm:

1. Polycystic kidneys.
2. Coarctation of aorta.
3. Arteriovenous malformations.
4. Ehlers-Danlos syndrome.
5. Marfan's syndrome.
6. Moyamoya disease.

Q. Common clinical features in SAH:

1. Sudden onset of excruciating occipital headache ('thunderclap headache').
2. Sudden transient loss of consciousness.
3. Vomiting, convulsions, collapse and coma may be present.
4. *Presence of neck rigidity and positive Kernig's sign.*
5. Features of increased intracranial tension.
6. Focal signs, e.g. visual field defect, IIIrd nerve palsy, hemiplegia are not common.
7. Fundoscopy reveals subhyaloid haemorrhage.
8. A bruit may be audible over the eyes or head in arteriovenous malformation.

- Poor risk in SAH: Coma and persistent severe neuro deficit.

Q. Common complications of SAH:

There are four major causes of delayed neurodeficit in SAH.

1. Rebleed: Risk of rebleeding is usual in first 7 days.
2. Vasospasm: May occur between 4 and 14 days (most frequent at 7th day) of initial event and may predispose to focal ischaemic deficit.
3. Hydrocephalus: Blockage of normal CSF may lead to acute, subacute or chronic hydrocephalus necessitating ventricular drainage.
4. Hyponatraemia: Usually occurs within first 2 weeks as a result of SIADH.
5. Others: Seizures, cardio-pulmonary complications.

- Delayed cerebral ischaemia is prevented by controlling hypotension, hyponatraemia, hypovolaemia, hyperglycaemia and hyperthermia.

Q. Investigations performed to diagnose SAH:

1. CT scan (high-quality non-contrast): Shows blood in the subarachnoid space, hydrocephalus, associated brain ischaemia and sometimes the site of aneurysm itself.
2. Lumbar puncture and CSF analysis (the hallmark of diagnosis is blood in the CSF): Done, if CT scan is indecisive.
3. MRI scan.
4. Magnetic resonance angiography (MRA): Usually in patients who are fit for surgery (awake and <65 years).
5. Digital subtraction angiography (DSA), or cerebral angiography (i.e. four-vessel conventional X-ray

angiography involving both carotids and both vertebral arteries) or CT angiography.

- Nowadays, CT imaging is the first investigation of choice and subsequently lumbar puncture is done, if CT remains inconclusive.

Q. Why the supernatent fluid (CSF) in SAH is yellow on prolonged standing?

The uniformly sanguineous CSF develops yellow supernatent fluid on prolonged standing or centrifugation. This is known as **xanthochromia**. In the early stages. It is due to oxyhaemoglobin formation but lately bilirubin (spectophotometry may estimate bilirubin) is responsible for.

Q. Prevention of vasospasm and rebleeding:

a. Vasospasm (due to vasoconstrictor substances released from activated platelet, RBC or cerebral tissue): It is prevented by slow calcium-channel inhibitors, e.g. nimodipine (30 mg/tab) is given as 2 tab 4 hourly to be started within 3–4 days of SAH and is usually continued for 3 weeks. It reduces mortality.
   Though nimodipine is first-line therapy against vasospasm, maintenance of euvolaemia and treatment of comorbidities (e.g. hypertension) are equally important.
b. Rebleeding (due to fibrinolysis): Use of antifibrinolytic agent, e.g. epsilon amino-caproic acid (EACA) is often considered. EACA is infused 24–48 g/day in 5% dextrose-saline over 24 hours with the help of a micro-drip apparatus. It is not routinely used as it increases the risk of delayed cerebral infarction. Another antifibrinolytic agent tranexamic acid (1 g, IV stat, followed by 1 g, QDS) may be useful.
   Coiling and clipping: Surgical treatment to prevent rebleeding is done by clipping the ruptured berry aneurysm though endovascular treatment, i.e. coiling is an increasingly practiced alternative to surgical clipping.

- In treatment of SAH, immediate treatment is done by bed rest and supportive care with control of hypertension. If angiography demonstrates an aneurysm, endovascular treatment by placing platinum coils for ablation of the aneurysm is the first line of surgical treatment.

XANTHOCHROMIA

Naked-eye Examination

Pressure	Low
Appearance	Yellowish
On standing	Formation of big coagulum

Chemical Examination

Protein	1200 mg%
Sugar	65 mg%
Chloride	730 mg%

Microscopic Examination

Total cells	4/mm^3
Polymorphs	Nil
Lymphocytes	100%
RBC	Nil

Bacteriological Examination

Ordinary culture shows no growth (sterile).

Queckenstedt's Test

Positive.

Interpretation

1. Low pressure in the CSF with yellowish appearance (probably indicates xanthochromia) suggests spinal subarachnoid block.
2. Total cell count is within normal limit though the protein content is high, indicating 'albumino-cytological dissociation'.
3. Positive Queckenstedt's test, i.e. no rise in CSF pressure on compression of internal jugular vein along with the above features confirm the diagnosis of complete spinal subarachnoid block.

Inference

This is a chart of complete spinal subarachnoid block.

Q. What is xanthochromia?

Xanthochromia is yellowish discolouration of the CSF. It is always an abnormal feature in the CSF and is commonly due to:

1. Old subarachnoid haemorrhage (due to oxyhaemoglobin and bilirubin).
2. Guillain-Barré syndrome (due to high protein).
3. Acoustic neurofibroma (due to high protein).
4. Froin's loculation syndrome (spinal block and is chiefly due to high protein).
5. Deep Jaundice (due to high bilirubin).
6. Massive old intracerebral bleed or haemorrhagic infarction (same as subarachnoid haemorrhage).
7. Subdural haematoma (rare).

- Xanthochromia occurs within 12 hours of SAH and remains detectable for 2 weeks.

Q. Causes of spinal subarachnoid block:

1. Spinal tumours, e.g. meningioma, neurofibroma.
2. Patchy arachnoiditis.
3. Spinal epidural abscess.

Q. What is Froin's loculation syndrome?

This syndrome develops as a result of spinal cord compression (spinal block). CSF examination shows:

1. Low CSF pressure.
2. Xanthochromia.
3. Clot formation on standing.

4. High protein content.
5. Positive Queckenstedt's test.

Q. What is Queckenstedt's test?

Vide the chapter on 'Lumbar puncture needle' from 'Instruments and bedside procedures' section.

Q. What do you mean by albumino-cytological dissociation?

It means, there is raised protein content in the CSF without any rise in the total cell count. The probable causes are:

1. Guillain-Barré syndrome.
2. Froin's loculation syndrome.
3. Acoustic neurofibroma.

Q. How the patient with spinal block presents?

The patient usually presents with features of spastic paraparesis or paraplegia (compressive myelopathy). Spinal block may result from spinal epidural abscess, haematoma or tumour.

CHARTS ON TEMPERATURE

Introduction

At first, one may read the chapter on 'Abnormal temperature' from 'Bedside Clinics in Medicine, Part I' where the temperature patterns are disscused in details. However, a gist is given below:

Normal body temperature and its variations are:

1. Normal: 98–99°F (with a diurnal variation of 1.5°F; the temperature is lowest in the morning and is highest in the evening); normal temperature is known as euthermia.
2. Subnormal: Below 98°F
3. Pyrexia or febrile: Above 99°F
4. Hypothermia: Below 95°F
5. Hyperpyrexia: Above 106.7°F

Rectal or vaginal temperature > oral temperature > axillary temperature.

- **Temperature taken under the tongue is more reliable** than axillary temperature. Electronics thermometer are more accurate and gradually replacing mercury thermometer. Tympanic membrane (TM) thermometers measure radiant heat from the tympanic membrane and is lower than rectal temperature.
- Recently fever or pyrexia has been defined like this: AM temperature (oral) of >98.9°F and PM temperature (oral) of >99.9°F. Roughly assess patient's temperature by touching the body by using your dorsum of the hand (more sensitive than palmar aspect).

Clinical Wisdom

Methods of taking body temperature: 1. oral, 2. axillary or groin, 3. rectal, 4. temporal (i.e. on forehead), 5. on tympanic membrane.

Types of Fever

1. Intermittent: Fever is present only for several hours and always touches the baseline sometime during the day. It has three subdivisions:
   a. Quotidian: When the paroxysm of fever occurs daily (i.e. daily rise and daily fall).
   b. Tertian: When the paroxysm occurs on alternate days (i.e. a gap of 48 hours).
   c. Quartan: When two days intervene between consecutive paroxysmal attacks (i.e. a gap of 72 hours).
2. Continued (or continuous): Fever does not fluctuate more than 1°C (1.5°F) during the 24-hours period and it never touches the baseline.
3. Remittent: Daily fluctuation of fever is more than 2°C (3°F) during the 24-hours period and it never touches the baseline.

Appearance of Rash in a Febrile Patient

Mnemonic: 'Very sick person must take double tea' stands for:

1st day	Varicella (chickenpox)
2nd day	Scarlet fever
3rd day	Pox (smallpox, eradicated globally)
4th day	Measles
5th day	Typhus
6th day	Dengue
7th day	Typhoid or enteric fever

Onset of pyrexia may be

a. Sudden, e.g. Malaria, lobar pneumonia.
b. Gradual, e.g. Enteric fever.

- Drug rash may appear any time/any day.

Diseases Spread by Pets and Rodents

a. Dogs: Rabies, hydatid disease, bronchial asthma (by allergy); *Campylobacter*, *Salmonella*, *Giardia*, *Cryptosporidium* infection, brucellosis, leptospirosis, ringworm, tetanus.
b. Cats: Toxoplasmosis, rabies, bronchial asthma (by allergy), cat-scratch disease (*Bartonella henselae*), tularaemia, campylobacter infection.
c. Rats: Plague, leptospirosis, rat bite fever (*Streptobacillus moniliformis*), Hantavirus pulmonary syndrome, murine typhus, Lassa fever, lymphocytic choriomeningitis, monkeypox, bronchial asthma (by allergy), Weil's disease.

Epidemiological Clues to Fever/Rash

1. Male homosexuals: HIV, hepatitis B, amoebiasis
2. Travel abroad: Malaria, typhoid, giardiasis, hepatic amoebiasis
3. Cats: Toxoplasmosis, tularaemia
4. Dogs: Leptospirosis
5. Sewerage workers/water sports: Leptospirosis

6. Hunting: Tularaemia, Lyme disease
7. Hiking: Giardiasis, Rocky Mountain spotted fever
8. Raw meat: Brucellosis
9. Raw milk: Bovine tuberculosis, toxoplasmosis, brucellosis
10. Raw egg: Typhoid
11. IV drug abuser: HIV, hepatitis B and C, infective endocarditis, thrombophlebitis.

- The term 'fastigium' is the period of highest rise in a temperature curve.
- In the clinical thermometer, an arrow is marked at 98.6°F or 37°C indicating normal body temperature (axillary temperature).

QUOTIDIAN TEMPERATURE (Fig. 7.9)

Inference

The chart shows daily rise of temperature with daily fall. So, this is the quotidian variety of intermittent temperature.

Q. Causes of quotidian temperature:

1. Double infection of *P. vivax*.
2. Pent-up pus anywhere in the body.
3. Tuberculosis.
4. Urinary tract infection.
5. Amoebic liver abscess.
6. Septicaemia.
7. Pyaemia.
8. Filariasis.

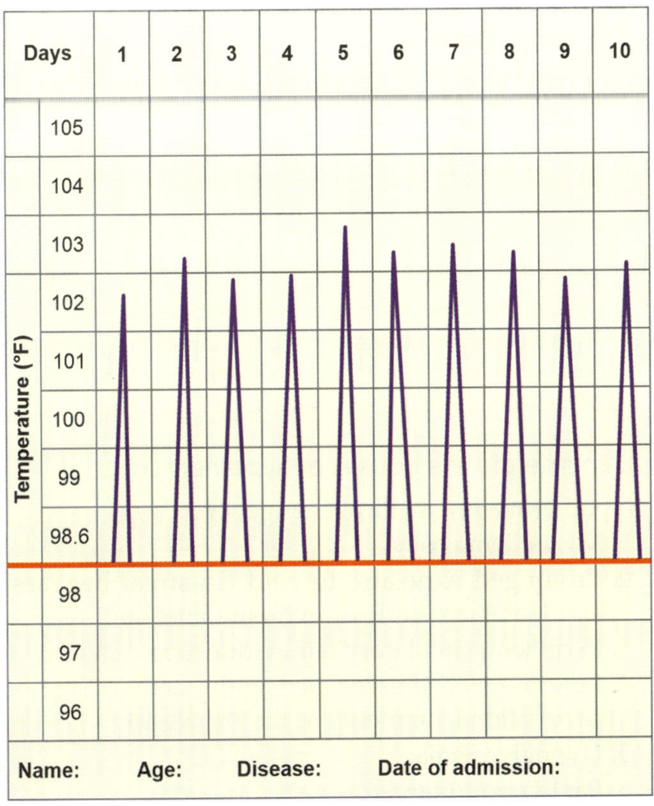

Fig. 7.9: Quotidian temperature

Q. Is it the common type of temperature in *P. vivax* infection?

No. Tertian variety of intermittent temperature is commonly seen in *P. vivax* malaria.

Q. What is meant by 'double infection' of *P. vivax*?

It is the infection by two different *P. vivax* types having different life cycles.

Often different species of malaria parasites develop in the same mosquito and may transmit the infection to man giving rise to 'mixed infection', the commonest being *P. vivax* and *P. falciparum* species. This type of mixed infection may also give rise to quotidian temperature.

Q. Temperature pattern in 'pent-up pus' anywhere in the body:

It is known as **'hectic' temperature**. There is wide swings in the temperature and the temperature rises with chill and rigor (often with facial flushes), then persists for few hours, and suddenly falls with profuse perspiration. Common examples are lung abscess, pyogenic liver abscess, empyema thoracis, empyema of gallbladder, subdiaphragmatic abscess, acute osteomyelitis. Hectic temperature may also be seen in septicaemia or pyaemia.

Q. Importance of 'thick' and 'thin' film blood smear in malaria:

A. Thick film:
   a. For screening
   b. Helpful in low parasitaemia
B. Thin film:
   a. For confirmation of diagnosis
   b. Identification of the species
   c. Quantity load in *P. falciparum*

Q. What are pyrogens?

Pyrogens are substances that produce fever. It may be of two types: exogenous and endogenous.

The *exogenous pyrogens* are microorganisms, their products, or toxin; chemically they are lipopolysaccharides. The *endogenous pyrogens* are chemically polypeptides, produced primarily by macrophages/monocytes; common examples are interleukin-1, interleukin-6, tumour necrosis factor (TNF)-α, interferon-α (in a general sense, collectively known as **cytokines**).

Q. What is 'periodic fever'?

It is the periodic attacks of pyrexia alternating with a period of apyrexia, and is commonly seen in:

1. Hodgkin's disease (Pel-Ebstein fever).
2. Brucellosis (undulant fever).
3. Relapsing fever.
4. Malaria.
5. Rat bite fever.
6. Dengue.

TERTIAN TEMPERATURE (Fig. 7.10)

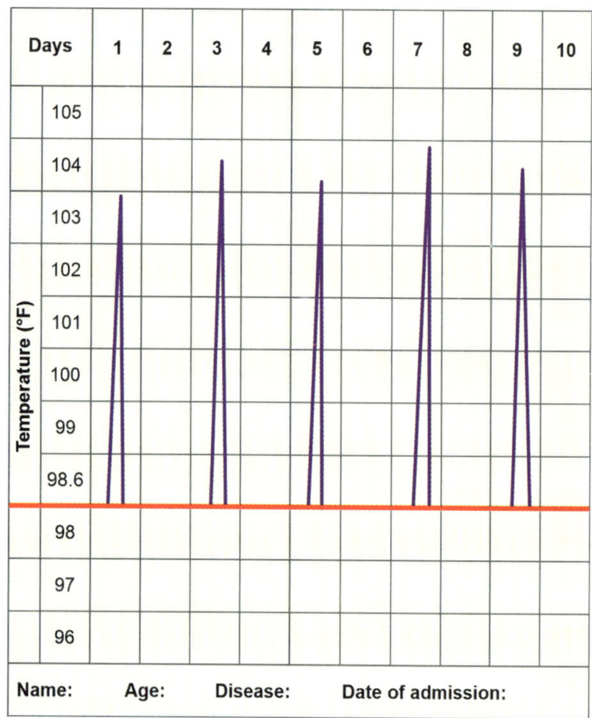

Fig. 7.10: Tertian temperature

Inference

As the temperature comes on alternate days and touches the baseline, this is the tertian variety of intermittent temperature (i.e. the temperature shoots on 1st, 3rd, 5th, 7th, 9th days and so on).

Q. Causes of tertian temperature:

1. Benign tertian malaria (commonly by *P. vivax*, and rarely by *P. ovale* or *P. malariae*).
2. Malignant tertian malaria (*P. falciparum*).

Q. Asexual cycle in different types of *Plasmodium*:

i. *P. vivax* and *P. ovale*: 48 hours
ii. *P. falciparum*: Less than 48 hours.
iii. *P. malariae*: 72 hours.

This determines the temperature pattern in different types of *Plasmodium* infection.

Q. Different stages in 'malarial paroxysm':

There are 3 stages:

1. Cold stage (chill, shivering, rigor, teeth chattering, goose flesh),
2. Hot stage (feels hot, hot flush, throbbing headache, prostration, vomiting), and
3. Stage of sweating (drenching sweat, defervescence of fever, exhaustion).

The patient usually remains afebrile in between paroxyams.

- Infected female anopheline mosquito → sporozoites inoculated in man → goes into liver → merozoites leave the liver → Invades RBC → produce schizonts → rupture of schizonts releases many merozoites into the blood and produces fever.

Q. Pathogenesis of chill, rigor and sweating:

Normal temperature is maintained in health by regulating a balance between heat gain and heat loss, governed by the hypothalamus.

It should be looked upon in the setting of 'thermostat'. When the temperature is rising to a higher level, heat is being conserved, the cutaneous vessels are constricted (so the patient feels cold/chill) and the patient may even shiver violently. The shivering is known as 'rigor', and is often associated with piloerection and teeth chattering.

When the higher temperature is reached, heat loss starts and the cutaneous vessels starts dilating for dissipation of heat. The patient feels hot and sweating starts.

The presence of chill and rigor is modestly predictive of bacteraemia.

Q. Causes of quartan temperature:

It is found in quartan malaria (*P. malariae*), which is rare in India.

Q. Causes of hyperpyrexia:

Hyperpyrexia is a life-threatening emergency that needs urgent medical attention.

1. Malaria.
2. Septicaemia.
3. Encephalitis.
4. Pontine haemorrhage.
5. Lobar pneumonia.
6. Heat stroke.
7. Dhatura poisoning.
8. Malignant hyperthermia (halothane-induced).
9. Thyroid storm.
10. Neuroleptic malignant syndrome (haloperidol-induced).
11. Rabies, pyogenic meningitis.
12. Drug-induced (e.g. amphetamines, cocaine).
13. Serotonin syndrome (SSRI/MAOI-induced).

- Fever is due to elevated set-point of the thermostat, whereas hyperpyrexia results from inadequate heat dissipation.
- **Hyperthermia** occurs when the body absorbs or generates more heat than it can release. Hyperthermia does not involve pyrogen molecules (e.g. heat stroke).

Q. Enumerate the causes of hypothermia:

Hypothermia is a medical emergency.

1. Myxoedema coma.
2. Prolonged exposure to cold (in street beggars, accidental in elderly or in mountaineering).
3. Peripheral circulatory failure due to any cause.
4. Enteric fever, if associated with haemorrhage or perforation (commonly in the 3rd week).
5. Hypoglycaemia.
6. Panhypopituitarism.
7. Adrenal insufficiency.

8. Artificial hypothermia induced in open heart surgery.
9. Extreme wasting as in starvation, terminal stage of malignancy.
10. Near-drowing.
11. Alcohol intoxication.
12. Autonomic dysfunction.

Q. Causes of fever with chill and rigor:

1. Malaria.
2. Urinary tract infection.
3. Pent-up pus anywhere in the body, e.g. sub-diaphragmatic abscess.
4. Septicaemia or pyaemia.
5. Cholangitis.
6. Subacute bacterial endocarditis.
7. Thrombophlebitis.
8. Acute pyelitis or acute pyelonephritis.
9. Acute lobar pneumonia.
10. Pyrogen reaction after fluid infusion or blood transfusion.
11. Filariasis.
12. Agranulocytosis.

Q.D/D of severe falciparum malaria:

The list of most likely diseases are:

1. Meningitis.
2. Viral encephalitis.
3. Septicaemia.
4. Enteric fever.
5. Leptospirosis.
6. Fulminant hepatitis.
7. Dengue fever.
8. Rickettsial infection

Q. Drug-induced fever:

1. Allupurinol.
2. Sulphonamides.
3. Carbamazepine.
4. Iodides, bromides.
5. Barbiturates.
6. Rifampicin ('flu syndrome').
7. Phenolphthalein.
8. Phenytoin.
9. Quinidine.
10. Nevirapine.

Q. Essential enquiries in a case of 'pyrexia':

A detailed enquiry about fever needs a good clinical skill and the points stressed are:

1. H/o contact.
2. Medications.
3. Substance abuse.
4. Immunosuppression.
5. Travel.
6. Duration.
7. Types of pyrexia.
8. Localising symptoms.
9. Loss of weight.
10. Joint pain.

CONTINUED TEMPERATURE (Fig. 7.11)

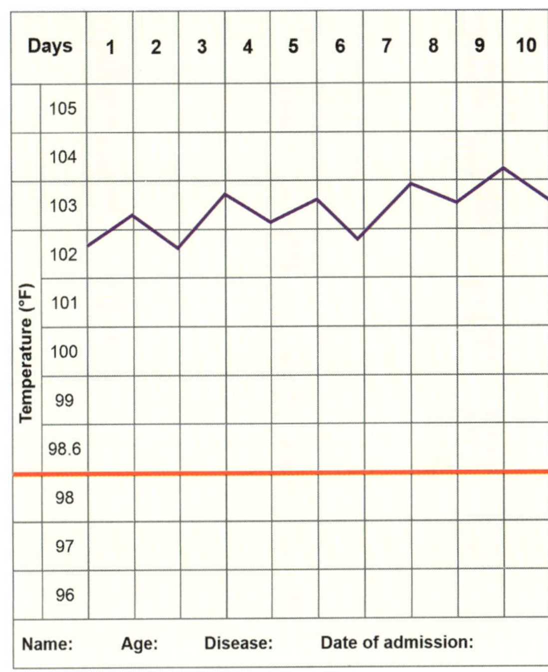

Fig. 7.11: Continued temperature

Inference

The fluctuation of temperature is limited within 1.5°F and it does not touch the baseline. This is a chart showing continued type of pyrexia.

Q. Causes of continued temperature:

1. Lobar pneumonia
2. Second week of enteric fever.
3. Miliary tuberculosis.
4. Meningococcal meningitis.
5. Acute rheumatic fever.
6. Subacute bacterial endocarditis (SBE).
7. Untreated urinary tract infection.
8. Collagen vascular diseases (e.g. SLE).
9. Lymphoma or leukaemias.
10. Typhus.

Q. Features of enteric fever in the 'second week':

A. Symptoms:

1. Disappearance of headache.
2. Continued type of high pyrexia.
3. Constipation is usually replaced by 'pea-soup diarrhoea' (loose, greenish stool).
4. Lethargy and apathy appear.
5. Abdominal distention (meteorism).
6. Cough may be present (due to bronchitis).

B. Signs:

1. Pulse: Tachycardia appears, dicrotic pulse usually disappears. Pulse is of low volume.
2. Tongue remains dry and coated.
3. Soft and mildly tender splenomegaly. Abdomen is distended and may be tender.
4. Rose spots may appear on 7–10th day (in 30% patients).
5. Lungs may shows features of bronchitis/bronchopneumonia.

Q. What is 'Typhoid facies'?

Classically the description goes like this: the face is thin and flushed; bright eyes and a dull, heavy, staring, apathetic expression. This type of facial appearance is characteristic of a patient of enteric fever who is progressing into the third week.

Q. Aetiology of enteric fever:

1. Transmitted by faecal-oral route through the contamination of milk, food or water.
2. The bacilli may persist in the gallbladder of chronic carriers for months or years.
3. Incubation period is 10–14 days.
4. a. Typhoid fever is caused by *Salmonella typhi*.
   b. Paratyphoid fever is due to *S. paratyphi* A and B (course is shorter and milder).

Q. Diagnosis of enteric fever:

A. First week:
   a. Though in most patients the WBC count is normal, 15–25% patients may have leucopenia and neutropenia.
   b. Blood culture (90%): Often clot culture is done.
   c. Culture of bone marrow aspirates will yield the organism (55–90%) even earlier than blood culture: Not used routinely is clinical practice.
   d. Culture of intestinal secretions.

B. Second week:
   a. Widal test (95%).
   b. Blood culture (60%).

C. Third week:
   a. Stool culture (75%).
   b. Widal test (95% in high titre).
   c. Blood culture (50%).
   d. Urine culture (70%).

D. Fourth week:
   a. Urine culture (70%).
   b. Stool culture (50%).
   c. Widal test.
   d. Blood culture (25%).

Mnemonic: **BASU**, i.e. the most efficacious test in first week—**B**lood culture, second week—**A**gglutination test (Widal test), third week—**S**tool culture, and in fourth week—**U**rine culture. Figure within the bracket indicates positivity in percentage of cases.

- The hallmark of enteric fever is prolonged and persistent pyrexia, if remains untreated. Leucopenia and relative bradycardia are typical.

Q. Newer diagnostic tests in enteric fever:

Slide agglutination test, indirect haemagglutination test, ELISA or typhidot test (IgG and IgM), counter immunoelectrophoresis, enzyme immunoassay, PCR, IgM capture, monoclonal antibodies, DNA probes, etc. Though highly sensitive, the tests are costly.

Q. Leucocytosis in enteric fever:

If enteric fever is complicated by perforation or bronchopneumonia, leucocytosis may be observed.

Q. What are rose spots?

These are sparse, small rose-red, blanching, slightly raised macules mainly present over upper abdomen and chest during the end of the first week of illness (2–4 mm in diameter and about 6–10 in number). It is usually visible only on fair-skinned persons. The lesions last only 2–3 days and result from bacterial embolism in skin capillaries. *Salmonella* can be cultured from punch biopsy of rose spots.

Q. What is Widal test?

1. It is an agglutination reaction where agglutinating antibodies develop against O (somatic), H (flagellar) and Vi (capsular)-antigens.
2. It is usually positive from 7 to 10 days and onwards.
3. **The O-agglutinins are more valuable in active disease than H-agglutinins.** H-agglutinins may develop as a result of previous inoculation or there may be an anamnestic rise. Vi-agglutinin develops after 3–4 weeks of illness and thus not used routinely for early diagnosis (important in diagnois of carriers).
4. A four-fold 'rising titre' is very suggestive of enteric fever. The titre has no correlation with the severity of illness.
5. A titre (against O-antigen) above 1:160 is suggestive and **a titre above 1:640 is often very significant of enteric fever** in a non-immunised person.
6. It is not a very reliable test and should be interpreted with caution, especially in typhoid vaccinated patients. Due to high rates of false positivity and false negativity, misinterpretation is very common. Nowadays, Widal test is not preferred by the clinicians.

Q. What is 'typhoid state'?

The untreated enteric fever patient may enter into severe toxaemic state along with high rise of temperature usually at the end of second week or onset of the third week of illness, and is manifested by some neurological (encephalitis-like) features such as:

1. Semiconsciousness or unconsciousness.
2. Low muttering delirium.

3. Coma vigil: Patient lies with half-open eyes but ignorant of his surroundings (staring stupor).
4. Subsultus tendinum: Involuntary movements of fingers and wrists due to muscular twitching.
5. Carphology: Agitated plucking of the bed sheets, and
6. Convulsions rarely.

This is a moribund situation and should be tackled immediately with intravenous dexamethasone or hydrocortisone hemisuccinate along with parenteral antimicrobials (chloramphenicol, ceftriaxone).

- Steroids should not be used in the third or fourth week in classical enteric fever as there is chance of precipitation of intestinal haemorrhage or perforation.
- Features like meningism may be present in typhoid state.

Q. Life-threatening complications in enteric fever:

1. Typhoid state.
2. Intestinal haemorrhage or perforation (usually in the 3rd or 4th week).
3. Acute pancreatitis (rare).
4. Acute peripheral circulatory failure; endotoxic shock.
5. Myocarditis.
6. DIC (Disseminated intravascular coagulation).
7. Septicaemia, pyaemia.
8. Meningitis, nephritis and osteomyelitis.
9. Haemophagocytic syndrome or macrophage activation syndrome (MAS).
10. Haemolytic-uraemic syndrome.

- Two other important complications (late) are carrier state (1–4%) and chronic cholecystitis.

Q. Immunisation against enteric fever:

a. Oral: Contain life attenuated *S. typhi*. Four (4) doses: One capsule to be taken 1 hour prior to meal with cold or lukewarm water on every alternate days (on days 1, 3, 5 and 7). Totally 4 capsules are required (Typhoral). Booster dose to be repeated after every 5 years. The minimum age for vaccination is 6 years.
b. Parenteral: Purified Vi-polysaccharide inactivated vaccine prepared from bacterial capsule (Vi CPS). Single dose: One injection of 0.5 mL (Typhim Vi) given IM or deep SC. Booster dose is to be repeated every 2 years. The minimum age for vaccination is 2 years.

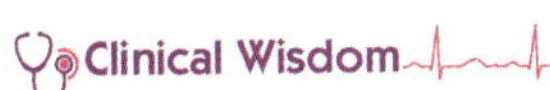

The old parenteral whole-cell typhoid/paratyphoid A and B vaccine is no longer used.

REMITTENT TEMPERATURE (Fig. 7.12)

Inference

The fluctuation of temperature is more than 3°F and it does not touch the baseline. There is a special feature in this chart, i.e. double rise of temperature on the same

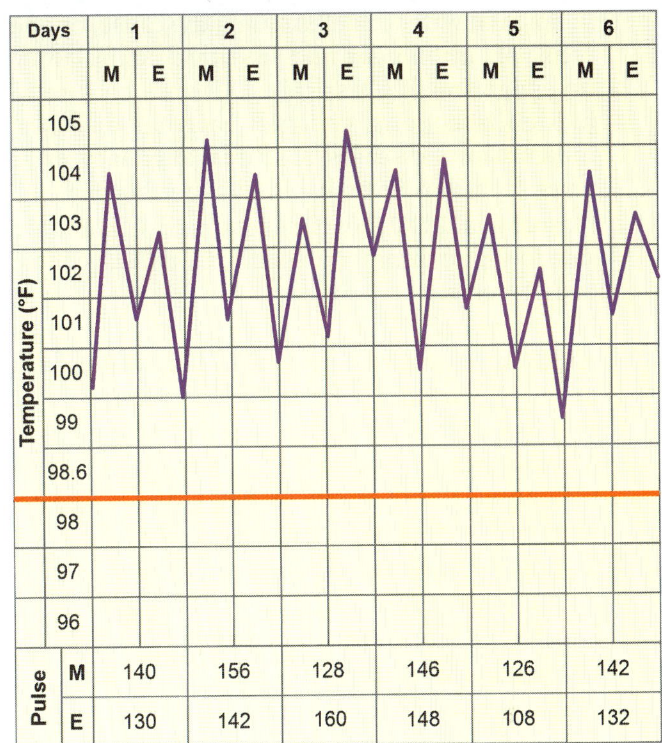

Fig. 7.12: Remittent temperature

day and is known as double quotidian temperature. Basically, the chart deals with remittent type of pyrexia.

Q. Causes of remittent temperature:

1. Amoebic liver abscess.
2. Sometimes in urinary tract infection.
3. Third week of enteric fever.
4. Acute bronchopneumonia.
5. Acute tonsillitis.
6. Bacteraemia, septicaemia, pyaemia.

Q. Probable causes of double quotidian (camel hump fever) pyrexia:

It is the double fever spike in a single day and is seen in:

1. Kala-azar (20%, commonest cause).
2. Gonococcal perihepatitis or endocarditis.
3. Sometimes in acute bacterial endocarditis.

- This type of fever is often known as 'rabbit-ear patten' pyrexia.

Q. What is pyrxia of unknown origin (PUO)?

a. It is also known as fever of unknown origin (FUO). Criteria to diagnose PUO are (Petersdorf and Beeson, 1961):
   1. Fever higher than 101°F on several occasions.
   2. A duration of fever for more than 3 weeks.
   3. Failure to reach a provisional diagnosis after one week of inpatient investigations.
b. From 1991, PUO is classified as (Durack and Street, 1991):
   1. Classical PUO (as previous definition, except the time frame which is 3 outpatient visits or 3 days

in hospital without determining the cause, or one week of 'intelligent and invasive' ambulatory investigations): Classical PUO may be due to hidden infections, collagen vascular diseases, inflammatory diseases, obscure malignancy, drug fever, factitious fever, habitual hyperthermia.

2. Nosocomial PUO (hospital-acquired): Commonly due to septic thrombophlebitis, *Cl. difficile* colitis, drug fever, etc.
3. Neutropenic PUO: The neutrophil count is <500/mm^3 and is commonly due to perianal infection, *Candida* or *Aspergillus* infection.
4. HIV-associated PUO: As a result of tuberculosis, *Mycobacterium avium* intracellulare (MAI), toxoplasmosis, *Pneumocystis jiroveci*, cryptococcosis, non-Hodgkin's lymphoma, drug fever.

c. **The most recent classification of PUO** has been further modified as:

1. Fever >101°F on at least 2 occasions.
2. Duration of fever ≥3 weeks.
3. No known immunocompromised state.
4. Diagnosis still remains uncertain after a thorough history taking, meticulous clinical examination, and some obligatory investigations like TC, DC, Hb%, ESR, CRP, platelet count, AST, ALT, LDH, CK, RF, ANF, chest X-ray, blood culture, urine analysis, abdominal USG, etc.

- In the present era of antipyretics and antibiotics, it is difficult to diagnose the classical types of fever.

Q. Common causes of PUO in India:

1. Tuberculosis, amoebic liver abscess, SBE, chronic kala-azar, malaria, cryptococcosis, cysticercosis, AIDS; many a time enteric fever presents as PUO.
2. Acute rheumatic fever, SLE, vasculitis, thrombophlebitis.
3. Lymphomas, leukaemias, multiple myeloma, hypernephroma.
4. Drug fever, faulty thermometer, factitious fever.

- The success in diagnosing PUO rests on meticulous history taking (with special reference to family, occupational and recent travel history), repeated interview with the patient, thinking about the patient and careful physical examination with specific investigations.

Q. Probable causes of 'aseptic fever' (i.e. fever without infection):

1. Heat stroke.
2. Lymphoma, leukaemia or disseminated malignancy.
3. Collagen vascular disease, e.g. SLE.
4. Pontine haemorrhage.
5. Thyroid storm.
6. Drug fever, e.g. rifampicin or sulphonamide.
7. Acute myocardial infarction.
8. Gout.
9. Crush injury.
10. Over-atropinisation.
11. Radiation sickness.
12. Porphyria.
13. Acute pancreatitis.

- A patient of SBE may not have fever (i.e. infection without fever) in the presence of CCF, CRF, severe sepsis, in elderly patients and with prior antimicrobial therapy.

STEP-LADDER PATTERN PYREXIA (Fig. 7.13)

Inference

The chart shows gradually increasing pattern of pyrexia for first 7 days of illness and may be called 'step-ladder pattern' pyrexia. The rise in the pulse rate shown in the chart is not corresponding to the elevated temperature, and relative bradycardia is noted. The temperature pattern from 8th to 10th day is of continued in type.

The temperature pattern deals with pyrexia due to enteric fever/typhoid fever.

Q. Features of enteric fever in its 'first week':

1. Step-ladder pattern of pyrexia.
2. Frontal headache.
3. Constipation (diarrhoea, vomiting and pain abdomen may be seen in children).

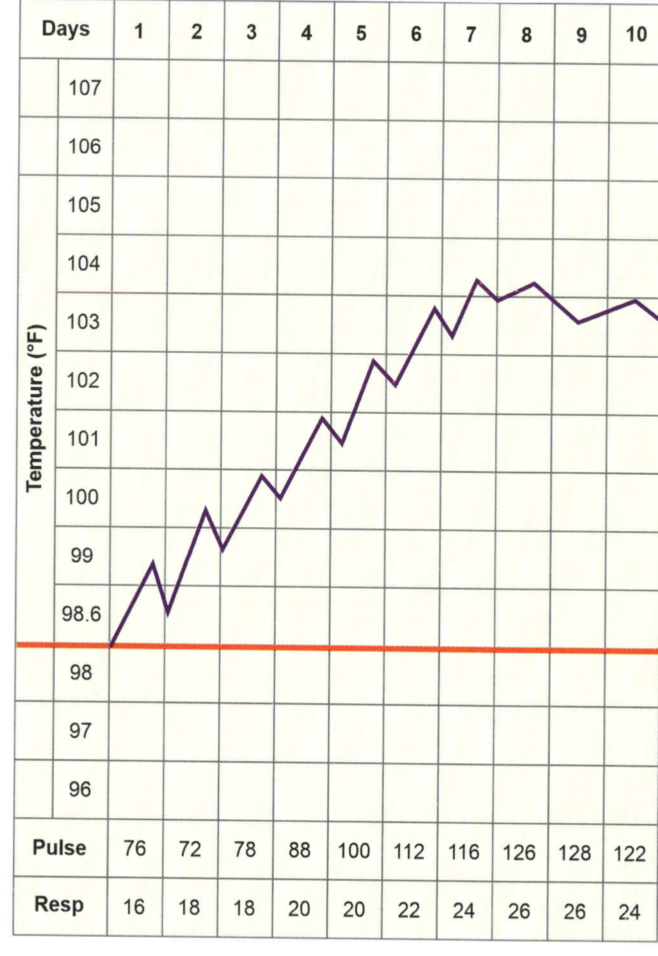

Fig. 7.13: Step-ladder pattern pyrexia

4. Anorexia, nausea, cough and epistaxis.
5. Flushed face with toxic look.
6. Angry looking tongue: Central coating with red tip and margins.
7. Caecal gurgling (due to presence of fluid faeces and air)—palpate the right iliac fossa.
8. Relative bradycardia and rarely dicrotic pulse.
9. Rose spots appearing on the 7th day (usually appears on 7th–10th day).
10. There may be just palpable, soft and tender spleen at the end of first week.

- It needs immense clinical acumen to diagnose enteric fever in the first week.

Q. What is 'step-ladder pattern' pyrexia?

1. The temperature of today always exceeds that of previous day.
2. Usually the temperature rises (2°F) in the evening and falls (1°F) in the next morning.
3. It is basically continued or remittent type of pyrexia (i.e. not touching the baseline).

Q. Pattern of pyrexia in different weeks of enteric fever:

1. 1st week: Step-ladder pattern.
2. 2nd week: Continued type.
3. 3rd week: Continued or remittent type with fluctuation of 3–4°F. There may be 'fall by crisis' of temperature as a result of haemorrhage or perforation.
4. 4th week: Reverse step-ladder pattern, i.e. temperature 'falls by lysis'.

Q. What is relative bradycardia?

It is known that with per degree (°F) rise of temperature in an adult, the pulse rate increases by 10 beats/minute. If the increase in pulse rate is less than 10 beats/minute with per degree (°F) rise of temperature, the condition is known as relative bradycardia. It is commonly found in:

1. Any viral illness (e.g. in yellow fever—known as Faget's sign; and dengue).
2. First week of enteric fever.
3. Sometimes in pyogenic meningitis.
4. Brucellosis, psittacosis, Weil's disease.
5. Drug fever, factitious fever.

Clinical Wisdom

In **relative tachycardia**, pulse rate is increased by more than 10 beats/minute with per degree (°F) rise of temperature. The common examples are acute rheumatic fever, tuberculosis and diphtheritic myocarditis.

Q. What is meant by 'fall by crisis' and 'fall by lysis'?

Fall of temperature is also known as **defervescence**. They are:

a. ***Fall by crisis:*** When the pyrexia falls to normal or subnormal level very quickly within 6–12 hours and is associated with severe sweating, it is known as fall by crisis. It is usually found in:
   1. Acute lobar pneumonia.
   2. Enteric fever complicated by intestinal haemorrhage or perforation.
   3. Adrenal crisis (seen in meningococcal meningitis).
   4. Septicaemic shock.
   5. Dengue.

b. ***Fall by lysis:*** When the temperature falls gradually in steps over several days, it is known as fall by lysis. It is usually found in:
   1. Uncomplicated enteric fever.
   2. Acute rheumatic fever.
   3. Acute bronchopneumonia.

- Most of the raised temperature falls by lysis. Use of antipyretics (paracetamol) may precipitate fall by crisis.

TEMPERATURE CHART ON MEASLES (Fig. 7.14)

Inference

The temperature shoots up to 100.5°F on the first day and then persists for next 2 days as continued in type. The chart shows that on the 4th day, the temperature again elevates up to 104°F with the appearance of rash in the body. Thereafter, pyrexia gradually **falls by lysis** on next 5 days, making the patient afebrile on the 10th day.

The pattern of pyrexia as well as the appearance of rash on the fourth day strongly indicate the diagnosis of measles.

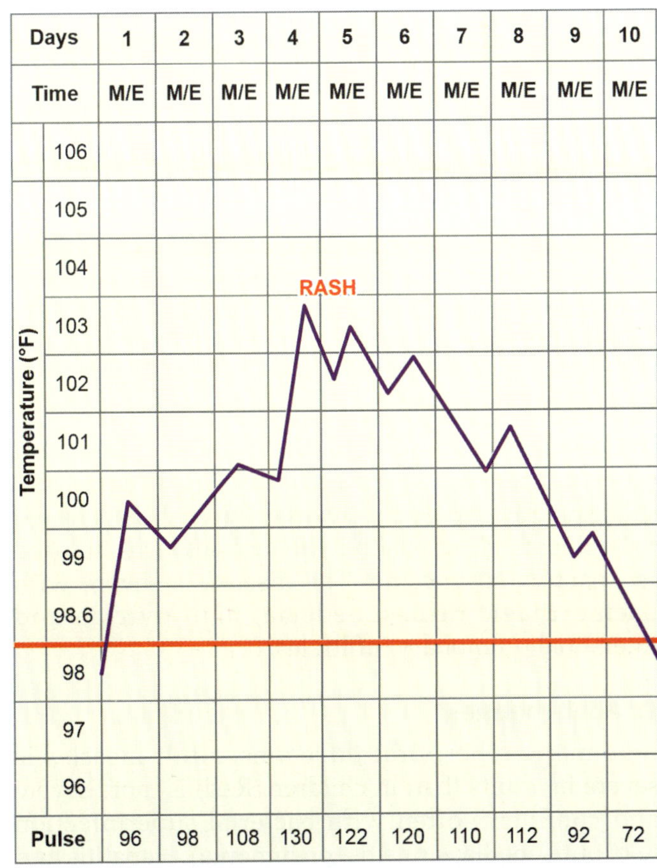

Fig. 7.14: Temperature chart on measles

Q. Aetiology:

Synonym: Rubeola.
Infective agent: Paramyxovirus (RNA virus).
Age: Young children are mostly affected.
Spread: By droplet infection.
Route of infection: Nasopharynx.
Incubation period: 7–14 days (mean 10 days).

Q. Stages of illness in measles:

1. Catarrhal or pre-eruptive stage.
2. Exanthematous or eruptive stage.
3. Recovery stage.

Q. Describe the characteristic rash in measles (exanthem):

1. Usually appears on the fourth day, maculo-papular in type. Rash first appears at the back of the ears, and at the junction of skin and hair on the forehead; ultimately face, neck, trunk, limbs up to palms and soles may be affected. The density of rash is found to be greatest on the forehead.
2. Rashes are discrete, pink, and blanch on pressure. Later they become confluent giving rise to characteristic blotchy appearance. Measles' rash is also known as **morbilliform rash**.
3. Rash disappears in the reverse order of appearance giving rise to a faint brown staining of the skin followed by fine desquamation.

Q. What is Koplik's spot (enanthem)?

1. **Koplik's spots are virtually pathognomonic of measles.** Usually appears on the second day of illness and disappear before the appearance of exanthem (true rash).
2. These are tiny white or bluish-white spots surrounded by a narrow zone of inflammation around the opening of the parotid duct, i.e. in the buccal mucous membrane (inner aspect of cheek) opposite the crown of upper second molar teeth. This stage is highly infectious (stage of viraemia).

Q. Atypical measles:

It is seen in persons who has taken formalin-inactivated measles vaccine (not used after 1970) and were subsequently exposed to measles virus. It is believed to be due to hypersensitivity to measles virus induced by inactivated vaccine. The disease is severe with haemorrhagic rashes, oedema, high pyrexia and interstitial pulmonary infiltrates.

Q. Adult measles:

Like many other viral infections, adult measles is severe in adults than in children. Rash is more severe and confluent, often with bacterial superinfection (e.g. otitis media, sinusitis, pneumonia). Hepatitis and bronchospasm are more common.

Q. Period of infectivity in measles:

The catarrhal stage and up to 5 days after appearance of morbilliform rash is highly infectious. The total duration of illness in a classical case is 10 days or less.

Q. Immunological changes in a sufferer of measles:

1. Transient loss of PPD (Mantoux test becomes negative).
2. Improvement of eczema and bronchial asthma.
3. Remission of leukaemia, lipoid nephrosis and Hodgkin's disease.

Q. Major complications of measles:

a. Three 'tubes' are mainly affected like:
   1. Otitis media (eustachian tube),
   2. Bronchopneumonia (bronchus), and
   3. Gastroenteritis (intestine).
b. Bronchitis and bronchiolitis, croup, giant cell pneumonia, conjunctivitis, myocarditis, generalised purpura, reactivation of tuberculosis, viral encephalitis, acute post-measles encephalomyelitis, subacute sclerosing panencephalitis (SSPE, develops after several years), keratitis.

Q. Prophylaxis against measles:

a. Active: Single dose (0.5 mL) of life-attenuated viral vaccine (by Enders and colleagues) given by SC route at 9 months of age (may be given in combination with mumps and rubella vaccine, as 'MMR' vaccine) with booster dose at 1½ years of age. MMR vaccine is likely to be replaced by MMR-V (V for varicella) vaccine. Many countries recommend measles vaccine at 6–15 months of age.
b. Passive (post-exposure prophylaxis): Human normal immunoglobulin is given within 6 days of exposure, by IM route for attenuation of measles in contacts with the dose of:
   i. 0.25 mL/kg: For healthy persons, and
   ii. 0.5 mL/kg: For immunocompromised individuals.

Clinical Wisdom

Other causes of **fever and rash like measles (D/D)** are rubella, scarlet fever, dengue, infectious mononucleosis, roseola (exanthem subitum), Rocky Mountain spotted fever, Still's disease, Kawasaki disease, meningococcaemia, adenovirus and enterovirus infection. Measles is a very serious disease in immunocompromised (typical rash may be absent) and malnourished patients.

TEMPERATURE CHART ON VARICELLA INFECTION (Fig. 7.15)

Inference

There is acute pyrexia on the 1st day reaching 103.8°F with the appearance of rash. Thereafter, pyrexia gradually **falls by lysis** for next 8 days and the patient becomes afebrile on the 9th day.

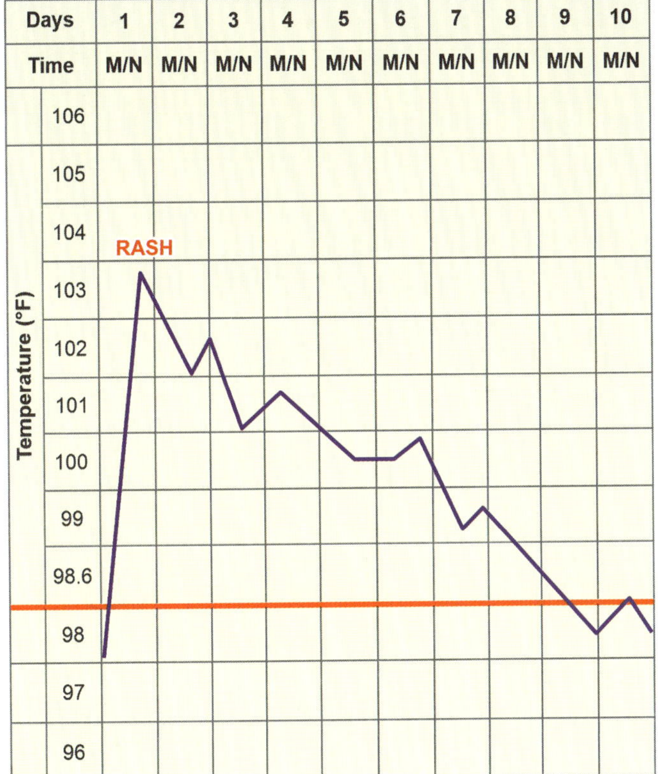

Fig. 7.15: Temperature chart on varicella infection

The pattern of pyrexia as well as the appearance of rash on the 1st day strongly indicate the diagnosis of varicella infection.

Q. Aetiology:

Infective agent: Varicella-zoster virus (DNA virus).

Spread: By droplet infection.

Route of infection: Nasopharynx.

Incubation period: 12–21 days (mean 17 days).

Period of infectivity: Usually about a week, starting probably a day before the appearance of rash and continues up to next 6 days. **The crusts are not infective.** Chickenpox is highly contagious and spreads easily from person to person. The patients are most infective during the prodromal period.

Q. Describe the characteristic rash in chickenpox:

1. True rash appears on the first day of the illness. They are more dense on the trunk than on the face and limbs (centripetal). At first, it is macular in type and then rapidly passes over to papule, vesicle or even pustule.
2. Rash is mostly present on flexor surfaces. Axilla may be involved. Palms and soles are seldom affected. They are oval, superficial and likely to be ruptured very easily by simple pressure. **Rash is pleomorphic**, i.e. at a given time, different stages of rash are seen.
3. Vesicular rashes are **unilocular** and **not umbilicated**; often surrounded by erythema. There is complete collapse on pricking. Rise of temperature occurs with appearance of each fresh crop of rash. Scabs begin to form usually 4–7 days after the appearance of rash and totally fall off within 14 days. Scar remains after separation of the crusts, which is usually not permanent.

- The total duration of illness in a classical case is 10 days.

Q. Complications after varicella infection:

1. Secondary bacterial infection of the skin lesion which may lead to septicaemia.
2. Interstitial pneumonia (most serious complication and commonly occurs in adults).
3. Encephalitis, transverse myelitis, optic neuritis, cerebellar syndrome, meningitis.
4. Orchitis.
5. Myocarditis, hepatitis.
6. Acute glomerulonephritis.
7. Maternal infection in early pregnancy results in fetal damage.

- High risk for complications: Infants, pregnant women and immunosupressed persons (e.g. AIDS).

Q. Differential diagnosis of chickenpox rash:

1. Herpes zoster.
2. Impetigo contagiosa.
3. Dermatitis herpetiformis.
4. Bullous impetigo.
5. Infected scabies.
6. Rickettsialpox.
7. Disseminated vesiculo-papular lesions associated with echovirus, coxsackievirus and atypical measles.
8. Smallpox (eradicated world-wide).

- Though eradicated globally, concern about smallpox has increased recently because of the threat of bioterrorism. The lesions of **smallpox** are larger than chickenpox and are: monomorphic (all are at same stage of evolution at a point of time). The rash of smallpox appears on the third day of fever.
- **Bioterrorism:** Biological agents, used in 'biological warfare' are: anthrax, botulinum toxin, smallpox, plague, tularaemia, encephalitis and haemorrhagic fever viruses (Ebola and Marburg), influenza, swine flu, and brucellosis (Fig. 7.16).

The World Health Organization declares that "swine flu" (strain H1N1, spreading from Mexico), has reached the status of a pandemic

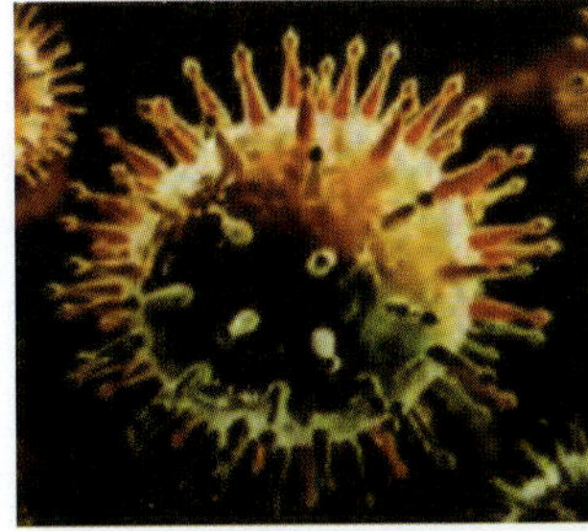

Fig. 7.16: **Swine flu** is now pandemic

Q. Prophylaxis against chickenpox:

a. Active: 0.5 mL of life-attenuated vaccine (varilrix) is given in subcutaneous route. Two doses are recommended for children, i.e. first at 12–15 months of age and the second is at 4–6 years of age. Above 13 years, two doses of vaccine are given at an interval of 4–8 weeks.
b. Passive: Varicella-zoster Immunoglobulin (VZIG) is given within 72 hours of exposure. A dose of 1.25 mL to 5 mL is administered by IM route.

Q. Vesicles/bullae In skin:

Cutaneous blisters are known as vesicle (<0.5 cm) or bulla (>0.5 cm). Blistering (vesicle/bulla) diseases of skin are:

1. Insect bites, burn, contact dermatitis.
2. Pemphigus vulgaris.
3. Bullous pemphigoid.
4. Dermatitis herpetiformis.
5. Stevens-Johnson syndrome.
6. Toxic epidermal necrolysis.
7. Bullous impetigo.
8. Staphylococcal scalded skin syndrome.
9. Varicella or herpes zoster infection.
10. Epidermolysis bullosa.
11. Bullous diabeticorum.
12. Behcet's syndrome.
13. Bullous SLE.
14. Porphyria cutanea tarda.
15. Herpangina (Coxsackie virus),
16. Hand, foot and mouth disease.

- **Pemphigus:** An autoimmune blistering disease with intraepidermal thin-walled, flaccid, easily ruptured bullae; affects apparently normal skin and mucous membrane with less tendency to heal. Mostly seen in scalp, face and flexures though may be generalised. Nikolsky's sign (extension of the blister on application of pressure to the affected skin) is positive.
- **Pemphigoid:** Subepidermal tense bullae with less chance of rupture, and a positive tendency to heal without scarring. Mucosa of mouth and conjunctiva are rarely involved. Mostly seen in trunk, limbs and flexures. A relatively benign condition though pemphigoid may be associated with (occult) lymphoma. Nikolsky's sign is negative.

TEMPERATURE CHART ON LOBAR PNEUMONIA (Fig. 7.17)

Inference

Acute pyrexia on the 1st day where temperature shoots up to 103°F and remains continued in type for next 6 days. On the 7th day, temperature suddenly **falls by crisis**.

The pulse: Respiration ratio is diminished as a result of high respiratory rate. The pulse: temperature ratio is not altered (i.e. absence of relative bradycardia or tachycardia).

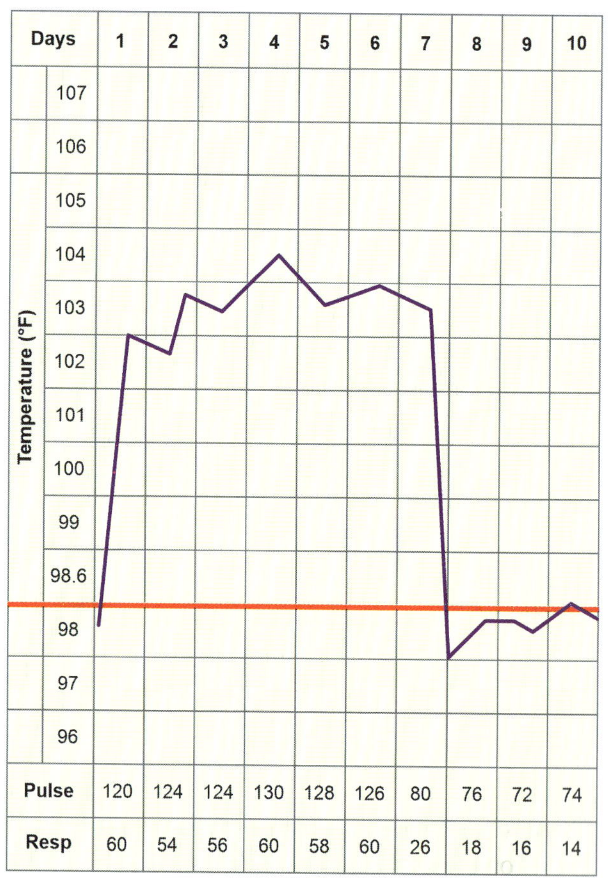

Fig. 7.17: Temperature chart on lobar pneumonia

The pattern of pyrexia is typically seen in acute lobar pneumonia.

Q. What is pulse: respiration ratio?

It is seen that with per degree (°F) rise of temperature, there is an increase in respiratory rate by 2–3/minute. The pulse: respiration ratio goes like this:

a. Normal pulse: respiration 4:1(72:18).
b. Increased pulse: respiration, e.g. 12:1 (72: 6) is seen in narcotic poisoning.
c. Decreased pulse: respiration, e.g. 2:1 (112: 56) is seen in acute lobar pneumonia.

- In a treated case of acute lobar pneumonia, temperature may fall by lysis or crisis on the 3rd or 4th day of illness.

Q. Causes of tachypnoea:

Tachypnoea is increased rate of respiration (normal respiratory rate in an adult is 14–18 breaths/min). The common causes are:

1. Nervousness, exertion, anxiety.
2. Fever due to any cause.
3. Acute lobar pneumonia.
4. Left ventricular failure.
5. Acute pulmonary thromboembolism.
6. COPD.
7. Shock.
8. Acidosis.
9. ARDS or acute lung injury.
10. Hysterical hyperventilation.

TEMPERATURE CHART ON DENGUE (Fig. 7.18)

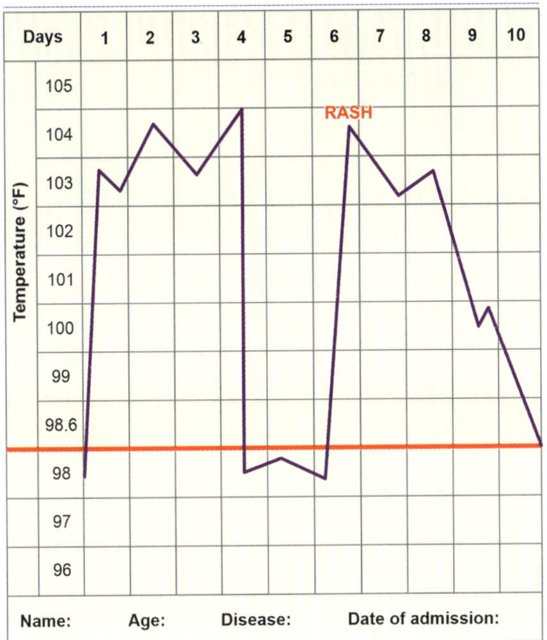

Fig. 7.18: Temperature chart on dengue

Inference

There is acute pyrexia on the 1st day which gradually increases on the next 3 days. Then the temperature **falls by crisis** and remains near normal for 2 more days only to reappear on the 6th day along with the development of rash. From 8th day onwards, temperature falls gradually and the patient is afebrile on the 10th day.

This pattern of biphasic or **'saddle-back' pyrexia** is classical of dengue.

Q. Type of pyrexia in dengue:

It is continued or saddle-back in type, with a break usually on the 4th or 5th day. Fever persists for 7–9 days.

Q. Aetiology:

Causative agent: Arbovirus (flavivirus).

Principal vector: Aedes aegypti (mosquito).

Incubation period: 2–7 days.

Usual course of the disease: 7–9 days (usually does not cross 10 days).

Serotypes: Four (4) antigenically different serotypes are DEN-1, DEN-2, DEN-3 and DEN-4.

Q. Describe the characteristic rash in dengue:

a. *Primary or initial rash:* Appears on the 1st–2nd day. Rash is erythematous (diffuse flushing) and present over face, neck and shoulder.
b. *Secondary or true rash:* Measly or morbilliform rash which appears on the 6th day of illness and is usually present over the dorsum of hands and feet. Ultimately the rash becomes generalised (mostly over the trunk) including the face. The rash may persist from 2 hours to several days and terminates by desquamation.

Q. Other features in dengue fever:

1. Pyrexia, generalised lymphadenopathy, intense headache, severe backache (**'break-bone fever'**), retro-orbital pain, arthralgia, scleral injection, cough, epistaxis, scattered petechiae (may be with positive tourniquet test), relative bradycardia, extreme prostration.
2. Delirium, agitation, transient loss of accommodation, GI haemorrhage and splenomegaly may be found.

- Severe fatigue and depression are common after remission of fever.
- Chikungunya rash is of similar type but arthralgia or arthritis is commonly associated with.

Q. Types of dengue:

a. **Classic dengue fever:** Described above.
b. **Dengue haemorrhagic fever (DHF):** DHF is a severe form of dengue and is thought to be due to two or more sequential infections with different serotypes of dengue. DHF is diagnosed on the basis of following triad—haemorrhagic manifestations (into skin, epistaxis, haematemesis, melaena), a platelet count<100000/mm^3 and objective evidence of plasma leakage (shown either by fluctuation of packed cell volume >20%, or evidence of pleural effusion, ascites or hypoproteinaemia). This develops into **'dengue shock syndrome'** which is characterised by a rapid and weak pulse with narrow pulse pressure (<20 mm of Hg), or profound hypotension. Immediate volume-replacement therapy is mandatory, otherwise the mortality rate is 40%.

Q. Important points to be remembered in the treatment of dengue:

1. Don't use NSAIDs or aspirin. Paracetamol should be used for bodyache.
2. Volume replacement (by N. saline and/or Ringer's lactate) and blood transfusion in dengue shock syndrome (capillary leak syndrome).
3. Platelet transfusion in symptomatic thrombocytopenia.

Q. Do you know the 'formula of 20' in dengue?

Dengue is the most important emerging tropical viral disease in humans today (there are no specific antiviral treatment till now). Management of classic dengue fever is supportive with adequate fluid replacement. The 'formula of 20' helps to diagnose and manage a severe form of diseases (e.g. DHF) in the hospital setting. They warn about the worse bedside signs of dengue, and are:

1. Rise in pulse rate by 20/minute.
2. Fall in systolic BP by 20 mm of Hg.
3. Pulse pressure <20 mm of Hg.
4. Rapid rise of haematocrit by 20% and rapid fall in platelet count to <20000/mm^3.
5. Appearance of >20 new petechiae in the 'tourniquet test'.

6. Intervention: Give 20 mL/kg IV fluid stat and fluid replacement amounting to 20 mL/kg/hour with crystalloid or colloid solution.

- Only one dengue vaccine is currently available for use (approved for use in USA though has not been licenced in India, named DENGVAXIA) in individuals of 6–16 years of age with laboratory-confirmed previous dengue infection and living in endemic areas. It is a live-attenuated tetravalent vaccine.

Q. Causes of haemorrhagic fever:

1. Dengue haemorrhagic fever (flavivirus).
2. Yellow fever (flavivirus).
3. Meningococcaemia.
4. Gram-negative septicaemia.
5. Relapsing fever (by Spirochaetes).
6. Rocky Mountain spotted fever (by Rickettsiae).
7. Plague.
8. African trypanosomiasis (protozoa).
9. Viral haemorrhagic fever (Lassa fever, Marburg/Ebola virus, yellow fever viruses).
10. Disseminated gonococcal infection.
11. Hantavirus infection.

Q. Fever associated with rash and/or thrombocytopenia:

1. Dengue.
2. Rickettsial infections (e.g. *Orientia tsutsugamushi*).
3. Meningococcal infection.
4. Malaria (especially *P. falciparum*).
5. Leptospirosis.
6. Measles, rubella and other viral exanthems.

Q. Causes of febrile encephalopathy:

1. Encephalitis (e.g. H. simplex, Japanese B).
2. Meningitis (*S. pneumoniae, N. meningitidis, H. influenzae*).
3. Enteroviruses.
4. Scrub typhus.
5. Cerebral malaria.
6. Typhoid encephalopathy.
7. Sepsis-associated encephalopathy.

Q. Fever with acute respiratory distress syndrome (ARDS):

1. Falciparum malaria.
2. Scrub typhus.
3. Swine flu (H1N1 virus strain).
4. Leptospirosis.
5. Hantavirus infection, melioidosis.
6. Severe community-acquired pneumonia (e.g. *Legionella* spp.)
7. Diffuse alveolar haemorrhage (e.g. SLE).

Q. Fever with multiple organ dysfunction syndrome (MODS):

1. Bacterial sepsis.
2. Falciparum malaria.
3. Leptospirosis.
4. Dengue.
5. Scrub typhus.
6. Hantavirus infection.
7. Hepatitis with fulminant hepatic failure.
8. Macrophage activation syndrome (MAS).
9. Systemic inflammatory response syndrome (SIRS).

CHARTS ON LIVER FUNCTION TESTS (LFT)

Introduction

These tests (LFT) do not point to a specific disease but indicate the underlying pathological process. The tests for liver function are:

1. Serum bilirubin: The normal serum bilirubin level is 0.3–1.0 mg/dL; the conjugated fraction is 0.1–0.3 mg/dL and the unconjugated fraction remains as 0.2–0.7 mg/dL.

   When chemical analysis reveals more than 50% conjugated bilirubin, it is considered to have predominantly conjugated hyperbilirubinaemia; and when the unconjugated bilirubin is more than 80% of the total bilirubin, the patient is considered to have primarily unconjugated hyperbilirubinaemia. Majority of hepatobiliary disorders lead to conjugated hyperbilirubinaemia. Conjugated hyperbilirubinaemia indicates impairment of secretion into the bile while unconjugated hyperbilirubinaemia points towards impaired conjugation.

   In hepato-cellular diseases, e.g. viral hepatitis or cirrhosis of liver, usually there is interference in all the three steps of bilurubin metabolism, i.e. uptake, conjugation and excretion. As excretion is the rate-limiting step and is usually hampered to the greatest extent, it is the conjugated hyperbilirubinaemia which predominates in hepato-cellular disorders.

   Clinically, serum bilirubin level up to 6 mg/dL, in between 6–15 mg/dL, and greater than 15 mg/dL, is believed to be known as **mild, moderate and severe jaundice,** respectively.
2. Aminotransferases (transaminases): There are mainly two enzymes (SGPT and SGOT) which indicate hepato-cellular damage or injury to liver. Normal blood level of each enzyme is 10–40 IU/L.
   - SGPT: Serum glutamic pyruvic transaminase is nowadays known as ALT (alanine aminotransferase).
   - SGOT: Serum gluamic oxaloacetic transaminase is nowadays known as AST (aspartate aminotransferase).

   Although raised SGPT (ALT) and SGOT (AST) levels may be observed in other non-hepatic diseases like acute myocardial infarction or skeletal muscle disorders, **SGPT (ALT) is more specific in hepato-cellular disorders than SGOT (AST).**

SGPT (ALT) is exclusively found in the cytosol, while SGOT (AST) exists in both mitochondria and cytosol. Elevated levels are found in hepatic necrosis due to any aetiology (viral hepatitis, toxin or drug-induced hepatic injury). Low level may be seen in fulminant hepatitis (due to exhaustion) or uraemia (spurious). AST: ALT >2 may be found in alcoholic hepatitis.

3. Alkaline phosphatase: Normal serum value is 35–130 IU/L or 3–13 KA unit (King-Armstrong)/dL. The enzyme is found in liver, bone (↑ level reflects osteoblastic activity), intestine and placenta.
   - Mild to moderate elevation: In parenchymal hepatic disorders like hepatitis and cirrhosis of liver.
   - Striking increase (3–10 times) occurs in biliary obstruction (extrahepatic or intrahepatic cholestasis).

   Common causes of raised serum alkaline phosphatase are pregnancy, adolescence, rickets, osteomalacia, bony metastasis, healing fracture of bone, sarcoidosis, hyperparathyroidism, tumours of GI tract, Paget's disease of bone and obstructive jaundice. The concomitant elevation of GGT (see below) and 5'-nucleotidase confirm the source of alkaline phosphatase as liver.
4. Serum proteins: They reflect the hepatic transport and synthetic function (serum bilirubin also reflects the same).

   Normal value of serum albumin is 3.5–5.5 g/dL and that of serum globulin is 2–3.5 g/dL. Albumin is synthesized by the liver. Serum globulins include alpha, beta and gamma globulin fractions (separated on electrophoresis). In cirrhosis of liver, globulin level increases (polyclonal) due to stimulation of reticulo-endothelial system as the Kupffer cells cannot clear all the antigens presented to the liver. Though albumin and globulin ratio has no physiologic significance, the ratio is often altered, i.e. from 2:1, it tends to become 1:2 in cirrhosis of liver.

   A falling serum albumin in hepatic disorder is a bad prognostic sign.
5. Prothrombin time (PT): The liver synthesizes six coagulation factors, i.e. factor I, II, V, VII, IX and X. Determination of prothrombin time efficiently reflects the abnormality of these factors. As factor VII is the rate-limiting pathway in the coagulation cascade, it has the greatest influence on prothrombin time. **Prothrombin time is a very important 'prognostic marker' of hepato-cellular damage** (i.e. a sensitive indicator of acute or chronic hepatic disorder). The normal prothrombin time is 12–16 seconds. In hepato-cellular injury, prothrombin time is increased and does not return to normal level with vitamin K therapy. Acutally, prothrombin time assesses the severity of hepatic damage.
6. Serum ammonia: Normal serum ammonia level is 10–80 µg/dL. A very high level reflects severe hepato-cellular damage. Highest level is found in hepatic encephalopathy.
7. Serum lipids: These are sensitive but non-specific indicators of hepato-cellular diseases. In cirrhosis of liver, serum cholesterol level is low. Acute parenchymal liver disorders may have high triglycerides and low cholesterol esters level. Cholestasis (intra- or extrahepatic) is associated with raised unesterified cholesterol and serum phospholipids.
8. Bromsulphthalein (BSP) excretion test: Not used nowadays and its only value remains in the diagnosis of Dubin-Johnson syndrome (double rise).
9. Other enzymes:
   a. 5'-nucleotidase: Increased in hepatic necrosis. Elevated level of 5'-nucleotidase indicates that raised alkaline phosphatase is of hepatic in origin (elevated alkaline phosphatase level in pregnancy, bone metastasis or of intestinal origin do not have associated raised 5'-nucleotidase level).
   b. γ-glutamyl transpeptidase (GGT): It is the **most sensitive indicator of hepatobiliary disorders.** Though elevated in hepato-cellular damage, it is rather non-specific because elevated GGT level may be found in pancreatic, renal, cardiac or pulmonary disorders. **GGT is a potential marker of alcohol abuse.** GGT level is raised in hepato-cellular damage and cholestasis. The normal serum level is 9–58 U/L.
   c. LDH and OCT (ornithine carbamoyltransferase) levels may be elevated in viral hepatitis, cirrhosis of liver and hepatic metastasis. These are not routinely performed.

- Hepato-cellular disease and cholestasis are associated with conjugated hyperbilirubinaemia while haemolysis results in raised level of unconjugated bilirubin. An isolated rise in serum bilirubin without SGPT or SGOT elevation may be due to haemolysis or familial. Increase in SGOT and SGPT level with a striking elevation of >1000 IU/L are obtained in extensive hepatic damage by acute viral hepatitis, drug or toxin-induced liver injury, or ischaemic liver injury (e.g. prolonged hypotension or acute heart failure). The alkaline phosphatase level rises much in cholestasis and to a lesser extent in hepato-cellular injury.
- **'Severity assessment of hepatic injury' is reflected mainly by prothrombin time, and partly by serum albumin** and factor V levels.
- Prothrombin time (PT) measures the extrinsic pathway while activated partial thromboplastin time (aPTT) reflects the intrinsic pathway of coagulation cascade.

ACUTE VIRAL HEPATITIS

Bilirubin	8.7 mg/dL
Conjugated	6.3 mg/dL
Unconjugated	2.4 mg/dL

SGPT (ALT)	296 IU/L
Alkaline phosphatast	145 IU/L
Total protein	7.4 g/dL
Albumin	4.5 g/dL
Globulin	2.9 g/dL
Prothrombin time	17 seconds
Australia antigen (HB_SAg)	Positive

Interpretation

1. Serum bilirubin level is elevated (moderate jaundice) and the conjugated fraction is raised more. SGPT is raised by more than 7 times of upper limit of normal. Alkaline phosphatase level is slightly raised.
2. Total protein with albumin and globulin fractions are within normal limit (i.e. indicating the absence of chronic hepato-cellular dysfunction). Prothrombin time is just high.
3. Australia antigen (HB_SAg) is present.

Inference

Predominant conjugated hyperbilirubinaema with raised SGPT level reflects hepato-cellular damage or acute parenchymal liver disease. Presence of Australia antigen suggests acute viral hepatitis due to type B virus infection. The patient is now in the icteric stage.

- Often 'history' is very important to interpret the data.

Q. Causes of conjugated hyperbilirubinaemia:

1. Viral or drug-induced hepatitis.
2. Cholestasis (drug-induced or pregnancy induced).
3. Cirrhosis of liver.
4. Extrahepatic biliary obstruction (gallstones, carcinoma of the head of pancreas).
5. Dubin-Johnson syndrome.
6. Rotor syndrome.
7. Secondary carcinoma of liver.

Q. Serology in different types of acute viral hepatitis:

Type A: IgM anti-HAV
Type B: HB_SAg and IgM anti-HBc
Type C: Anti-HCV
Type D: Coinfection: Anti-HDV plus IgM anti-HBc
Superinfection: Anti-HDV plus IgG anti-HBc
Type E: IgM anti-HEV

Q. Drugs producing hepato-cellular jaundice:

1. Rifampicin.
2. INH.
3. Halothane (anaesthetic).
4. Alcohol.
5. Paracetamol overdose (>10 g/day).
6. Phenytoin.
7. Ketoconazole.
8. Zidovudine.
9. Carbamazepine.
10. Social drugs (e.g. 'Ecstasy').

UNCONJUGATED HYPERBILIRUBINAEMIA

Bilirubin	5.8 mg/dL
Conjugated	1.1 mg/dl
Unconjugated	4.7 mg/dL
SGPT (ALT)	36 IU/L
Alkaline phosphatase	109 IU/L
Total protein	7 g/dL
Albumin	4 g/dL
Globulin	3 g/dL
Prothrombin time	13 seconds
Australia antigen	Negative

Interpretation

1. Serum bilirubin is elevated (mild jaundice). Unconjugated bilirubin is raised by more than 80% of total bilirubin. SGPT (ALT), alkaline phophatase are within normal limit.
2. Total protein, prothrombin time are normal. Australia antigen is absent.

Inference

The chart reflects mild, predominantly unconjugated hyperbilirubinaemia without any hepato-cellular damage. The possibilities are **(predominant unconjugated hyperbilirubinaemia)**:

1. Haemolysis (thalassaemia, spherocytosis, immune haemolysis, G_6PD deficiency).
2. Ineffective erythropoiesis.
3. Prolonged fasting (<300 cal/day).
4. Sepsis.
5. Gilbert's syndrome and rarely, Crigler-Najjar syndrome.
6. Neonatal jaundice.

Q. How to come to a definitive diagnosis from here?

1. Detailed history.
2. Meticulous clinical examination: Haemolytic jaundice will have splenomegaly. Gilbert's syndrome shows no physical abnormality except mild jaundice. In the presence of sepsis, patient will present with pyrexia.
3. Blood for routine examination as well as the peripheral blood film will point towards haemolytic jaundice (e.g. thalassaemia). Reticulocytosis suggests haemolysis; Hb concentration will reflect the degree of anaemia in haemolysis.
4. **Fasting test:** When a patient of Gilbert's syndrome is placed on 300 calorie per day for 2 days, he will show increase in bilirubin level by 1.5 mg/dL after 2 days of fasting.

Q. Prognosis in Gilbert's syndrome:

The disease is benign in nature and the prognosis is good. The life-span is normal.

Q. Congenital non-haemolytic hyperbilirubinaemia—spectrum of diseases:

1. Gilbert's syndrome (unconjugated).
2. Crigler-Najjar syndrome (type I and type II: unconjugated).
3. Dubin-Johnson syndrome (conjugated).
4. Rotor syndrome (conjugated).

Q. Common examples of haemolytic jaundice in city hospitals:

1. Thalassaemia.
2. Snake bite (Viperidae group).
3. Malaria (especially falciparum malaria).
4. Rh incompatibility.
5. Mismatched blood transfusion.
6. Autoimmune (SLE, drug-induced).

- In haemolytic jaundice, bilirubin is usually less than 6 mg/dL, and there is presence of reticulocytosis.

CIRRHOSIS OF LIVER

Bilirubin	4.9 mg/dL
Conjugated	3.1 mg/dL
Unconjugated	1.8 mg/dL
SGPT (ALT)	62 IU/L
Alkaline phosphatase	173 IU/L
Total protein	7.2 g/dL
Albumin	2.9 g/dL
Globulin	4.3 g/dL
Prothrombin time	18 seconds
Australia antigen	Negative

Interpretation

1. Total bilirubin is high (mild jaundice) and there is conjugated hyperbilirubinaemia. SGPT (ALT) is just elevated and alkaline phosphatase is slightly raised.
2. Total protein is normal with hypoalbuminaemia and hyperglobulinaemia. Albumin and globulin ratio is 1: 1.5 (i.e. altered); prothrombin time is raised by 2 seconds over the highest limit of normal. Australia antigen is negative.

Inference

High bilirubin level, just raised SGPT (ALT) and alkaline phosphatase (excludes acute hepatic parenchymal injury and cholestasis respectively), low albumin as well as high globulin level clinch the diagnosis of chronic liver disease or CLD (e.g. cirrhosis of liver). Increased prothrombin time reflects hepato-cellular damage (e.g. failure) and certainly indicates a bad prognostic sign.

Q. Causes of hyperglobulinaemia (polyclonal gammopathy):

1. Chronic liver disease, e.g. cirrhosis of liver.
2. Chronic infection, e.g. chronic kala-azar, disseminated tuberculosis.
3. SLE and other collagen vascular diseases.
4. AIDS (polyclonal).
5. Multiple myeloma.

Q. Causes of hypoglobulinemia:

1. Primary: Hereditary forms (X-linked hypogammaglobulinaemia, severe combined immunodeficiency).
2. Secondary origin: Use of corticosteroid, immunosuppressants, chemotherapy, nephrotic syndrome, nutritional disorders.
3. Chronic lymphatic leukaemia.

Q. Can it be a chart of carcinoma of liver?

No. Primary hepato-cellular carcinoma (hepatoma) 'usually' does not raise the bilirubin level. Secondary metastasis in liver may produce jaundice but globulin level remains normal. Moreover, in carcinoma of liver the alkaline phosphatase level would have been more high.

Q. How to confirm your diagnosis?

Liver biopsy confirms the diagnosis of cirrhosis of liver.

Q. How a patient of cirrhosis of liver usually presents?

Apart from the features peculiar to the aetiology, cirrhosis of liver results in two major events: hepatocellular failure and portal hypertension, the tempo of which determines the clinical presentation. The patient may be in the 'compensated' or 'decompensated' form.

Usually the patient presents with undue fatigability, flatulent dyspepsia, anorexia, swelling of legs or abdomen, jaundice, haematemesis or melaena, poor health, ascites or in the stage of hepatic pre-coma.

CHOLESTASIS

Bilirubin	18 mg/dL
Conjugated	14.6 mg/dL
Unconjugated	3.4 mg/dL
SGPT (ALT)	58 1U/L
Alkaline phosphatase	1362 IU/L
Total protein	7 g/dL
Albumin	4.2 g/dL
Globulin	2.8 g/dL
Prothrombin time	19 seconds
Australia antigen	Negative

Interpretation

1. There is very high bilirubin level (severe jaundice) with predominant conjugated hyperbilirubinaemia. SGPT (ALT) level is slightly raised. Alkaline phosphatase is 10 times more than the upper limit of normal.
2. Total protein with alburnin and globulin fractions show no abnormality (suggesting absence of chronic hepato-cellular damage as well as reflecting normal protein metabolism). Prothrombin time is raised by

3 seconds above normal. Australia antigen is absent (i.e. playing no role).

Inference

Conjugated hyperbilirubinaemia with very high alkaline phosphatase signifies cholestasis. As SGPT (ALT) level is not much altered, probably it is a case of extrahepatic cholestasis.

Q. Causes of obstructive jaundice:

When the flow of bile from the liver is reduced or blocked, it is called **cholestasis**, which may be intrahepatic or extrahepatic.

A. Intrahepatic (medical):

1. Viral hepatitis (cholestatic variety).
2. Chronic hepatitis.
3. Cirrhosis of liver (especially primary biliary cirrhosis).
4. Lymphoma.
5. Recurrent cholestasis of pregnancy.
6. Drugs like chlopromazine, chlorpropamide, erythromycin estolate, oral contraceptive pills, methimazole, anabolic steroids, methyl testosterone.
7. Secondary carcinoma of liver.

B. Extrahepatic (surgical):

1. Gallstone impaction in common bile duct (CBD).
2. Carcinoma of the head of pancreas, periampullary carcinoma.
3. Carcinoma of the gallbladder.
4. Enlarged glands at porta hepatis.
5. Stricture of CBD.
6. Sclerosing cholangitis from ulcerative colitis.
7. Cholangiocarcinoma.

- Features of chronic cholestasis are pruritus, xanthoma, bruising and bone pain.

Q. How the prothrombin time is corrected in cholestasis?

It is known that vitamin K-dependent coagulation factors are II, VII, IX and X (produced in the liver). Vitamin K is a fat-soluble vitamin and its deficiency is seen most commonly as a result of cholestasis, either intra- or extra-hepatic. Thus, coagulopathy may occur from cholestasis.

In 'extrahepatic cholestasis', parenteral replacement of vitamin K usually corrects the prothrombin time rapidly to normal (within 24–48 hours). But if the coagulopathy is due to 'parenchymal hepatic disorders', the prothrombin time may not improve or may improve but not to normal. In the liver, vitamin K is required for a complex conversion to produce the different coagulation factors (II, VII, IX, X), and protein C and protein S. Thus in hepatic disorders (e.g. intrahepatic cholestasis), coagulopathy is usually not corrected after administration of vitamin K (the complex conversion in the liver is hampered). The usual dose of vitamin K is 10 mg, IM daily for consecutive 3 days.

Q. Modalities adopted in treating pruritus in cholestasis:

Pruritus in cholestasis is often violent leading to intense scratching, sleep deprivation and even suicidal ideations. Conventional belief is that pruritus is due to irritation of the free nerve ending by bile acids; the recent view is in favour of upregulation of opioid receptors and increased level of endogenous opioids.

1. Cholestyramine (a bile salt sequestering agent): 12 g/day orally in divided doses, before as well as after meals with orange juice.
2. Ursodeoxycholic acid (UDCA): 13–15 mg/kg/day orally.
3. Antihistaminics (e.g. tab cetrizine 10 mg daily).
4. Phenobarbitone: May be tried in resistant cases.
5. Ondansetron: This 5-HT type 3 receptor antagonist may be of some value; 4–8 mg, BID/TID.
6. Naloxone (opiate antagonist), naltrexone or propofol (hypnotic): May be tried.
7. Methyl testosterone: 25 mg daily sublingually. Anabolic steroid, i.e. stanazolol may be of some help.
8. Rifampicin 300–450 mg/day orally may relieve pruritus within one week. It is a hepatotoxic drug (recently introduced in the therapeutic armamentarium of refractory pruritus in cholestasis).
9. Biliary drainage (internal or external).
10. Phototherapy: UV radiation for 9–12 minutes/day improves pruritus.
11. Plasmapheresis (or PLEX): Rarely utilised in severe intractable itching.
12. Liver support device (molecular absorbent recirculating system): MARS, may be considered.
13. Miscellaneous: Use creams, lotions, gels that sooth and cool the skin; use moisturiser daily. Avoid scratching the skin (trim the fingernails) and may take a lukewarm bath, use lightweight clothing.
14. Hepatic transplantation: Probably the only answer in chronic intractable pruritus.

Q. What is hepatic granuloma?

These are aggregates of macrophages, often transformed to an epitheloid appearance, in the hepatic parenchyma. They may be an incidental finding in liver biopsy (2–35%). Usually granulomas are asymptomatic.

Bilirubin level remains normal but alkaline phosphatase level is usually high. The causes are:

1. Tuberculosis.
2. Sarcoidosis.
3. Histoplasmosis.
4. Leprosy.
5. Primary biliary cirrhosis (PBC).
6. Lymphomas.
7. Berylliosis.
8. Brucellosis.
9. Drugs (e.g. allopurinol).

10. Schistosomiasis.
11. Viral infection (e.g. Hep B or C).
12. Drug-induced (e.g. quinidine).

CHRONIC HEPATITIS

Bilirubin	7.1 mg/dL
Conjugated	5.2 mg/dL
Unconjugated	1.9 mg/dL
SGPT (ALT)	370 IU/L
SCOT (ASI)	324 IU/L
Alkaline phosphatase	142 IU/L
Total protein	5.9 g/dL
Albumin	2.9 g/dL
Globulin	3 g/dL
Prothrombin time	17 seconds
Australia antigen	Positive
IgG anti-HBC	Positive
HB_eAg	Positive
Anti-HCV	Negative
Antinuclear factor (ANF)	Negative

Interpretation

1. Serum bilirubin is moderately increased with predominant conjugated hyperbilirubinaemia. Both SGPT (ALT) and SGOT (AST) are raised but ALT level is >AST level. Serum alkaline phosphatase is also elevated.
2. Total protein is a bit subnormal probably as a result of hypoalburninaemia. Serum globulin is within normal limit. Albumin : globulin ratio is approximately 1 : 1; prothrombin time is just elevated by 1 second over the highest limit of normal.
3. Australia antigen is found with evidence of (IgG anti-HBc) chronic infection by type B hepatitis virus. Hb_eAg is also positive. Marker of type C virus is not found. ANF is absent.

Inference

There is conjugated hyperbilirubinaemia. Serum transaminases are 8–9 times more than normal. Serum alkaline phosphatase is slightly elevated. Hypoalbuminaemia with raised transaminases and just raised prothrombin time indicate hepatocyte damage.

Positive HB_SAg and IgG anti-HBc indicate chronic HBV infection. Presence of HB_eAg indicates replication of HBV (i.e. highly infective). Markers of HCV and auto-immunity (ANF) are not found.

Thus, it seems that the patient is suffering from chronic hepatitis as a result of type B virus infection of high infectivity.

- If cirrhosis develops from chronic hepatitis, SGOT (AST) tends to exceed SGPT (ALT). Classically, in type B-induced chronic hepatitis, SGPT (ALT) tends to be elevated more than SGOT (AST).

Q. Aetiology of chronic hepatitis:

1. Hepatitis B, C, and D.
2. Autoimmune hepatitis (lupoid hepatitis).
3. Drugs, e.g. methyl dopa, oxyphenisatin, INH, nitrofurantoin, ketoconazole.
4. Wilson's disease.
5. Alcoholic liver disease, non-alcoholic steatohepatitis (NASH), α_1-antitrypsin deficiency, ulcerative colitis.
6. Cryptogenic.

Q. Common types of chronic hepatitis:

Chronic hepatitis is the chronic inflammatory reaction in the liver **continuing without improvement for 6 months or longer. Liver biopsy confirms the diagnosis.** The types are:

1. Chronic lobular hepatitis (milder form): Histology resembles unresolved acute viral hepatitis.
2. Chronic persistent hepatitis (milder form): The limiting plate between hepatocytes and portal zones remain intact, and piecemeal necrosis is not seen. There is expansion of the portal zone by infiltration with mononuclear cells.
3. Chronic active hepatitis (severe form): Prognostically grave. There is erosion of limiting plate, presence of piecemeal necrosis, formation of 'rosette' and bridging necrosis. This type can lead to cirrhosis of liver.

This classification is not helpful for prognostication. The new classification of chronic hepatitis is based on 1. Aetiology, 2. Histological activity or grade (evidences of inflammation and necrosis), and 3. The stage (extent of fibrosis and reflects the level of progression of the disease).

Q. Significance of serological markers in type B infection:

- HB_eAg → Acute hepatitis B; persistence indicates infectivity and ongoing viral replication
- IgG anti HBc → Past exposure to hepatitis B or chronic HBV infection
- IgM anti Hbc → Acute HBV infection
- DNA polymerase and HBV DNA → Indicates ongoing viral replication
- Anti-HBe → Late acute or chronic hepatitis B of low infectivity
- Anti-HBs → Immunity to HBV (i.e. vaccinated or previous exposure).

Q. Autoimmune hepatitis:

The aetiology is unknown but prominent immunological changes are noted in liver and blood. The patient is usually a female in the age group of 15–25 years or at menopause.

Serum transaminases are 10 times high with gamma globulin level 2 times more than normal. Serum ANF is positive; anti-smooth muscle and anti-LKM_1 antibody may be positive. The patient shows dramatic response to corticosteroid.

Q. Outline of treatment in HVB/HCV-induced chronic hepatitis:

Chronic hepatitis is not curable but it is manageable with treatment. The newer antiviral drugs are promising.

1. Treatment of hepato-cellular failure.
2. Pegylated α-interferon is used to prevent ongoing viral replication.
3. Other antiviral drugs like lamivudine, famciclovir, adefovir dipivoxil, tenofovir, entecavir, telbivudine, fialuridine or ribavirin may be tried.
4. A patient of chronic hepatitis or cirrhosis of liver should be screened at 6 monthly interval for the development of hepato-cellular carcinoma (hepatoma) by serial measurement of serum α_1-fetoprotein.

"Just one small positive thought in the morning can change your whole day."

—**14th Dalai Lama (born on 1935)** *Spiritual leader in Tibet*

Appendix

IMPORTANT LABORATORY REFERENCE VALUES

Lipid Profile

Normal range:
Total cholesterol: <200 mg/dL (desirable)
Low density lipoprotein (LDL): <100 mg/dL (optimal)
High density lipoprotein (HDL): 40–60 mg/dL
Very low density lipoprotein (VLDL): 35–100 mg/dL
Triglycerides (TG): <165 mg/dL

Lactate Dehydrogenase (LDH) Isoenzymes

LDH_1: 14–26% (cardiac, RBCs)
LDH_2: 29–39% (cardiac, RBCs)
LDH_3: 20–26% (pulmonary)
LDH_4: 8–16% (striated muscle, liver)
LDH_5: 6–16% (striated muscle, liver)

Protein Electrophoresis

Albumin: Normal range 3.5–5.5 g/dL
Globulin: Normal range 2–3.5 g/dL
α_1: Normal range 0.2–0.4 g/dL
α_2: Normal range 0.5–0.9 g/dL
β: Normal range 0.6–1.1 g/dL
γ: normal range 0.7–1.7 g/dL

Immunoglobulins

Normal range of:
IgG: 700–1700 mg/dL
IgA: 70–360 mg/dL
IgM: 50–300 mg/dL
IgD: 0–14 mg/dL
IgE: 1–87 IU/mL (high >150 IU/mL)

Serum/Urine Values

- eGFR
  Male: 90–140 mL/min
  Female: 80–125 mL/min
- Albumin (mg)/Creatinine (mmol) (ACR)
  Female: <3.5
  Male: <2.5

Haemoglobin Electrophoresis

HbA: 95–98% (97%)
HbA_2: 1.5–3.5% (2.5%)
HbF: <2%
HbC and HbS: Absent

Creatine Kinase (CK, CPK) Isoenzymes

CK-MB (mainly in cardiac muscles), CK-MM (mainly in skeletal muscles) and CK-BB (in brain and smooth muscles) are 3 subsets of CK, which are described below.

a. CK-MB: Increased in AMI, myocarditis, pericarditis, cardiac defibrillation, cardiac surgery, cardiomyopathy, severe rhabdomyolysis, strenuous exercise (e.g. marathon runners).
   CK-MB has two subforms: MB_1 and MB_2 (MB_2 is released from cardiac cells and converted in the blood to MB_1). CK-MB_2 ≥1.0 U/L, with a ratio of CK-MB_2/ CK-MB_1 ≥1.5 diagnoses AMI within 6 hours of onset of symptoms.
b. CK-MM: Increased in crush injury, convulsions, rhabdomyolysis, polymyositis and dermatomyositis, IM injections, muscular dystrophy (myopathy), drugs (e.g. statins, colchicine).
c. CK-BB: Increased in CVA, meningitis, severe shock; neoplasm of breast, prostate and lung.

C-reactive Protein (CRP)

Normal range: <5 mg/L

It is a trace plasma protein which increases in response to infection, trauma, tissue necrosis and inflammation. The CRP level correlates better than the ESR with the changing disease activity in different rheumatic diseases.

It is elevated in: Rheumatoid arthritis, rheumatic fever, bacterial infections, inflammatory bowel disease, third trimester of pregnancy, different inflammatory and neoplastic diseases, AMI. In SLE, the CRP is not elevated and thus the concentration of CRP is often used to distinguish infection in SLE (high) from disease activity (not high).

High sensitivity C-reactive protein (hs-CRP or cardio-CRP) is a new test to diagnose pateint with silent atherosclerosis. The risk of cardiovascular event increases, if it is >1.1 mg/L.

Procalcitonin

Normal range: <0.1 ng/mL

It is a peptide precursor of calcitonin. It can be measured as a marker of severe sepsis (or septic shock), especially of bacterial origin (e.g. bacterial pneumonia or bacterial meningitis).

Rheumatoid Factor

Normally: Negative

Titres >1:40 are considered significant and are found in (i.e. rheumatoid factor is elevated in) rheumatoid arthritis, Sjögren's syndrome, SLE, vasculitis, e.g. polyarteritis nodosa, old age, infections (e.g. SBE, syphilis, leprosy), chronic liver disease, sarcoidosis, pulmonary fibrosis.

Antinuclear Antibody (ANA)

Normal range: <1:20 titre

ANA is positive in SLE (more significant if titre is >1: 160), drug-induced lupus, mixed connective tissue disease, scleroderma, rheumatoid arthritis, chronic autoimmune hepatitis, Sjögren's syndrome, necrotizing vasculitis, old age (>80 yrs), HIV infection, bacterial endocarditis, interstitial pulmonary fibrosis.

International Normalised Ratio (INR)

The INR is a comparative rating of prothrombin time (PT) ratios. The INR represents the observed PT ratio (i.e. patient's prothrombin time divided by normal pooled plasma prothrombin time) adjusted by the International Reference Thromboplastin. This method was adopted by WHO in 1982 and is used to standardize the reporting of PT. That means the INR is the PT ratio that would be obtained if the WHO reference thromboplastin, which by definition has an ISI (International Sensitivity Index) of 1.0 were used to assess PT.

The recommended INR range in different disorders after treatment are:

Disorder	Recommended INR range
TIA	2–3
Atrial fibrillation	2–3
Pulmonary embolism	2–3
Deep vein thrombosis	2–3
Mechanical prosthetic valves	3–4.5
Recurrent venous thromboembolism	3–4.5

Leucocyte Alkaline Phosphotase (LAP) Score

Increased in: Leukaemoid reaction, neutrophilic leucocytosis from infections, after steroid administration, Hodgkin's disease, polycythemia vera, myelosclerosis, hairy cell leukaemia.

Decreased in: Chronic myeloid leukaemia, paroxysmal nocturnal haemoglobinuria, thrombocytopenic purpura, aplastic anaemia, hypophosphataemia.

Antineutrophil Cytoplasmic Antibodies (ANCAs)

p-ANCA ('p' stands for perinuclear pattern) or antimyeloperoxidase (anti-MPO): Found in microscopic polyarteritis, crescentic glomerulonephritis, Churg-Strauss syndrome, inflammatory bowel disease, primary sclerosing cholangitis, primary biliary cirrhosis, autoimmune chronic active hepatitis.

c-ANCA ('c' stands for cytoplasmic pattern) or antiproteinase-3 (anti-PR_3): Found in Wegener's granulomatosis (i.e. granulomatosis with polyangiitis).

α_1-fetoprotein:

Normal range: 0–8.5 ng/mL.

Increased in: Hepato-cellular carcinoma (usually with values >1000 ng/mL), germinal neoplasia (ovary, testis, retroperitoneum), hepatic disorders (alcoholic cirrhosis, chronic active hepatitis), anencephaly of fetus or neural tube defect, spina bifida, ataxia telangiectasia, pancreatic carcinoma, retinoblastoma, atresia of oesophagus.

APPROXIMATE CONVERSION CHART

1 ounce (oz)	28 mL
1 gallon (gal)	4.5 litres
1 inch (in)	2.54 cm
1 foot (ft)	0.3 meter
1 pound (lb)	0.45 kg
1 calorie (cal)	4.2 J
1 milliliter (fluid)	15 drops

BASIC SYSTEM INTERNATIONAL (SI) UNITS

Base quantity	Name and symbol
Length	Meter (m)
Mass	Kilogram (kg)
Pressure	Pascal (Pa)
Energy	Joule (J)
Frequency	Hertz (Hz)
Amount of substance	Mole (mol)
Volume	Liter (L)

INCUBATION PERIOD OF SOME IMPORTANT INFECTIONS

AIDS (HIV infection)	12–26 weeks (up to 12 years)
Amoebiasis	3–4 weeks
Bacillary dysentery (shigellosis)	1–7 days
Brucellosis	1–3 weeks
Chickenpox	12–21 days
Cholera	Few hours to 5 days
COVID-19	2–14 days (average 5–6 days)
Dengue	2–7 days
Diphtheria	2–5 days
Encephalitis (Japanese)	9–12 days
Enteric fever	10–14 days
Gonorrhoea	2–10 days

Hepatitis A	2–6 weeks
Hepatitis B	6 weeks to 6 months
Influenza	2–3 days
Kala-azar	Usually 3–6 months
Leprosy	2–6 years (few months –20 years)
Leptospirosis	4–20 days
Malaria	Usually 10–21 days (rarely up to months)
Measles	7–14 days
Meningitis (meningococcal)	2–10 days
Mumps	2–3 weeks
Plague	1–7 days
Poliomyelitis	3–21 days
Rabies	Usually 1–3 months
Rubella	2–3 weeks
Syphilis	9–90 days
Tetanus	3 days to 3 weeks
Tuberculosis	Months to years
Whooping cough	7–14 days

THERAPEUTIC AND TOXIC BLOOD LEVELS OF COMMONLY USED DRUGS

	Therapeutic level	Toxic level
Amitriptyline	120–250 ng/mL	>500 ng/mL
Carbamazepine	4–10 μg/mL	>20 μg/mL
Chlordiazepoxide	500–3000 ng/mL	>5000 ng/mL
Diazepam	200–1000 ng/mL	>2000 ng/mL
Digoxin	0.5–1.2 ng/mL	>2.4 ng/mL
Ethanol (legal limit)	—	≥80 mg/dL
Levetiracetam	12–46 mg/L	>46 mg/L
Lithium	0.5–1.3 mEq/L	>2 mEq/L
Phenobarbital	15–40 μg/mL	>60 μg/mL
Phenytoin	10–20 μg/mL	>40 μg/mL
Quinidine	2–5 μg/mL	>6 μg/mL
Salicylate	2–29 mg/dL	>40 mg/dL
Theophylline	10–20 μg/mL	>30 μg/mL
Valproic acid	50–100 μg/mL	>100 μg/mL

IMPORTANT HAEMATOLOGICAL DATA

RBC count:	
Males	4.5–6.3 million/mm^3
Females	4.2–5.4 million/mm^3
Reticulocyte	0.2–2% of RBC
Red blood cell volume:	
Males	30 mL/kg of body weight
Females	25 mL/kg of body weight
Osmotic fragility of RBC:	
Slight haemolysis	at 0.45–0.39 g/dL NaCl
Complete haemolysis	at 0.33–0.30 g/dL NaCl
Haemoglobin:	
Males	13–17 g/dL
Females	12–15 g/dL
Haematocrit (PCV):	
Males	42–52%
Females	37–47%
MCH	29.5 ± 2.5 pg
MCHC	35 ± 3 g/dL
MCV	87 ± 7 cubic microns
WBC count (total)	4.3–10.8 × 10^9/L
Differential WBC count:	
Neutrophils	45–74% of total WBC
Lymphocytes	16–45% of total WBC
Monocytes	4–10% of total WBC
Eosinophils	0–7% of total WBC
Basophils	0–1% of total WBC
Platelet count	1.5–4 lac/mm^3
Bleeding time (Ivy)	2.5–10 minutes
Coagulation time (glass tubes)	9–15 minutes
Prothrombin time	12–16 seconds
Partial thromboplastin time (activated)	32–46 seconds
Clot retraction time	onset–1 hour, completion–6 hours
ESR (Westergren)	
Males	0–15 mm/hour
Females	0–20 mm/hour
pH (arterial blood)	7.38–7.44
Red cell life span	120 days
Red cell life span T½ (^{51}Cr)	25–35 days
Anaemia:	
Male	Hb <13 g/dL
Female	Hb <12 g/dL
Polycythemia:	
Male	Hb >18 g/dL
Female	Hb >16 g/dL

DECIMAL MULTIPLES AND SUBMULTIPLES IN SI UNITS

Multiple	Prefix	Symbol
10^9	Giga	G
10^6	Mega	M
10^3	Kilo	K
10^{-1}	Deci	d
10^{-2}	Centi	c
10^{-3}	Milli	m
10^{-6}	Micro	μ
10^{-9}	Nano	n
10^{-12}	Pico	p
10^{-15}	Femto	f

NORMAL INTRACARDIAC AND VASCULAR PRESSURE (mm of Hg)

Right atrium	1–5
Left atrium	2–12
Right ventricle	25/5

Left ventricle	120/10
Pulmonary artery	25/10
Aorta	120/80

BLOOD GAS ANALYSIS (BREATHING AMBIENT AIR)

	Normal values
O_2 saturation (SpO_2)	95–100%
Arterial O_2 tension (PaO_2)	80–100 mm of Hg
Arterial CO_2 tension ($PaCO_2$)	35–45 mm of Hg
pH (arterial blood)	7.38–7.44
Plasma HCO_3	22–26 mEq/L

IMPORTANT SERUM BIOCHEMICAL VALUES

Albumin	3.5–5.5 g/dL
Aminotransferases:	
AST (SGOT)	10–40 IU/L
ALT (SGPT)	10–40 IU/L
Ammonia	10–80 µg/dL
Amylase	20–96 U/L (method-dependent)
Bicarbonate	22–26 mEq/L
Bilirubin:	0.3–1.0 mg/dL
Conjugated	0.1–0.3 mg/dL
Unconjugated	0.2–0.7 mg/dL
Calcium (total)	9–11 mg/dL
Calcium (ionised)	4.5–5.6 mg/dL
Chloride	98–106 mEq/L
Cholesterol (total)	Up to 200 mg/dL
CK-MB	<6% of total CK
Copper	70–140 µg/dL
Cortisol:	
8 AM–12 noon	5–25 µg/dL
8 PM–8 AM	0–10 µg/dL
C-reactive protein (CRP)	<5 mg/L (varies lab to lab)
Creatinine	0.6–1.2 mg/dL
Creatine kinase (CK, CPK)	55–170 U/L
D-dimer (plasma)	220–740 ng/mL
Ferritin	30–300 ng/mL
Fibrinogen (plasma)	200–400 mg/dL
Folate	5.4–18 ng/mL
Globulin	2–3.5 g/dL
Glucose (fasting)	75–100 mg/dL
Glucose (2-hour postprandial)	<140 mg/dL
HbA_{1C} (glycated Hb)	4–6% of total Hb
Insulin	2–20 µU/mL
Iron	70–140 µg/dL
Lactate dehydrogenase	100–190 U/L
Lipase	3–43 U/L (method-dependent)
Osmolality (blood)	280–300 mOsmol/kg
Oxygen content:	
Arterial blood	17–21 volume%
Venous blood	10–16 volume%
Phosphatase:	
Acid	1–5 U/L
Alkaline	35–130 U/L
Phosphate	3–4.5 mg/dL
Potassium	3.5–5 mEq/L
Prolactin	2–15 ng/mL
Protein (plasma)	5:5–8.0 g/dL
Sodium	136–145 mEq/L
Triglyceride	<165 mg/dL
TSH	0.3–5 µU/mL
T_3 (triiodothyronine)	80–150 ng/dL
T_4 (thyroxine)	4–12 µg/dL

Table A.1: Serum 'tumour markers'

Carcinoma	Tumour markers
a. Testicular (germ cell)	a. Alpha-1-fetoprotein (AFP), β-human chorionic gonadotrophin (β-HCG)
b. Ovary	b. CA-125
c. Prostate	c. Prostate specific antigen (PSA)
d. Choriocarcinoma	d. β-HCG
e. Hepato-cellular	e. AFP
f. Colorectal	f. Carcinoembryonic antigen (CEA)
g. Breast	g. CA—15-3
h. GI tract carcinoma, especially pancreas	h. CA—19-9
i. Early recurrence of treated breast carcinoma	i. CA—27-29
j. Melanoma, astrocytoma	j. S-100
k. Medullary carcinoma of thyroid	k. Calcitonin
l. Many cancers including mesothelioma	l. Osteopontin

- **Tumour markers** are intracellular proteins or cell surface glycoproteins released into the circulation from internal malignancy, and detected by immunoassays. They may be hormones, enzymes, oncofetal antigens or tumour-associated proteins.

Urea	20–40 mg/dL
Uric acid	2–7 mg/dL
Vitamin B_{12}	200–600 pg/mL
Vitamin D (25-hydroxycholecalciferol)	30–100 ng/ml

YOUR ORAL/VIVA TABLE (IMPORTANT TIPS)

1. You should look smart and confident. It is often said that 'first impression is the best impression', and thus be alert about your own appearance.
2. Always be well-dressed with a clean shave; having a smile on your face will definitely pay you.
3. Have a clean apron with ID card bearing university roll number.
4. Avoid all sorts of casual attitude. Maintain etiquettes of the examination hall.
5. Do not chew any type of masala or chewing gum. Switch off your mobile phone.
6. Listen the question carefully and then answer 'to the point'. Speak out clearly, slowly and precisely but always try to keep the flow.
7. Try to answer in the order of presentation, i.e. from more common to less common causes, and avoid rare ones. Do not hurry, rather show patience.
8. It is better to say, 'I cannot recollect' or 'I am not sure' instead of going on thinking indefinitely.
9. Never argue with your examiner. 'Good morning', 'Thank you', 'Sorry' are magic words—be courteous and use them properly.
10. Most of the examiners ignore minor mistakes. Answering simple questions usually gives guarantee for 'passing'. So do not be biased, do not guess and do not cheat.

INSTRUMENTS TO CARRY FOR MEDICINE PRACTICAL EXAMINATION (CHECK-LIST)

1. Stethoscope (preferably double-tube).
2. Sphygmomanometer (mercury or aneroid type)—It is better to have your own instrument.
3. Hammer (preferably round head with flexible shaft).
4. Pencil torch (with fully charged batteries).
5. Pins (for testing of pain sensation and blanching reaction in spider naevi).
6. Cotton (for testing of corneal reflex and touch sensation).
7. Measuring tape (for measurement of expansion of chest, abdomen in ascites, neck in thyroid enlargement, height, head circumference in hydrocephalus and assessment of nutrition).
8. Tuning fork (128 or 256 cycles/second for vibration sense, and 256 or 512 cycles/second for cochlear function).
9. Skin pencil and rulers/scales (e.g. two small 15-cm rulers for measurement of JVP).
10. Divider or compass (for two point discrimination)—Optional.
11. Tongue depressor.
12. Clinical thermometer.
13. Two one-rupee coin (for coin percussion in the chest and test for stereognosis).
14. Glass slides (for examination of capillary pulsation, spider naevi and haemorrhagic spots).
15. Wrist watch (not digital and with a 'second hand')—A must.
16. Cotton wrapped in a broom-stick or throat swab stick (for gag reflex).
17. Test tubes (two) for hot and cold sensation (optional), goniometer (optional).
18. Four small glass containers for taste sensation (containing solutions of sugar, common salt, vinegar and quinine), soap/clove/coffee or camphor balls for smell sensation, ribbons (red, green and blue-coloured) for colour vision, gloves (e.g. to palpate an ulcer or per rectal examination) — Optional.
19. Cardboard or clipboard (for history writing), two pieces of cardboard for AP and TR diameter of chest.
20. Ophthalmoscope, log book, thesis/dissertation (for postgraduate students).
21. Admit card (hall ticket/call letter), apron (with clearly visible nameplate, roll number or ID card), pen, pencil, sharpener, eraser, a blunt-ended key (for eliciting plantar response), face mask and small hand sanitizer bottle. **Positive attitude** and **self-confidence** are your shield in examination hall.
22. Try to follow—wear formal clothes with polished shoes, clean and neat apron with a clean shave (if you are a boy) and hair tied up in a ponytail (if you are a girl).

Clinical Wisdom

Do not hesitate to ask for a back-rest (for neck vein examination), gauze pieces (for examination of tongue or penis), or weighing machine. Switch off your mobile phone or all electronic gadgets while in the examination hall.

THE 'MODEL' DISTRIBUTION OF MARKS IN GENERAL MEDICINE (MBBS)

The basic format is described below. This may vary from university to university:

General Medicine: Full marks 300

1. Theory: Paper I + II = 60 + 60 (total 120)
2. Internal assessment: 60 (theory 30+ practical/oral 30)
3. Oral (including instruments, X-ray, CT scan, ECG, emergency medicine, charts, flying oral): Usually 4 oral tables, carrying 5 marks in each: Total 20
4. Clinical/practical (bedside): total 100 (one long case 60 + one short case 30+ two spot cases 10)

- Marks distributed in long case (60) as follows: History taking 15+ demonstration of signs 30+ discussion 15

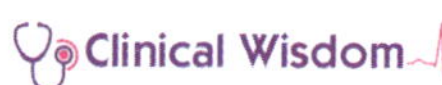

Criteria to pass in the examination:

- Aggregate 50%, i.e. 150 marks
- Theory and oral (including internal assessment) 50%, i.e. 100 marks
- Practical (bedside clinics) 50%, i.e. 50 marks

- One should get 50% in internal assessment (theory plus oral combined) to pass in the examination. Each theory paper usually contains 2 long questions (one deals with basic and allied, and other, with clinical problem), short questions and short notes. In many universities, MCQs have been added.
- Theory paper:
  Paper I: Cardiology, gastrointestinal and hepatobiliary system, genitourinary, deficiency disorder, tropical diseases, rheumatology, genetics and immunology.
  Paper II: Respiratory system, endocrinology, haematology, neurology, infectious diseases including HIV, psychiatry, dermatology including STD.
- Acute cases like acute severe asthma, LVF are usually not given in the examination.

Long case (45 minutes) comprises history writing + demonstration of signs + relevant discussion.

Short case (15 minutes) means general survey and examination of one particular system (nothing to be written).

Spot cases (1–3 minutes each) means spotting the diagnosis (with examiner observing) and mentioning the justification.

ADDENDUM

OSCE (Objective Structured Clinical Examination) to judge 'clinical skills' by giving a clinical senario, which is a common practice in MD, DNB and MRCP examination. UGs (MBBS group) should start the rehearsal with their teachers (yet to be started).

In **DNB** examination there are OSCE (25 stations), viva voce (4 stations: on drugs, ECG, ABG, EEG, X-ray, PFT, capnography, instruments, emergency, therapeutics, recent advances, research methodology), ward round cases (4 real case scenarios) and clinical cases (2). In **MD** examination, semilong cases are given.

NExT (National Exit Test) will start soon and has two parts: NExT 1 and 2. NExT 1 is the online theory examination (with 540 MCQs) which will give entry to internship and to get a PG seat; the theory examination will be governed by Central Board of NMC (National Medical Commission). NExT 2 is purely a practical/clinical/*viva voce* examination controlled by respective Health University, which will give the license to practice Medicine with an MBBS certificate. OSCE is included in NExT 2. The subjects to be dealt with in NExT examination are Medicine, Surgery, Gynae and Obstetrics, Pediatrics, Orthopedics, Eye and ENT (total 7).

Artificial Intelligence (AI) looks to be the future of the world. It is the human intelligence processes by machines, especially computer system. AI seems to be very promising in healcare system. Try to built-up some idea about it.

Route of success: Try to practice mock examination in front of your teacher/mentor or even a friend. Be systematic, plan ahead, set realistic goals and keep motivating yourself.

THE REFERENCES/SUGGESTED READING

1. Textbook of Radiology and Imaging by David Sutton.
2. Principles of Clinical Electrocardiography by MJ Goldman.
3. Manual of Medical Procedures by MJ Ford, CE Robertson and JF Munro.
4. Conn's Current Therapy.
5. Data Interpretation for Medical Students by P Hamilton and IC Bickle.
6. Kumar and Clark's Medical Management and Therapeutics.
7. Hutchison's Clinical Methods.
8. Macleod's Clinical Examination.
9. Harrison's Principles of Internal Medicine.
10. Davidson's Principles and Practice of Medicine.
11. Kumar and Clark's Clinical Medicine.
12. Talley and O'Connor's Clinical Examination.
13. Bates' Guide to Physical Examination and History Taking.
14. Sapira's Art and Science of Bedside Diagnosis.
15. Chamberlain's Symptoms and Signs in Clinical Medicine: An Introduction to Medical Diagnosis.
16. Charles Seward's Bedside Diagnosis.
17. Ferri's Clinical Advisor.
18. Oxford Handbook on Clinical Medicine by JJ Murray Longmore.
19. Pappworth MH's A Primer of Medicine.
20. DeGowin & DeGowin's Bedside Diagnostic Examination.
21. Cecil Textbook of Medicine.
22. Bedside Cardiology by Jules Constant.
23. Bickerstaff's Neurological Examination in Clinical Practice.
24. Neurological Differential Diagnosis by John Pattern.
25. Adams and Victor's Principles of Neurology.
26. The Washington Manual of Medical Therapeutics.
27. Sherlock's Diseases of the Liver and Biliary System.
28. Crofton and Douglas: Respiratory Disease.
29. Oxford Textbook on Medicine.
30. Colour Atlas of Dermatology by LK Bhutani.
31. CURRENT Medical Diagnosis and Treatment (CMDT).
32. Color Atlas and Text of Clinical Medicine by Charles Forbes and William Jackson.
33. Medicine update [published every year by Association of Physicians of India (API)].
34. Progress in Medicine (published every year by Association of Physicians of India (API)].
35. API Textbook of Medicine.

Index